STAY FIT FOR LIFE

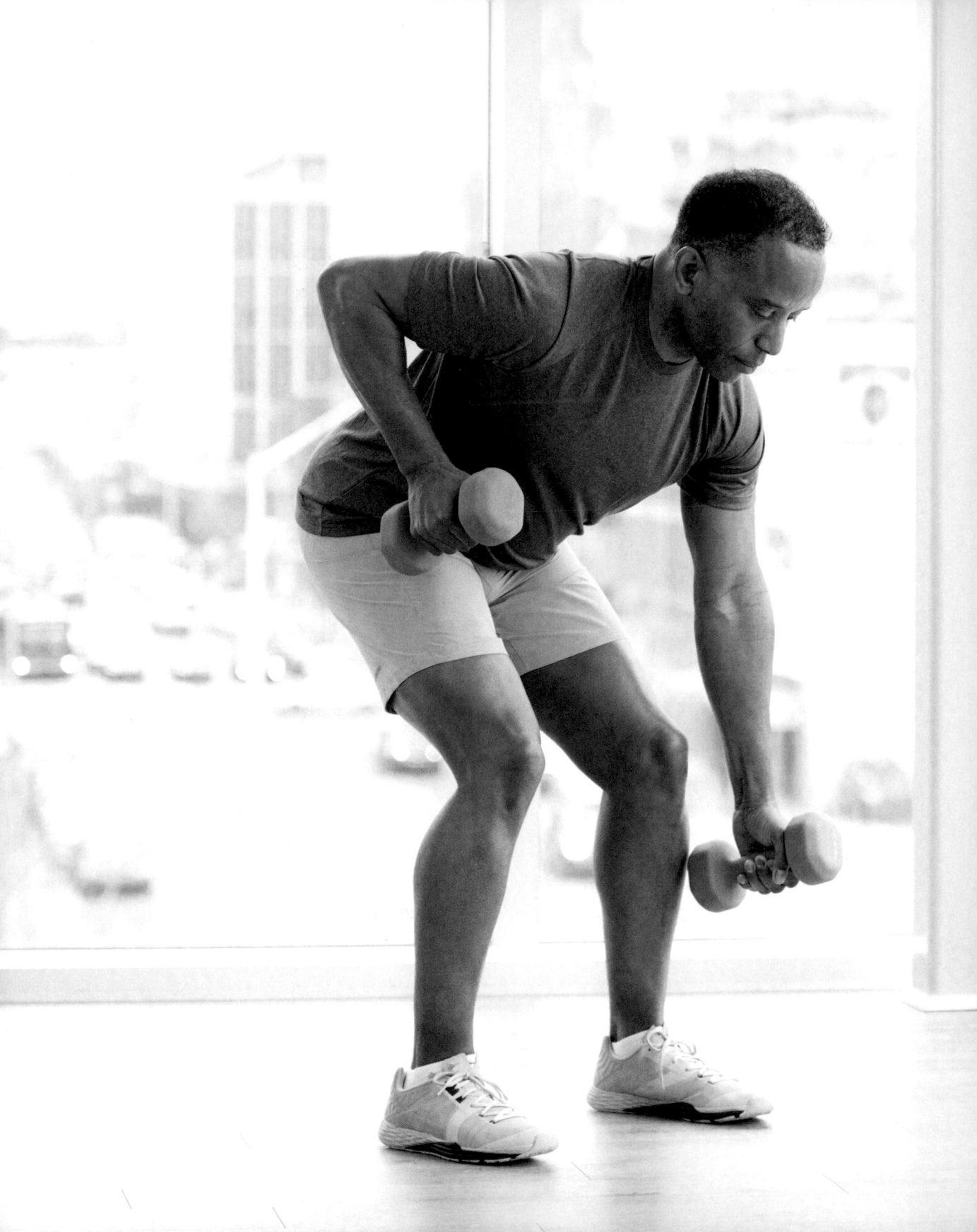

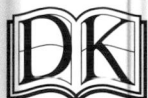

STAY FIT FOR LIFE

JOSHUA KOZAK

Contents

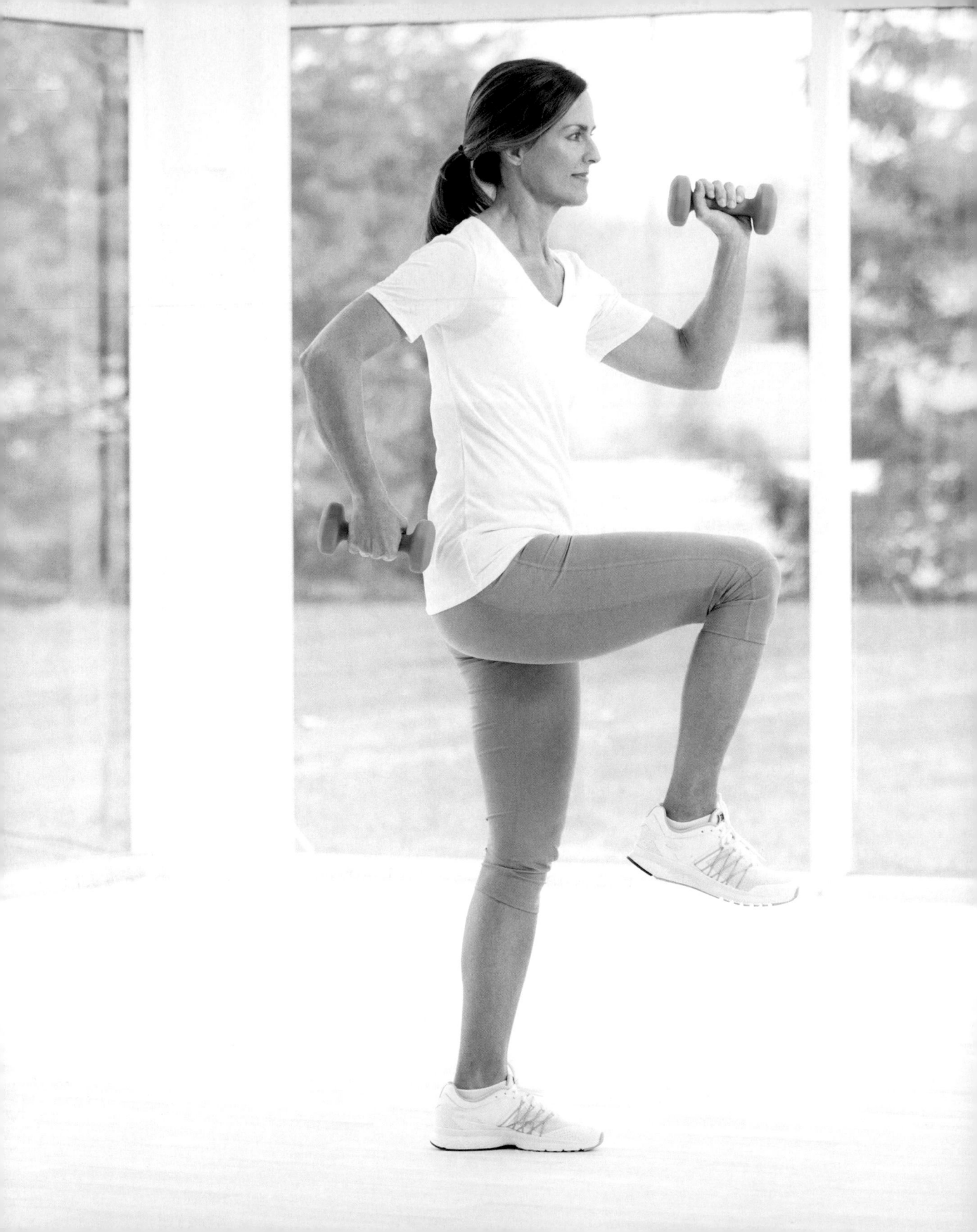

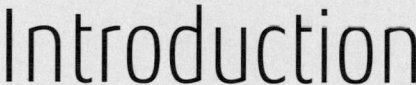

Introduction

We're all aging, but not necessarily at the same rate. Have you ever wondered why one 70-year-old has a hard time making it out of bed in the morning, while another is running half marathons? More often than not, it's because the marathon runner has kept all the parts of his or her body moving on a daily basis. That's what functional training is all about—engaging all parts of your body so you can still perform everyday activities with efficiency, no matter your age.

So what is your goal? Maybe you want to be able to pick up your grandkids with ease, get back in the pool, or take those long hikes you used to enjoy. Whatever it is, the moment you realize the direct correlation between improving your fitness and improving your life is the moment you will find all the motivation you need to stick with a fitness program. The functional training method is the key to staying fit and active for life.

Use this book to future-proof your body with 62 step-by-step exercises (each with modifications to meet your ability level), 20 unique workout routines, and 3 easy-to-implement, one-month fitness programs. *Stay Fit for Life* will empower you to do more of the things you love with confidence and ease for years to come.

FUNCTIONAL FITNESS BASICS

Functional training is a total-body approach to fitness that mimics your daily activities and enables you to live a healthier, more dynamic lifestyle. Life is unpredictable and unstable, so why should your training be full of predictable and stable movements?

Why train functionally?

By mimicking the way your body naturally moves, functional exercise strengthens your body's connections so you can move with ease and confidence and continue to do the things you love as you age.

Prepare for daily life

Improving your body's efficiency through functional exercise lets you more safely perform your daily activities and substantially reduces your risk of injury as you age.

Improved posture

Functional training restores your body to its natural, upright state by improving flexibility in the spine, chest, and hips, while strengthening the back and glutes.

Greater strength

Strengthening your muscle groups makes it easier to perform daily tasks with more confidence and less pain. For example, functional training teaches your muscles to safely and effectively lift a heavy box.

Increased stability

Training your core with full-body movements improves balance and reduces the risk of falling. Strengthening the abdomen and back stabilizes your torso and gives you better control of your arms and legs.

Better mobility

Functional exercises enable you to move more freely and smoothly by increasing the range of motion of joints, improving flexibility, and helping you perform actions such as reaching and bending.

More endurance

Dynamic movements improve both cardiovascular and muscular endurance, which reduces your risk of developing chronic diseases, helps you control your weight, and preserves heart and lung health.

The benefits

Each exercise in this book tags the functional areas that it benefits in the Improves box. Follow a fitness program to grow in all five areas.

IMPROVES

//// **Posture**
//// **Strength**
//// **Stability**
//// **Mobility**
//// **Endurance**

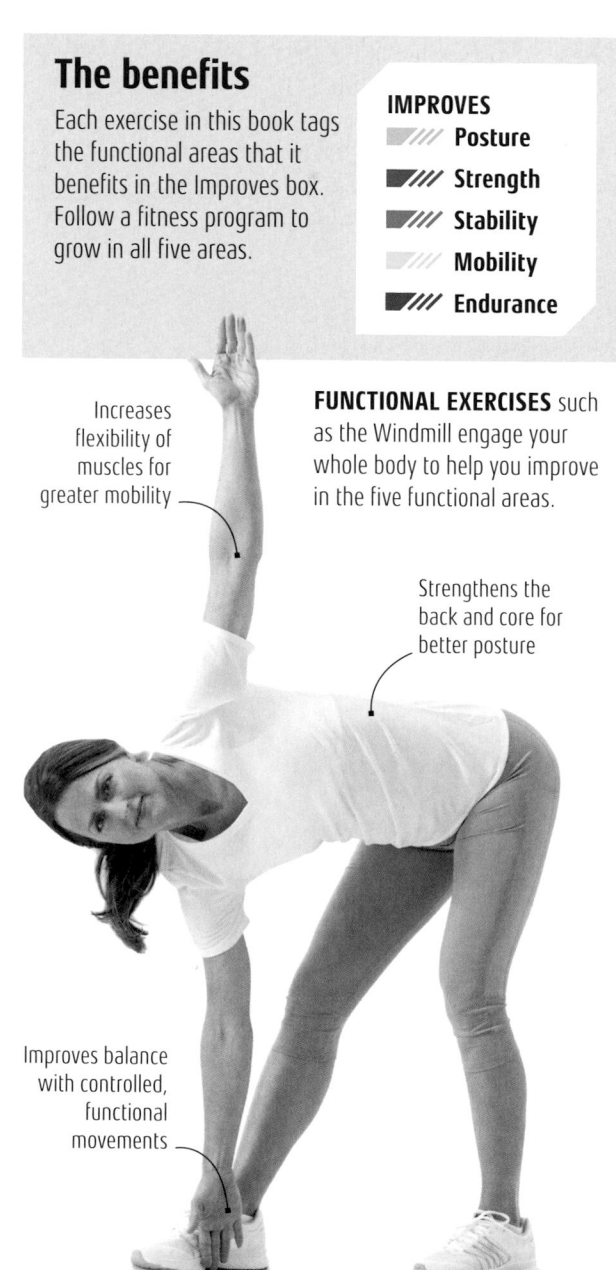

Increases flexibility of muscles for greater mobility

FUNCTIONAL EXERCISES such as the Windmill engage your whole body to help you improve in the five functional areas.

Strengthens the back and core for better posture

Improves balance with controlled, functional movements

The foundational movements

The human body can lift, flex, twist, and stretch in seemingly countless ways, but human movement can be distilled into five foundational types of movement: locomotion, pushing, pulling, rotation, and raising and lowering. Functional exercises require multiple joints and muscles to work together in the same way your everyday activities do, which improves your efficiency in these five movement patterns. A simple task such as picking up groceries involves your ankles, knees, hips, core, shoulders, and elbows; functional training mimics movements like this to help make everyday activities easier and safer to perform.

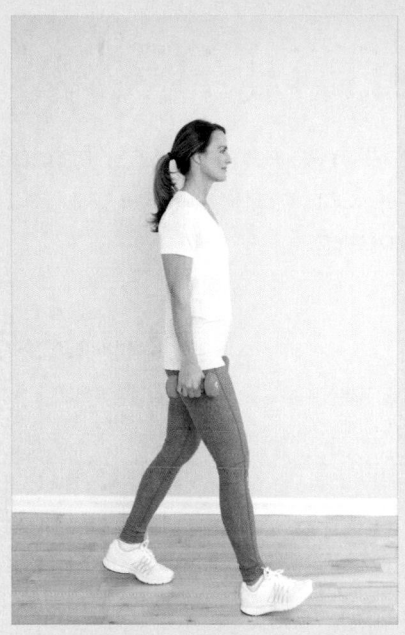

LOCOMOTION is the ability to move your body from one place to another. Activities such as walking, running, or climbing stairs all require locomotive skills.

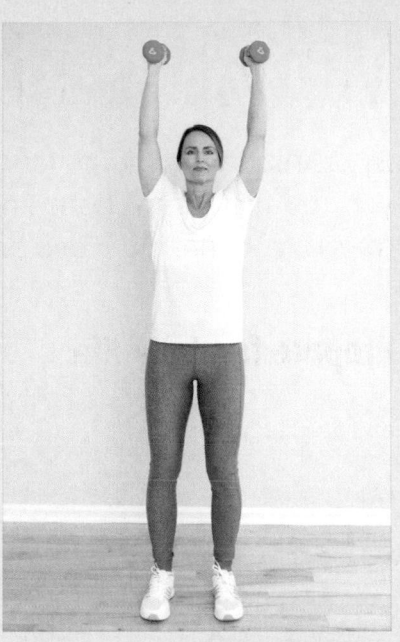

PUSHING involves activities that take your arms away from the body. Activities such as using a shovel or moving a cart full of groceries require efficient pushing.

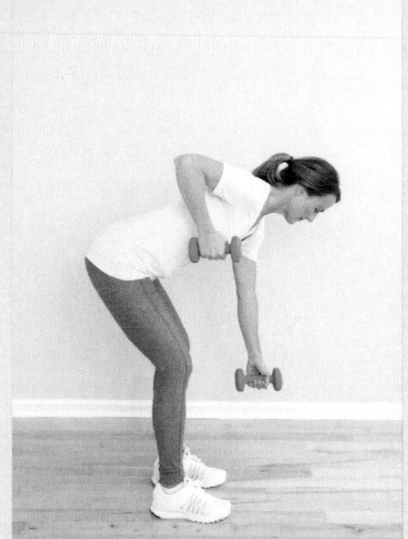

PULLING brings your arms toward your body or pulls your center of mass toward an object. Examples include starting a lawn mower or pulling your chair up to a desk.

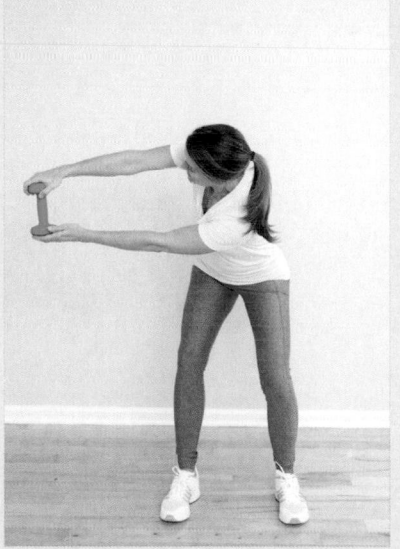

ROTATION requires the upper body to move in opposition to the lower body by twisting your hips and core. For example, swimming and throwing both use rotation.

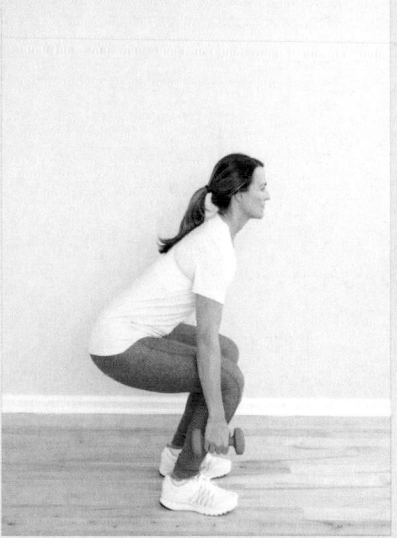

RAISING AND LOWERING the body's center of mass involves bending, squatting, and lunging, and can be found in everyday tasks such as getting into a car.

How the body moves

Daily movement is dynamic, requiring a complex orchestration of your entire body in multiple directions and angles. Functional exercises use compound movements to train your body for that purpose. By understanding how your lower-body, core, and upper-body systems work together as one unit, you can more efficiently and easily move throughout your daily life.

 ## Kinetic chain

Your individual muscles are useless without the kinetic chain—the body's system of joints, muscles, ligaments, and tendons that work together in a linear sequence to accomplish movement. For example, a throwing motion begins at your ankles and transfers force through the kinetic chain all the way to your wrists. Some links in the chain keep your joints stable, while others enable mobility; but if one link is not working properly, it will affect surrounding links, and ultimately the movement.

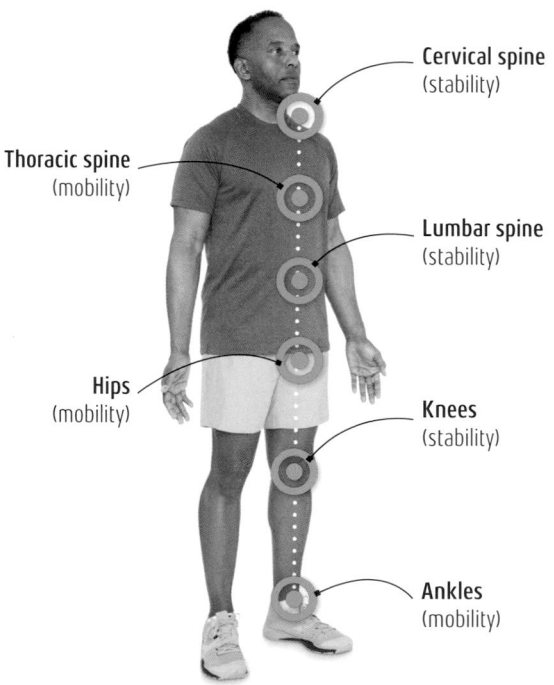

Cervical spine
(stability)

Thoracic spine
(mobility)

Lumbar spine
(stability)

Hips
(mobility)

Knees
(stability)

Ankles
(mobility)

Links of movement

 ## Planes of movement

Your body moves within three dimensions, called planes. If you imagine all the different movements your body can make, every one of them occupies at least one plane of movement. However, most actions are not performed precisely in one plane, but rather they use multiple planes at once—we move up and down and side to side in fluid motions. Functional training works your body in all 3 planes of movement to improve overall coordination and stability.

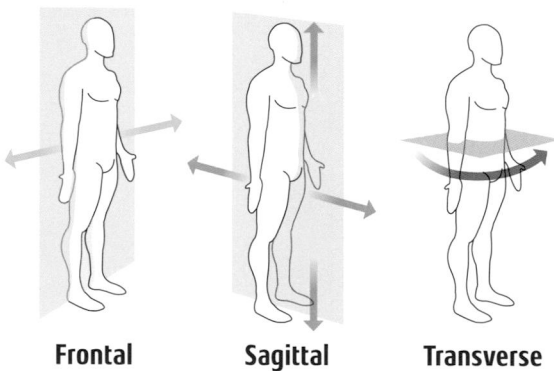

Frontal   **Sagittal**   **Transverse**

FRONTAL PLANE divides the front and back halves of the body. We move from side to side in this plane.

SAGITTAL PLANE splits the left and right sides of the body. We move up and down or forward and backward in this plane.

TRANSVERSE PLANE separates the top and bottom of the body at the hips. We rotate in this plane.

Compound exercise

Functional exercises are usually compound, meaning they use several muscle groups at once. By performing exercises that recruit your whole kinetic chain within multiple planes of movement, you effectively prepare your body for any movement challenge that an active life may throw your way.

A COMPOUND MOVEMENT, such as the Reverse lunge with twist, can use multiple planes of movement (the transverse and saggital planes, in this instance), while engaging the total kinetic chain.

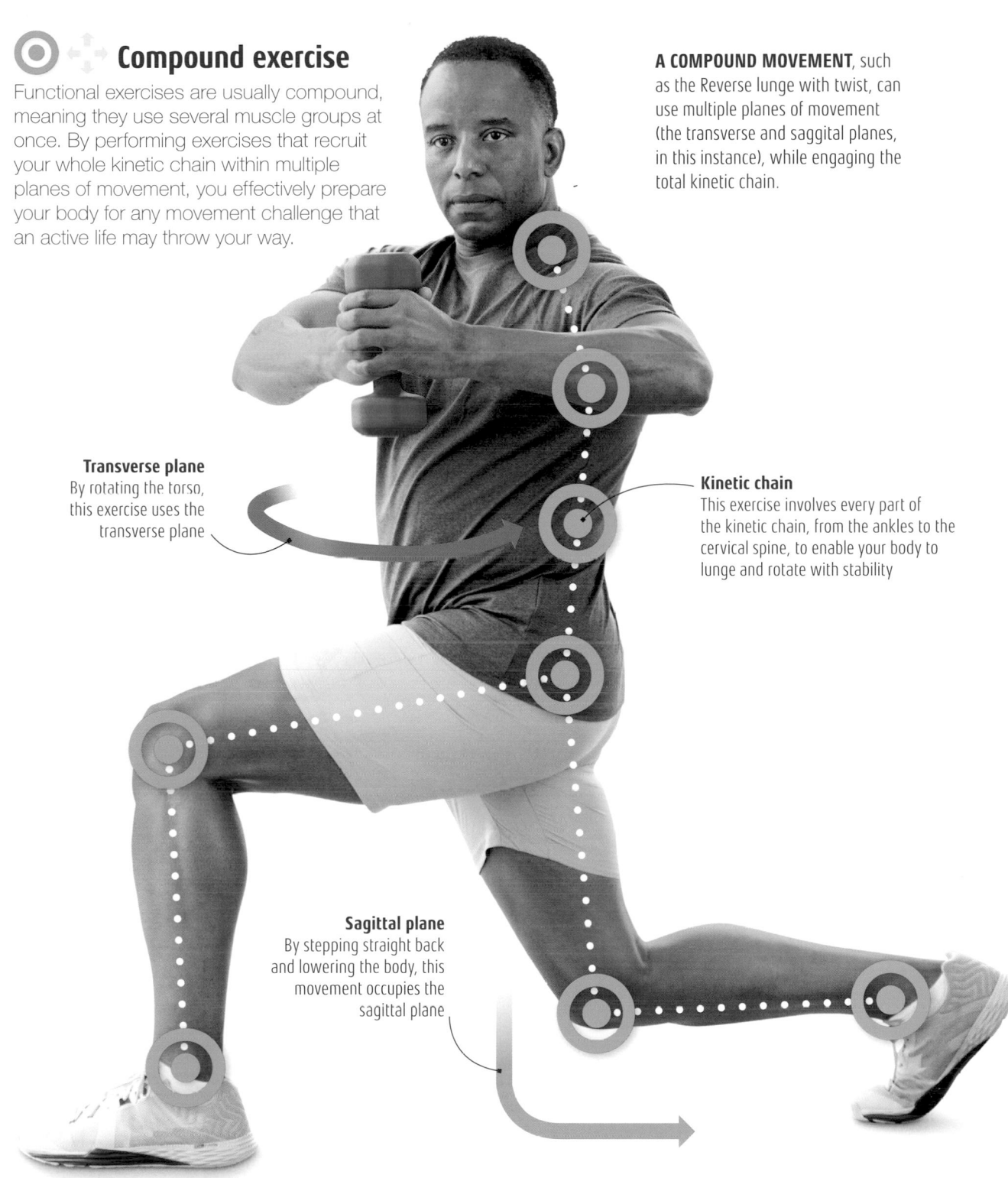

Transverse plane
By rotating the torso, this exercise uses the transverse plane

Kinetic chain
This exercise involves every part of the kinetic chain, from the ankles to the cervical spine, to enable your body to lunge and rotate with stability

Sagittal plane
By stepping straight back and lowering the body, this movement occupies the sagittal plane

How exercise helps the body

You've probably heard the axiom "move it or lose it," and it's true. Nothing will speed up the aging process quite like disuse and inactivity of the body, but performing functional exercise on a regular basis will improve your health and quality of life, and keep your body looking and feeling youthful.

STRENGTHENS BONES

1% Amount of bone density the average person loses each year after age **35**

Bones tend to weaken with age, but functional training uses weight-bearing exercises to slow down bone-density loss. By loading your bones with weight, you increase muscle mass, which is proven to directly increase bone cell growth and help prevent osteoporosis and fractures.

BUILDS LEAN MUSCLE

4% Amount of muscle mass the average person loses each decade after age **30**

With age and inactivity, the body can experience a significant loss of muscle mass, a condition called *muscle atrophy*. However, when you perform weight-bearing exercises, your body replaces damaged muscle fibers with new fibers that strengthen and build lean muscle tissue. Stronger muscles enable you to live a more confident and active lifestyle.

PRESERVES VITAL JOINT TISSUES

350 million

Estimated number of people worldwide who have arthritis

The breakdown of joint tissue over time can lead to pain, inflammation, stiffness, and often arthritis. Functional exercise stimulates blood flow to joint tissues so that the increased supply of oxygen and nutrients can lubricate your joints. This results in healthier, pain-free movement.

SHARPENS NERVOUS SYSTEM

11 seconds

Frequency at which US emergency rooms treat an older adult for a fall

Your nervous system and brain function inevitably decline with age, which impairs your ability to sense your body's movement and position in space—known as *proprioception*. Functional training focuses on movements that build a strong connection between your brain and body to improve your proprioception and increase your reaction time for safer and more agile movement.

IMPROVES HEART HEALTH AND BLOOD FLOW

31% Percentage of total deaths worldwide in **2015** due to heart disease

The aging heart can't pump out as much blood as a younger heart, but functional fitness boosts your heart's endurance, lowers your resting heart rate, and causes blood vessels to dilate, which means more oxygen reaches your organs and muscles. Increased flow of oxygen gives you the energy to move with more vitality.

IMPROVES MOOD AND CONFIDENCE

350 million Number of people worldwide who suffer from depression

When you're stressed, your body releases stress hormones, such as cortisol and adrenaline, that can produce inflammation in your body and lead to anxiety and depression. Functional training combats this by engaging your body to release feel-good hormones, or *endorphins*, that counter the negative effects of stress and anxiety to lift your mood and increase your confidence.

EXTENDS LIFE SPAN

7 minutes

Length of time your life is extended by every minute of exercise after age **39**

Study after study has shown that a sedentary lifestyle can have devastating effects on individual health, including a shortened life span. Functional training helps rebuild and re-energize weakened muscles and joints, strengthens the heart and lungs, and improves and extends your life. The benefit may level off as you age, but when you give a little, you always gain a little. It's never too late to start, so get moving!

INCREASES LUNG FUNCTION

1/3 Amount a person's lung capacity reduces from age **30** to **60**

The effects of aging on the respiratory system include weakened lungs and respiratory muscles, making you feel short of breath when you exercise. But increased fitness levels make your movement and heart more efficient, thus making it easier for your lungs to supply your body with oxygen. You'll notice increased stamina the more you work out.

BOOSTS METABOLISM

2% Amount a person's metabolism slows with each decade of life

Your basal metabolic rate (BMR) is the number of calories your body burns at rest. Functional training increases your BMR by increasing your lean muscle mass. Because muscle cells require energy in the form of calories, even when you're not exercising, increasing your muscle mass makes your body more efficient at burning calories to keep you leaner.

How to train effectively

Getting fit doesn't require spending long hours at the gym, but it does require taking good care of your body and observing some essential rules for effective training and living. To get the most out of your training, begin building healthy habits and follow this exercise and lifestyle guidance.

Q HOW MUCH WATER SHOULD I DRINK EVERY DAY?

A You should drink 2l of water, or about eight 8-ounce glasses, every day. Staying hydrated helps your heart and muscles work more efficiently. Drink water before the thirst sensation even arises—if you're already thirsty, then you're already dehydrated. It helps to carry a water bottle with you everywhere you go so you can drink throughout the day.

Q HOW DO I KNOW IF I'M DEHYDRATED?

A Listen to your body. Thirst, headaches, dizziness, and fatigue are all potential signs of dehydration. If you feel any of these symptoms, then it's possible you need more water. Urine color is also a good indicator. Ideally it's a pale straw color, but if it is dark yellow, then you're likely dehydrated. On the other hand, colorless urine might mean you're over-hydrated or drinking too quickly.

Q SHOULD I EAT BEFORE WORKING OUT?

A Yes! Eat a nutrient-rich meal between 1 and 3 hours before training. Eating before a workout provides essential nutrients to increase the effectiveness of your hard work. Whole foods are best—primarily low-fat proteins and low-glycemic carbohydrates such as eggs, oatmeal, chicken, and vegetables.

Q WHEN SHOULD I EAT AFTER WORKING OUT?

A Eat a post-workout meal within 15 to 20 minutes after working out. This meal should consist of a 3:1 ratio of carbohydrates to proteins to give your muscles the fuel to replenish glycogen, a substance that rebuilds and repairs muscle tissues. Good meal options include fish and brown rice, or turkey and sweet potatoes.

Q HOW CAN I SHOP SMARTER?

A Shop the perimeter of the grocery store and avoid center aisles. The perimeter of most stores is where you'll find whole foods, fruits and vegetables, dairy, and lean meats. By comparison, the center aisles tend to be where high-sugar and highly-processed foods are shelved. By avoiding center aisles, it is easier to fill your cart with healthful fuel options.

Q HOW SHOULD I BREATHE WHILE I'M EXERCISING?

A You should exhale through your mouth during the hardest part of a movement and inhale through your nose during the easier part, keeping a steady, mindful rhythm. Using a squat as an example, inhale on the way down and then exhale as you stand up. However, don't worry too much about exactly when to breathe—the most important thing is to remember not to hold your breath.

Q DO I REALLY NEED TO COOL DOWN AFTER A WORKOUT?

A Absolutely. It's essential to cool down at a controlled pace after every workout. After training, your heart rate is high, your blood vessels are dilated, and your body temperature is elevated. Stopping too fast can lead to passing out or feeling sick. Steadily slowing down lets your body comfortably transition back to a state of rest.

Q HOW CAN I LIMIT SORENESS AFTER TRAINING?

A Integrate foam rolling into your post-workout regimen. The sustained pressure to your muscle tissues deeply lengthens them, ensures they don't tighten up too quickly after exercise, and increases the range of motion of your joints. Use this method to release any of your soft tissues—including your glutes, thighs, calves, chest, or upper back—but never roll over bones or organs.

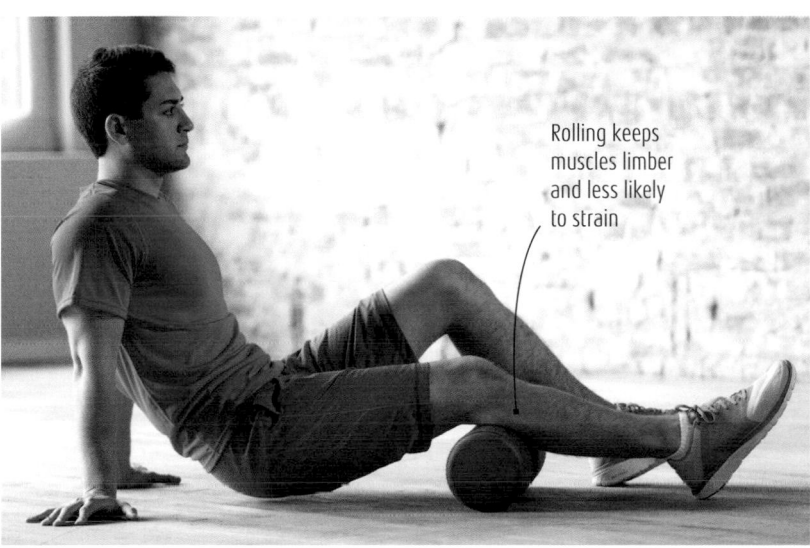

Rolling keeps muscles limber and less likely to strain

SLOWLY ROLL BACK AND FORTH over your soft tissues, applying pressure with body weight, for about 30 seconds.

Q DO I HAVE TO WORK OUT EVERY DAY?

A No. Your mind and body need time to recover, so always include two rest days during your exercise week. When you don't take your rest days, it can lead to mental burnout and an inability to sustain your fitness progress and achieve your goals. Time off also allows your muscles to relax and rebuild, which will make you stronger and less prone to injury. If you're feeling overly tired, or if your muscles and joints feel excessively stiff, it's a good time to take a rest day.

What does it take to stay fit for life?

Breathe consciously, even at rest
Breathing is so involuntary that some people are never really conscious of it until their bodies are starved of oxygen, such as during exercise. However, breathing deeply and deliberately—even while you're at rest—can improve your brain function, relax your body, and reduce stress.

Get quality sleep every night
Sleep is when your mind and body heal and recharge, so it is essential for a healthy lifestyle. Try to get 7 to 8 hours of quality sleep each night. For a more restful sleep, avoid drinking alcohol or large amounts of liquid at least two hours before bedtime, and try to go to bed at the same time each night.

Make time to exercise
It's easy to put off a workout, so always plan exactly when you'll do your workout routine, and try to make it consistent each day. A steady schedule helps you stay on track and ensures that you'll stick to your plan.

Be your own best coach
It's easy to stay motivated when you're in a groove, but it's normal to get off track sometimes. If you find yourself avoiding the gym or straying from a program, stay positive, don't be too hard on yourself, and jump right back in where you left off. Usually just completing that next workout is enough to help you regain lost momentum.

How to use this book

Stay Fit for Life is comprised of a collection of individual exercises, daily workout routines, and functional training programs that will help you get stronger and healthier. This simple method takes the guesswork out of your fitness regimen. Start by performing the fitness assessment, and the rest will fall into place—all you need is the motivation to stick with it.

1 >>> PERFORM THE ASSESSMENT TESTS

Perform each of the five assessment tests on the following pages and use your scores to calculate your fitness level: beginner, intermediate, or advanced. This tells you which exercise program to follow to get started with your training.

Score yourself on a scale of 1–4 for each test

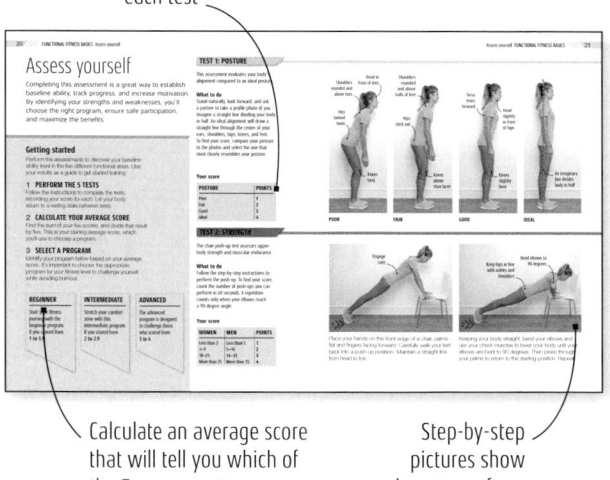

Calculate an average score that will tell you which of the 3 programs to use

Step-by-step pictures show how to perform the tests

2 >>> FIND YOUR FITNESS PROGRAM

Identify your fitness program based on your assessment results. Each 30-day program progresses in difficulty throughout the course of four weeks. The simple calendar design shows you exactly what to do each day.

Workout days specify the prescribed routine for that day, as well as which level to follow

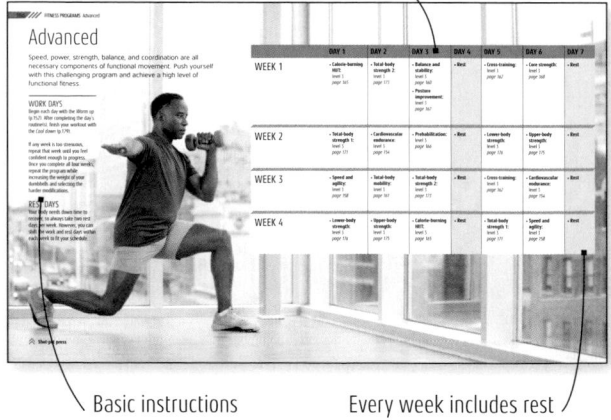

Basic instructions explain how to work through the programs

Every week includes rest days, which are essential for rejuvenating your body

What you need

Only a few simple pieces of equipment are needed to perform the exercises in this book.

Dumbbells

These help you get the most out of your exercise. We recommend having two pairs, one lighter and one heavier, so you can adjust the weight for difficulty.

Step

An aerobic step is used in some cardio and strength exercises. A stair step or low bench works well, too.

Mat

An exercise mat makes floor-based exercises more comfortable.

Chair

Use a sturdy, non-slip chair for some bodyweight exercises, for support to help you balance, or to do a movement while seated.

---

3 ›› FLIP TO THE DAILY WORKOUT ROUTINE

Find your assigned workout for the day, and identify the level prescribed by your program. Each workout routine is composed of five to ten individual exercises that work toward the routine's goal. Follow the directions to complete your level of the workout.

Purposefully chosen exercises work together to help you achieve each workout's goal

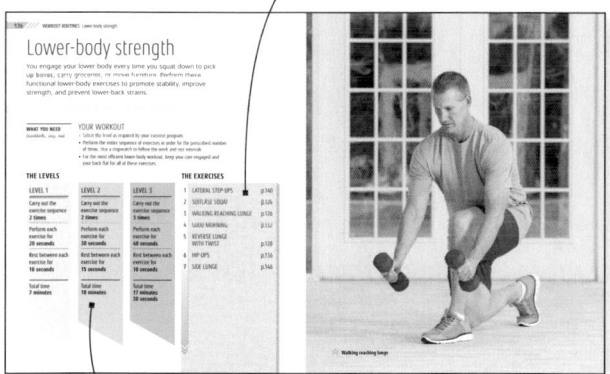

The level shows you how long to perform each exercise, then how long to rest between each exercise

4 ›› COMPLETE THE REQUIRED EXERCISES

Refer to the step-by-step instructional pages to help you execute the exercises in your workout. Each of the 62 exercises found in the routines has its own highly visual spread showing you how to perform the exercise using proper technique.

Each spread identifies which of the five foundational movements the exercise engages

Helpful annotations provide tips for performing the exercise correctly

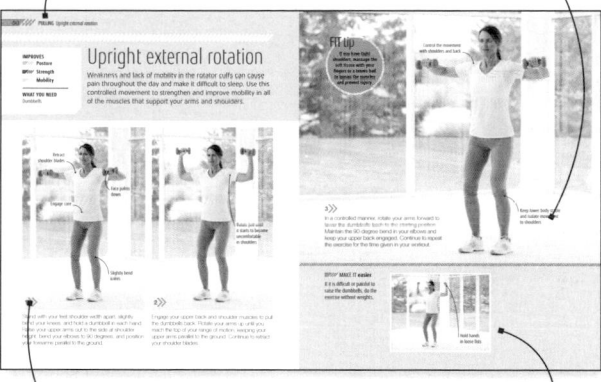

Detailed, step-by-step instructions and color photos show you exactly how to perform the exercise from start to finish

Whenever you want to make an exercise easier or more challenging, follow the directions for the modifications

Assess yourself

Completing this assessment is a great way to establish baseline ability, track progress, and increase motivation. By identifying your strengths and weaknesses, you'll choose the right program, ensure safe participation, and maximize the benefits.

Getting started

Perform the assessments to discover your baseline ability level in the five different functional areas. Use your results as a guide to get started training.

1 PERFORM THE 5 TESTS

Follow the instructions to complete the tests, recording your score for each. Let your body return to a resting state between tests.

2 CALCULATE YOUR AVERAGE SCORE

Find the sum of your five scores, and divide that result by five. This is your starting average score, which you'll use to choose a program.

3 SELECT A PROGRAM

Identify your program below based on your average score. It's important to choose the appropriate program for your fitness level to challenge yourself while avoiding burnout.

BEGINNER

Start your fitness journey with the beginner program if you scored from **1 to 1.9**

INTERMEDIATE

Stretch your comfort zone with this intermediate program if you scored from **2 to 2.9**

ADVANCED

The advanced program is designed to challenge those who scored from **3 to 4**

TEST 1: POSTURE

This assessment evaluates your body's alignment compared to an ideal posture.

What to do

Stand naturally, look forward, and ask a partner to take a profile photo of you. Imagine a straight line dividing your body in half. An ideal alignment will draw a straight line through the center of your ears, shoulders, hips, knees, and feet. To find your score, compare your posture to the photos and select the one that most closely resembles your posture.

Your score

POSTURE	POINTS
Poor	1
Fair	2
Good	3
Ideal	4

TEST 2: STRENGTH

The chair push-up test assesses upper-body strength and muscular endurance.

What to do

Follow the step-by-step instructions to perform the push-up. To find your score, count the number of push-ups you can perform in 60 seconds. A repetition counts only when your elbows reach a 90-degree angle.

Your score

WOMEN	MEN	POINTS
Less than 2	Less than 5	1
3–9	5–15	2
10–25	16–35	3
More than 25	More than 35	4

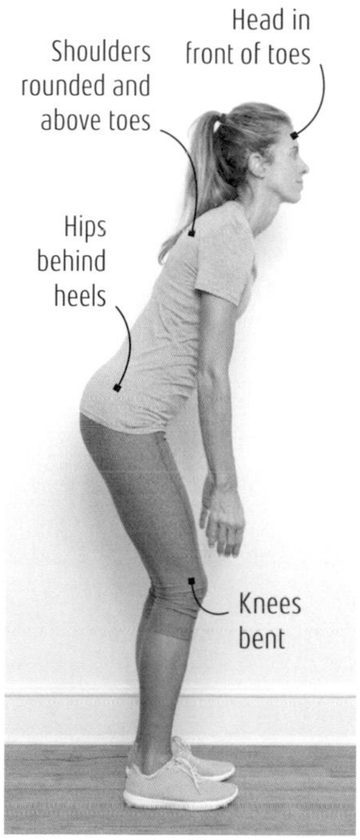

Shoulders rounded and above toes

Head in front of toes

Hips behind heels

Knees bent

POOR

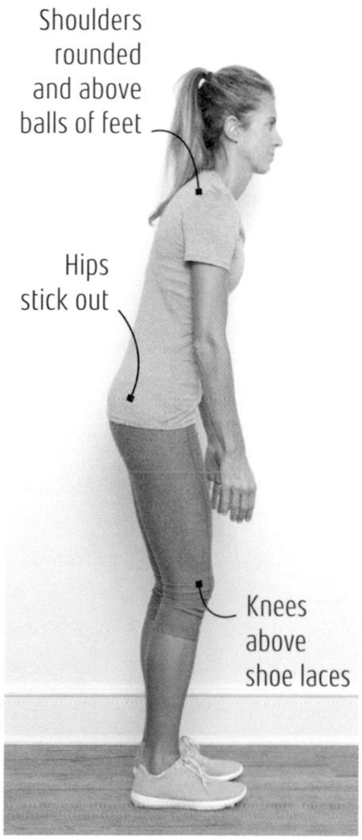

Shoulders rounded and above balls of feet

Hips stick out

Knees above shoe laces

FAIR

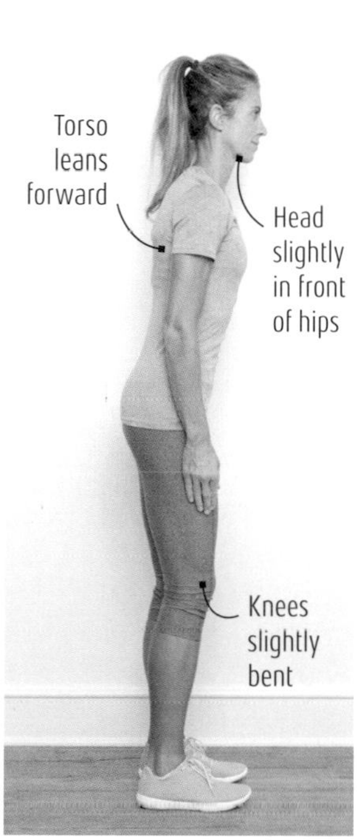

Torso leans forward

Head slightly in front of hips

Knees slightly bent

GOOD

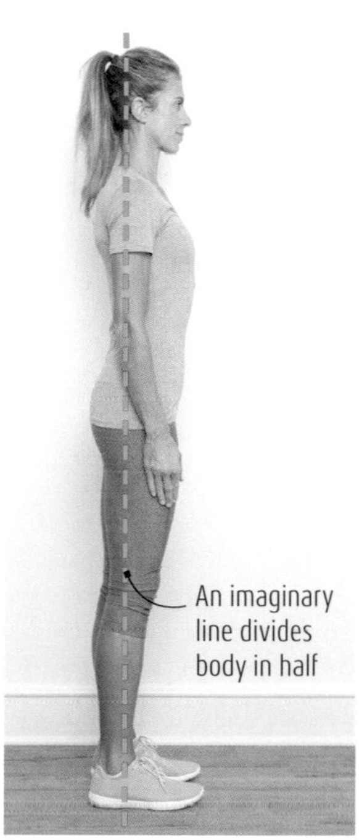

An imaginary line divides body in half

IDEAL

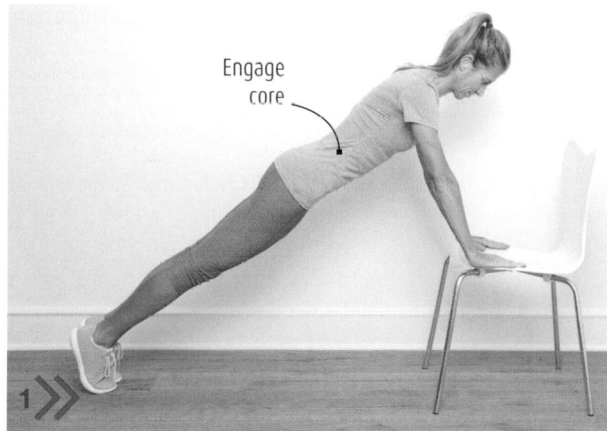

Engage core

Place your hands on the front edge of a chair, palms flat and fingers facing forward. Carefully walk your feet back into a push-up position. Maintain a straight line from head to toe.

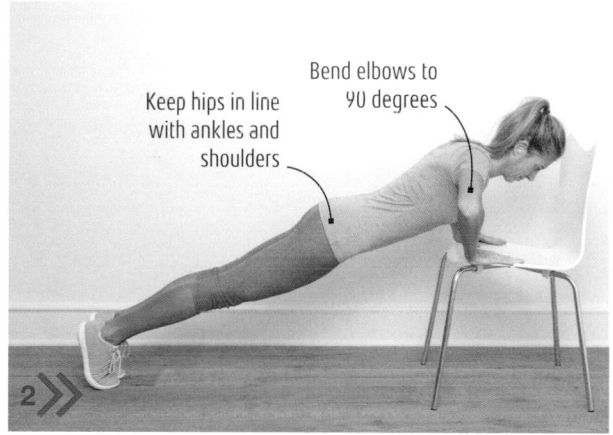

Keep hips in line with ankles and shoulders

Bend elbows to 90 degrees

Keeping your body straight, bend your elbows and use your chest muscles to lower your body until your elbows are bent to 90 degrees. Then press through your palms to return to the starting position. Repeat.

TEST 3: STABILITY

Use this test to evaluate your balance and stability while in a static position.

What to do

Follow the step-by-step instructions to get into position. Using a stopwatch, time how long you can balance on your left leg before your right foot touches the ground. Repeat on your right leg. To find your score, calculate the average of your two times.

Your score

ALL	POINTS
Less than 20 seconds	1
21–35 seconds	2
36–50 seconds	3
More than 50 seconds	4

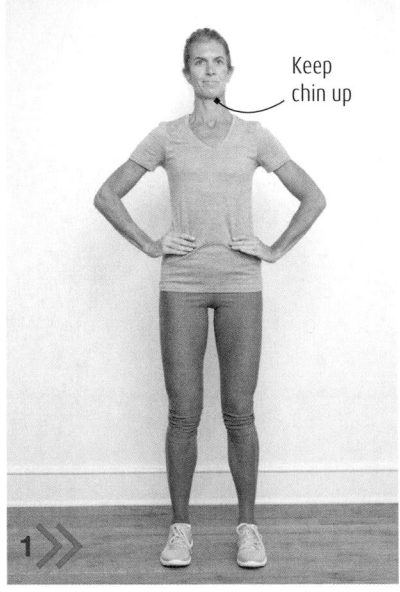

Keep chin up

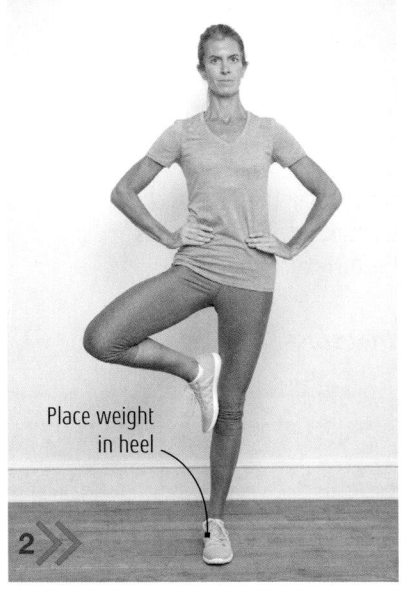

Place weight in heel

Stand with your feet shoulder-width apart and place your hands on your hips. Maintain an upright posture and engage your core. Retract your shoulder blades.

Lift your right leg and place the sole of the right foot against the side of your left knee. Time how long you can balance in this position. Repeat on your other leg.

TEST 5: MOBILITY

The overhead squat tests your flexibility and mobility on both sides of the body.

What to do

Stand with your feet shoulder-width apart and raise your arms straight overhead. Squat as deeply as you can, and ask a partner to take a profile photo of you. To find your score, select the photo that most closely resembles your position.

Your score

POSITION	POINTS
Poor	1
Fair	2
Good	3
Ideal	4

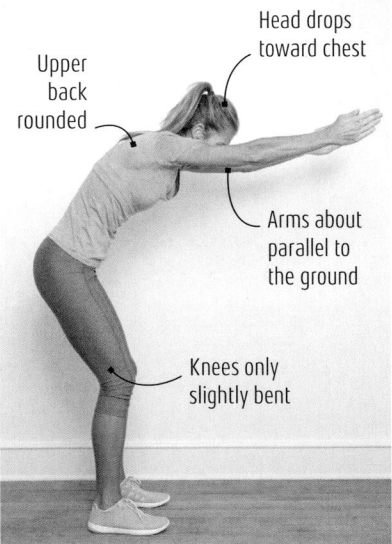

Upper back rounded

Head drops toward chest

Arms about parallel to the ground

Knees only slightly bent

POOR

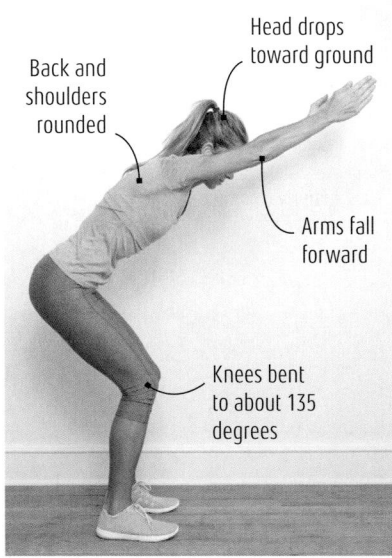

Back and shoulders rounded

Head drops toward ground

Arms fall forward

Knees bent to about 135 degrees

FAIR

TEST 4: ENDURANCE

This step test assesses your cardiovascular endurance.

What to do
Follow the step-by-step instructions. To find your score, count the number of times your left knee reaches the mark in 2 minutes.

Your score

WOMEN	POINTS
Less than 80	1
81–100	2
101–120	3
More than 120	4

MEN	POINTS
Less than 90	1
91–110	2
111–130	3
More than 130	4

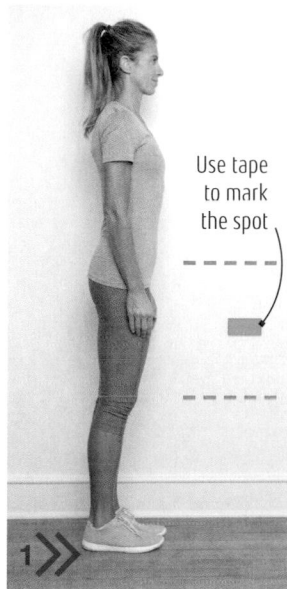

Use tape to mark the spot

1 Stand next to a wall and mark the spot that is halfway between your hip bone and knee.

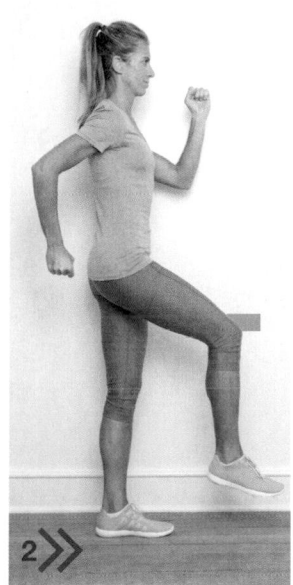

2 Lift your right knee until it reaches the mark on the wall. Swing your arms to help balance.

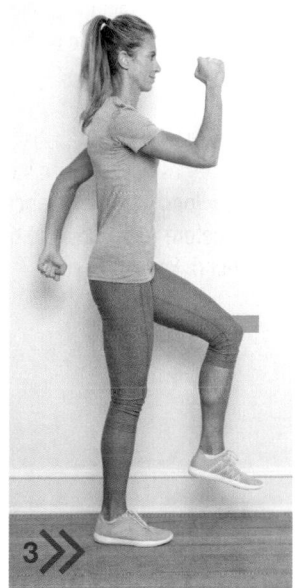

3 Lower your right leg to the ground, then raise your left knee to the mark. Continue to march in place.

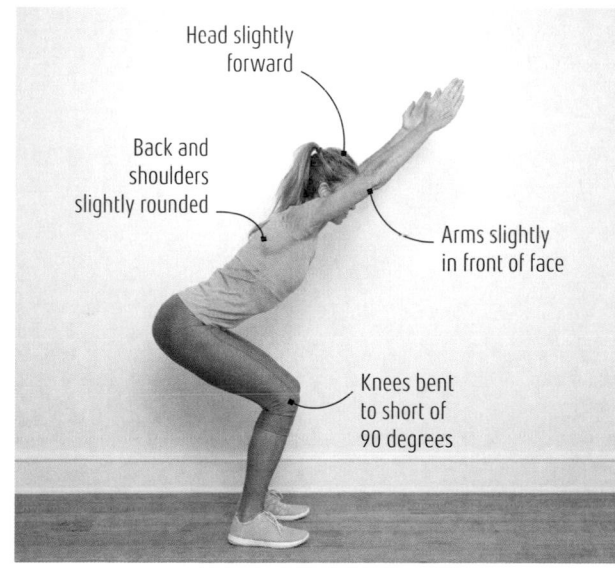

Head slightly forward

Back and shoulders slightly rounded

Arms slightly in front of face

Knees bent to short of 90 degrees

GOOD

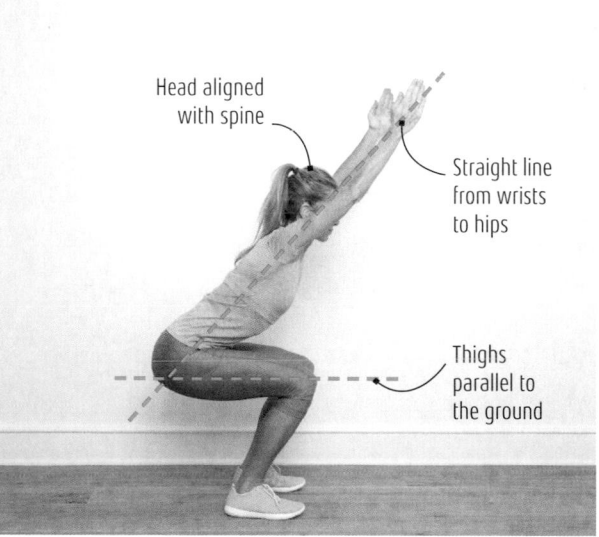

Head aligned with spine

Straight line from wrists to hips

Thighs parallel to the ground

IDEAL

EXERCISES

LOCOMOTION • PUSHING • PULLING • ROTATION • RAISING AND LOWERING

Living an active lifestyle requires a wide range of movements, so it is important to be prepared. By targeting your body's five foundational movements, this collection of functional exercises will make you stronger, more stable, and better equipped to tackle your everyday activities.

Fast feet

IMPROVES
Endurance

WHAT YOU NEED
No equipment needed

Strong communication between your brain and body is the key to moving quickly during walking activities. Run in place with this drill to improve your mind-body coordination and cardiovascular endurance.

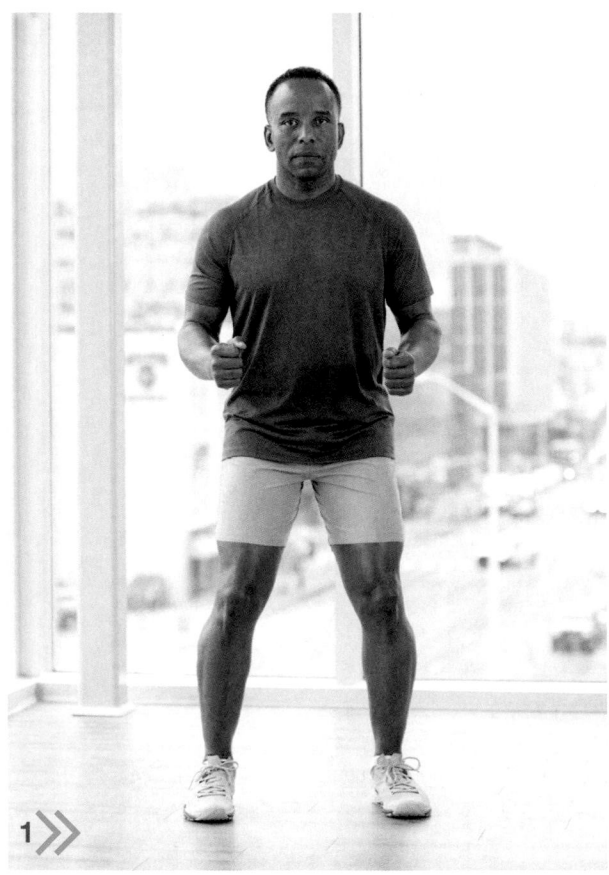

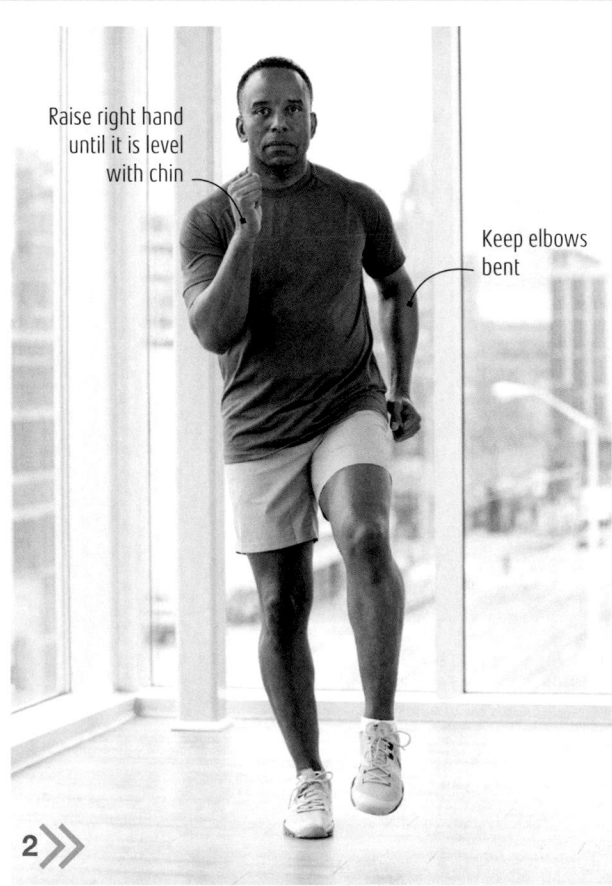

Raise right hand until it is level with chin

Keep elbows bent

1 »

Stand with your feet shoulder-width apart. Bend both elbows to 90 degrees, position your forearms in front of you, and hold your hands in loose fists. Engage your core and retract your shoulder blades.

2 »

Raise your left knee until your foot is about 3 inches (8cm) off the ground, and shift your weight to your right foot. Simultaneously raise your right hand toward your chin and pull your left hand toward your hip.

3 »

In a continuous motion, return your left foot to the ground, first making contact with the ball of your foot, and immediately lift your right foot about 3 inches (8cm) off the ground while raising your left hand toward your chin and pulling your right hand toward your hip. Continue to run in place for the time given in your workout.

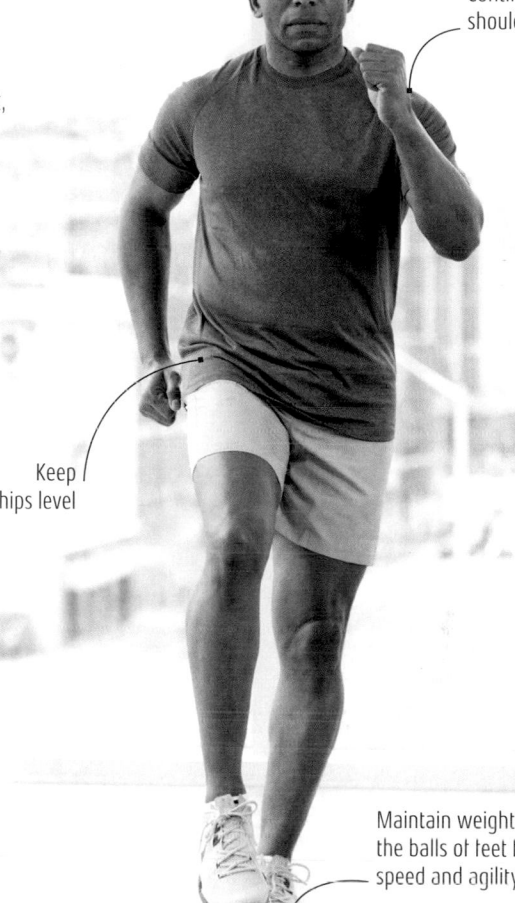

Continue to retract shoulder blades

Keep hips level

Maintain weight on the balls of feet for greater speed and agility

---

//// MAKE IT **easier**

If it is difficult to maintain balance, sit on the edge of a chair and run in place while seated.

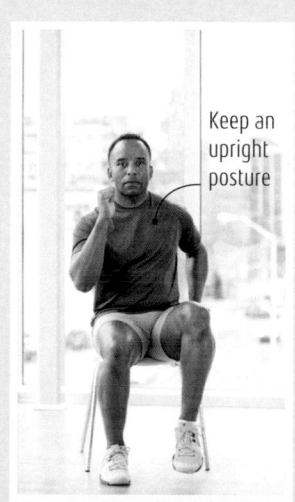

Keep an upright posture

//// MAKE IT **harder**

To increase intensity, raise your knee as high as you can with each step.

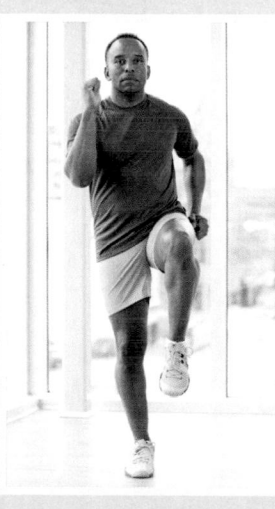

IMPROVES
■/// **Stability**
■/// **Endurance**

WHAT YOU NEED
No equipment needed

Side-to-side

Because life tasks often require you to move sideways, lateral exercises such as this one are essential to any fitness program. This fast-paced drill enhances your stability and coordination so you can move left and right with confidence.

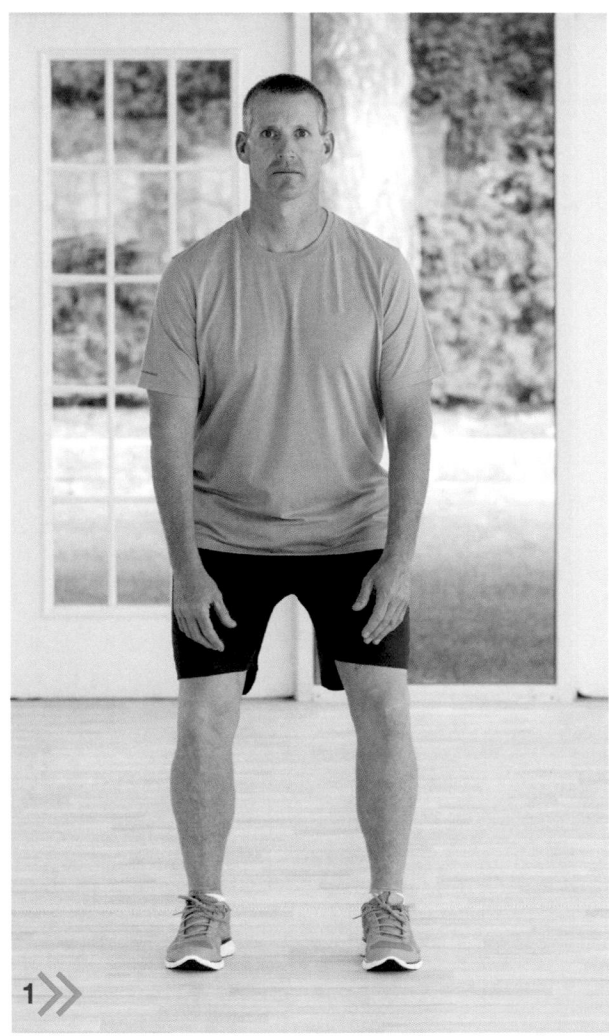

1 >>

Stand with your feet shoulder-width apart and relax your arms in front of you. Engage your core, slightly lean forward, retract your shoulder blades, and raise your head. Slightly bend your knees and hips.

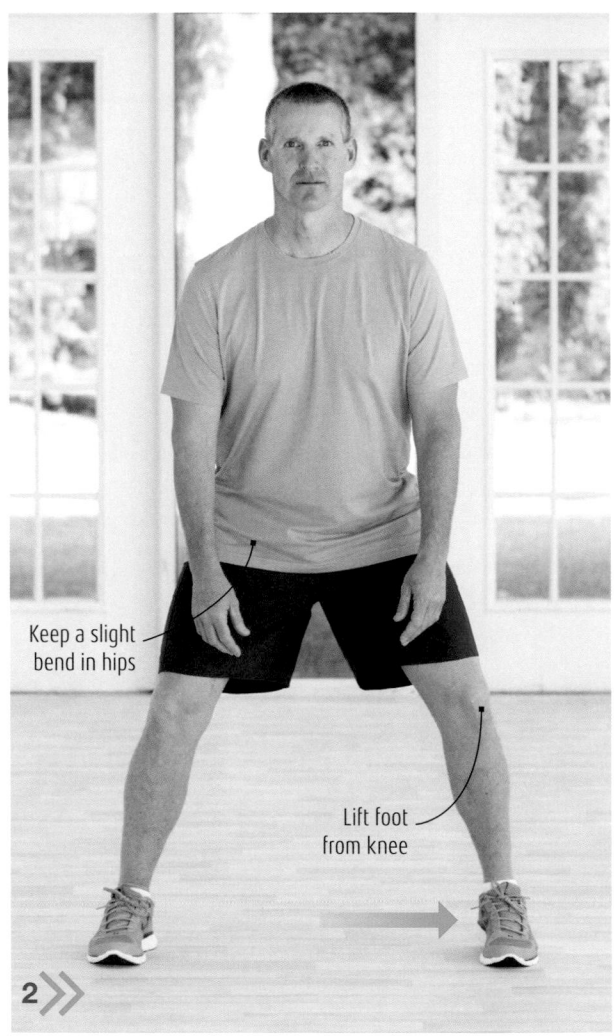

Keep a slight bend in hips

Lift foot from knee

2 >>

Raise your left foot off the ground and step to your left, first making contact with the ball of your foot, then with your heel. Step out slightly wider than shoulder-width apart.

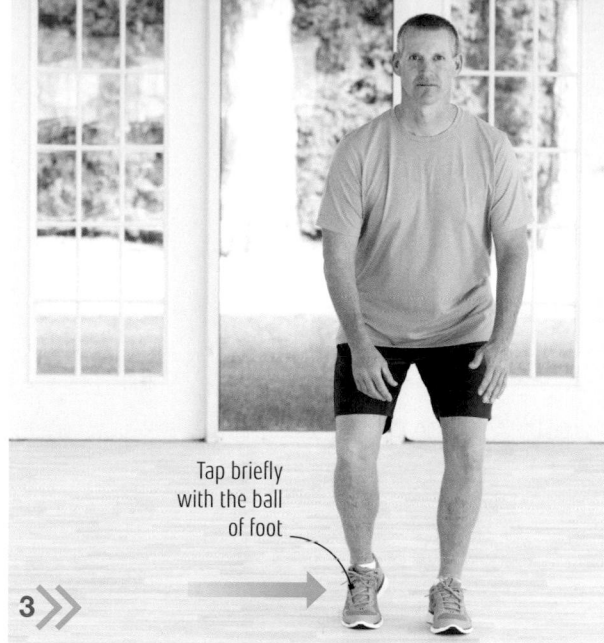

3 ›› Tap briefly with the ball of foot

Raise your right foot off the ground and tap it next to your left foot, transferring your weight to your left foot. Make light and brief contact with the ball of your right foot, and do not place your heel on the ground.

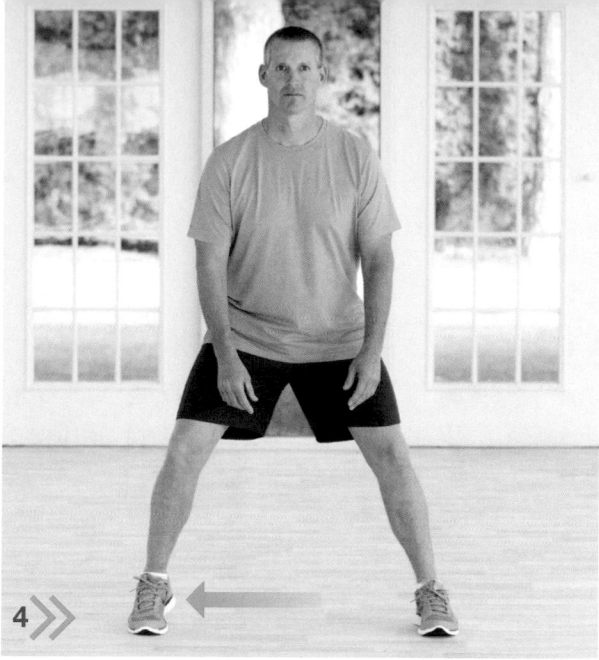

4 ››

Quickly step your right foot back to slightly wider than shoulder-width apart and shift your weight back to your right foot. Maintain a slight bend in your knees and hips for balance.

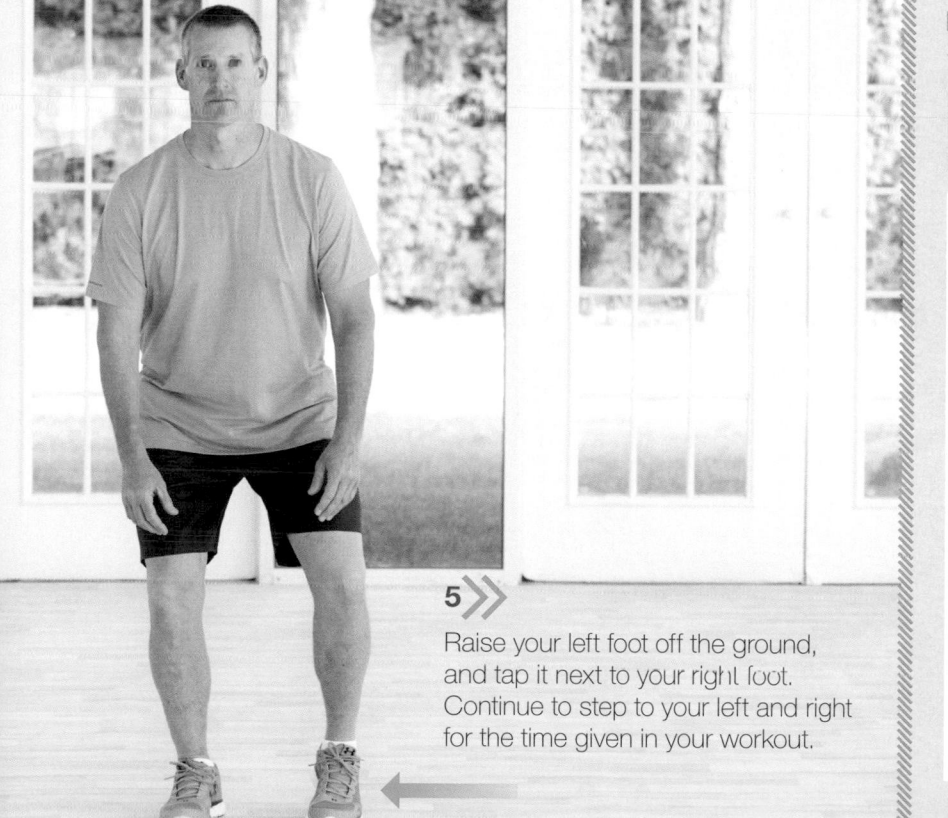

5 ››

Raise your left foot off the ground, and tap it next to your right foot. Continue to step to your left and right for the time given in your workout.

///// **MAKE IT harder**

To strengthen your legs, in step 1, squat until your thighs are parallel to the ground. Maintain the squat throughout the exercise.

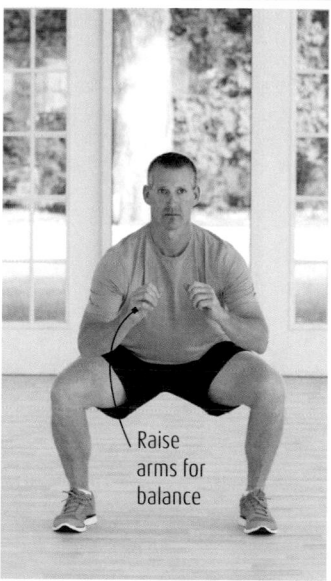

Raise arms for balance

Side shuffle

IMPROVES
//// **Strength**
//// **Stability**
//// **Endurance**

WHAT YOU NEED
No equipment needed

Lateral movements require agility, coordination, and stability. Shuffling quickly from side to side will improve your ability to perform these sideways motions while also strengthening your legs and glutes.

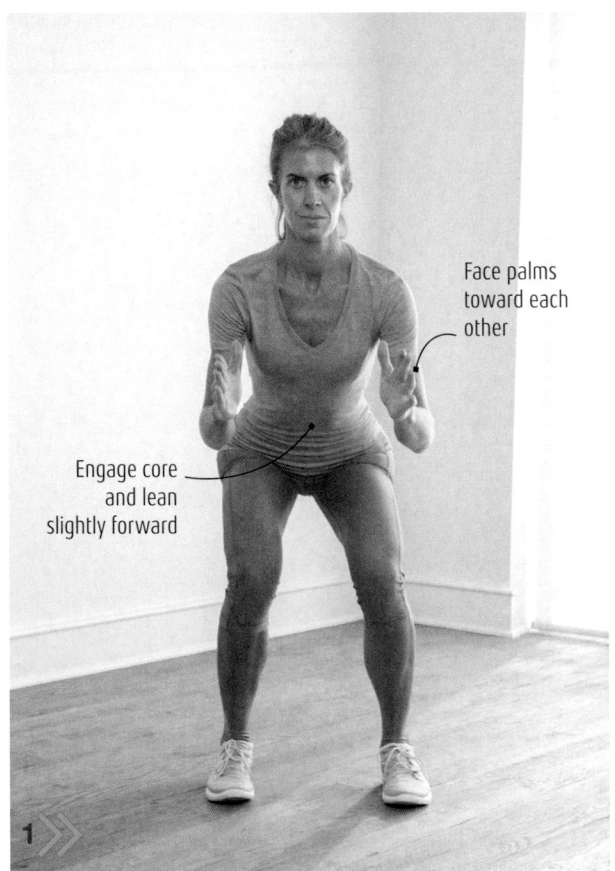

Face palms toward each other

Engage core and lean slightly forward

1

Stand with your feet shoulder-width apart and bend your knees and hips. Place your weight in your hips and heels. Raise your head and retract your shoulder blades. Hold your arms firmly in front of you.

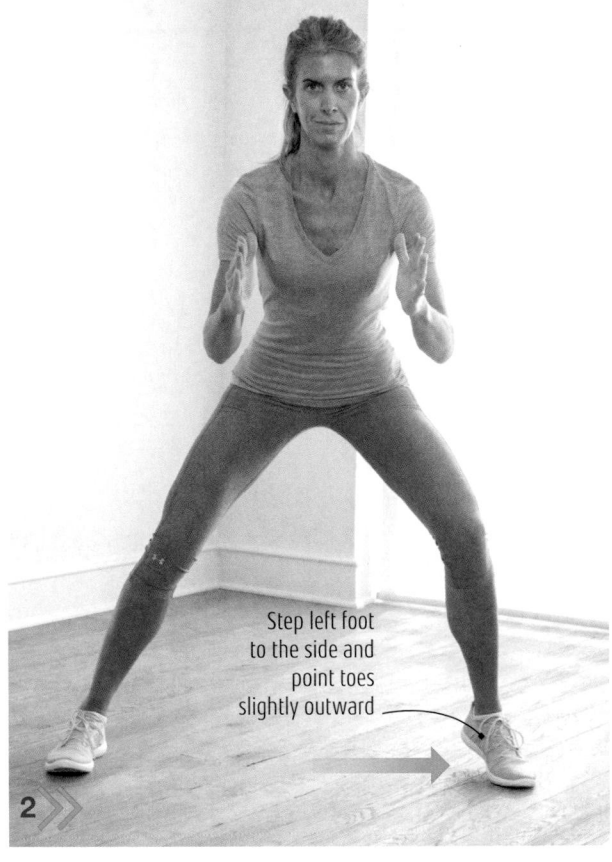

Step left foot to the side and point toes slightly outward

2

Push into the ground with your right foot and lift your left foot off the ground. Step to your left and place your left foot wider than shoulder-width apart. Transfer your weight to your left foot.

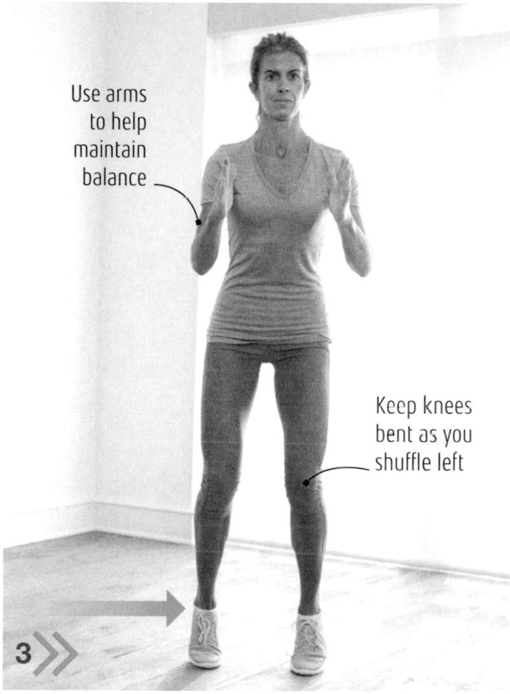

Use arms to help maintain balance

Keep knees bent as you shuffle left

Stay light on balls of feet to move quickly

3 »

Step your right foot next to your left foot and rise onto the balls of your feet. Step sideways again with your left foot and continue to shuffle rapidly to your left for 3 to 5 yards (2.5–4.5m), keeping your feet parallel. Keep your weight in the balls of your feet for balance.

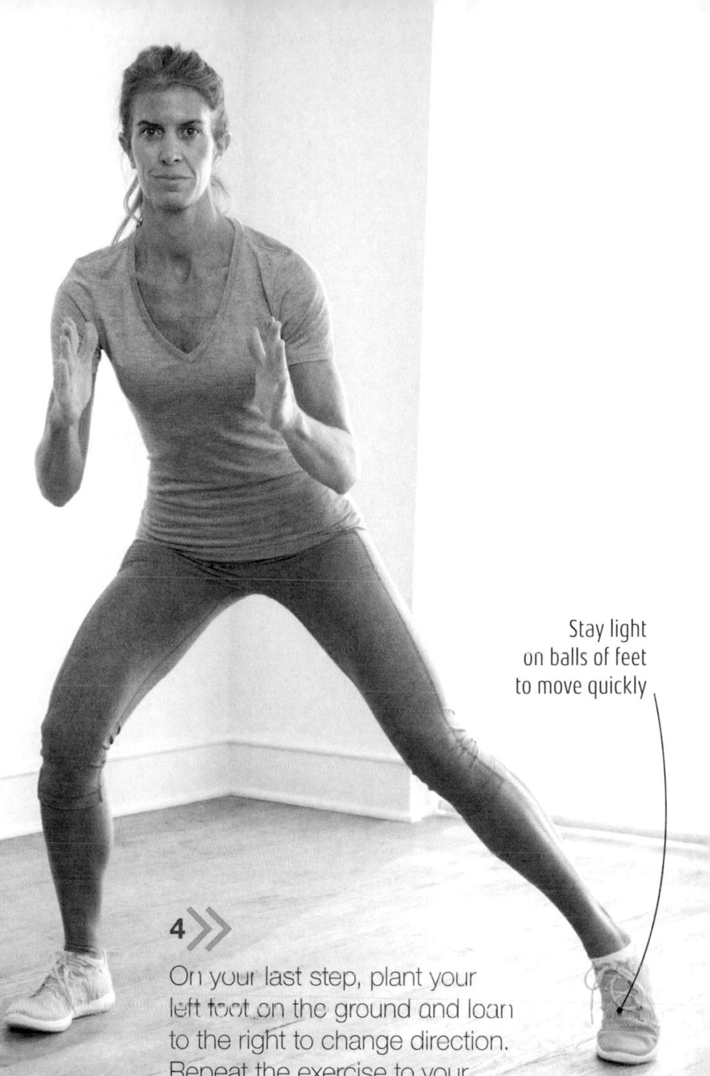

4 »

On your last step, plant your left foot on the ground and lean to the right to change direction. Repeat the exercise to your right. Continue to shuffle to your left and right for the time given in your workout.

MAKE IT **harder**
To strengthen your legs, in step 1, squat deep until your thighs are parallel to the ground. Maintain the squat throughout the exercise.

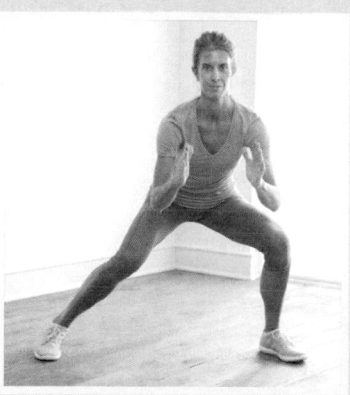

March in place

Running, hiking, and climbing stairs all demand your hips be flexible and strong. Perform this drill energetically to improve your endurance and balance while stretching and strengthening your hips.

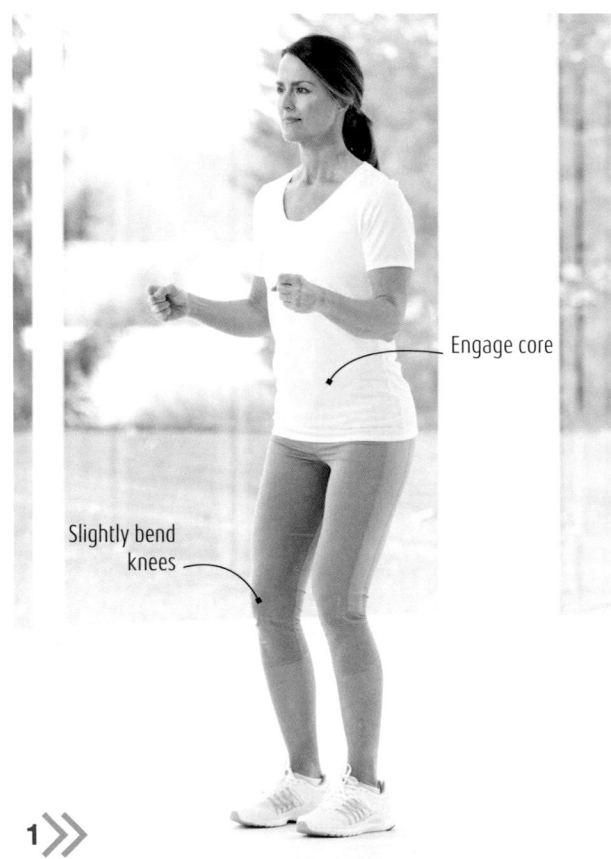

Engage core

Slightly bend knees

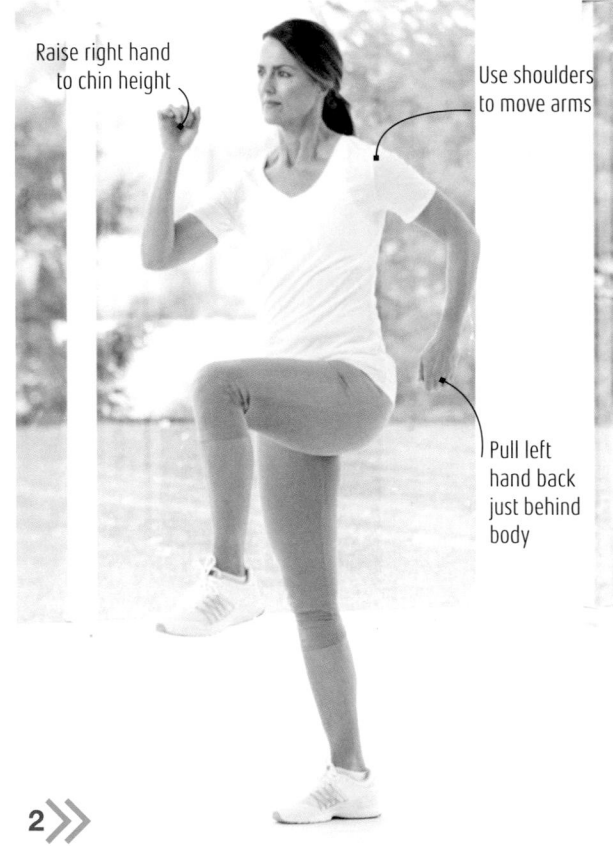

Raise right hand to chin height

Use shoulders to move arms

Pull left hand back just behind body

1 »

Stand with your feet shoulder-width apart. Bend both elbows to 90 degrees, position your forearms in front of you, and hold your hands in loose fists. Lengthen your spine and retract your shoulder blades.

2 »

Shift your weight to your right foot and raise your left knee until your thigh is parallel to the ground. Simultaneously swing your right arm up and your left arm back, maintaining the bend in your elbows.

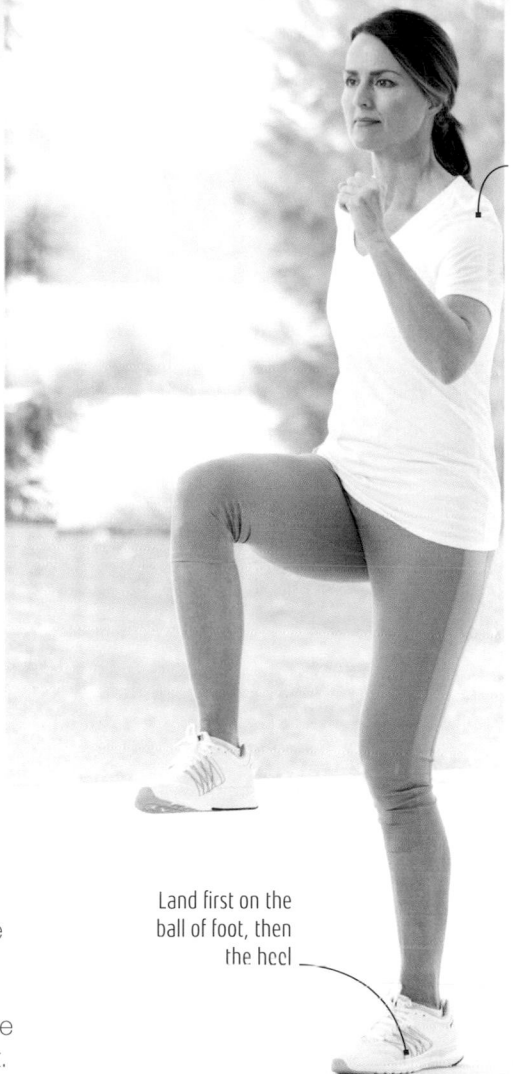

FIT tip

Increase intensity by lifting knees higher and marching faster, or decrease intensity by keeping knees lower and slowing down.

Maintain an upright posture

3 »

Quickly return your left foot to the ground and shift your weight to your left foot. Immediately raise your right knee and swing your arms in the opposite directions. Continue to march rapidly in place for the time given in your workout.

Land first on the ball of foot, then the heel

▰▰▱ MAKE IT **easier**

If it is difficult to maintain balance, sit on the edge of a chair and do the exercise by raising your feet about 6 inches (15cm) from the ground.

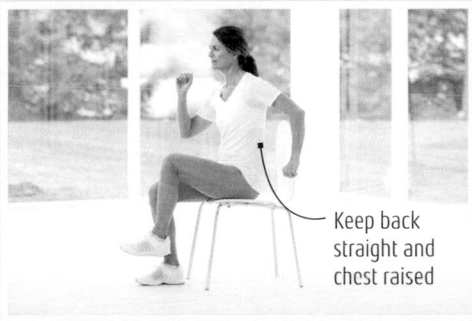

Keep back straight and chest raised

▰▰▱ MAKE IT **harder**

To strengthen your shoulders, hold a dumbbell in each hand as you do the exercise.

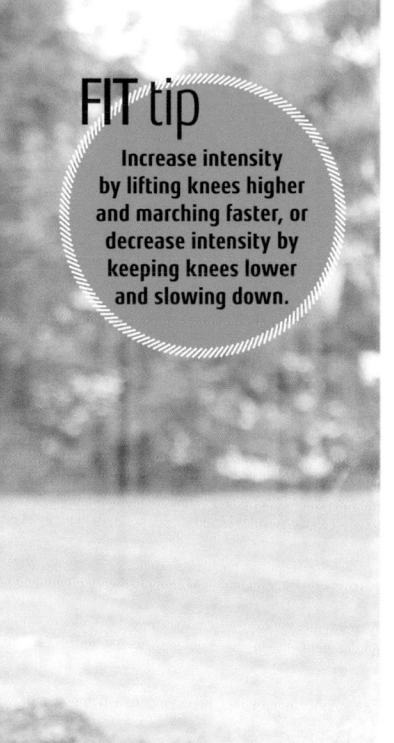

IMPROVES
■/// **Stability**
/// **Mobility**
■/// **Endurance**

WHAT YOU NEED
No equipment needed

High knee and reach

Perform this energy-intensive, total-body reach quickly to improve your stamina and stability. By dynamically engaging multiple muscle groups, you increase your body's endurance for powerful movement.

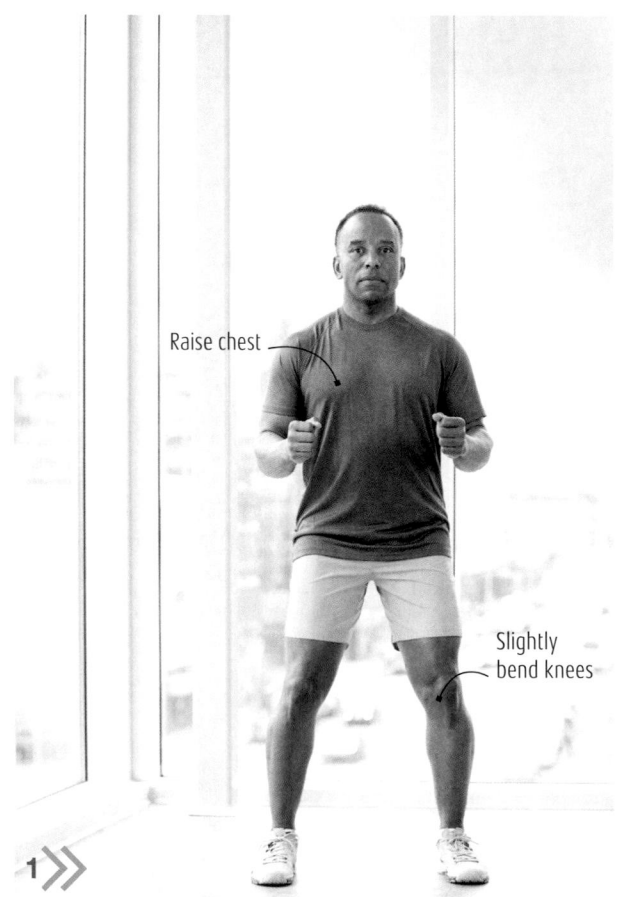

Raise chest

Slightly bend knees

1 ≫

Stand with your feet shoulder-width apart. Bend both elbows to 90 degrees, position your forearms in front of you, and hold your hands in loose fists. Engage your core and retract your shoulder blades.

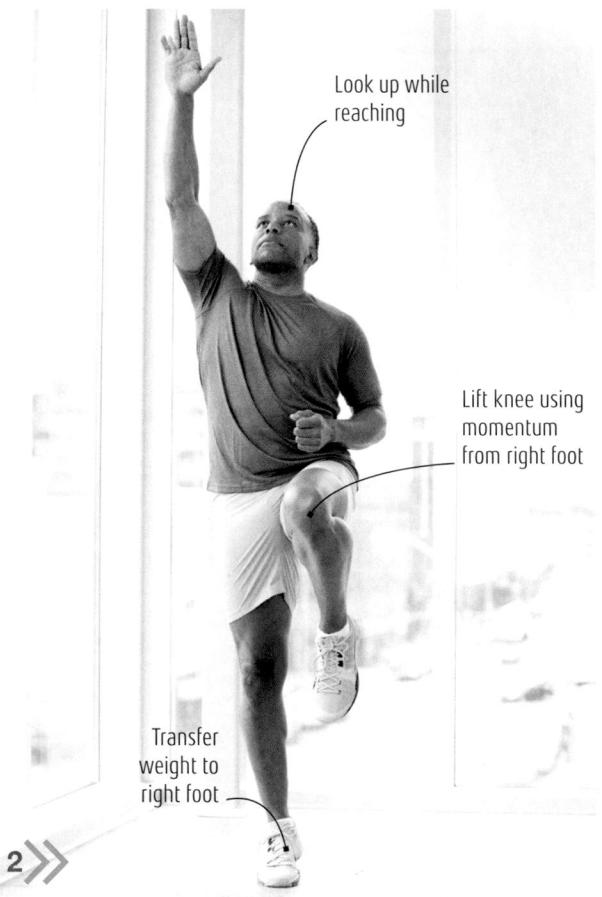

Look up while reaching

Lift knee using momentum from right foot

Transfer weight to right foot

2 ≫

Powerfully rise onto the ball of your right foot, letting your heel come off the ground, and raise your left knee until your thigh is parallel to the ground. Simultaneously reach overhead with your right hand as if you are grabbing something from a high shelf.

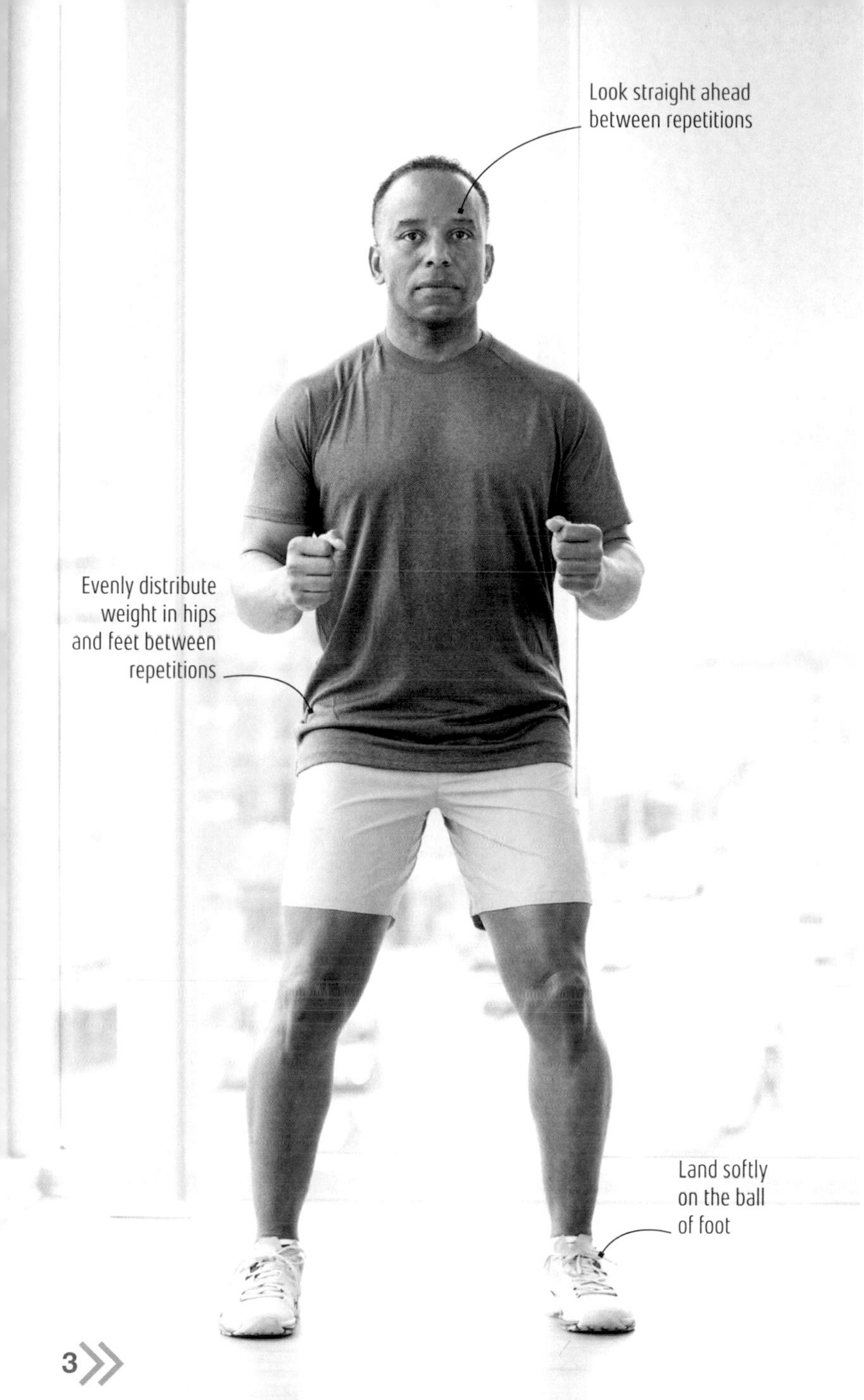

Look straight ahead between repetitions

Evenly distribute weight in hips and feet between repetitions

Land softly on the ball of foot

3 »

Lower both feet and your right arm to the starting position, and slightly bend your knees to absorb your weight. Quickly repeat the exercise by rising onto the ball of your left foot and raising your right knee and left hand. Alternate rapidly on each side for the time given in your workout.

///// MAKE IT easier

If it is difficult to maintain balance, sit on the edge of a chair and do the exercise by raising your feet about 3 inches (7cm) from the ground.

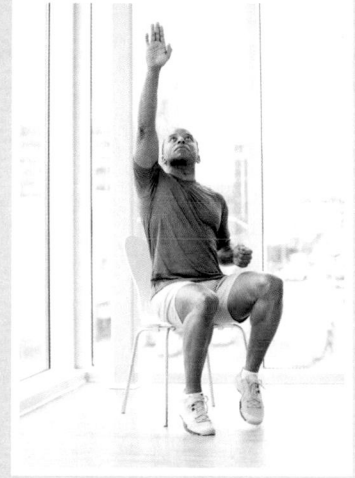

///// MAKE IT harder

To increase intensity, in step 2, jump off both feet, lift your left knee as high as you can, and let your right foot leave the ground completely.

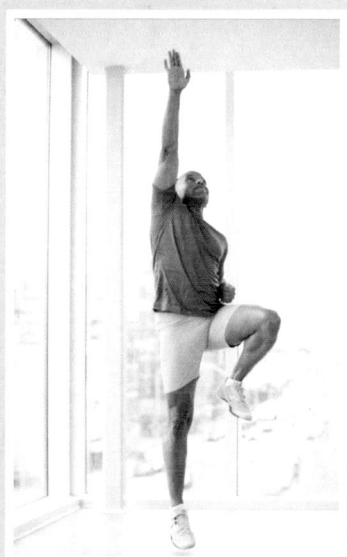

Farmer's walk

IMPROVES
▰/// **Strength**
▰/// **Stability**
▰/// **Endurance**

WHAT YOU NEED
Dumbbells

A full grocery bag sometimes weighs as much as 20 pounds (9kg). Carrying heavy items like this requires coordination, stability, and strength, and performing this controlled forward walk will prepare your body for weighted locomotion.

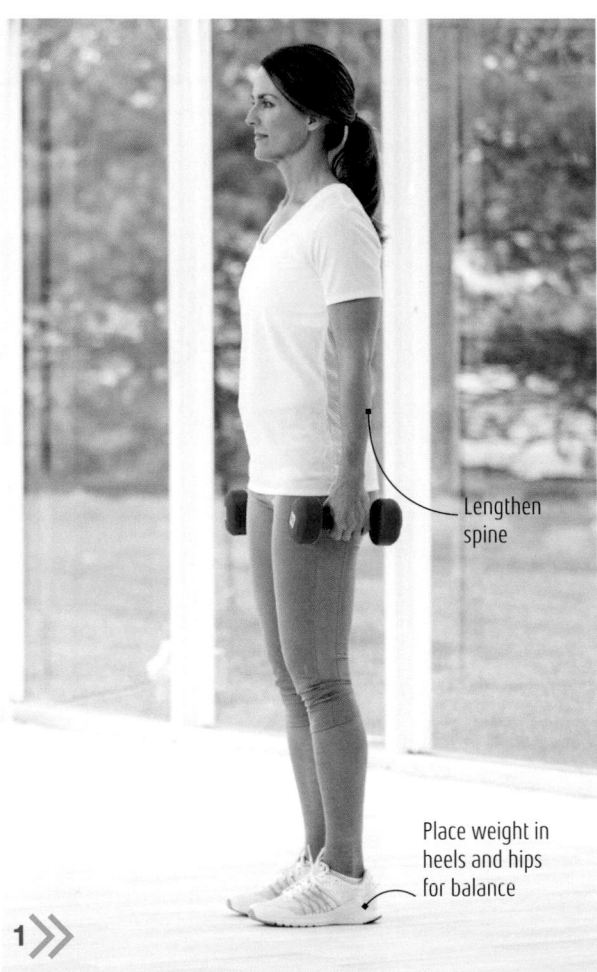

Lengthen spine

Place weight in heels and hips for balance

1 ⟫

Stand with your feet shoulder-width apart. Hold a dumbbell in each hand, palms facing inward, and let your arms hang at your sides. Engage your core and retract your shoulder blades.

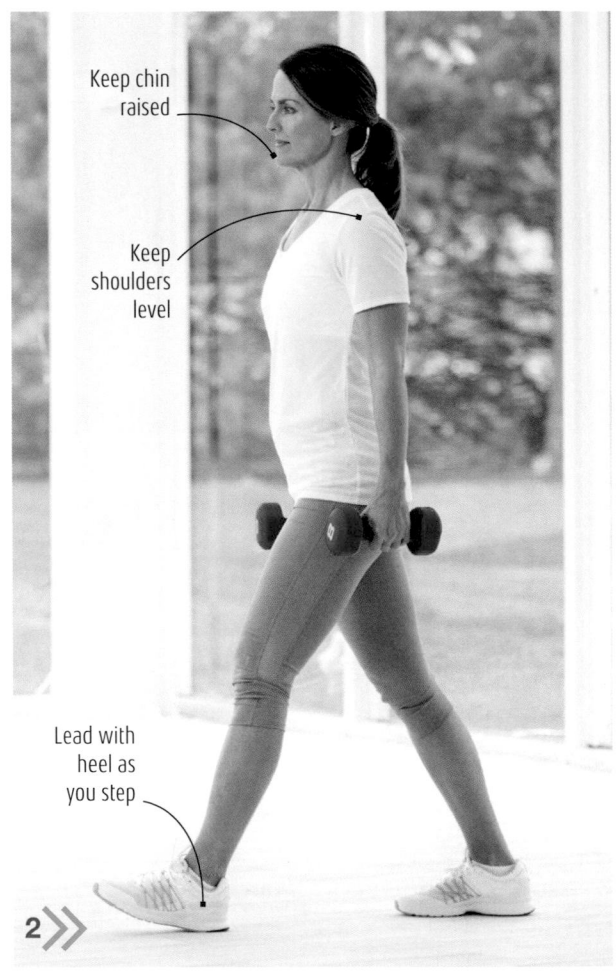

Keep chin raised

Keep shoulders level

Lead with heel as you step

2 ⟫

Take a long step forward with your left foot by engaging your hamstrings and glutes to pull your left heel forward. Land with your heel first. Maintain a stable, upright posture.

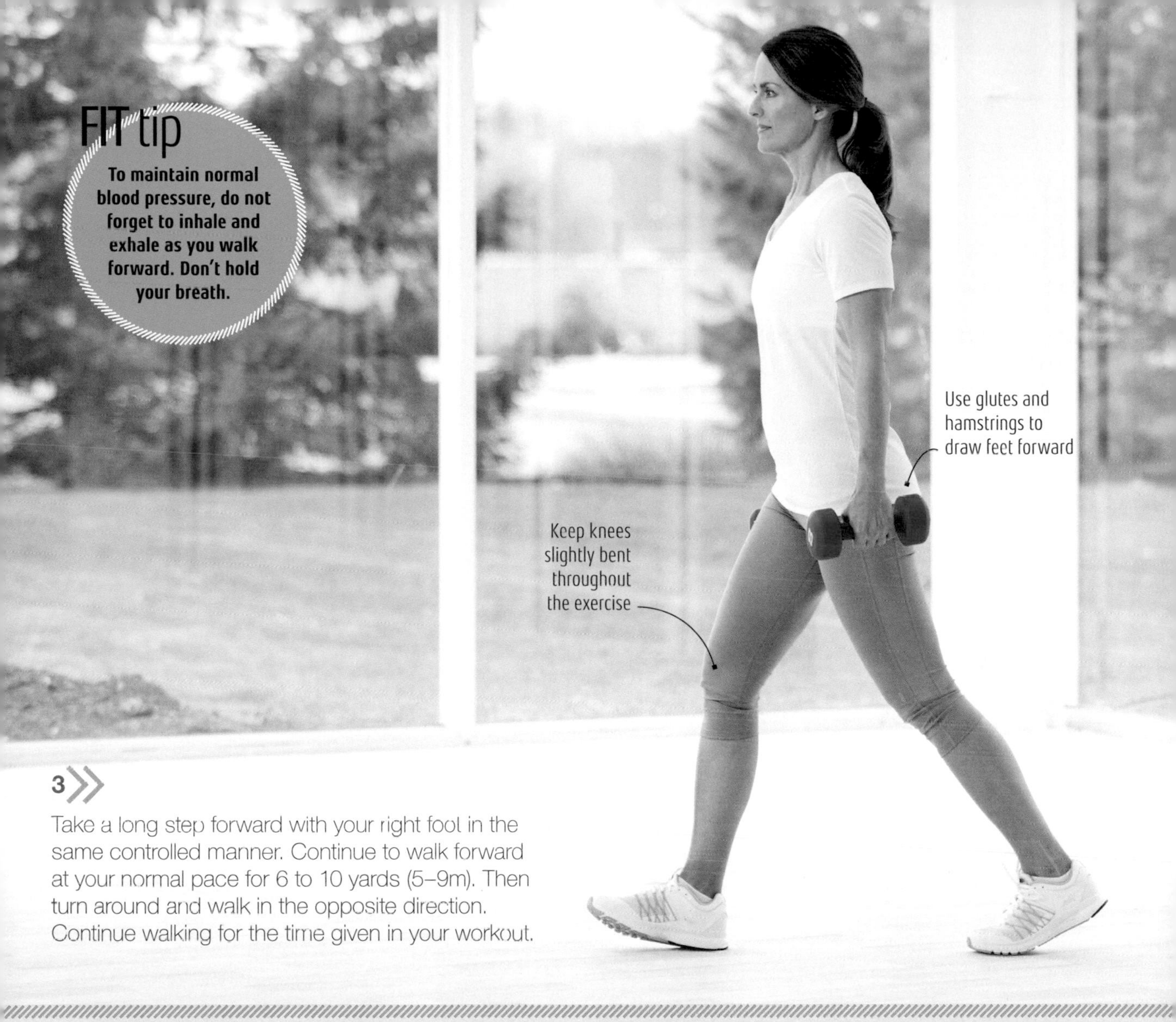

Use glutes and hamstrings to draw feet forward
Keep knees slightly bent throughout the exercise

FIT tip

To maintain normal blood pressure, do not forget to inhale and exhale as you walk forward. Don't hold your breath.

3

Take a long step forward with your right foot in the same controlled manner. Continue to walk forward at your normal pace for 6 to 10 yards (5–9m). Then turn around and walk in the opposite direction. Continue walking for the time given in your workout.

MAKE IT **easier**

If it is difficult to maintain balance, don't use dumbbells. March in place by raising your knee straight up until your thigh is parallel to the ground then lowering it to the starting position. Repeat with the opposite leg.

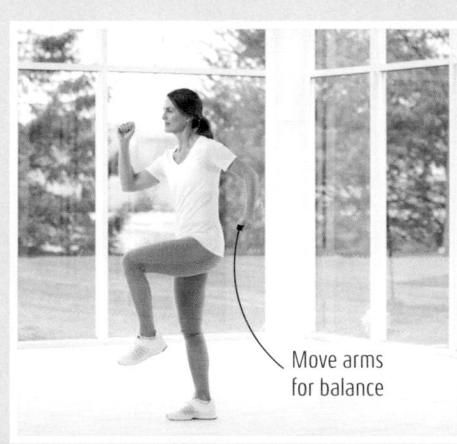

Move arms for balance

Skaters

Plyometric training, also known as jump training, involves rapidly stretching and contracting muscles to develop strength. Perform this quick plyometric drill to strengthen your legs and joints and improve your balance.

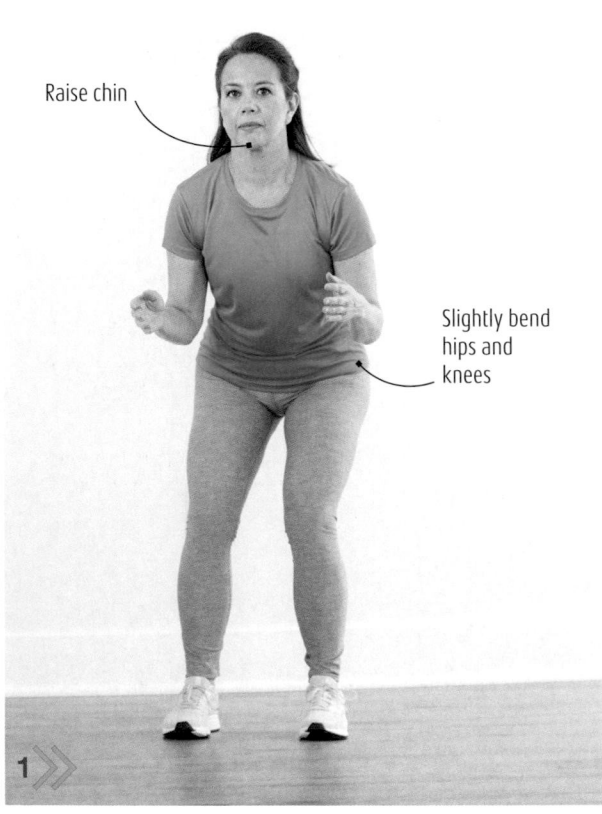

Raise chin

Slightly bend hips and knees

1 »

Stand with your feet shoulder-width apart. Bend your elbows to 90 degrees, position your forearms in front of you, and relax your hands. Slightly lean forward, engage your core, and retract your shoulder blades.

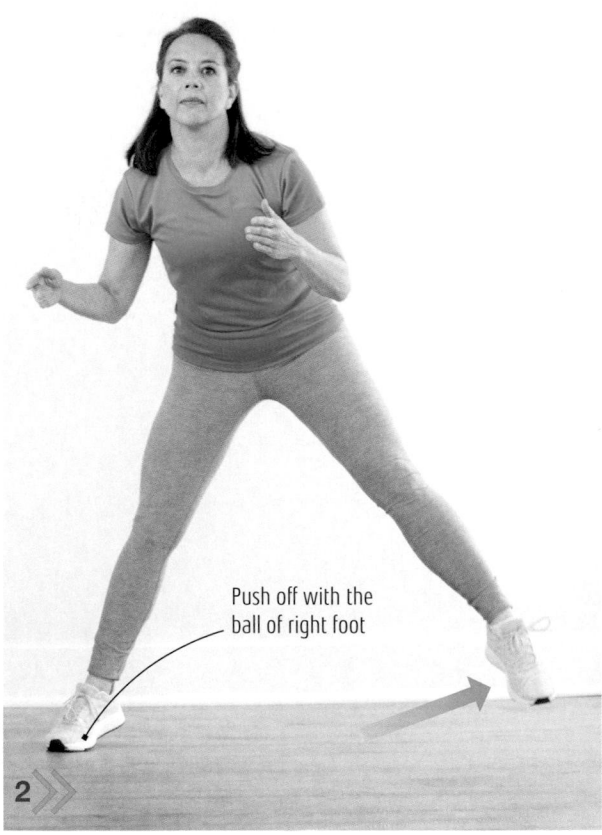

Push off with the ball of right foot

2 »

Push into the ground with your right foot, rising onto the ball of your foot, and extend your left leg out to the side to jump to your left. Keep your back lengthened and continue to lean slightly forward.

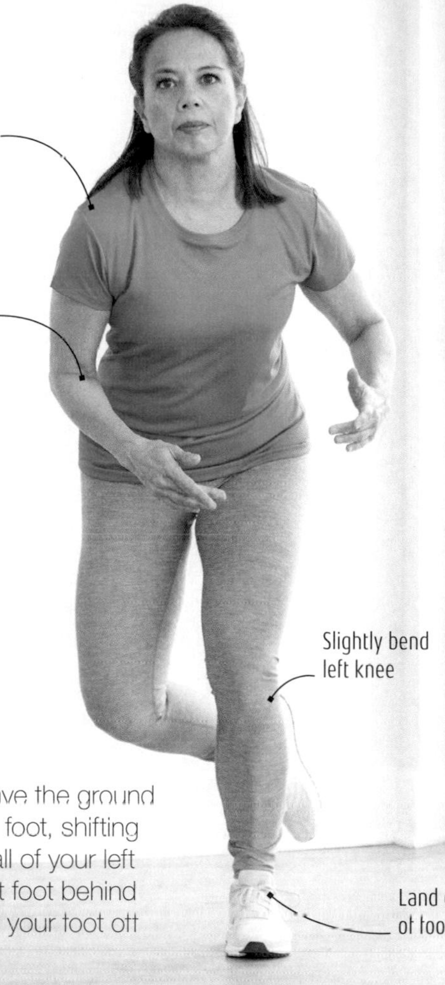

Keep back straight

Shift arms for balance

Continue to hold head up and retract shoulder blades

Slightly bend left knee

Stay light on feet by making quick contact with base foot

3 »
Let your right foot leave the ground and land on your left foot, shifting your weight to the ball of your left foot. Swing your right foot behind your left leg, keeping your foot off the ground.

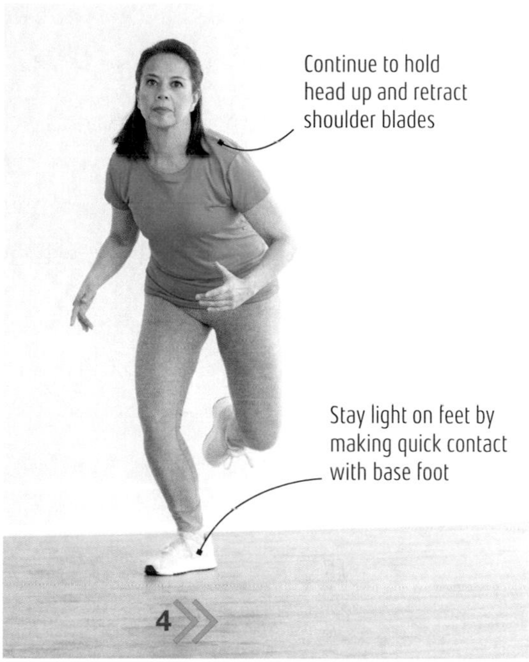

Land on the ball of foot first

4 »
Immediately bend your left hip and knee. Jump onto your right foot and swing your left leg behind your right leg. Continue to jump quickly to your left and right for the time given in your workout.

//// MAKE IT **easier**

To lessen the impact on your joints, in step 2, step your left foot to the side rather than jumping. In step 3, pull your heel up toward your glutes rather than behind your base leg. Continue to step quickly to your left and right.

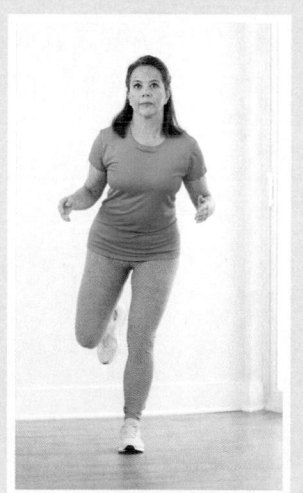

//// MAKE IT **harder**

To develop power in your lower body, in step 3, immediately upon landing on your left foot, squat down until your left thigh is parallel to the ground. Shift your arms for balance.

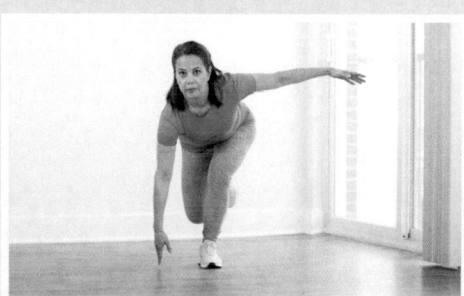

IMPROVES

▰//// **Strength**
▰//// **Stability**
//// **Mobility**
▰//// **Endurance**

WHAT YOU NEED
Step

Step-ups

A body with unhealthy knees is like a car with four flat tires—you can still run, but you will not go far. Briskly perform this elevated stepping exercise to develop stability and strength in the muscles and connective tissues surrounding your knees so you can run more efficiently.

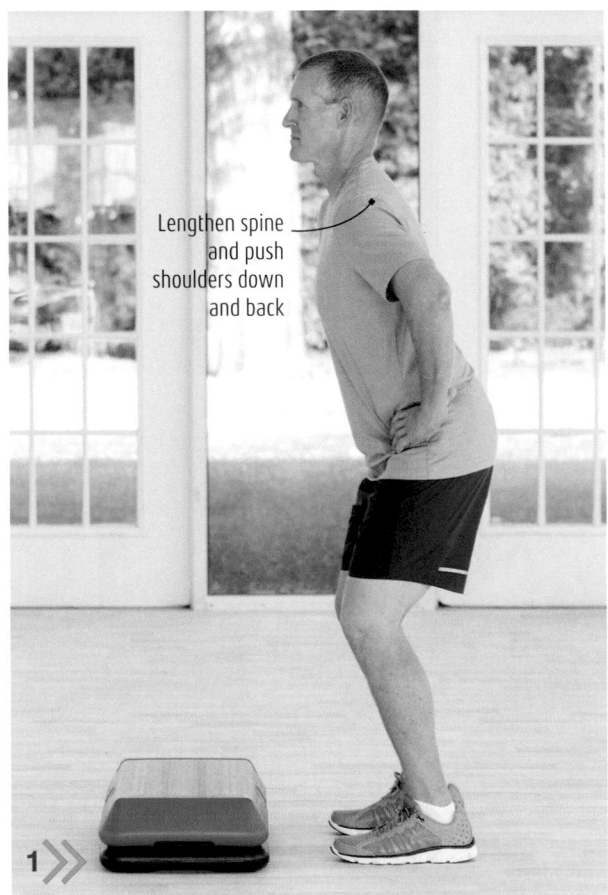

Lengthen spine and push shoulders down and back

1 ⟫ Stand behind a step or stair with your feet shoulder-width apart and place your hands on your hips. Slightly lean forward and bend your knees and hips. Engage your core and retract your shoulder blades.

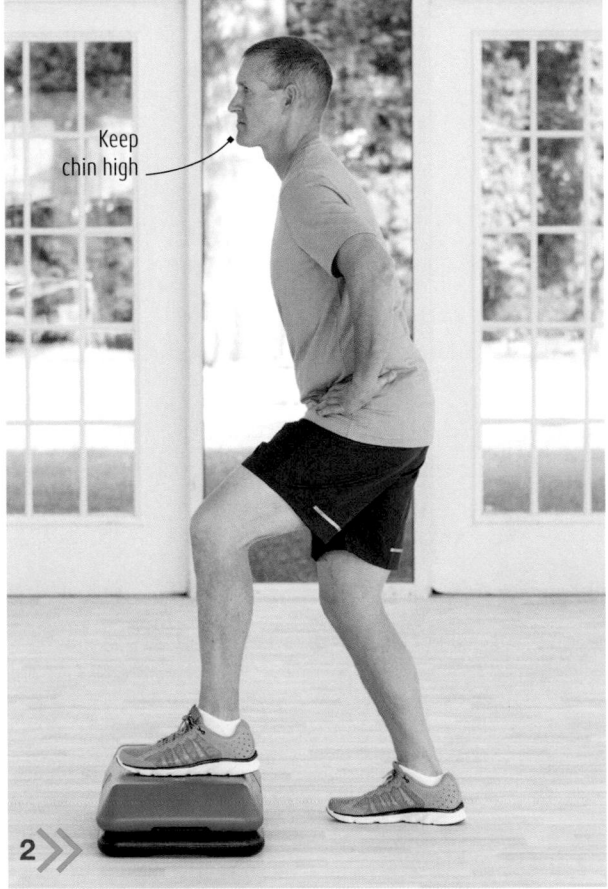

Keep chin high

2 ⟫ Lift your left leg from the knee until your left foot is about 2 inches (5cm) above the step, then place your foot fully on the step, maintaining a shoulder-width distance between your feet.

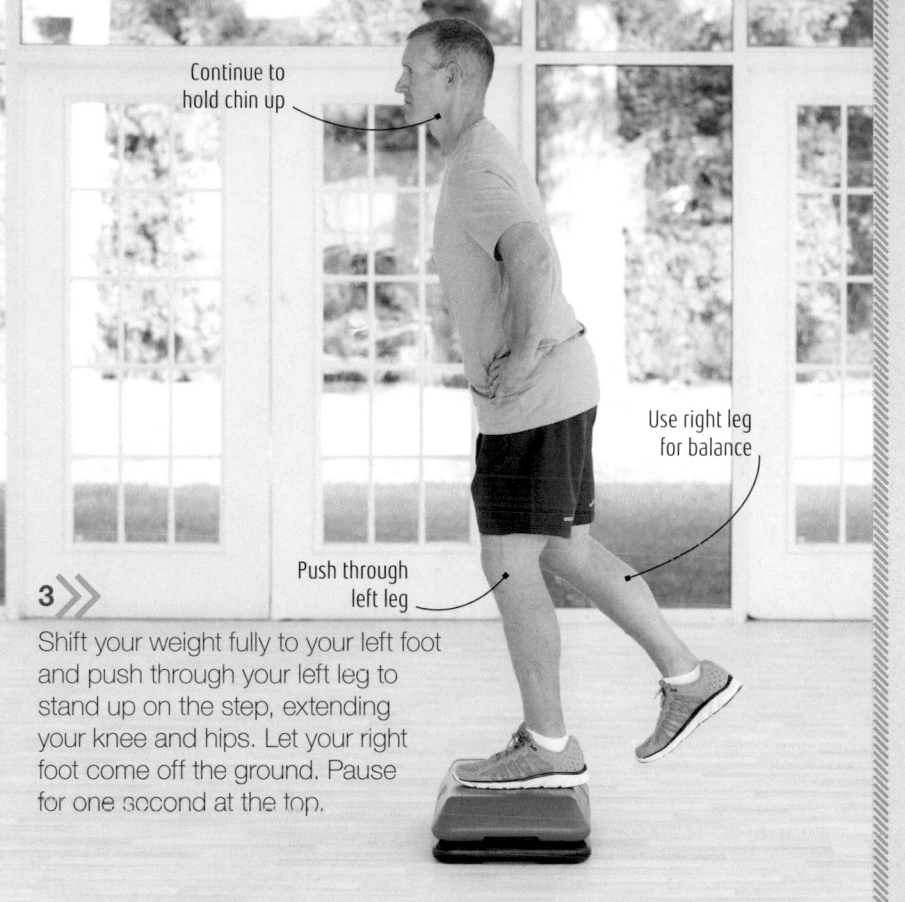

Continue to hold chin up

Use right leg for balance

Push through left leg

3 »

Shift your weight fully to your left foot and push through your left leg to stand up on the step, extending your knee and hips. Let your right foot come off the ground. Pause for one second at the top.

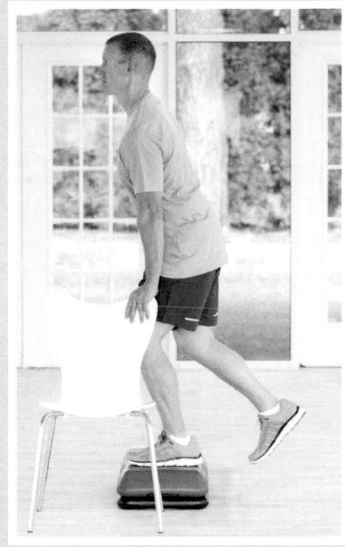

/// MAKE IT **easier**

If it is difficult to maintain balance, lightly rest your hand on a chair or rail for support.

/// MAKE IT **harder**

To increase resistance to your legs, hold a dumbbell in each hand and let them hang at your sides throughout the exercise.

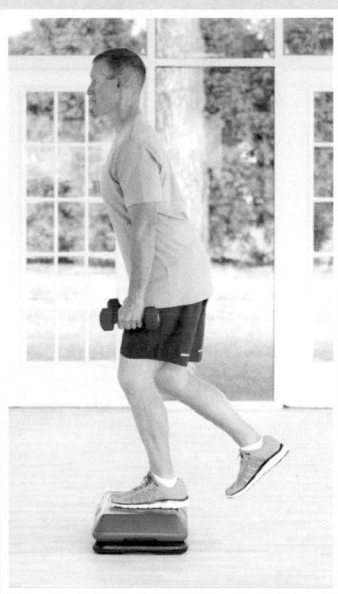

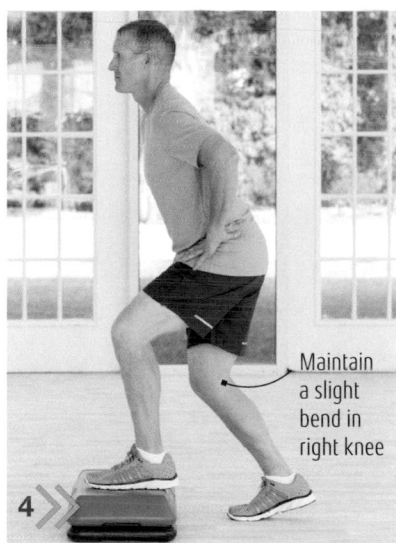

Maintain a slight bend in right knee

4 »

Lower your body back onto your right foot by bending your knees and hips. Shift your weight back to your right foot.

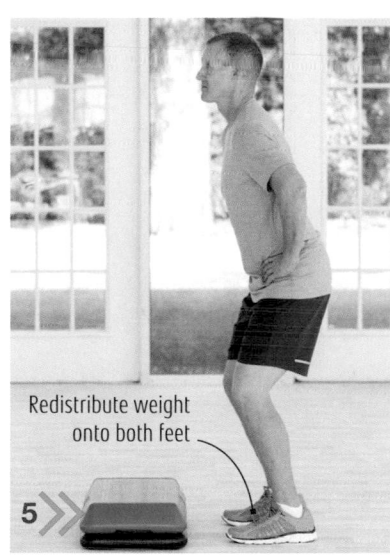

Redistribute weight onto both feet

5 »

Lift your left leg and return to the starting position. Alternate stepping with your left and right foot for the time given in your workout.

IMPROVES

///// Posture

///// Strength

///// Stability

///// Mobility

///// Endurance

WHAT YOU NEED
Dumbbells

Cross-country skiers

A strong, stable core better enables the nervous system to engage your muscles for functional movements. Your transverse abdominal, whose primary role is to stabilize your spine and pelvis, is the deepest abdominal muscle in your body. Use this fast-paced drill to strengthen this core muscle and protect your lower back.

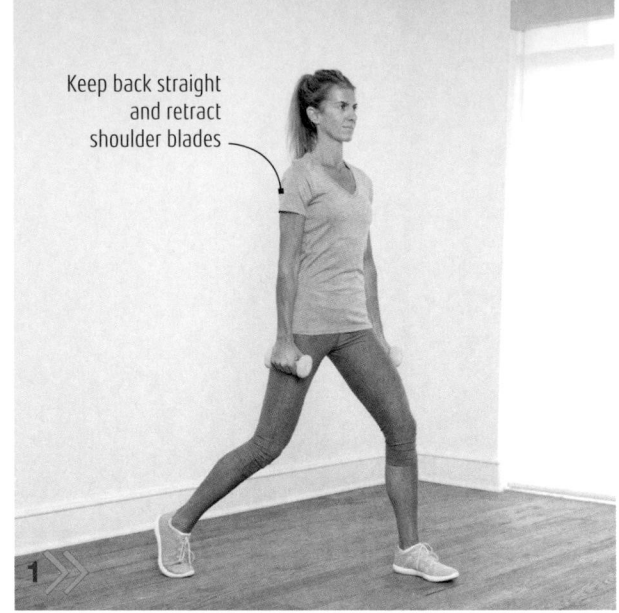

Keep back straight and retract shoulder blades

Hold a dumbbell in each hand and let your arms hang at your sides. Stand with your feet shoulder-width apart and step your right leg back into a staggered stance. Rise up onto the ball of your right foot and slightly bend your knees.

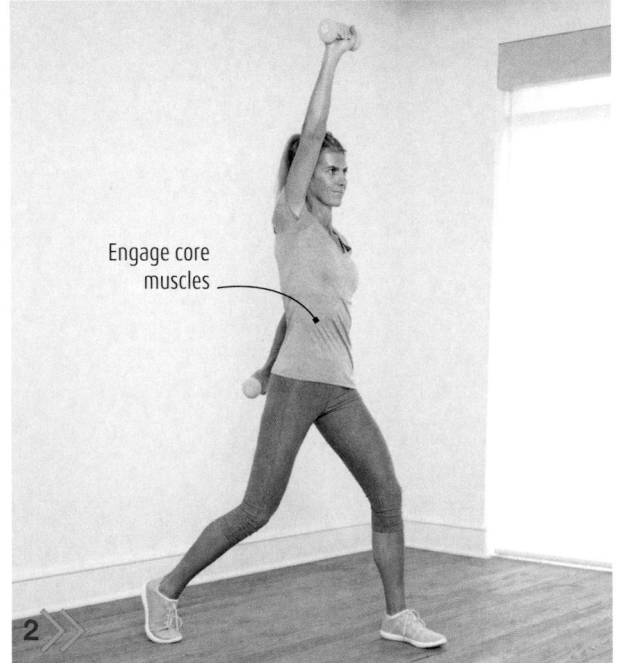

Engage core muscles

Swing your right arm forward from the shoulder and lift until your upper arm is near your ear. Pull your left arm behind your body. Keep both arms straight as you move them.

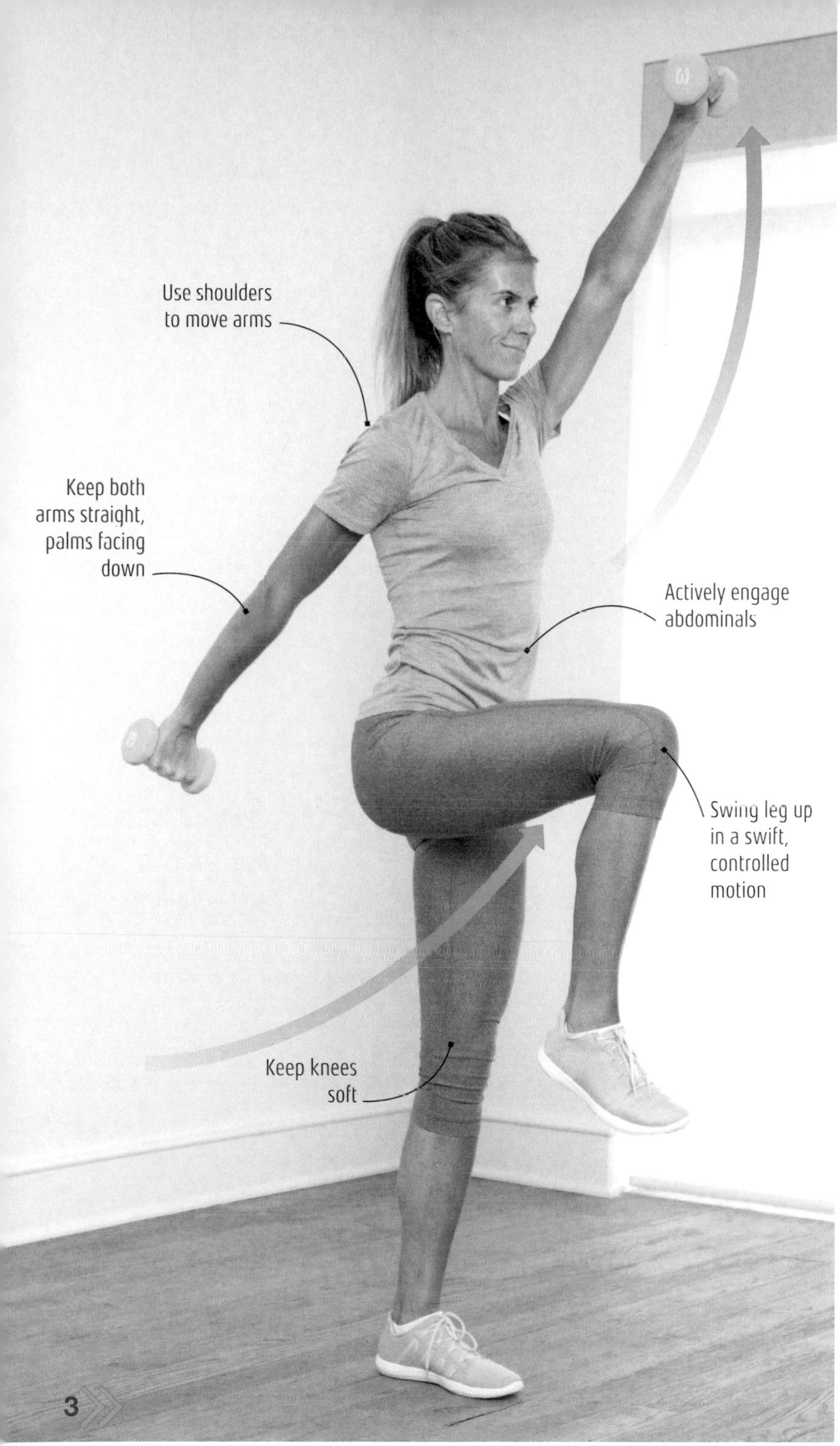

Use shoulders
to move arms

Keep both
arms straight,
palms facing
down

Actively engage
abdominals

Swing leg up
in a swift,
controlled
motion

Keep knees
soft

3

Shift your weight to your left foot and use your core
to raise your right knee until your thigh is parallel to the
ground. Simultaneously swing your left arm up and
forward, and swing your right arm down and back.

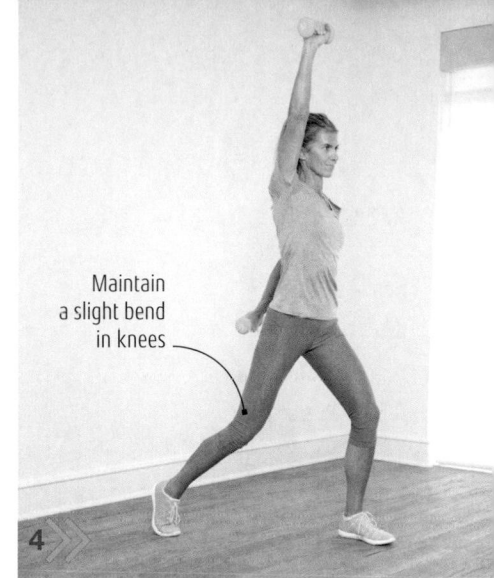

Maintain
a slight bend
in knees

4

In one swift motion, lower your right
leg and swing your arms to reverse
positions. Repeat the exercise for
the time given in your workout.
Spend half the time raising your
right leg, then reverse your stance
and raise your left leg.

///// MAKE IT **easier**

If it is difficult to maintain
balance, do the exercise
without dumbbells.

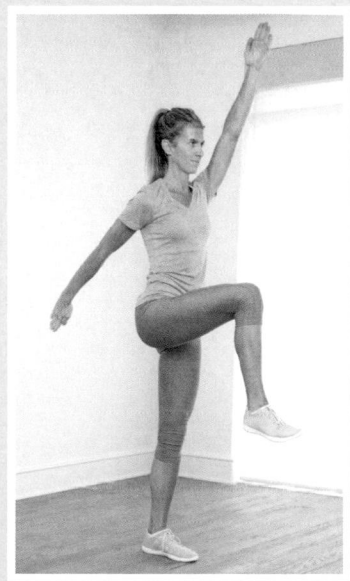

Faux jump rope

Jumping rope is excellent for increasing the bone density of your legs. Since both legs absorb each jump, it's easier on your joints than running, while the weight-bearing impact keeps bones healthy and stable. Try this rope-free version.

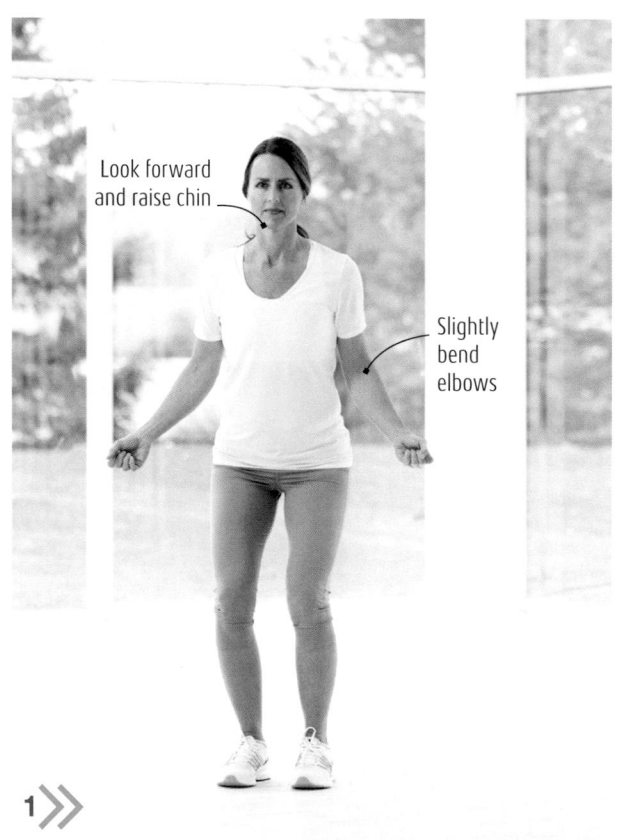

Look forward and raise chin

Slightly bend elbows

1 »

Stand with your feet shoulder-width apart and slightly bend your knees. Hold your hands in loose fists, palms facing forward, and bring them to waist height. Lengthen your torso and retract your shoulder blades.

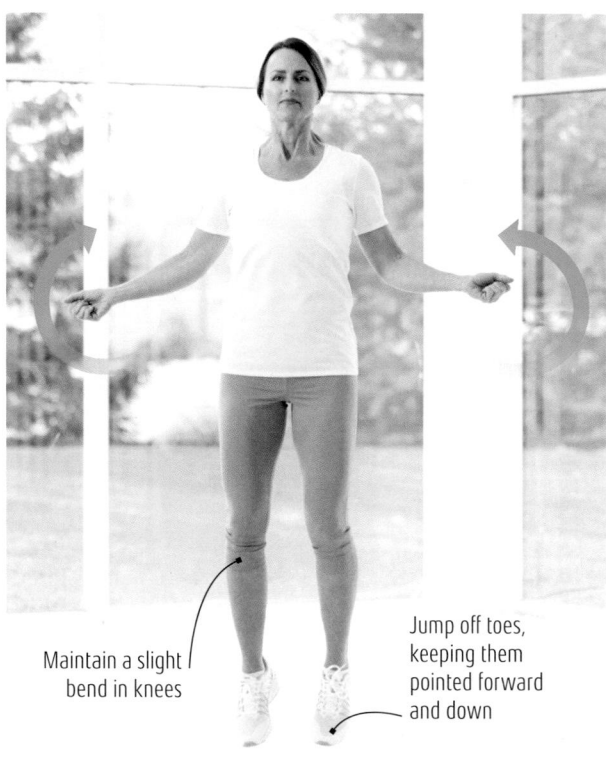

Maintain a slight bend in knees

Jump off toes, keeping them pointed forward and down

2 »

Powerfully jump off the balls of your feet, 1 to 3 inches (3–8cm) into the air. Simultaneously draw a small, forward circle with your wrists. Limit movement in your shoulders and elbows.

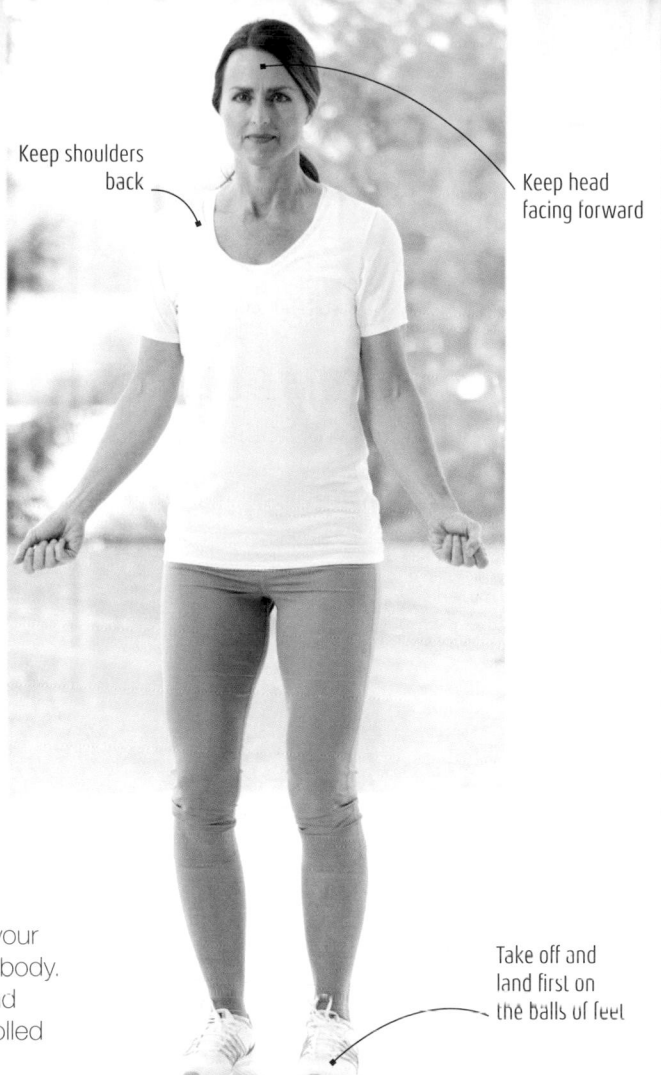

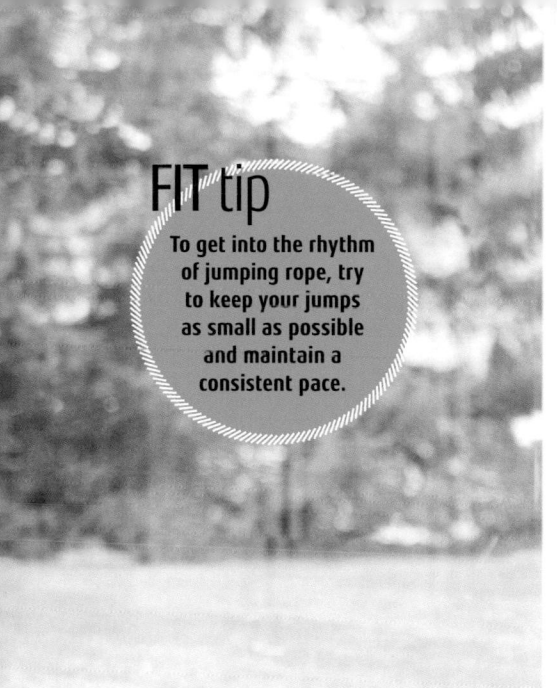

FIT tip

To get into the rhythm of jumping rope, try to keep your jumps as small as possible and maintain a consistent pace.

Keep shoulders back

Keep head facing forward

3 >>

Land softly on the balls of your feet and bend your knees to distribute the impact throughout your body. Quickly rebound back up into the next jump and wrist circle. Continue to jump with quick, controlled movements for the time given in your workout.

Take off and land first on the balls of feet

///// MAKE IT **easier**

To lessen impact, raise one foot off the ground at a time, alternating feet. Continue the sequence quickly with one wrist circle per step. Keep your heels off the ground.

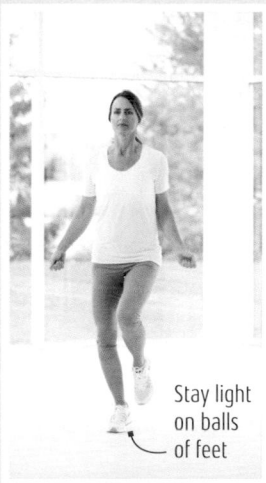

Stay light on balls of feet

///// MAKE IT **harder**

To improve reaction time, do the exercise with a jump rope. Hold a handle in each hand and place the rope behind your heels. Jump and use your wrists to swing the rope behind you, over your head, and then under your feet.

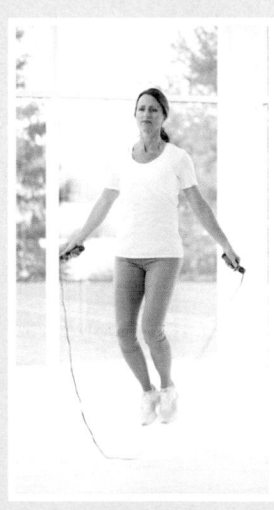

Chair mountain climber

This vigorous running exercise engages your whole body to improve your endurance and burn calories. Using only your bodyweight and a chair, the full-body movement increases the flexibility of your hips and strengthens your core and upper-body muscles.

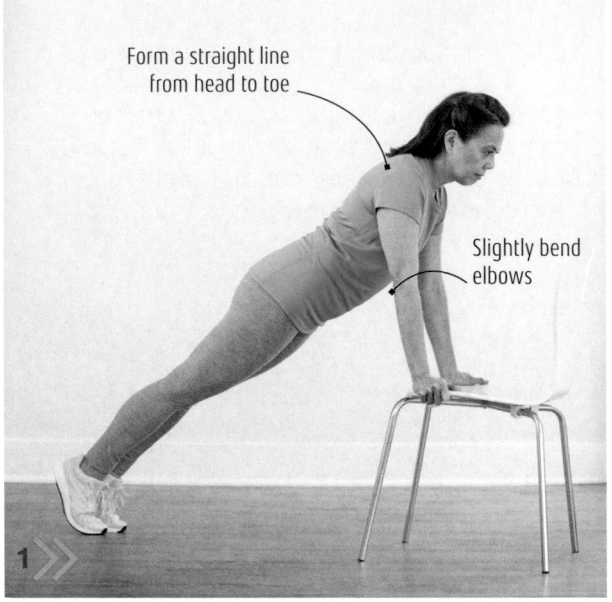

Form a straight line from head to toe

Slightly bend elbows

Stand facing the seat of a chair. Grip each side of the seat, step your feet back, and transfer your weight to your hands and the balls of your feet. Align your shoulders over your hands. Engage your core.

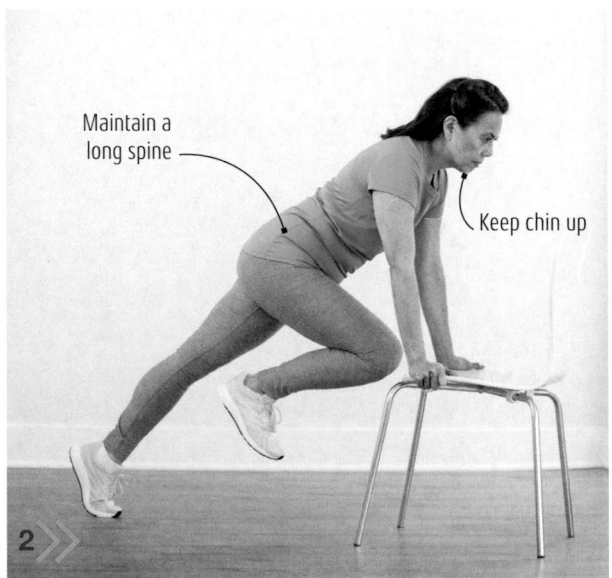

Maintain a long spine

Keep chin up

Push off the ball of your right foot and raise your right knee until your thigh is perpendicular to your left leg. Keep your core engaged and your shoulders square to the seat.

3 »

Keeping your body stable with both arms, return your right foot to the starting position, and shift your weight off your left foot and onto your right foot. Quickly push off from the ball of your left foot and raise your left knee. Alternate rapidly raising your left and right legs for the time given in your workout.

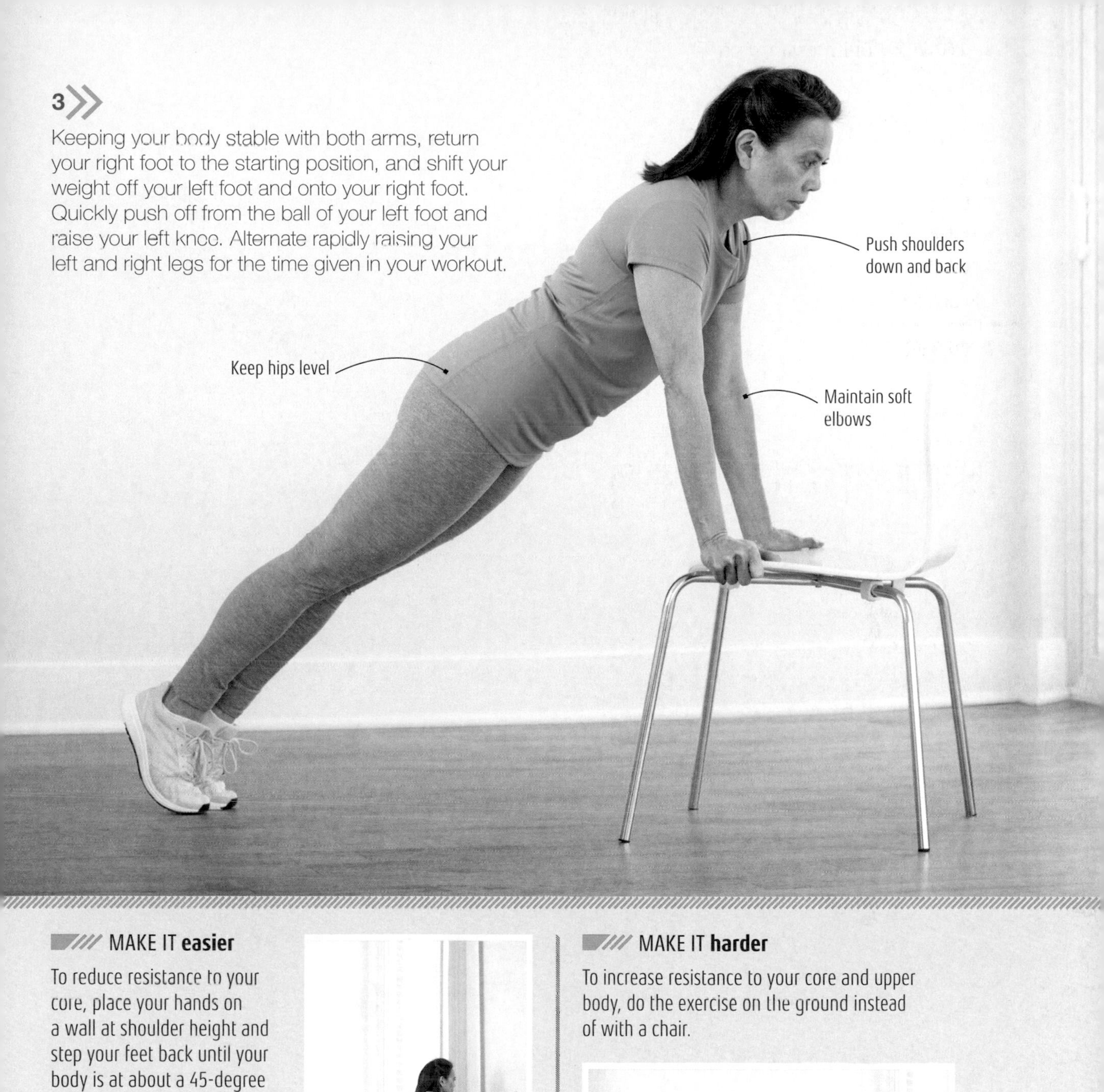

Push shoulders down and back

Maintain soft elbows

Keep hips level

///// MAKE IT **easier**

To reduce resistance to your core, place your hands on a wall at shoulder height and step your feet back until your body is at about a 45-degree angle to the ground. Do the exercise from this position.

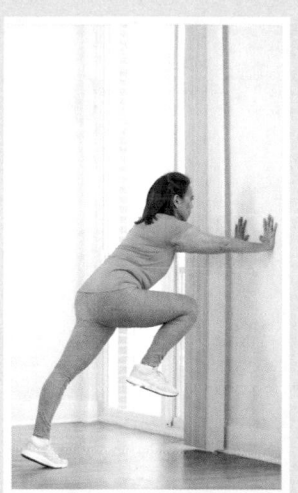

///// MAKE IT **harder**

To increase resistance to your core and upper body, do the exercise on the ground instead of with a chair.

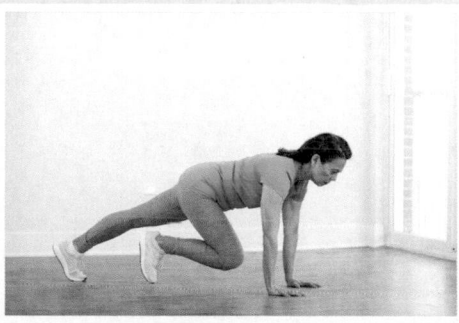

Switch jumps

Vigorous compound movements like this jumping exercise develop lower-body strength and power while improving your cardiovascular endurance. Use this dynamic drill to challenge your stability and make you more agile.

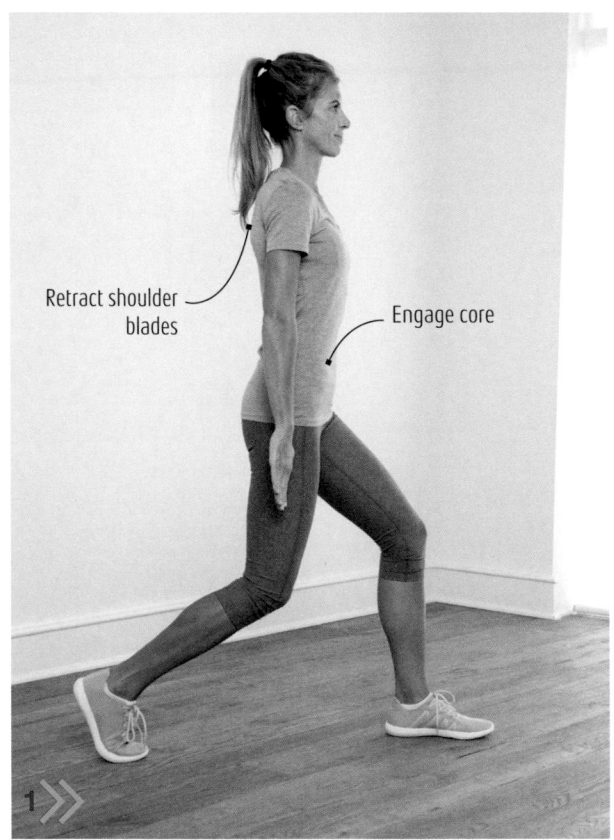

Retract shoulder blades

Engage core

1 »

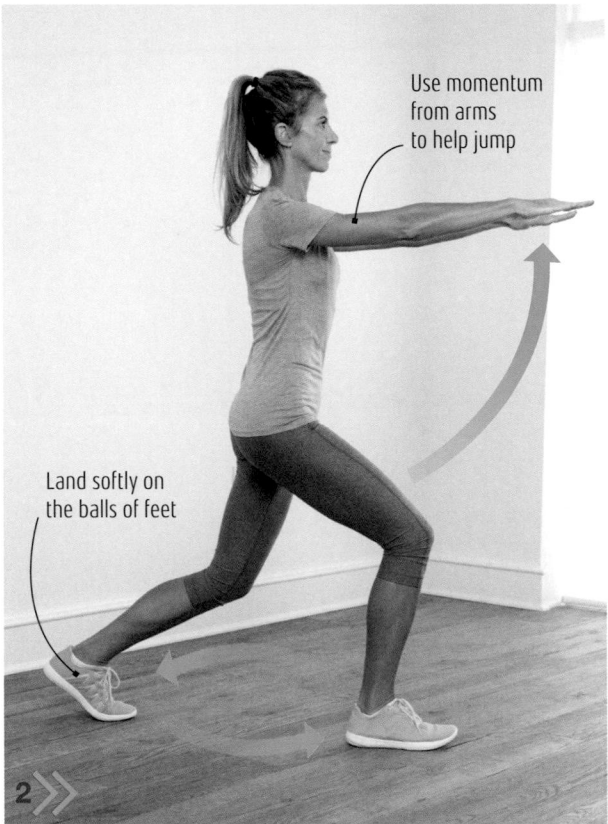

Use momentum from arms to help jump

Land softly on the balls of feet

2 »

Stand with your feet shoulder-width apart and straighten your arms at your sides with your palms facing behind you. Step your right leg back into a staggered stance and rise up onto the ball of your right foot. Slightly bend your knees.

Spring up off the balls of your feet to jump 1 to 2 inches (2–5cm) into the air, and switch your legs, bringing your right leg forward and left leg back. At the same time, swing your arms straight up so they are parallel to the ground.

Elongate spine

Keep torso
facing forward

3 »

Swing your arms back down to your sides and bend your hips and knees to build momentum for the next jump. Repeat the exercise to bring your right leg back and your left leg forward. Continue rapidly jumping for the time given in your workout, switching your legs and raising your arms with each jump.

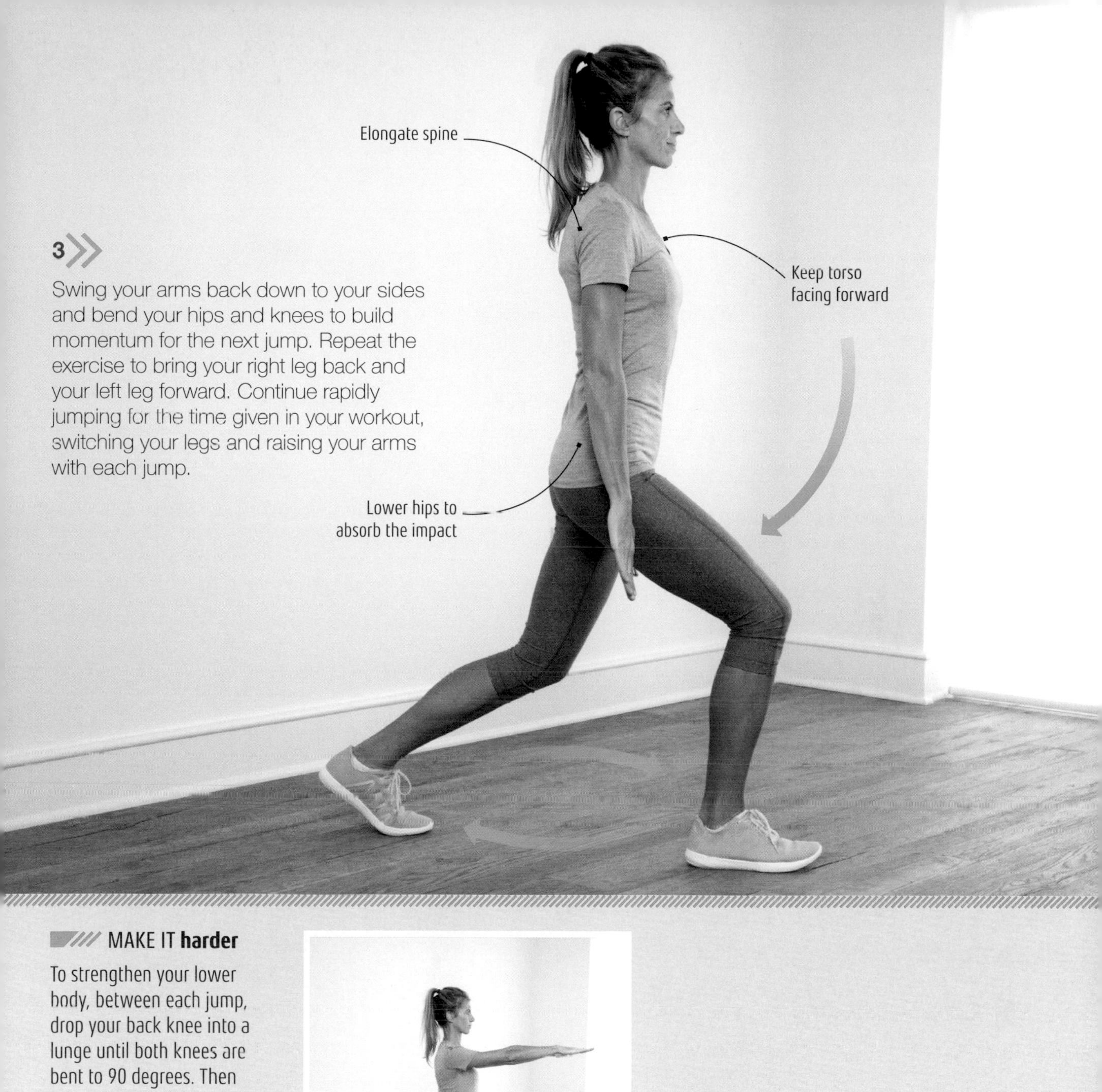

Lower hips to absorb the impact

///// MAKE IT **harder**

To strengthen your lower body, between each jump, drop your back knee into a lunge until both knees are bent to 90 degrees. Then jump off the balls of your feet and switch your legs.

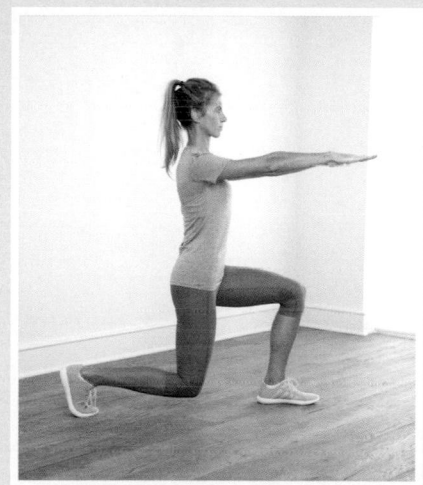

One-arm military press

This one-arm press teaches your body to transfer force from your core to your upper body. The controlled pushing movement challenges the stability of your entire body while strengthening the triceps and shoulders. By including this type of exercise in your regimen, you'll be better able to stand tall throughout your day.

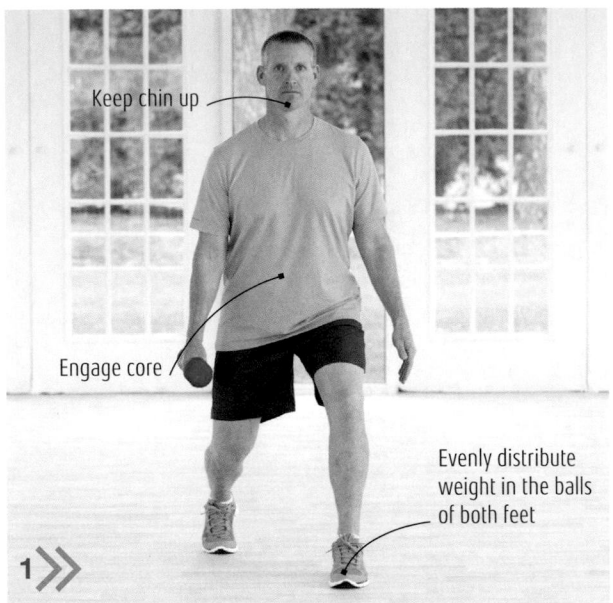

Keep chin up

Engage core

Evenly distribute weight in the balls of both feet

1 》

Hold a dumbbell in your right hand. Stand with your feet shoulder-width apart and step your right leg back into a staggered stance. Rise up onto the ball of your right foot. Slightly bend your knees.

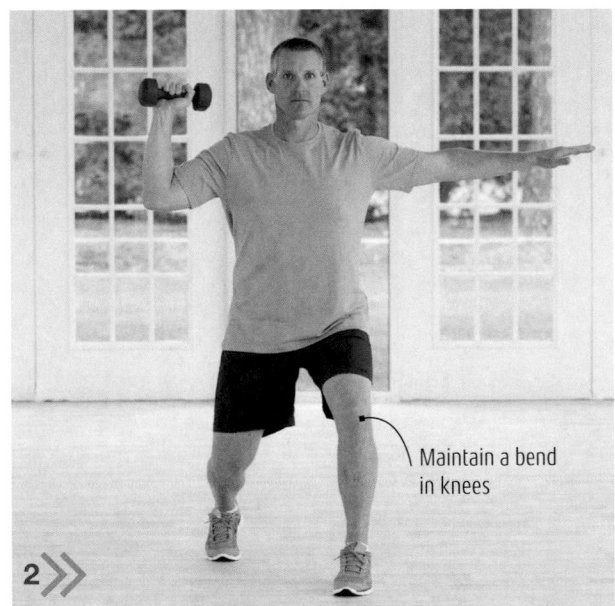

Maintain a bend in knees

2 》

Bend your right elbow to raise the dumbbell to chin height, palm facing forward and forearm perpendicular to the ground. Extend your left arm out to your side with your palm facing the ground.

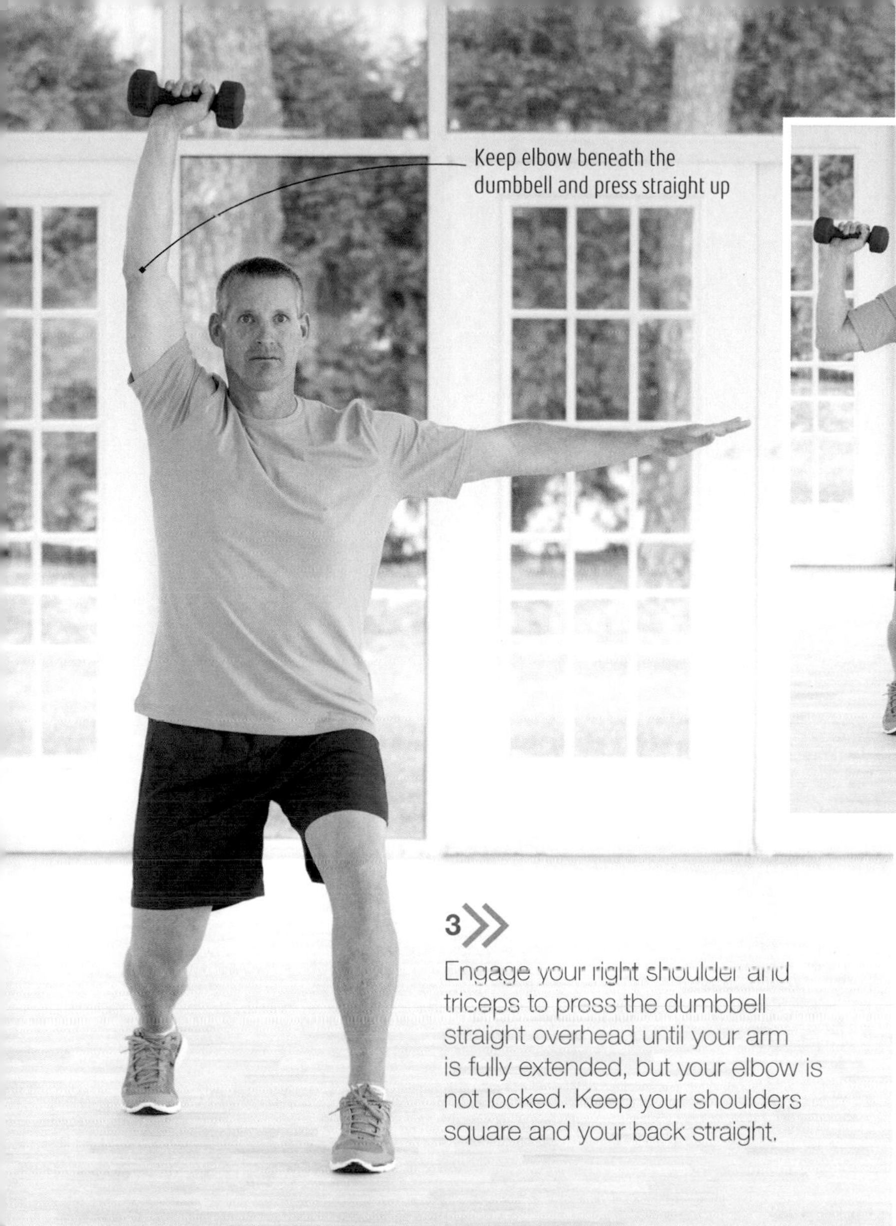

Keep elbow beneath the dumbbell and press straight up

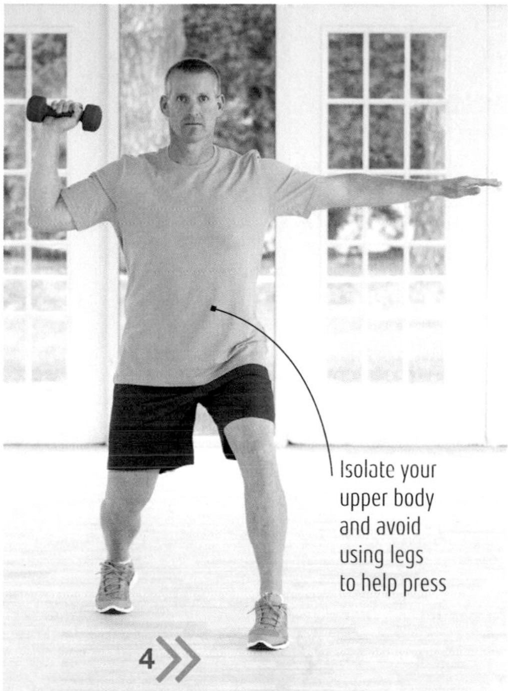

Isolate your upper body and avoid using legs to help press

4 »

In a controlled manner, lower the dumbbell back to chin height. Continue to press the dumbbell up and down for the time given in your workout. Spend half the time pressing with your right arm, then reverse your stance and press with your left arm.

3 »

Engage your right shoulder and triceps to press the dumbbell straight overhead until your arm is fully extended, but your elbow is not locked. Keep your shoulders square and your back straight.

//// MAKE IT **easier**

If it is difficult to maintain balance, sit on the edge of a chair while performing the exercise.

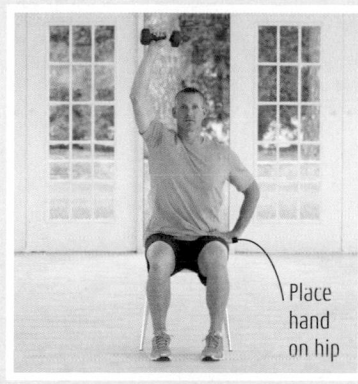

Place hand on hip

Chair dips

IMPROVES
▰//// **Strength**
//// **Mobility**
▰//// **Endurance**

WHAT YOU NEED
Chair

Many pushing activities, such as steering a stroller or shopping cart, require a strong upper body. Use this compound exercise to develop strength in your triceps, shoulders, chest, and back so you can perform these daily functions with ease.

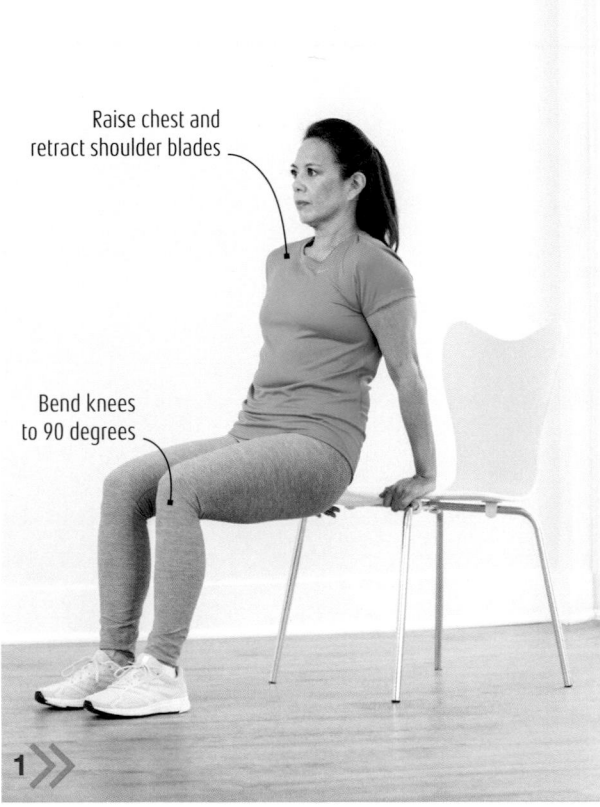

Raise chest and retract shoulder blades

Bend knees to 90 degrees

1 》》

Sit on a chair with your hands positioned shoulder-width apart and next to your hips on the edge of the chair. Extend your arms and press your body up onto the palms of your hands. Walk your feet out so your hips are suspended in front of the chair.

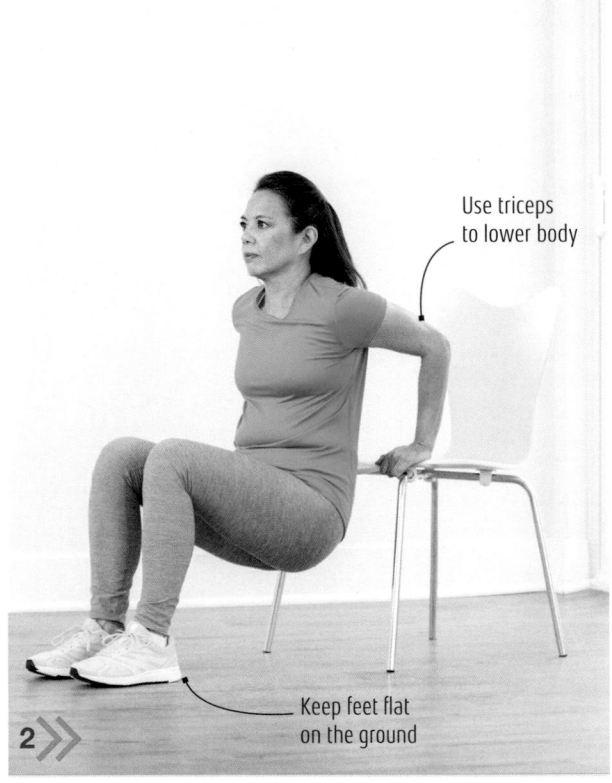

Use triceps to lower body

Keep feet flat on the ground

2 》》

Engage your triceps, chest, and shoulders and bend your elbows to lower your hips and torso straight down. Lower your body until your elbows are bent to 90 degrees. Keep your chin raised and your chest upright.

FIT tip

If you do not have a chair available, use any other sturdy object, such as a railing, low table, or the edge of a bathtub.

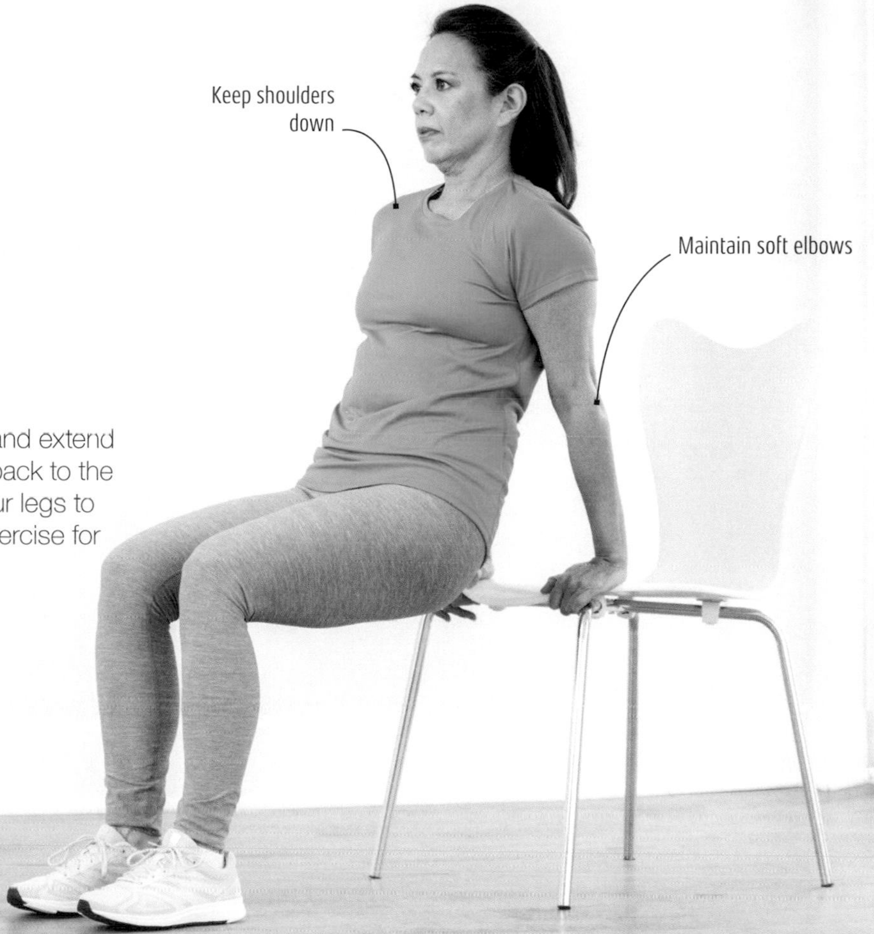
Keep shoulders down
Maintain soft elbows

3 »

Press your palms into the chair and extend your elbows to raise your body back to the starting position. Avoid using your legs to assist. Continue to repeat the exercise for the time given in your workout.

MAKE IT **easier**

To reduce resistance, do not walk your feet out in step 1 and keep your hips over the chair. In step 2, bend your elbows to lower your body back to a seated position.

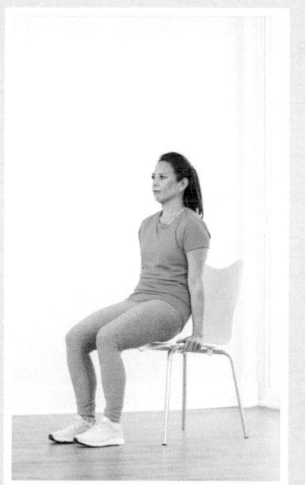

MAKE IT **harder**

To increase resistance, in step 1, walk your feet out until your legs are straight. Balance on your heels and keep your hips aligned under your torso.

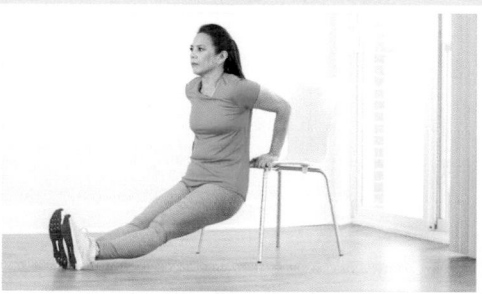

Inclined push-ups

Few exercises are more efficient and effective than the push-up. This foundational movement, made easier on a raised surface, activates nearly every muscle in your body to improve posture, strengthen the upper body, develop core stability, and enhance shoulder mobility.

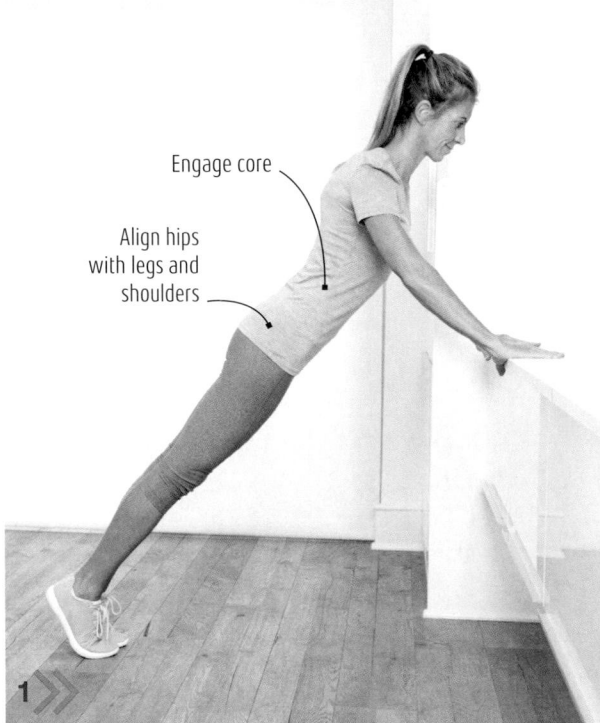

Engage core

Align hips with legs and shoulders

1

Stand facing a countertop, table, or other stable surface at about hip height. Place your hands shoulder-width apart on the edge of the surface. Step your feet back and transfer your weight to your hands.

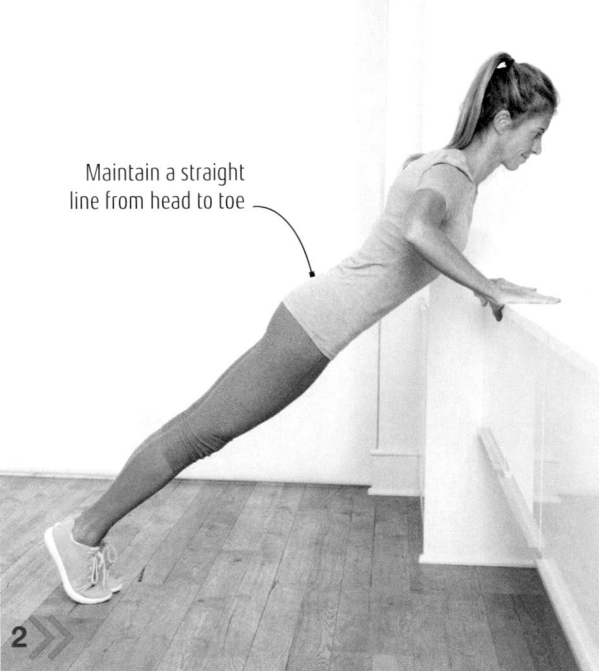

Maintain a straight line from head to toe

2

In a controlled manner, bend your elbows and use your triceps, chest, and shoulders to lower your body until your elbows are bent to 90 degrees. Maintain a flat back and keep your core tight.

FIT tip

If you can easily do 12 repetitions of this push-up, it is time to increase the resistance and try the harder modification.

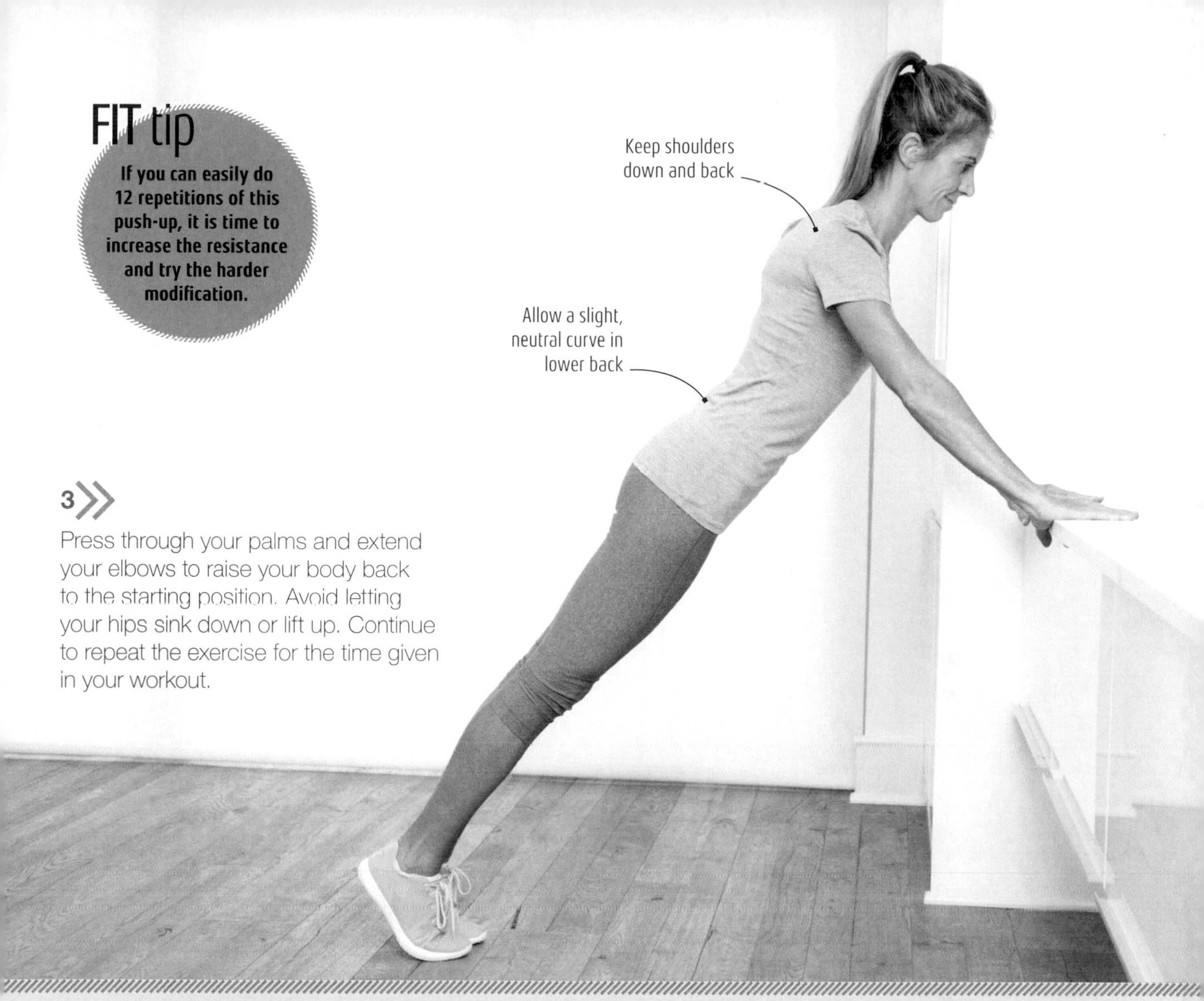

Keep shoulders down and back

Allow a slight, neutral curve in lower back

3 »

Press through your palms and extend your elbows to raise your body back to the starting position. Avoid letting your hips sink down or lift up. Continue to repeat the exercise for the time given in your workout.

▰/// MAKE IT **easier**

To reduce resistance to your upper body, place your hands on a wall at shoulder height and step your feet back until your body is at a 45-degree angle to the ground. Do the push-up from this position.

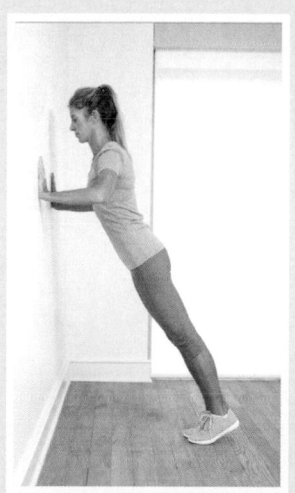

▰/// MAKE IT **harder**

To increase resistance to your core and upper body, do the exercise on the ground. Align your shoulders directly over your hands, fingers pointing forward.

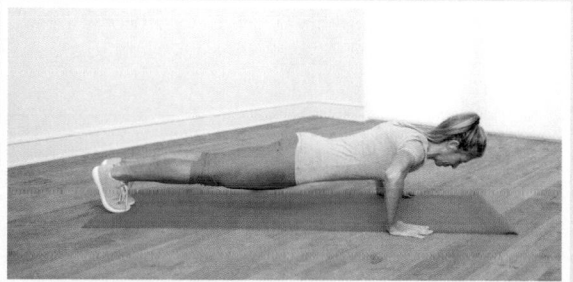

Curl and Arnold press and reach

Reaching overhead requires coordination and stability in your legs, core, and upper body. Perform this exercise so you are more prepared the next time you need to place an object on a high shelf or cabinet.

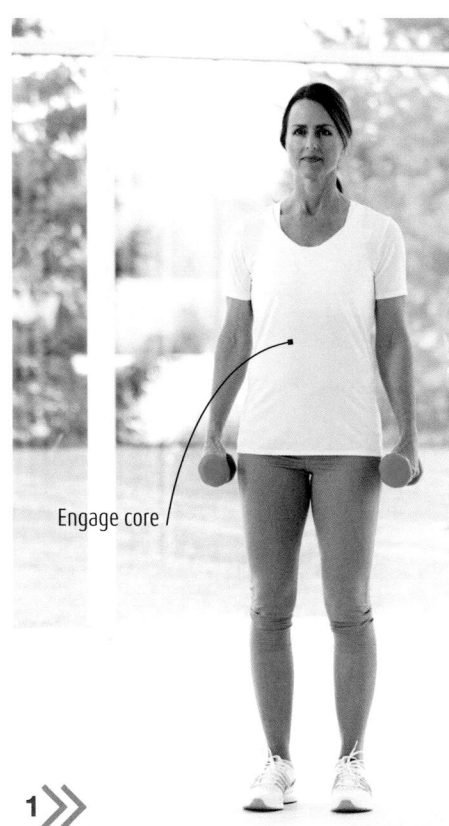

Engage core

1 ≫

Stand with your feet shoulder-width apart. Hold a dumbbell in each hand and let your arms hang at your sides. Slightly bend your knees. Lengthen your torso and retract your shoulder blades.

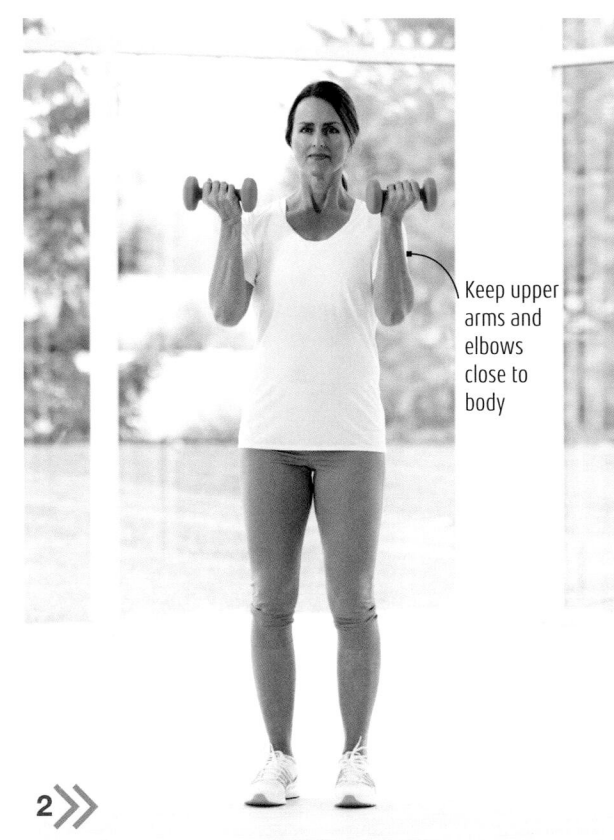

Keep upper arms and elbows close to body

2 ≫

In a controlled manner, with your palms facing forward, engage your biceps to curl the dumbbells to shoulder height. Raise them through your elbows, which act as hinges.

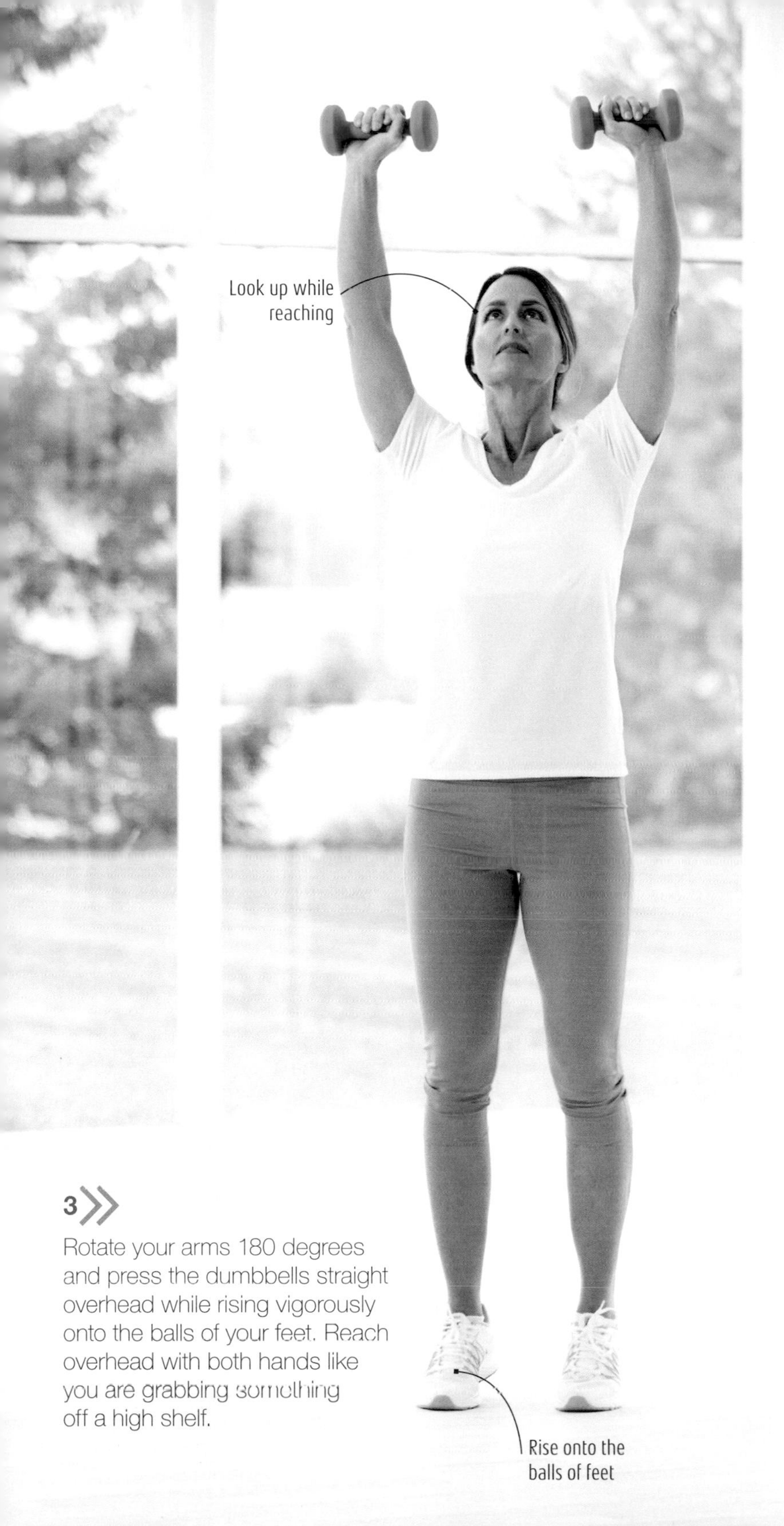

Look up while reaching

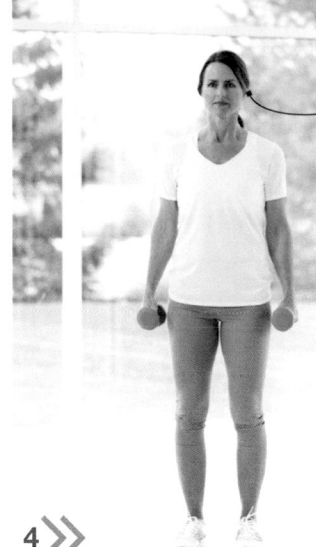

Lower head back down between repetitions

4 »

Lower your heels and return the dumbbells to the curl position, then back to the starting position. Continue to repeat the exercise for the time given in your workout.

///// MAKE IT **easier**

To decrease resistance, use a stability ball rather than dumbbells. Hold it down in front of you, curl it to shoulder height, then press and reach overhead.

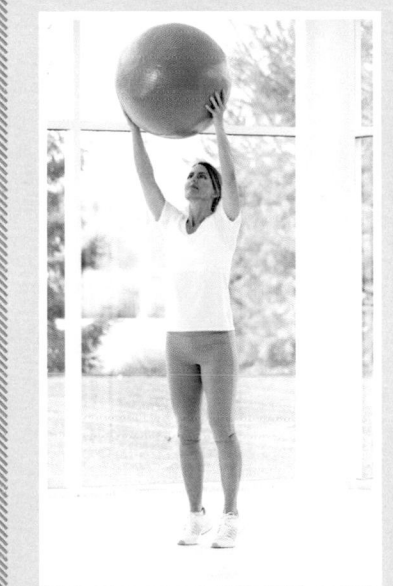

3 »

Rotate your arms 180 degrees and press the dumbbells straight overhead while rising vigorously onto the balls of your feet. Reach overhead with both hands like you are grabbing something off a high shelf.

Rise onto the balls of feet

IMPROVES
/// **Posture**
/// **Mobility**

WHAT YOU NEED
No equipment needed

Chest opener

Many daily activities require you to have your arms in front of you—lifting objects, holding a steering wheel, using your phone, or typing on a keyboard. Holding these positions for prolonged periods of time can result in tight shoulders and chest muscles. Use this chest stretch to loosen your upper-body muscles and improve your flexibility and posture.

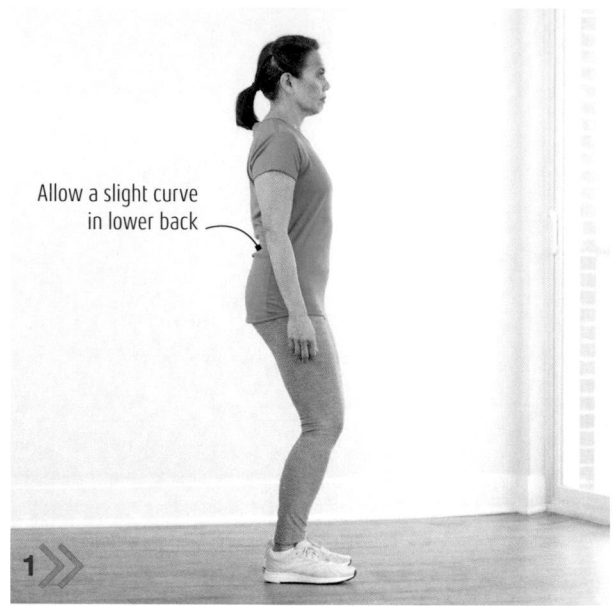

Allow a slight curve in lower back

Stand with your feet shoulder-width apart and let your arms hang at your sides. Lengthen your torso and retract your shoulder blades. Slightly bend your knees.

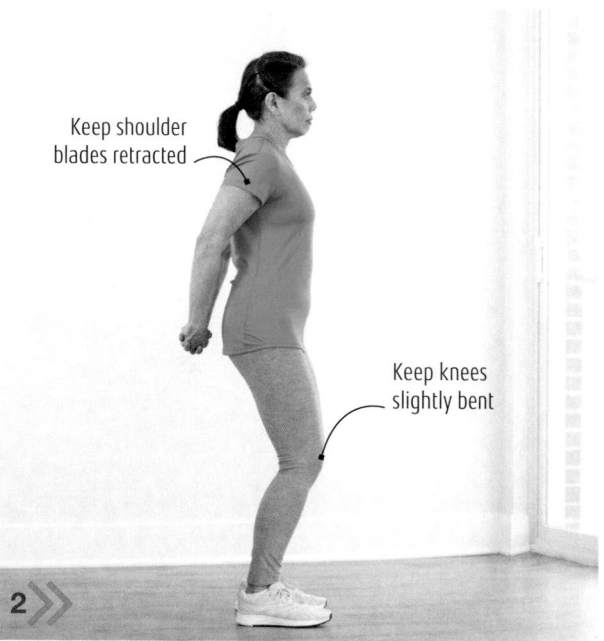

Keep shoulder blades retracted

Keep knees slightly bent

Bring your hands behind your back and interlock your fingers. Keep your head raised and shoulders back.

FIT tip

To get a deeper stretch, ask a partner to stand behind you and gently lift your arms upward.

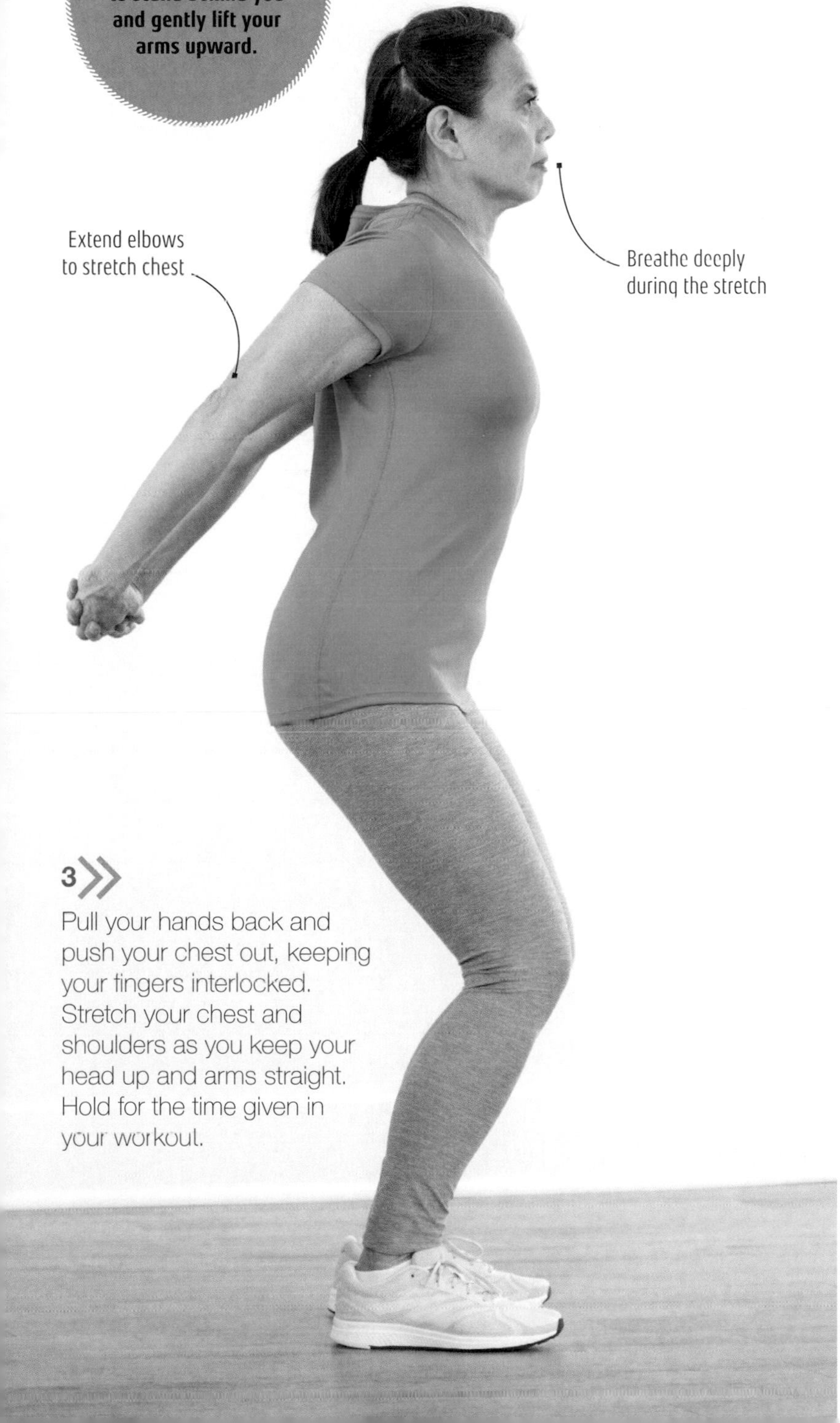

Extend elbows to stretch chest

Breathe deeply during the stretch

3 »

Pull your hands back and push your chest out, keeping your fingers interlocked. Stretch your chest and shoulders as you keep your head up and arms straight. Hold for the time given in your workout.

//// MAKE IT **easier**

If it is difficult to clasp your hands behind you, extend one arm behind you, parallel to the ground, and grab a stable surface. Turn your body away from your arm to open your chest. Repeat with the other arm.

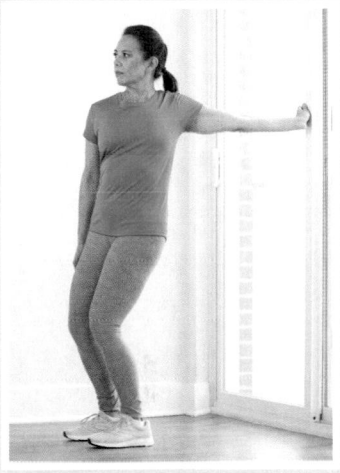

//// MAKE IT **harder**

To increase the intensity of the stretch, bend over at your waist, using your hips as a hinge, and pull your arms forward.

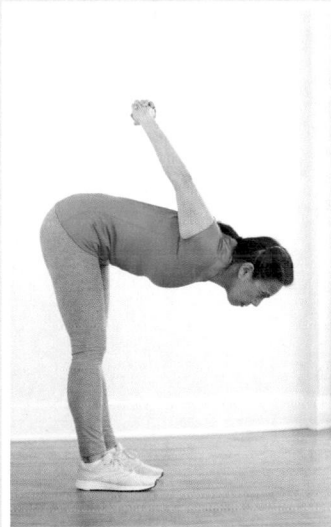

IMPROVES
/// **Posture**
/// **Strength**
/// **Stability**
/// **Mobility**
/// **Endurance**

WHAT YOU NEED
Dumbbells

Push press

Transferring weight from your lower to upper body requires immense central nervous system coordination. Use this dynamic overhead strength exercise to enhance your motor skills and improve your ability for actions such as lifting a box or suitcase overhead.

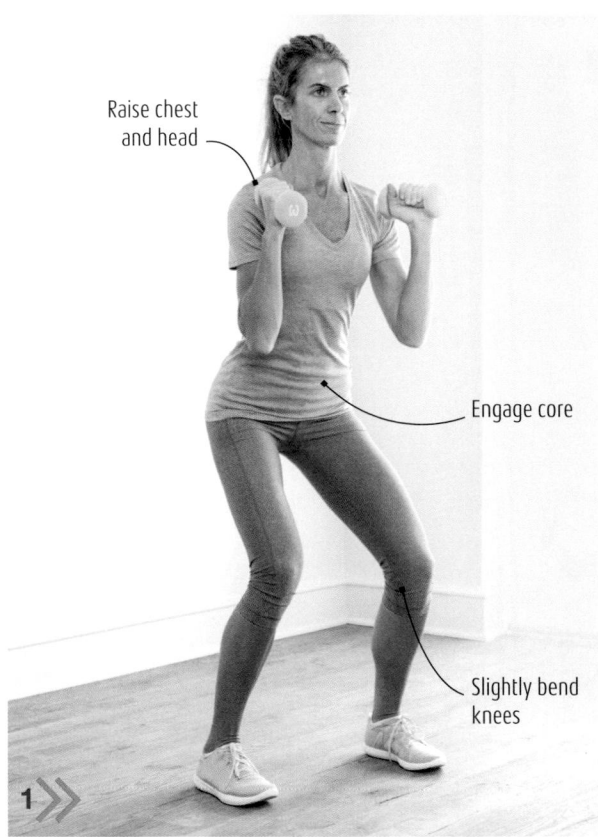

Raise chest and head

Engage core

Slightly bend knees

1

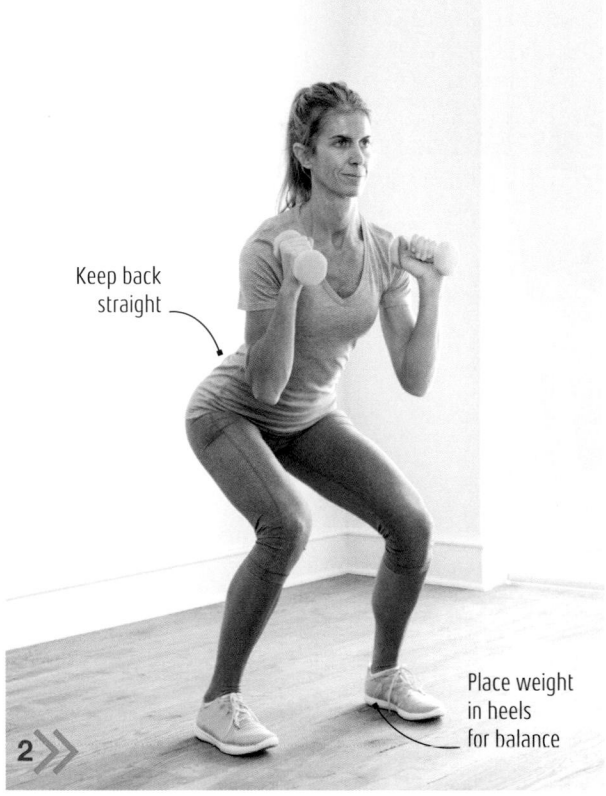

Keep back straight

Place weight in heels for balance

2

Stand with your feet slightly wider than shoulder-width apart and hold a dumbbell in each hand. Hold the dumbbells at shoulder height, palms facing each other, and keep your elbows close to your body.

Push your glutes back and bend at your hips and knees. Squat until your knees are bent to 45 degrees. Face your knees forward and keep your elbows close to your body.

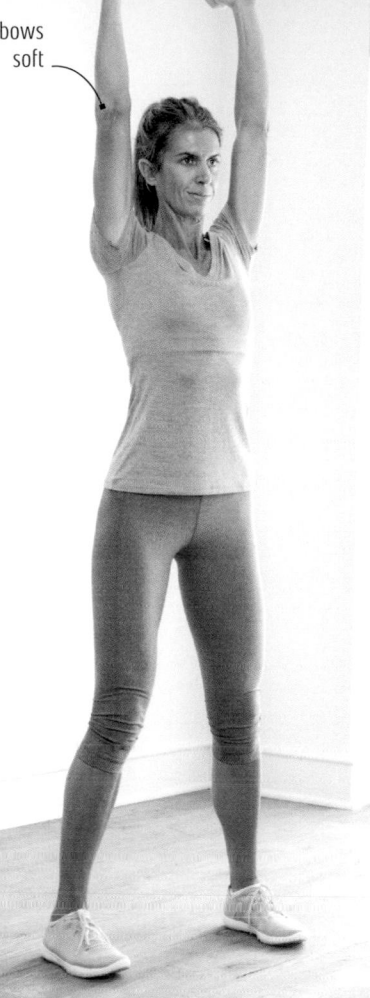

Keep elbows soft

3 »

Push through your heels and rise out of the squat until your legs are straight. Simultaneously use the momentum from your legs to press the dumbbells straight up until your arms are fully extended.

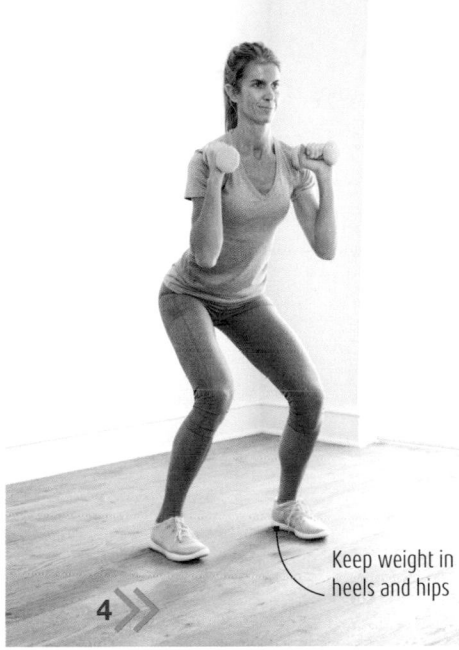

Keep weight in heels and hips

4 »

Lower the dumbbells back to your shoulders while bending your knees and hips to enter into the next squat. Continue to repeat the exercise for the time given in your workout.

/// MAKE IT **easier**

If it is difficult to maintain balance, sit on the edge of a chair while performing the exercise.

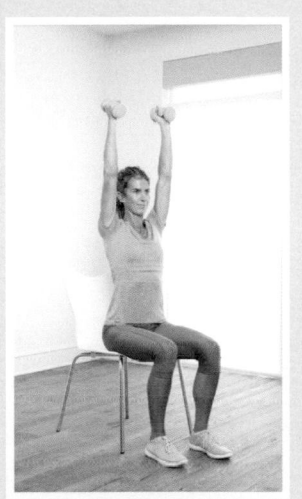

/// MAKE IT **harder**

To challenge your stability, in step 1, step your right leg back into a staggered stance. Rise up onto the ball of your right foot and slightly bend your knees. Drop your back knee and do a lunge between each press. Repeat with the opposite leg.

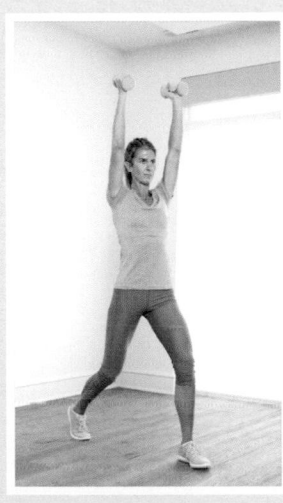

IMPROVES

/// **Posture**

/// **Strength**

/// **Stability**

/// **Endurance**

WHAT YOU NEED
Dumbbell

One-arm chest press

This balance exercise works one arm at a time, forcing your body to recruit your core muscles to keep your body stable and prevent you from tilting to the side. The controlled, unilateral movement is crucial for improving your core stability and correcting upper-body imbalances.

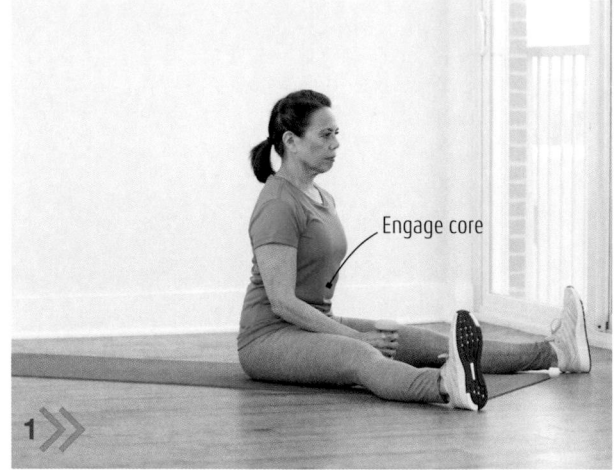

Engage core

Sit on the ground and extend your legs into a narrow v-shape. Firmly hold a dumbbell with your right hand and rest it between your legs. Rest your left hand on the ground for balance.

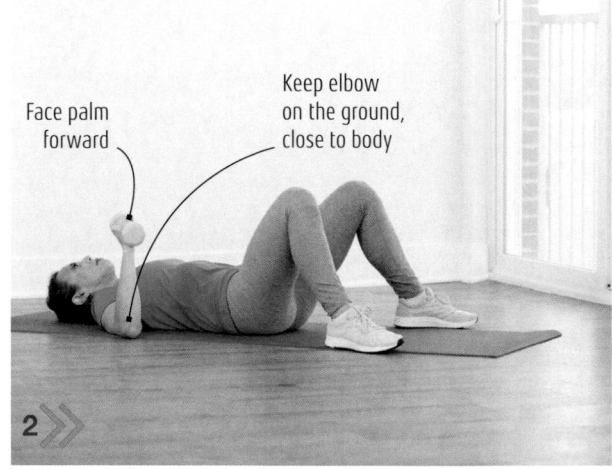

Face palm forward

Keep elbow on the ground, close to body

Lean back and lay your upper body flat on the ground. Bend your knees and plant your feet slightly wider than hip-width apart. Rest your right upper arm on the ground and raise your forearm. Extend your left arm out to your side, palm facing down.

3 »

In a controlled manner, engage your chest, triceps, and shoulder to press the dumbbell straight up, fully extending your right arm. Keep the dumbbell aligned directly over your elbow. Avoid arching your lower back by drawing your belly button into the ground.

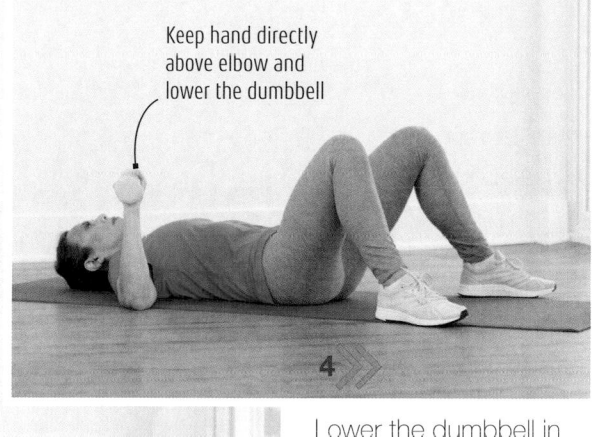

Keep hand directly above elbow and lower the dumbbell

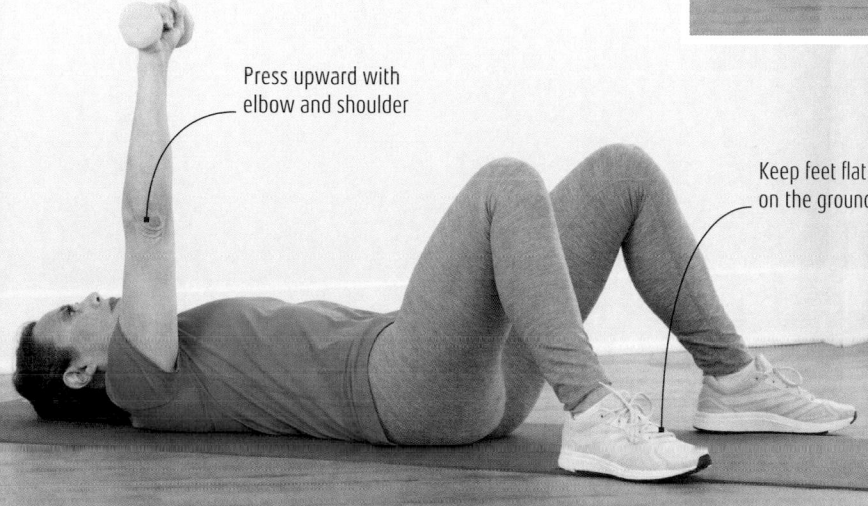

Press upward with elbow and shoulder

Keep feet flat on the ground

4 »

Lower the dumbbell in a controlled manner by bending your right elbow until your upper arm is flat on the ground. Repeat the press for the time given in your workout. Spend half the time pressing with your right arm, then switch to your left arm.

///// MAKE IT **easier**

If it is difficult to maintain balance, hold a dumbbell in each hand and press both dumbbells up at the same time. Keep the dumbbells aligned directly over your elbows.

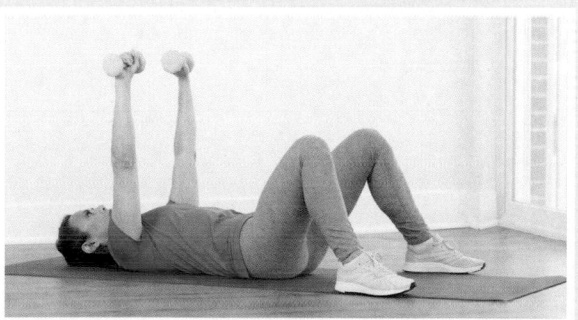

///// MAKE IT **harder**

To strengthen your glutes and hamstrings, drive your heels into the ground and lift your hips. Hold the position while you press and lower the dumbbell.

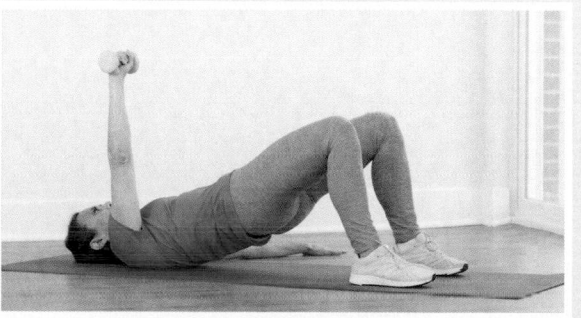

IMPROVES
/// **Posture**
/// **Strength**
/// **Stability**

WHAT YOU NEED
Dumbbell

One-leg arm raise

Balance is essential for safely performing most activities, such as enabling you to stand on one leg without falling over or maintain control while walking. Do this controlled, one-legged drill to improve your stability.

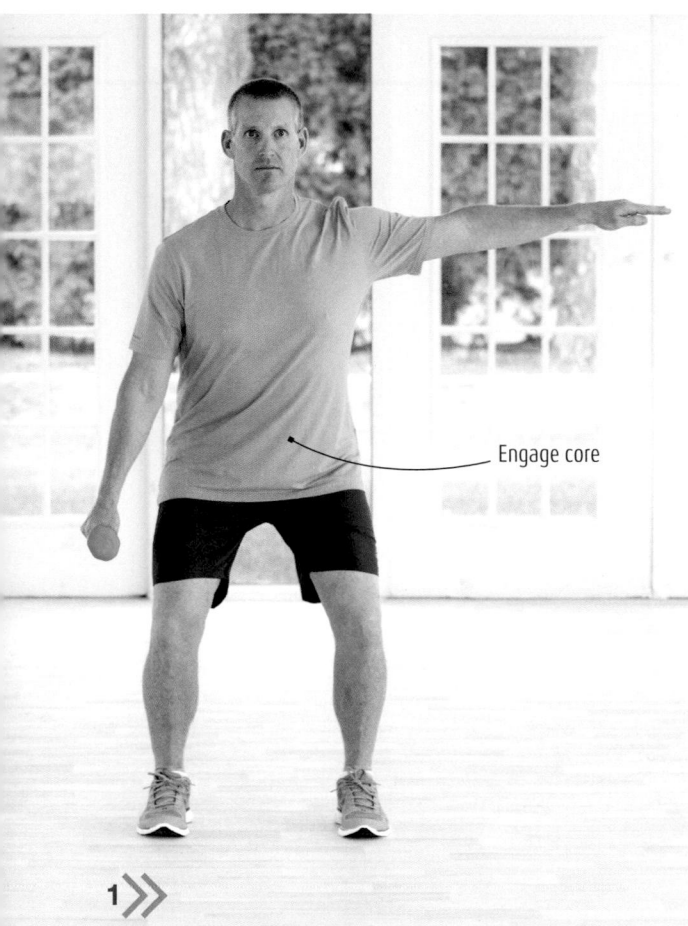

Engage core

1 »

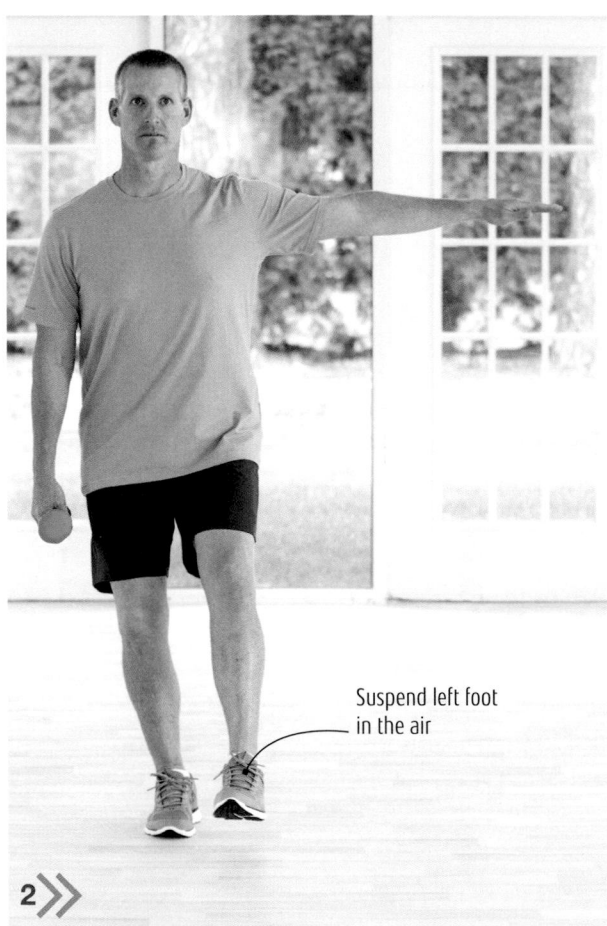

Suspend left foot in the air

2 »

Stand with your feet shoulder-width apart and slightly bend your knees. Hold a dumbbell in your right hand and let your arm hang at your side. Extend your left arm straight out to your side at shoulder height.

Raise your left knee until your foot is about 3 inches (8cm) off the ground, and transfer your weight to your right heel. Maintain a slight bend in both knees and keep your core engaged.

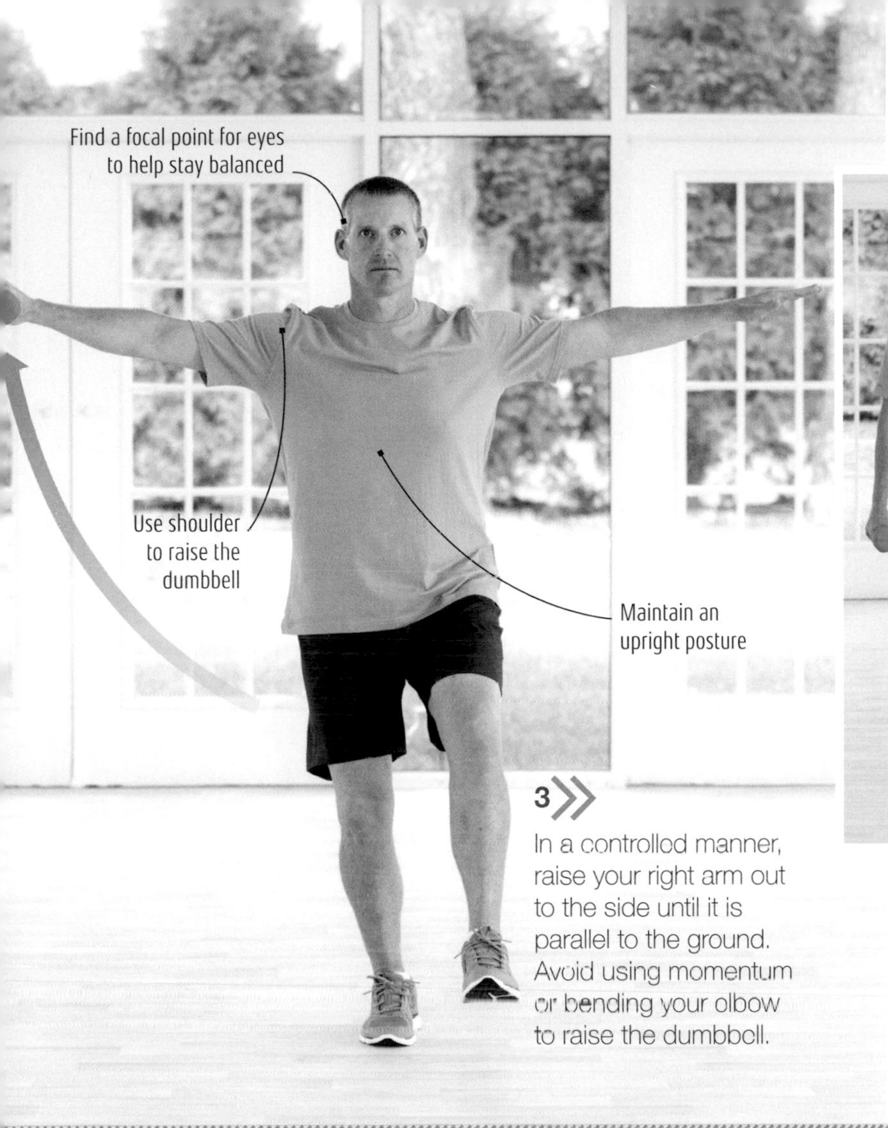

Find a focal point for eyes to help stay balanced

Use shoulder to raise the dumbbell

Maintain an upright posture

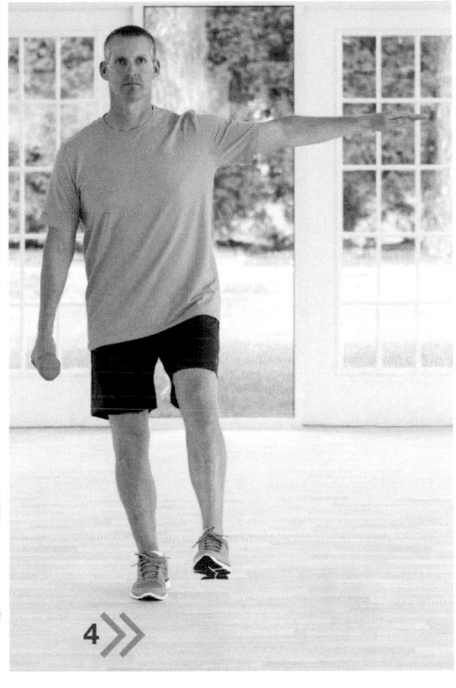

3 »
In a controlled manner, raise your right arm out to the side until it is parallel to the ground. Avoid using momentum or bending your elbow to raise the dumbbell.

4 »
Return the dumbbell to your side in a controlled manner. Keep your left foot raised and spend half the given time working your right arm. Then switch leg positions and repeat with the opposite arm.

/// MAKE IT **easier**

If it is difficult to balance, lightly rest your hand on a chair or wall for support, but avoid leaning into it or relying on it too much.

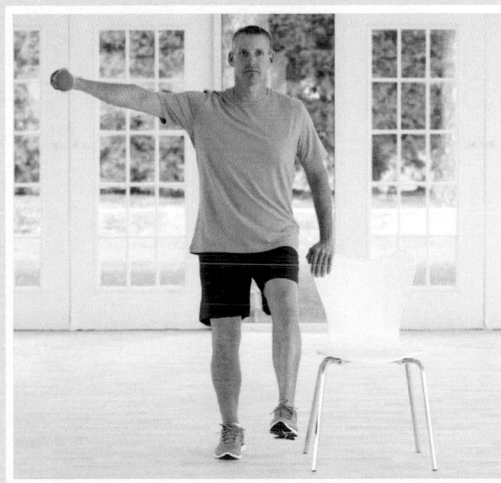

IMPROVES
- //// Posture
- //// **Strength**
- //// **Stability**
- //// Mobility
- //// **Endurance**

WHAT YOU NEED
Wall

Jumping wall push-ups

Add speed and explosive power to an inclined push-up by bursting off the wall between each repetition. Jumping exercises like this one develop the nervous system and improve your coordination, motor skills, and balance. The increased upper-body power generated by this exercise is especially beneficial for golfers, tennis players, and swimmers.

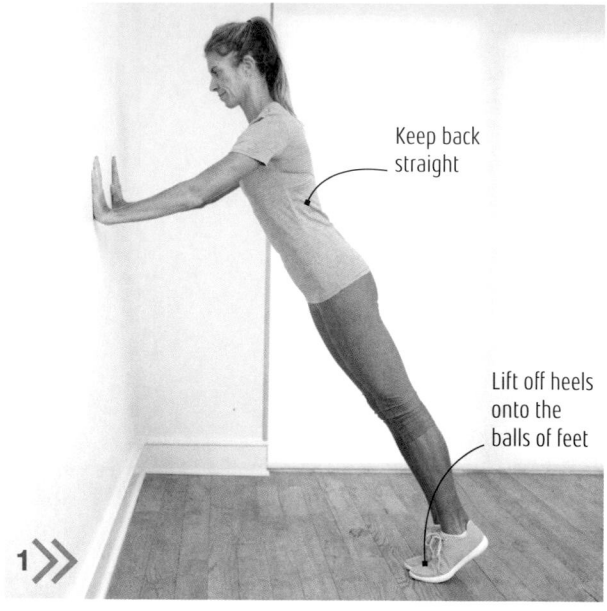

Keep back straight

Lift off heels onto the balls of feet

1 » Place your hands shoulder-width apart on a wall at chest height, and step your feet back until your body is about 45 degrees to the ground. Shift your weight to your hands and rise onto the balls of your feet.

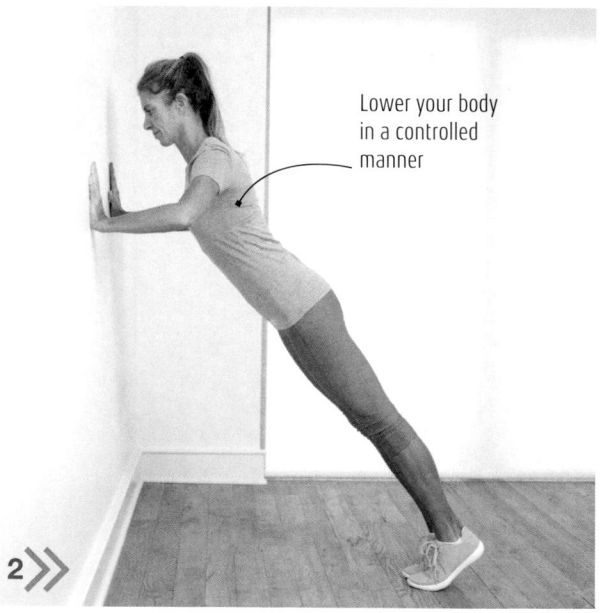

Lower your body in a controlled manner

2 » In a controlled manner, bend your elbows and use your triceps, chest, and shoulders to lower your body until your elbows are bent to about 90 degrees. Keep your core engaged and your back straight.

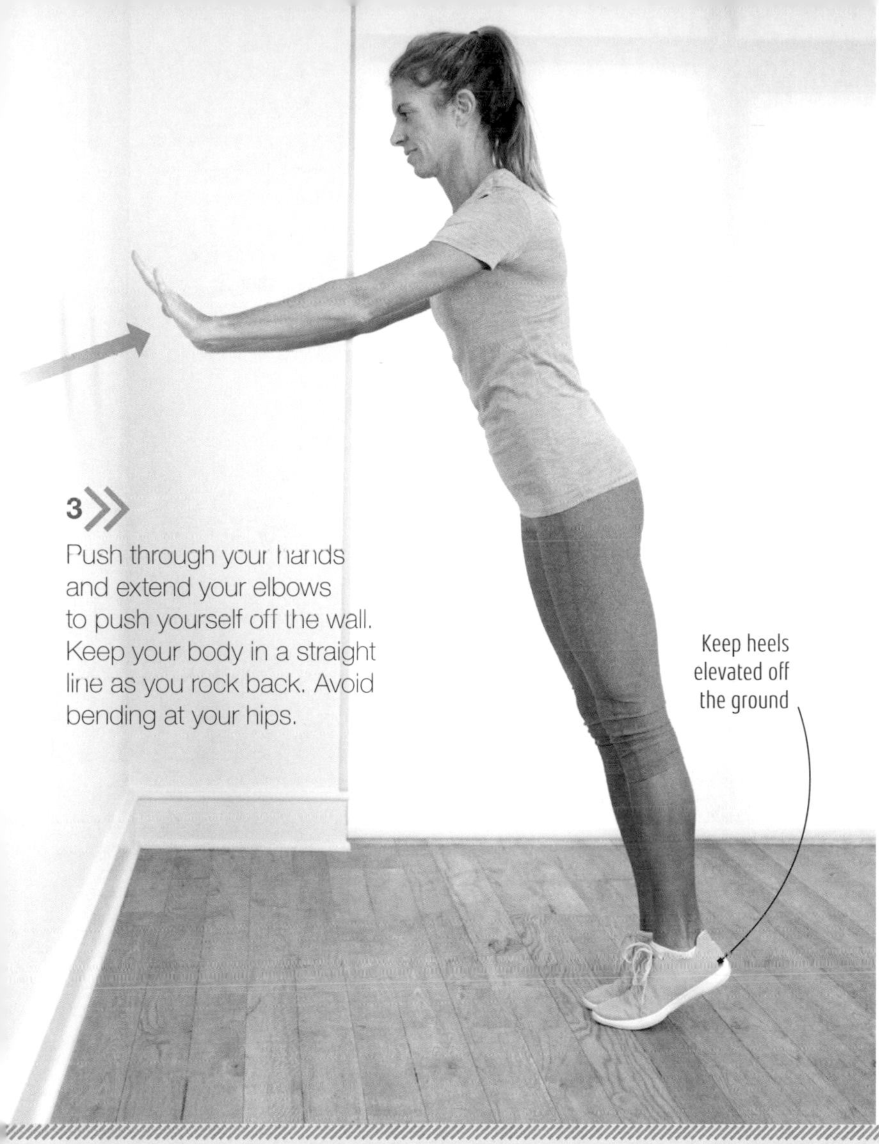

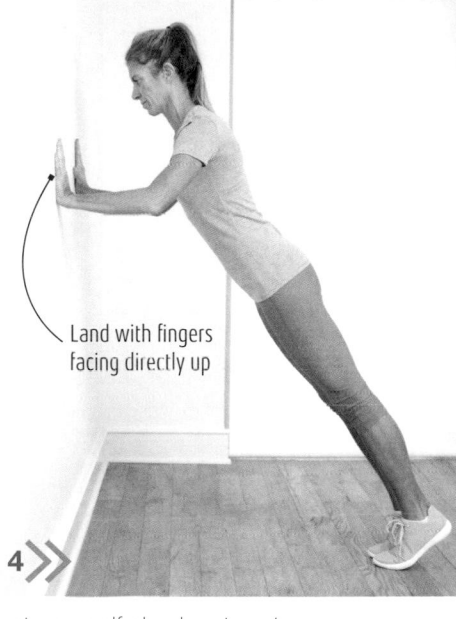

Land with fingers facing directly up

3 »

Push through your hands and extend your elbows to push yourself off the wall. Keep your body in a straight line as you rock back. Avoid bending at your hips.

Keep heels elevated off the ground

4 »

Let yourself slowly return to the wall. Catch yourself with your hands and bend your elbows to absorb the impact. Load your arms, chest, and shoulders for the next push-up, and repeat for the time given in your workout.

///// MAKE IT **easier**

To reduce the resistance to your upper body, stand closer to the wall. Step your feet back until your body is at about a 60-degree angle to the ground, and do the exercise from this position.

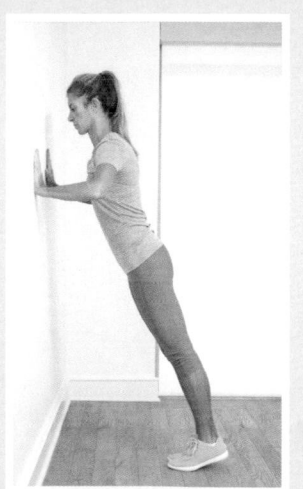

///// MAKE IT **harder**

To increase resistance to your core and upper body, do the exercise on the ground. Put your knees on the ground and lower your hips until your body is angled at about 45 degrees.

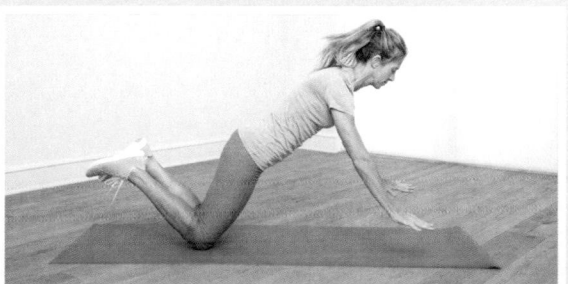

Gunslinger

Your core connects your upper and lower body, but a weak connection can lead to poor balance. This weighted pushing exercise strengthens your core and enhances your body's head-to-toe coordination.

IMPROVES
/// **Posture**
/// **Strength**
/// **Stability**

WHAT YOU NEED
Dumbbells

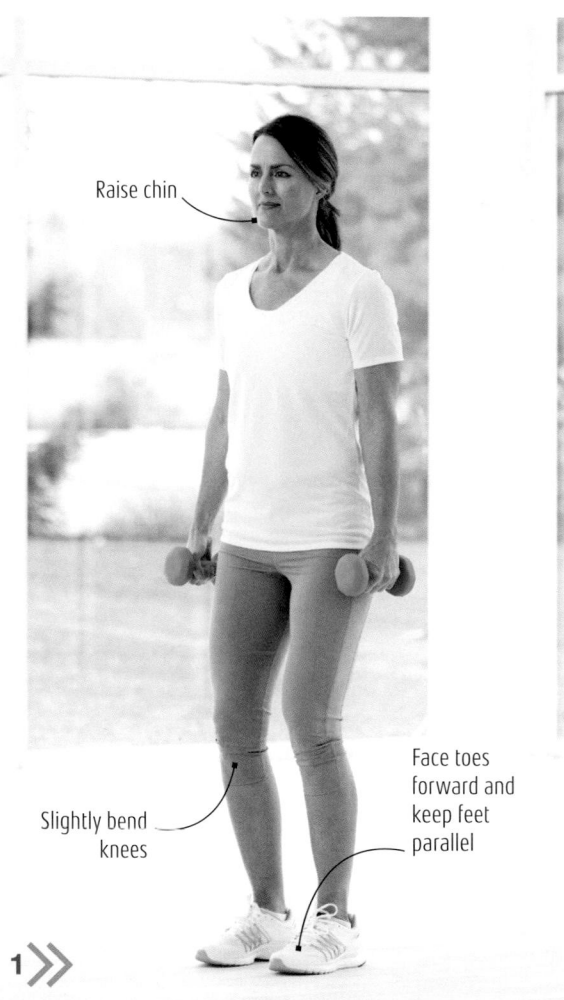

Raise chin

Slightly bend knees

Face toes forward and keep feet parallel

1 >>

Stand with your feet shoulder-width apart. Hold a dumbbell in each hand, palms facing inward, and let your arms hang at your sides. Engage your core and retract your shoulder blades.

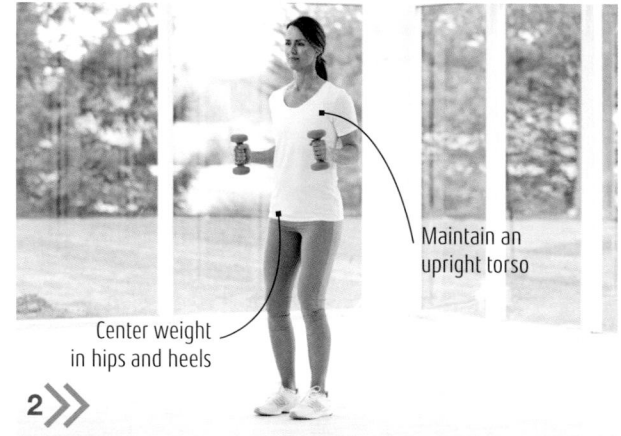

Maintain an upright torso

Center weight in hips and heels

2 >>

In a controlled manner, engage your biceps and forearms to curl the dumbbells until your forearms are parallel to the ground.

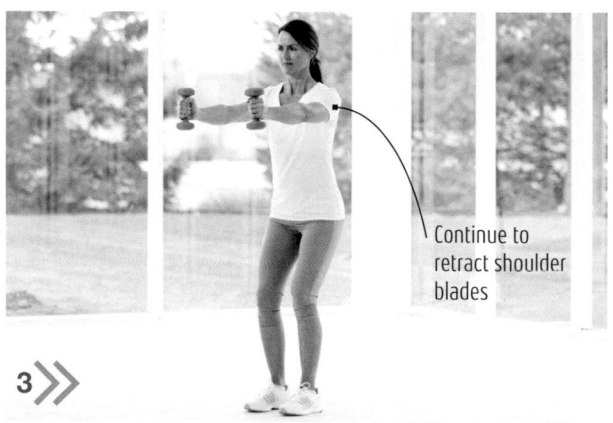

Continue to retract shoulder blades

3 >>

In the same controlled manner, engage your chest and shoulders to push the dumbbells straight out until your arms are fully extended in front of you and parallel to the ground.

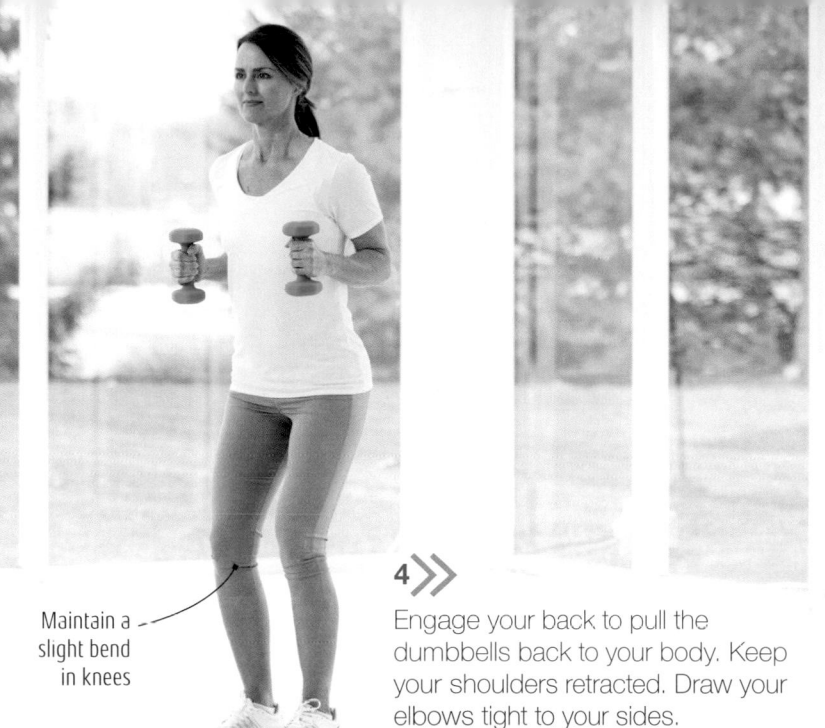

Maintain a slight bend in knees

4 »

Engage your back to pull the dumbbells back to your body. Keep your shoulders retracted. Draw your elbows tight to your sides.

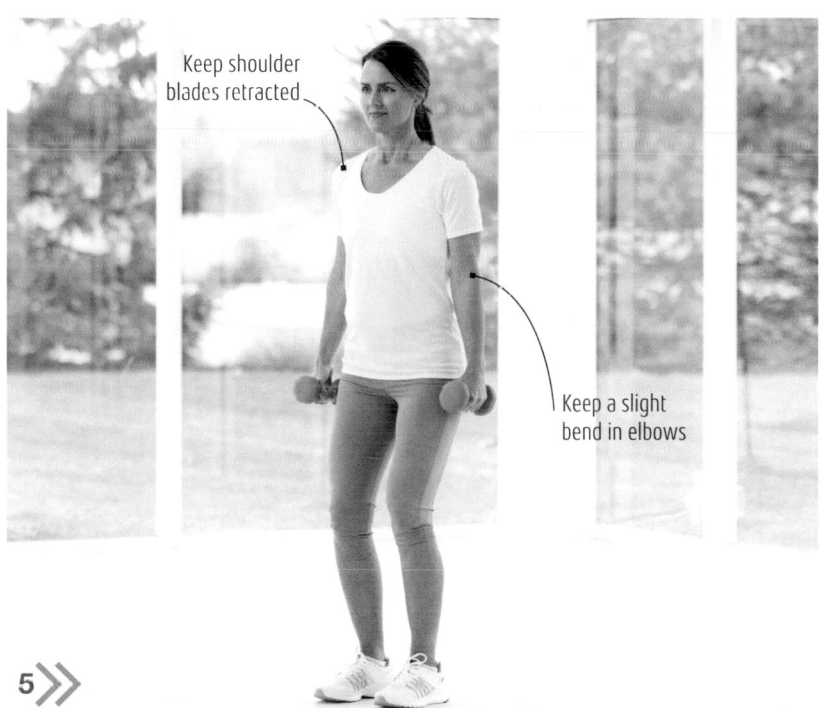

Keep shoulder blades retracted

Keep a slight bend in elbows

5 »

In a controlled manner, return the dumbbells to the starting position, and avoid hunching forward. Repeat the sequence for the time given in your workout.

//// MAKE IT **easier**

To decrease the load on your lower back, sit on the edge of a chair while performing the exercise.

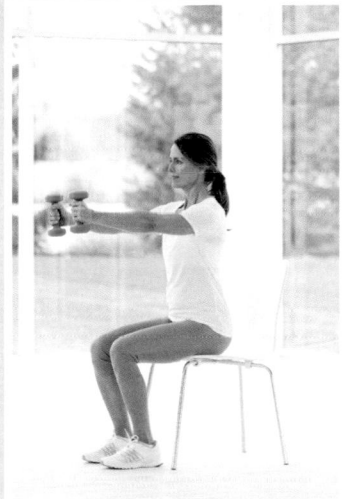

//// MAKE IT **harder**

To improve your balance, do the exercise from a staggered stance. In step 1, step your left leg back and rise up onto the ball of your left foot. Repeat in the opposite stance.

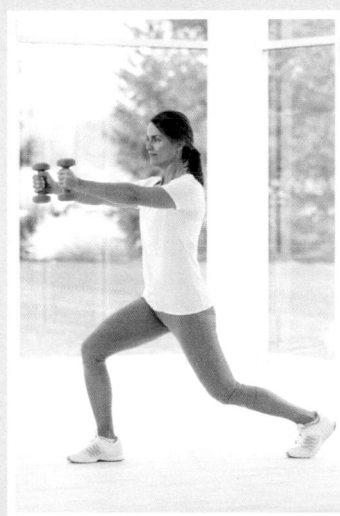

Shot-put press

You do not have to be an Olympic athlete to benefit from increased rotational power and stability. This swift and controlled throwing exercise improves your coordination for sports like baseball, golf, and tennis.

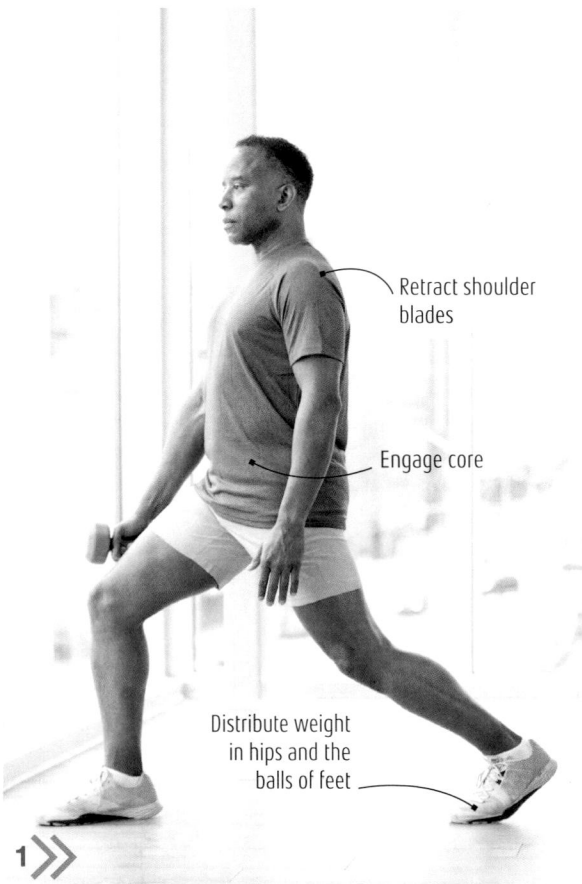

Retract shoulder blades

Engage core

Distribute weight in hips and the balls of feet

1 »

Stand with your feet shoulder-width apart. Hold a dumbbell in your right hand and let your arms hang at your sides. Step your left leg back into a staggered stance and rise up onto the ball of your left foot.

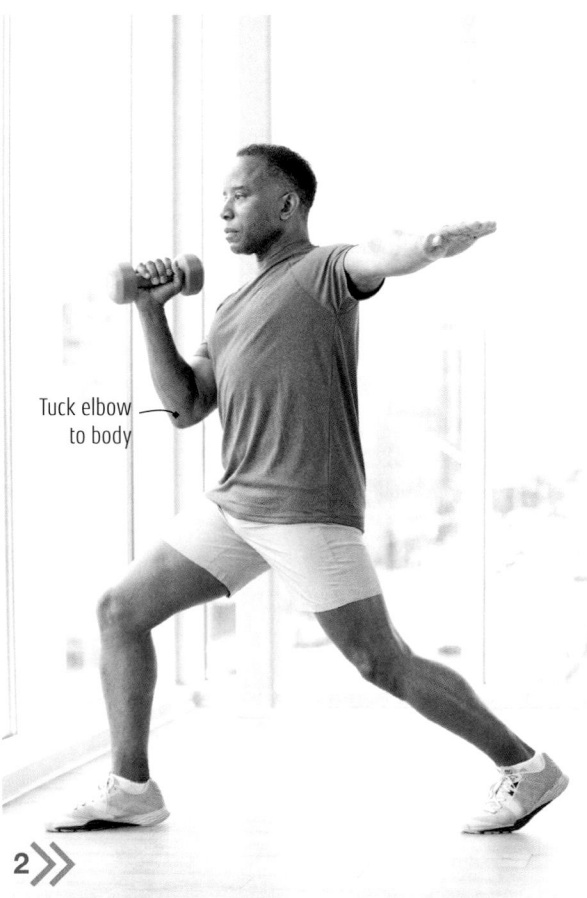

Tuck elbow to body

2 »

Bend your right elbow to raise the dumbbell near your chin, palm facing inward. Extend your left arm out to your side at a right angle to your body, palm facing the ground. Keep your core engaged.

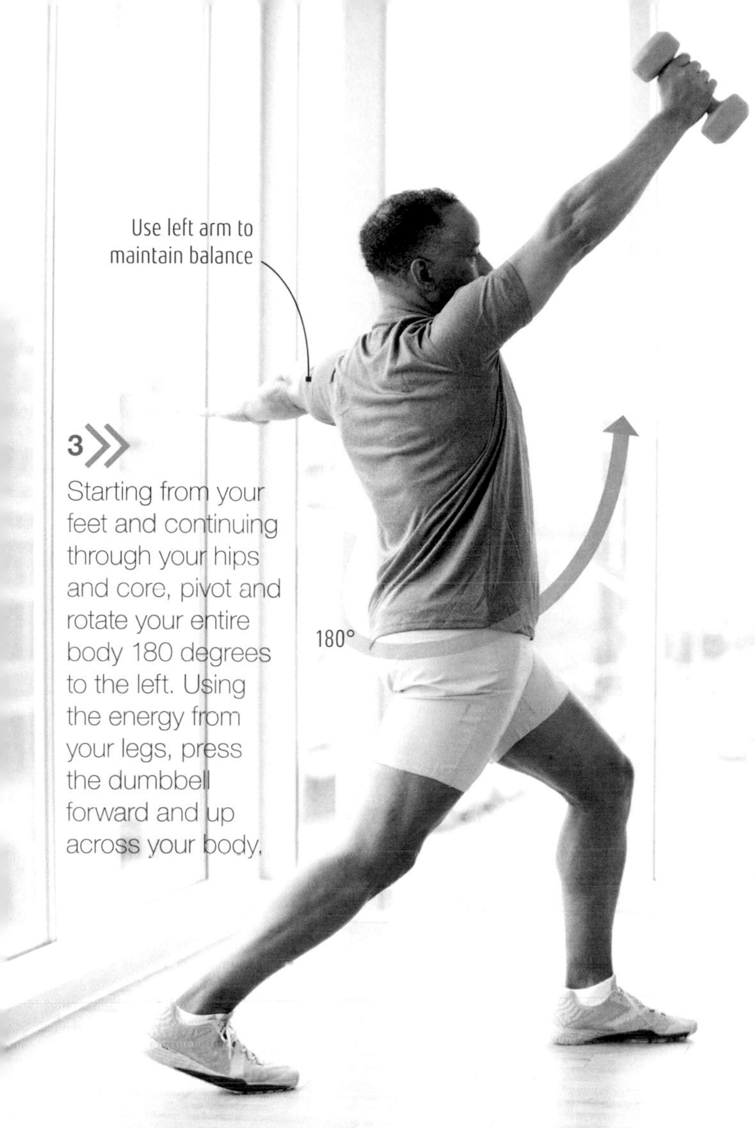

Use left arm to maintain balance

3 》》

Starting from your feet and continuing through your hips and core, pivot and rotate your entire body 180 degrees to the left. Using the energy from your legs, press the dumbbell forward and up across your body.

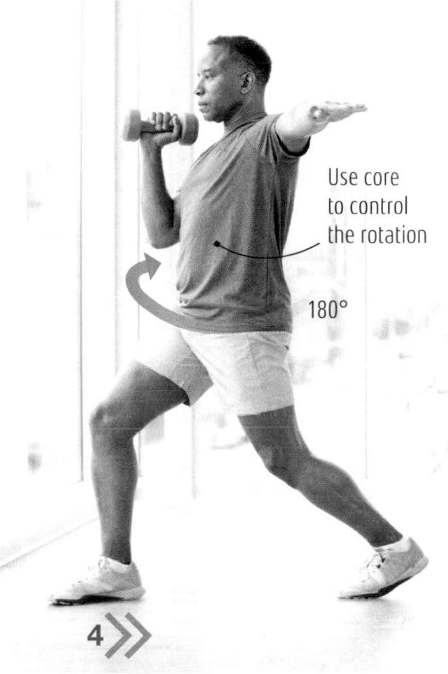

180°

Use core to control the rotation

180°

4 》》

Rotate back and return the dumbbell to the step 2 position. Repeat the sequence for the time given in your workout. Spend half the time with the dumbbell in your right hand, then switch hands and repeat on the opposite side, rotating to the right.

▰/// MAKE IT **easier**

If it is difficult to maintain balance, do the exercise without a dumbbell. Hold your hand in a fist.

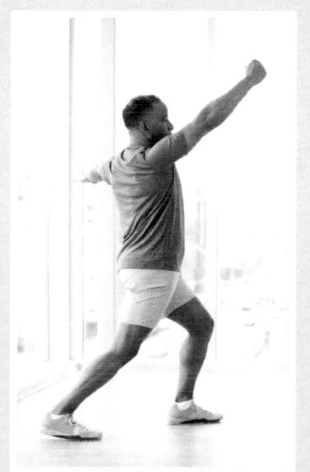

▰/// MAKE IT **harder**

To strengthen your legs, drop your back knee into a lunge before rotating in step 3. Rise back up into the staggered stance as you begin to rotate.

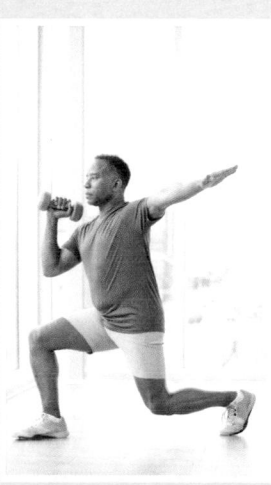

Suitcase row

Pulling with one arm at a time requires a strong and stable core. Use this quick and controlled unilateral movement to build back strength and improve stability for everyday activities such as pulling weeds and lifting luggage.

IMPROVES
/// **Posture**
/// **Strength**
/// **Stability**
/// **Endurance**

WHAT YOU NEED
Dumbbell

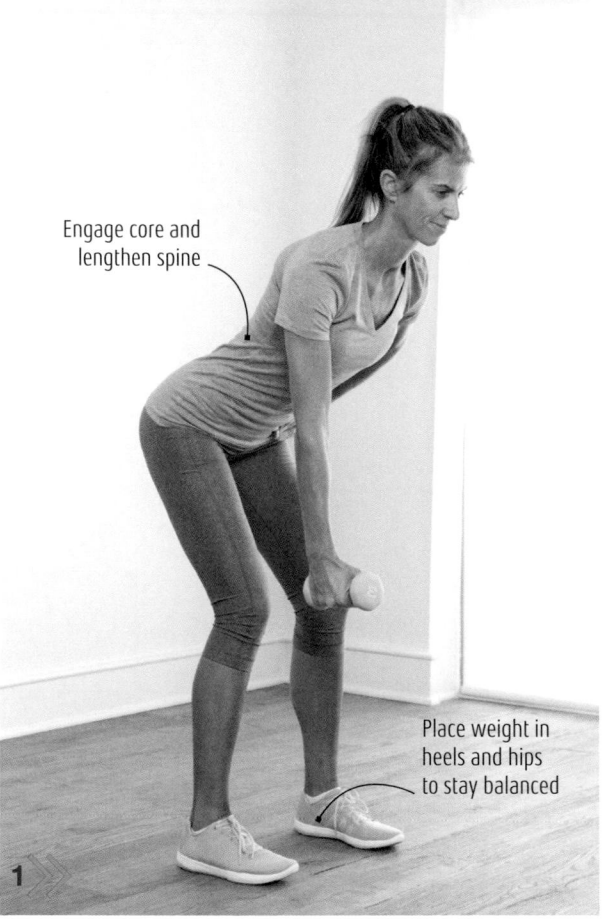

Engage core and lengthen spine

Place weight in heels and hips to stay balanced

1

Stand with your feet shoulder-width apart and bend over from the hips. Hold a dumbbell in your right hand and let your arm hang straight down. Put your left hand on your hip. Retract your shoulder blades.

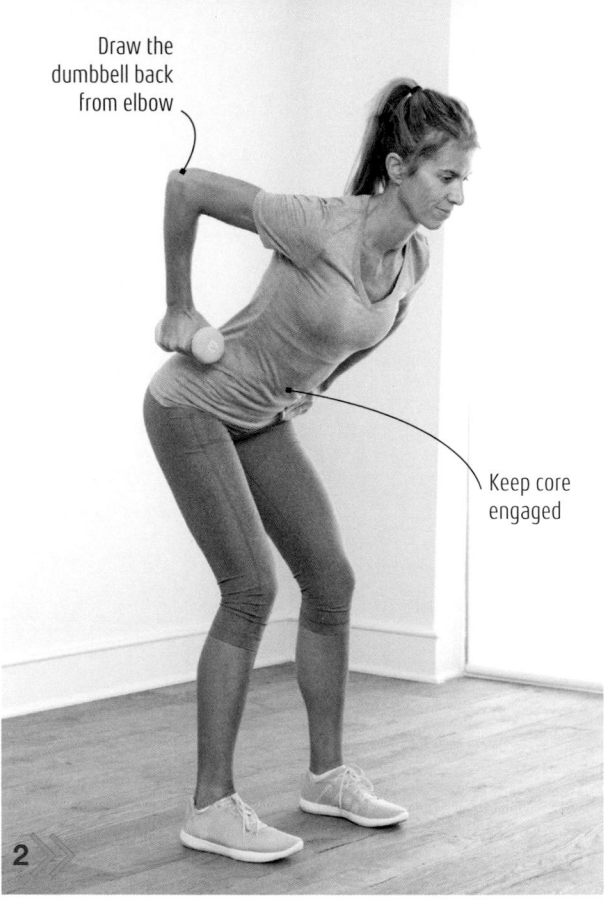

Draw the dumbbell back from elbow

Keep core engaged

2

Pull the dumbbell up and back from your elbow. Keep your shoulders square and your elbow tight to your body as you row. Contract your back at the top of the movement.

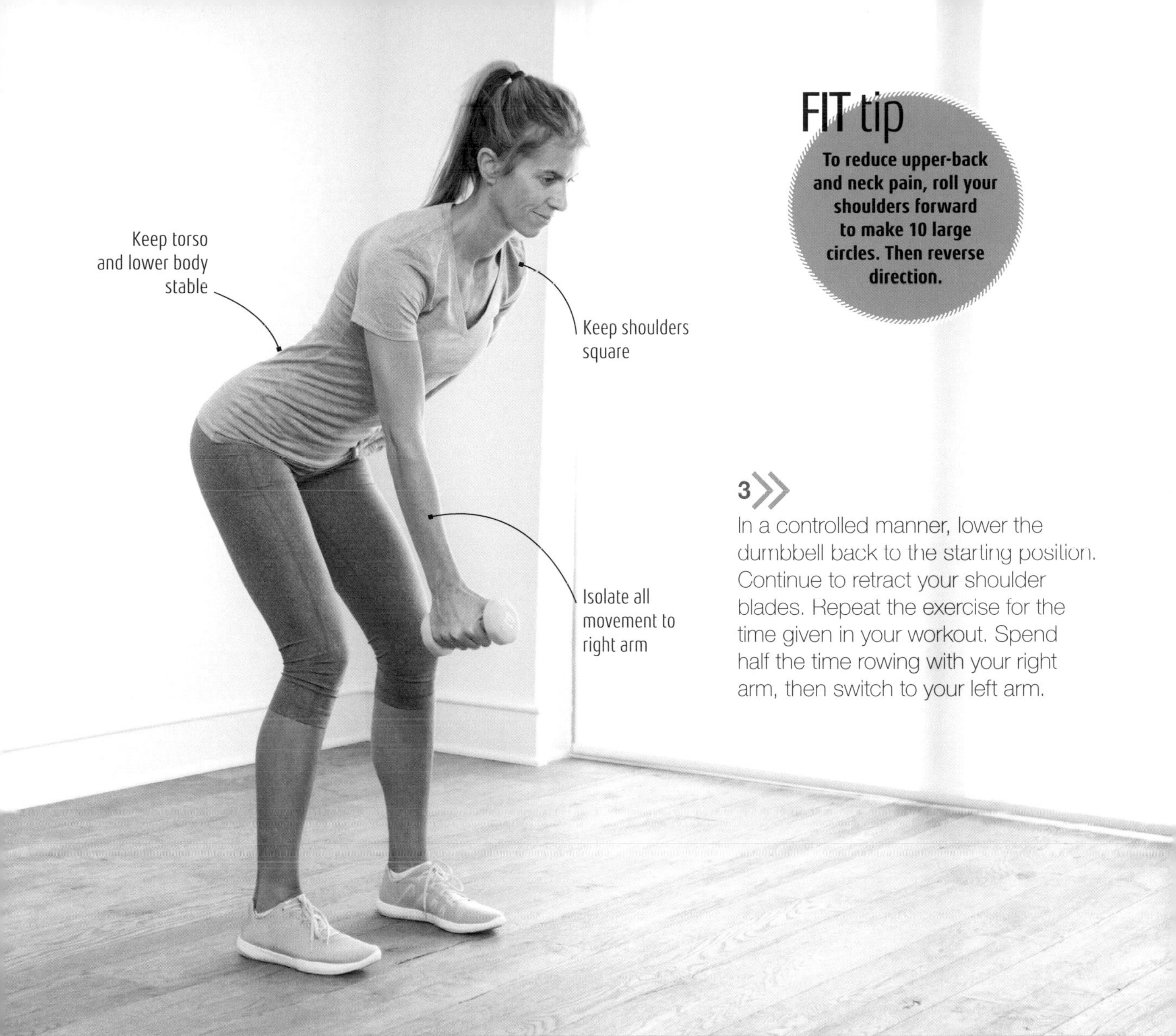

Keep torso and lower body stable

Keep shoulders square

Isolate all movement to right arm

FIT tip
To reduce upper-back and neck pain, roll your shoulders forward to make 10 large circles. Then reverse direction.

3 ❯❯

In a controlled manner, lower the dumbbell back to the starting position. Continue to retract your shoulder blades. Repeat the exercise for the time given in your workout. Spend half the time rowing with your right arm, then switch to your left arm.

///// MAKE IT easier

If it is difficult to maintain balance, sit on the edge of a chair and bend forward while performing the exercise.

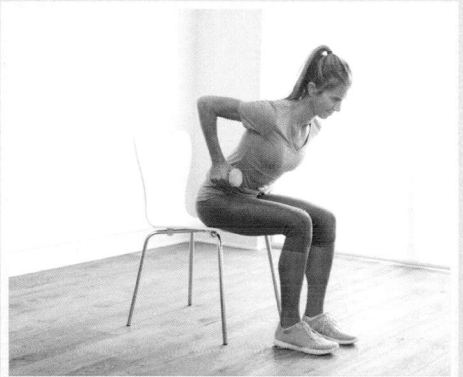

IMPROVES
▰//// Strength
▰//// Stability
//// Mobility
▰//// Endurance

WHAT YOU NEED
Dumbbell

Lawn mower row

Twisting and pulling to start a lawn mower is the type of compound movement life often demands. This quick and controlled exercise improves the rotational strength and total-body coordination needed for this kind of pulling activity.

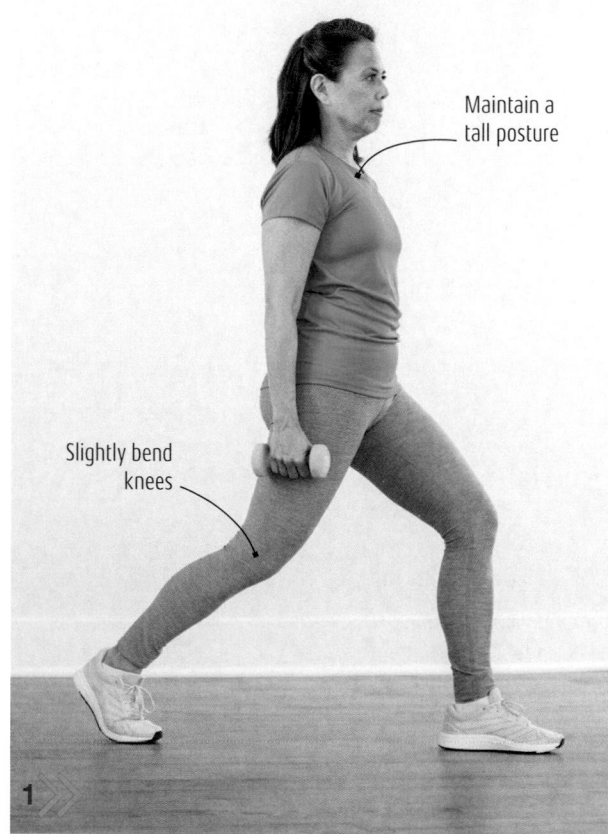

Maintain a tall posture

Slightly bend knees

1 >>

Stand with your feet shoulder-width apart. Hold a dumbbell in your right hand, and let your arms hang at your sides. Step your right leg back into a staggered stance and rise up onto the ball of your right foot.

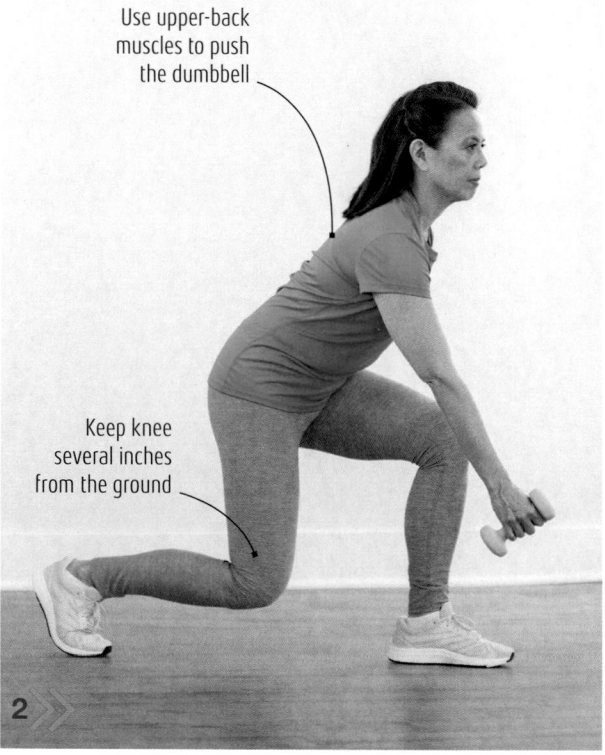

Use upper-back muscles to push the dumbbell

Keep knee several inches from the ground

2 >>

Drop your right knee down until both knees are bent to 90 degrees. Simultaneously push the dumbbell forward, toward your left toes, until your arm is fully extended. Center your weight in both feet and hips.

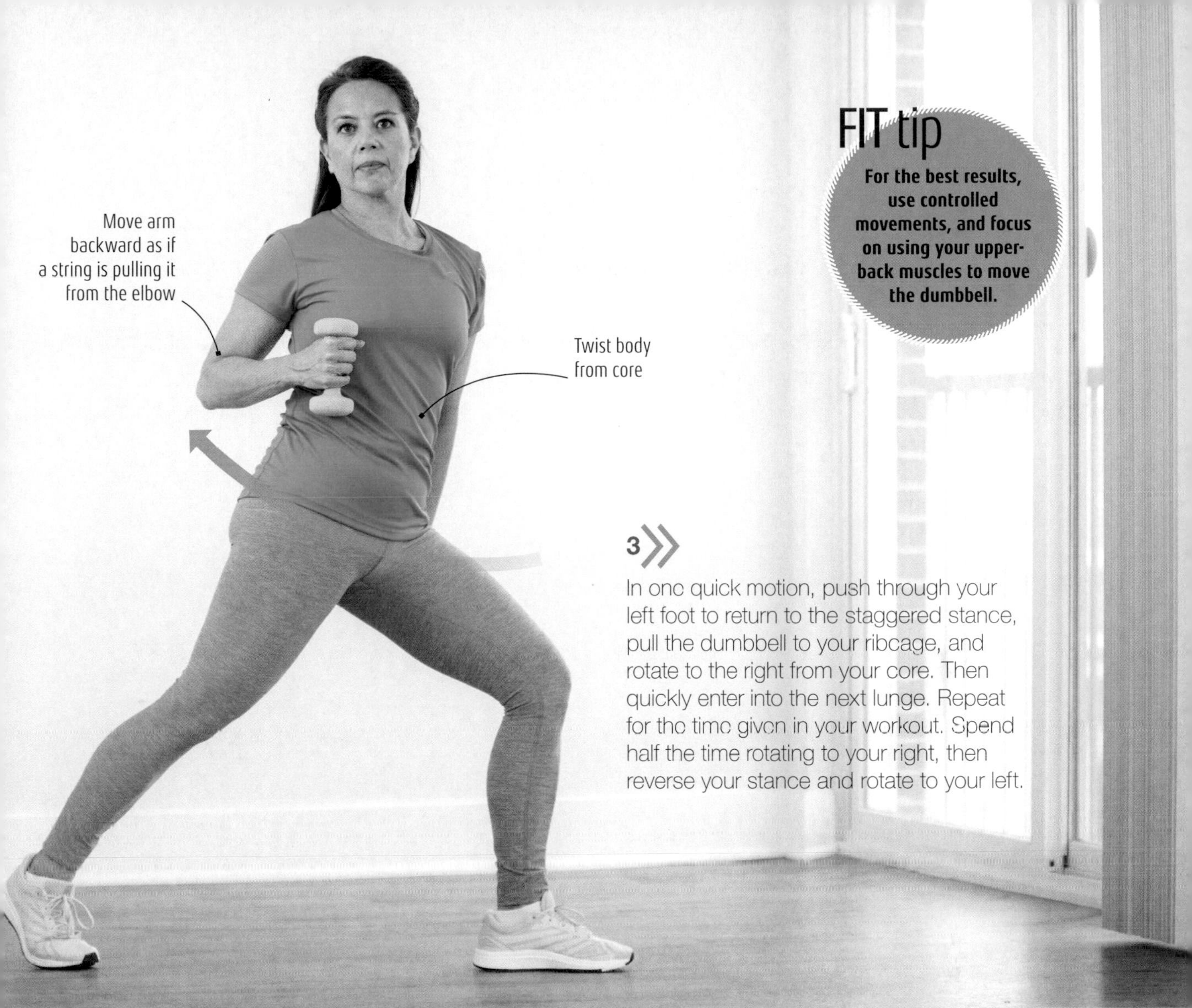

FIT tip

For the best results, use controlled movements, and focus on using your upper-back muscles to move the dumbbell.

Move arm backward as if a string is pulling it from the elbow

Twist body from core

3 »

In one quick motion, push through your left foot to return to the staggered stance, pull the dumbbell to your ribcage, and rotate to the right from your core. Then quickly enter into the next lunge. Repeat for the time given in your workout. Spend half the time rotating to your right, then reverse your stance and rotate to your left.

/// MAKE IT **easier**

To decrease the load on your legs, in step 1, keep your feet in a neutral stance. In step 2, rather than lunging, sit your hips back into a squat.

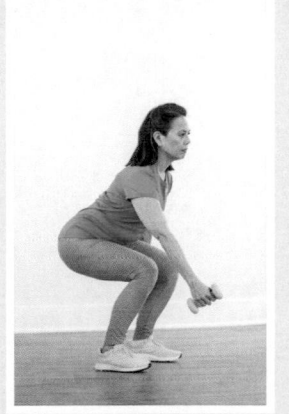

/// MAKE IT **harder**

To intensify the full-body coordination required, in step 1, step your left leg forward rather than stepping your right foot back. In step 2, drop into a lunge as you reach forward. In step 3, return your legs to the starting position by stepping your left leg back. Repeat on the opposite side.

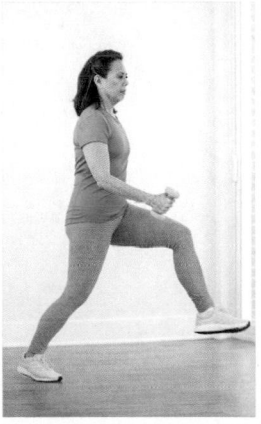

IMPROVES
//// Posture
//// Strength
//// Stability
//// Mobility

WHAT YOU NEED
Dumbbells

Staggered reverse fly

The human body is built to stand and move, so if you sit for many hours a day, it can lead to poor posture. Perform this quick upper-back exercise to improve your spinal alignment and strengthen your back.

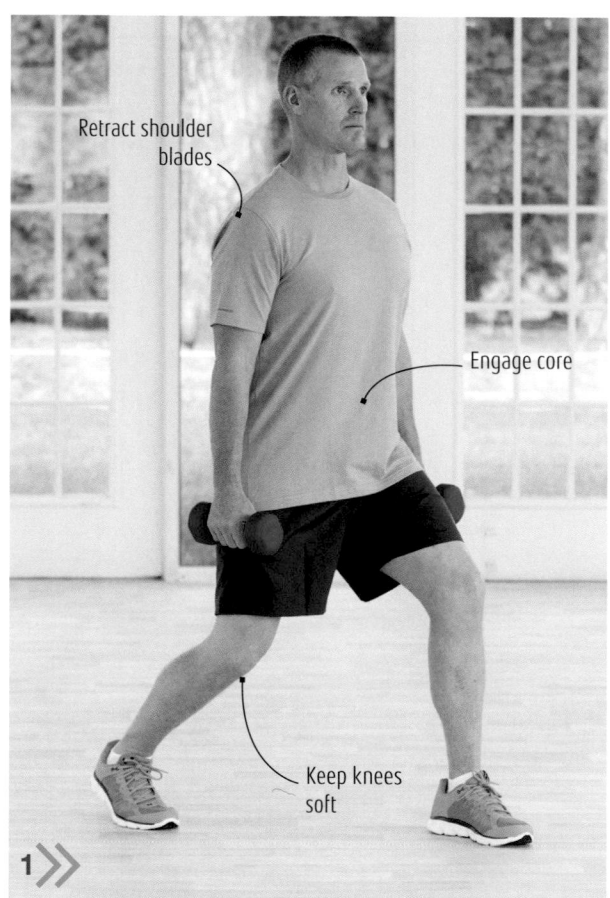

Retract shoulder blades

Engage core

Keep knees soft

1 >>

Hold a dumbbell in each hand. Stand with your feet shoulder-width apart and step your right leg back into a staggered stance. Rise up onto the ball of your right foot. Slightly bend your knees.

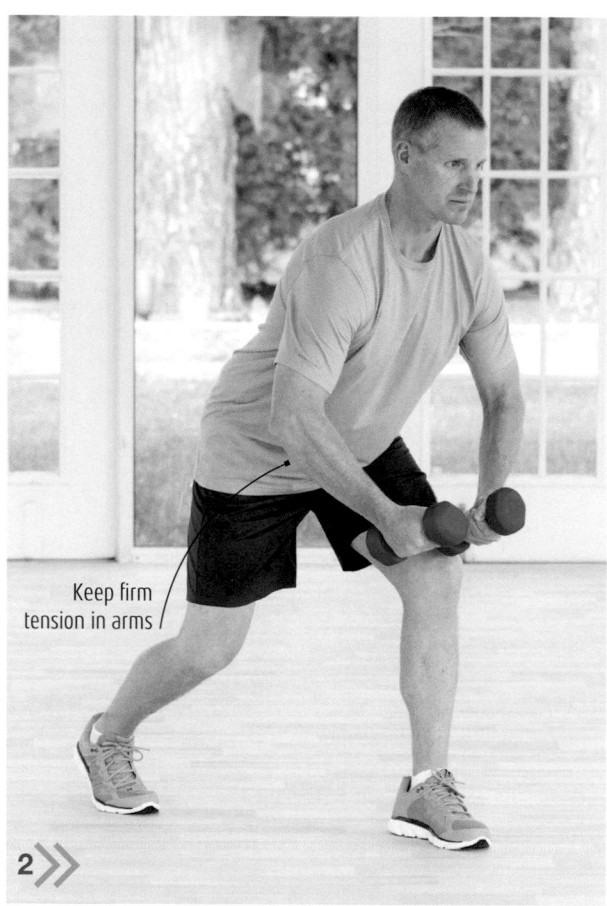

Keep firm tension in arms

2 >>

Bend over to 45 degrees from the hips and bring the dumbbells together. Slightly bend your elbows as if you are wrapping your arms around a tree trunk. Keep your back flat and your head raised.

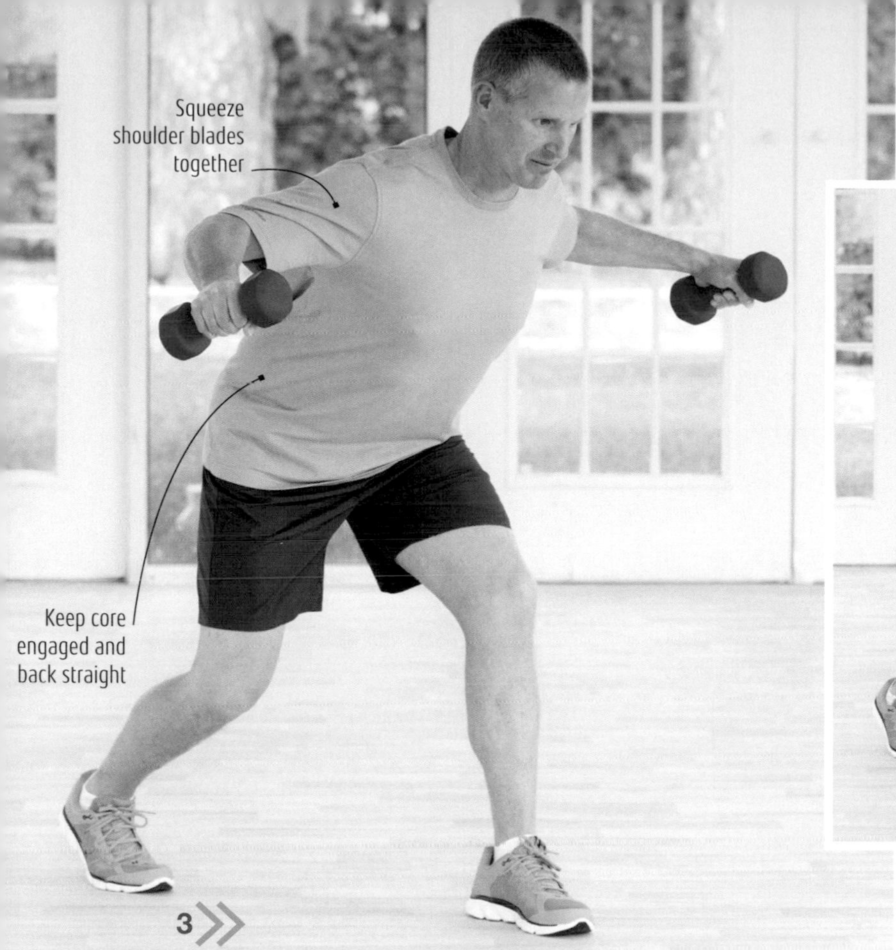

Squeeze
shoulder blades
together

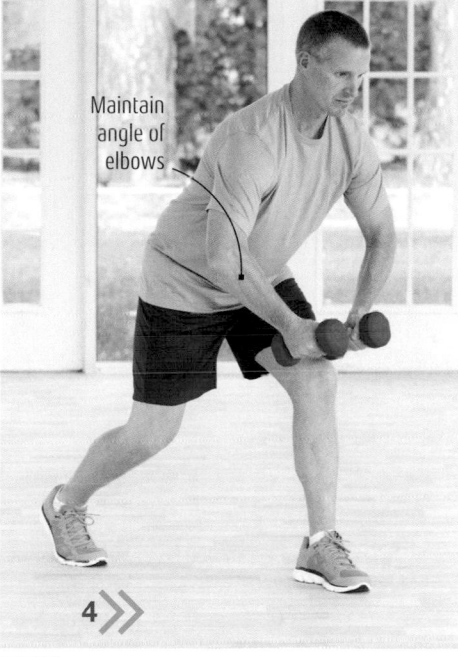

Maintain
angle of
elbows

Keep core
engaged and
back straight

3 ≫
Engage the muscles in your upper back to pull
the dumbbells apart, keeping your elbows bent.
Contract the middle of your back at the top of
the movement.

4 ≫
Using your back muscles, return
the dumbbells to the starting
position. Repeat the exercise in
a quick, controlled manner for the
time given in your workout. Switch
your stance halfway through.

////// MAKE IT **easier**

If it is difficult to maintain
balance, sit on the edge of
a chair and lean forward
at the hips while performing
the exercise.

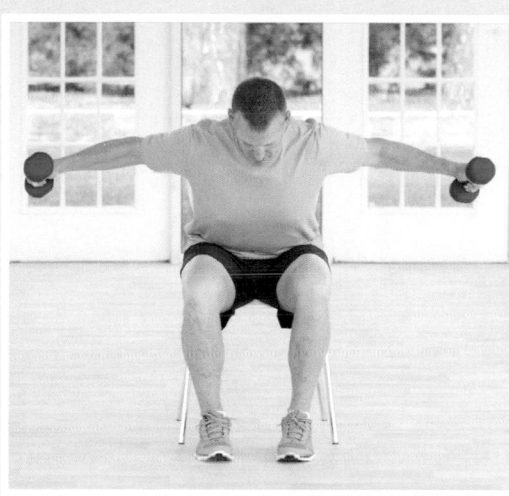

IMPROVES

//// Posture
//// Strength
//// Stability
//// Mobility
//// Endurance

WHAT YOU NEED
Dumbbells

Arm pullovers

Lack of shoulder mobility is one of the most common causes of upper-body injury. The rapid pulling motion in this exercise will help you to prevent injuries, improve mobility, and strengthen your shoulders and upper back for more functional movement.

FIT tip

If you do not have dumbbells at home, you can use soup cans, water bottles, or bags of fruit instead.

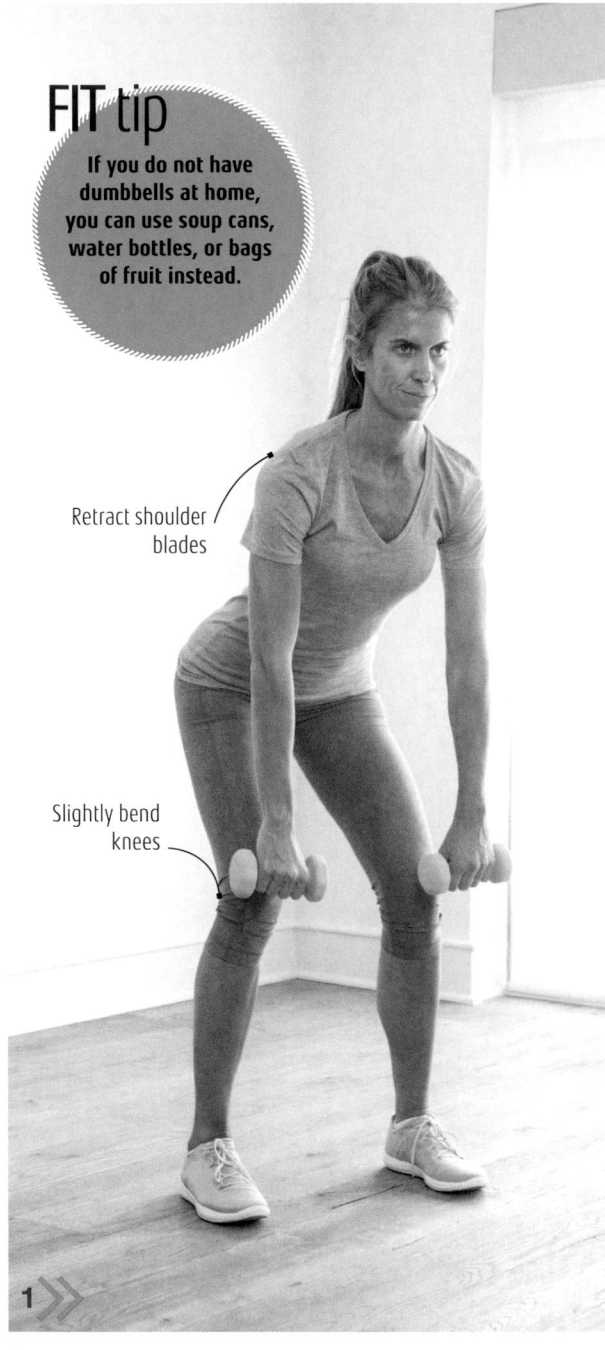

Retract shoulder blades

Slightly bend knees

1 »

Stand with your feet shoulder-width apart and hold a dumbbell in each hand. Engage your core and bend over to 45 degrees from the hips. Let your arms hang in front of you, palms facing your knees.

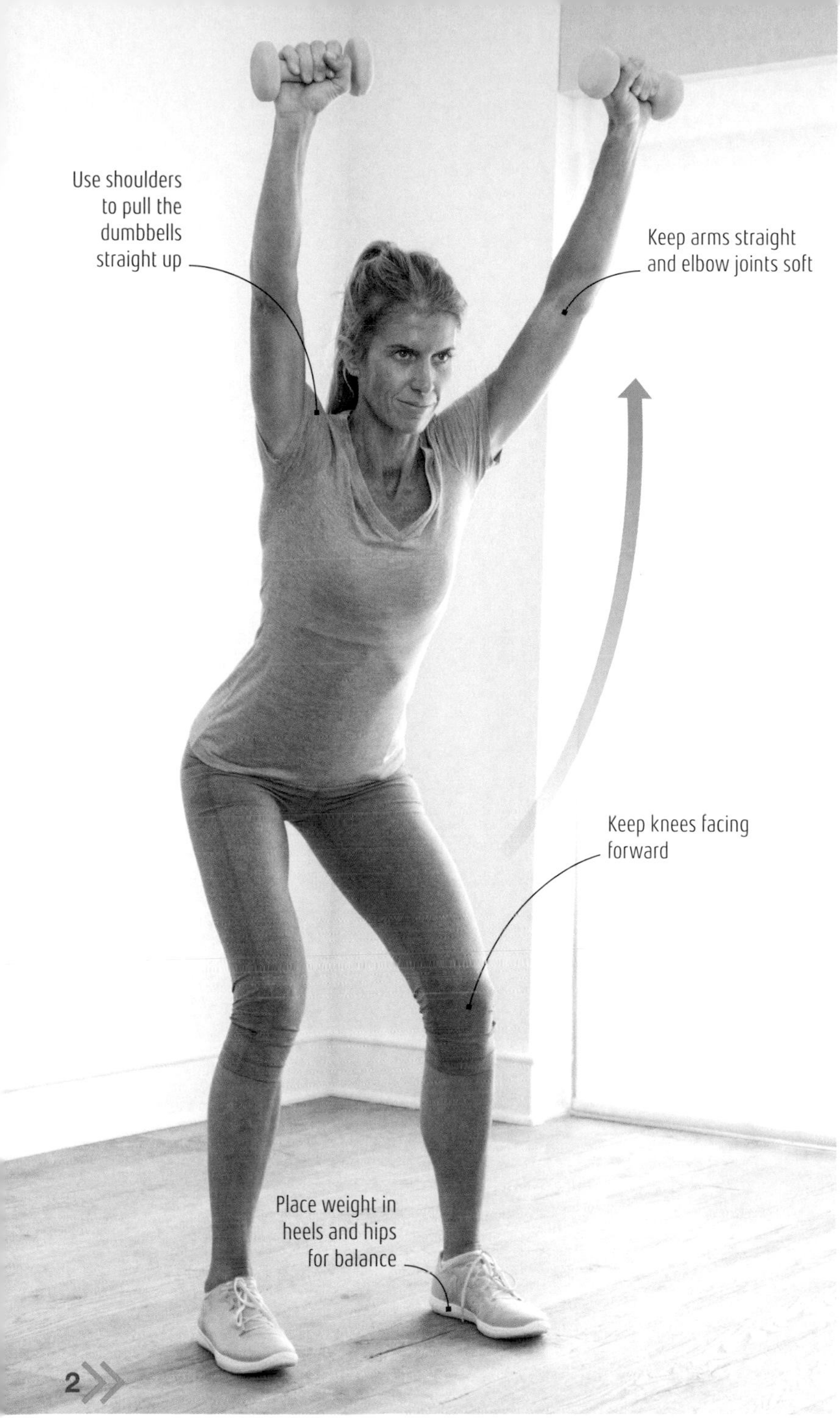

Use shoulders to pull the dumbbells straight up

Keep arms straight and elbow joints soft

Keep knees facing forward

Place weight in heels and hips for balance

2

Engage the muscles in your shoulders and upper back to raise the dumbbells straight up until your arms are aligned with your spine. Keep your arms straight and only move from the shoulder joints.

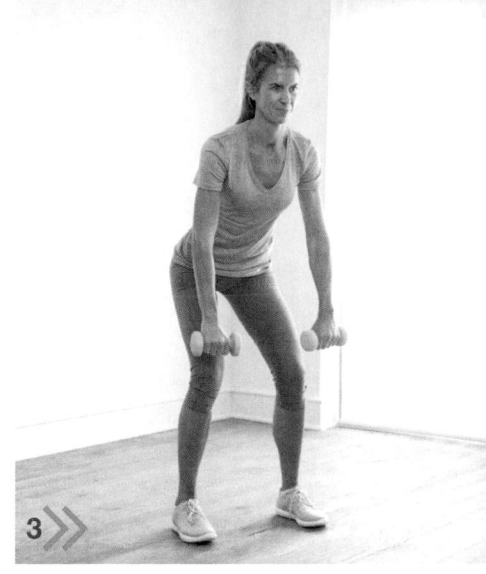

3

In a controlled manner, lower the dumbbells to the starting position, keeping your arms straight. Continue to repeat the exercise for the time given in your workout with quick, controlled movements.

//// MAKE IT **easier**

If it is difficult to raise the dumbbells overhead or if you feel pain in your shoulder joints, do the exercise without weights.

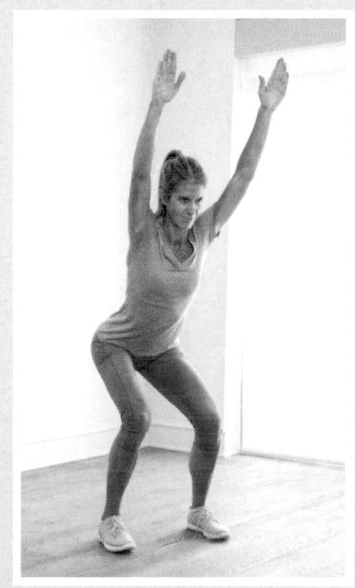

Upright external rotation

IMPROVES
//// **Posture**
//// **Strength**
//// **Mobility**

WHAT YOU NEED
Dumbbells

Weakness and lack of mobility in the rotator cuffs can cause pain throughout the day and make it difficult to sleep. Use this controlled movement to strengthen and improve mobility in all of the muscles that support your arms and shoulders.

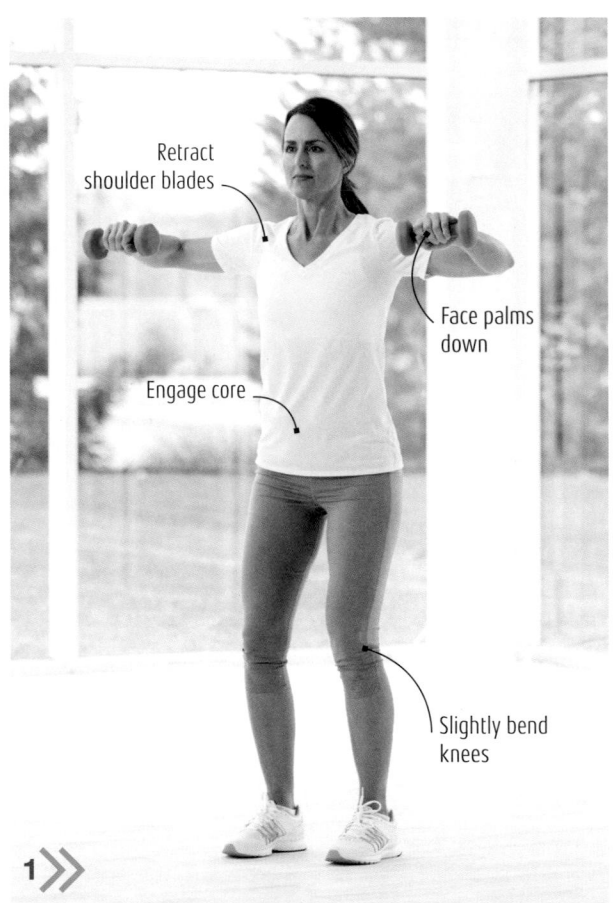

Retract shoulder blades

Face palms down

Engage core

Slightly bend knees

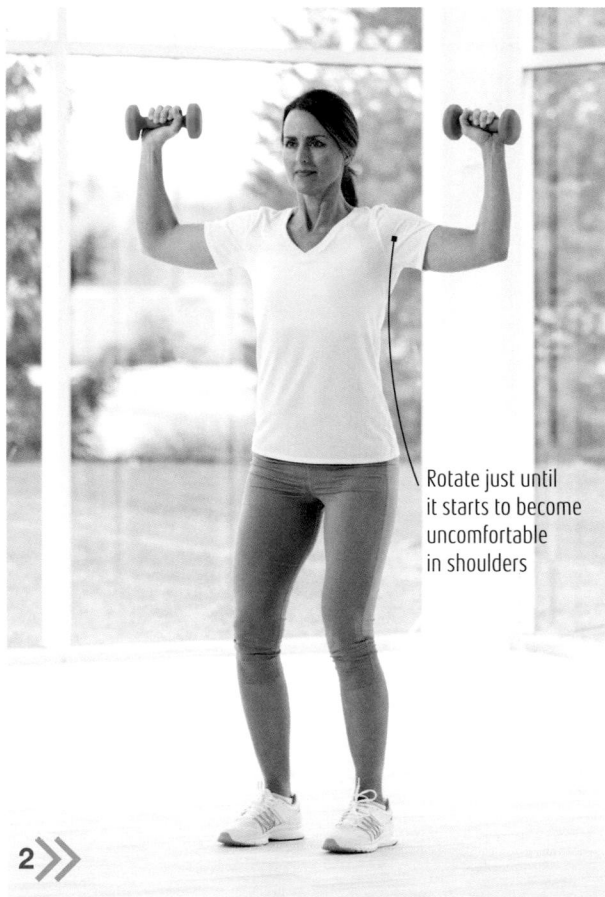

Rotate just until it starts to become uncomfortable in shoulders

1 》

Stand with your feet shoulder-width apart, slightly bend your knees, and hold a dumbbell in each hand. Raise your upper arms out to the side at shoulder height, bend your elbows to 90 degrees, and position your forearms parallel to the ground.

2 》

Engage your upper back and shoulder muscles to pull the dumbbells back. Rotate your arms up until you reach the top of your range of motion, keeping your upper arms parallel to the ground. Continue to retract your shoulder blades.

FIT tip

If you have tight shoulders, massage the soft tissue with your fingers or a tennis ball to loosen the muscles and prevent injury.

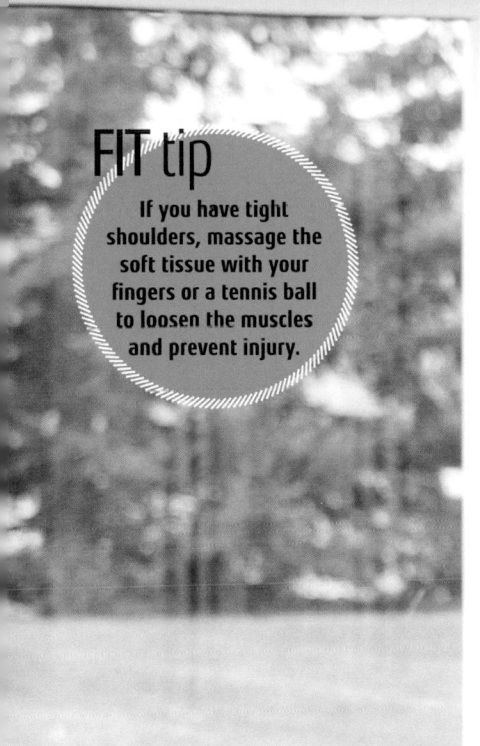

Control the movement with shoulders and back
Keep lower body stable and isolate movement to shoulders

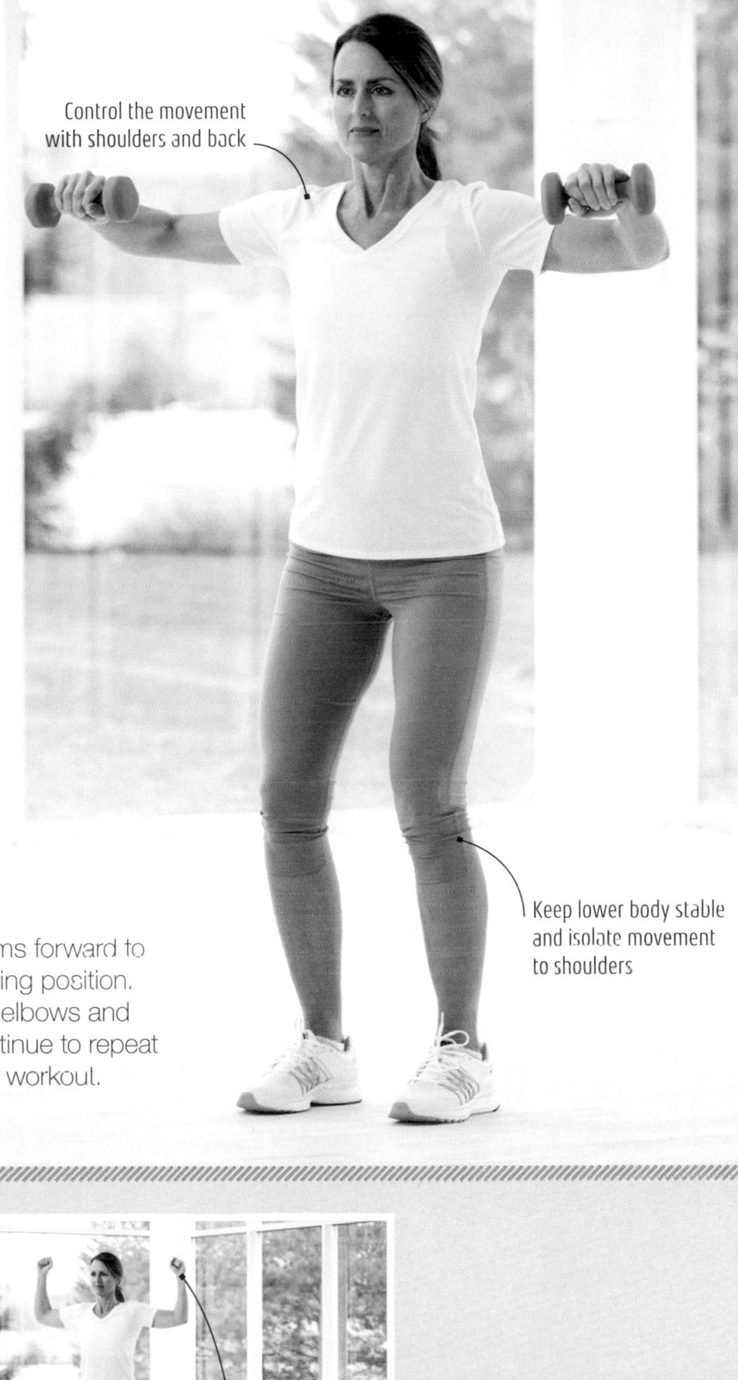

3

In a controlled manner, rotate your arms forward to lower the dumbbells back to the starting position. Maintain the 90-degree bend in your elbows and keep your upper back engaged. Continue to repeat the exercise for the time given in your workout.

MAKE IT **easier**

If it is difficult or painful to raise the dumbbells, do the exercise without weights.

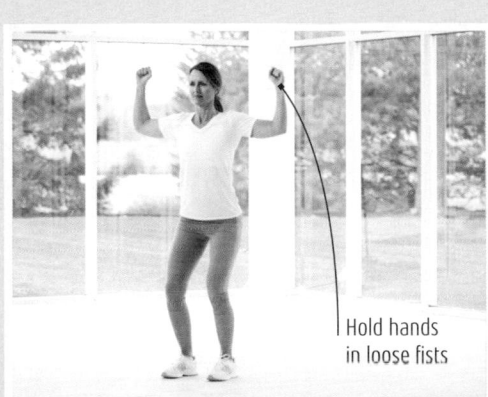

Hold hands in loose fists

IMPROVES
//// Posture
//// Strength
//// Stability

WHAT YOU NEED
Dumbbells

Bent row and hammer curl

Activities such as playing with children require you to bend over and pick up weight. Prepare for these movements with this quick and controlled compound exercise that improves total-body stability and strengthens your back and biceps.

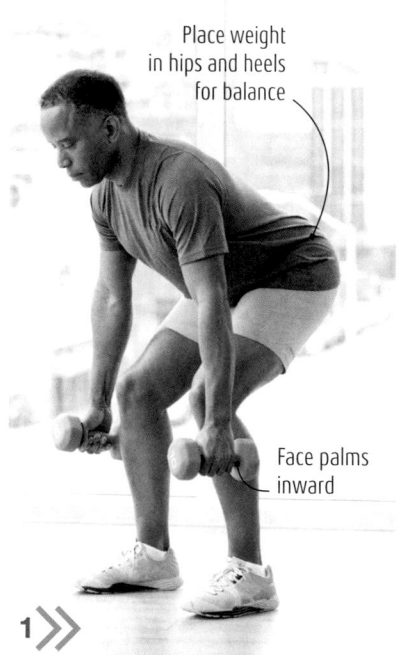

Place weight in hips and heels for balance

Face palms inward

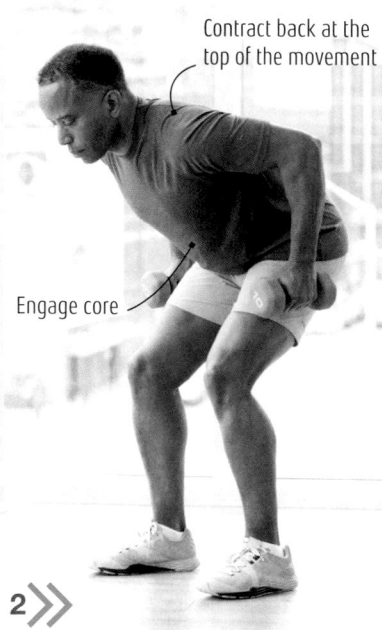

Contract back at the top of the movement

Engage core

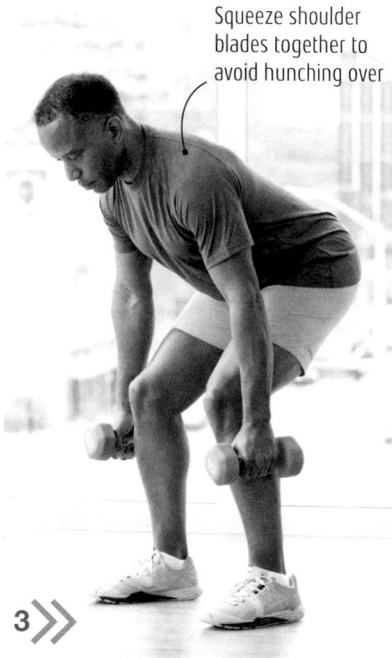

Squeeze shoulder blades together to avoid hunching over

1 >>
Stand with your feet shoulder-width apart and hold a dumbbell in each hand. Bend over to 45 degrees from the hips and slightly bend your knees. Let your arms hang straight down.

2 >>
Retract your shoulder blades and pull the dumbbells up and back from your elbows until your arms are parallel to the ground. Keep your elbows tight to your body.

3 >>
In a controlled manner, lower the dumbbells back to the starting position, keeping your back muscles engaged. Allow a slight bend in your elbow joints and keep your core firm.

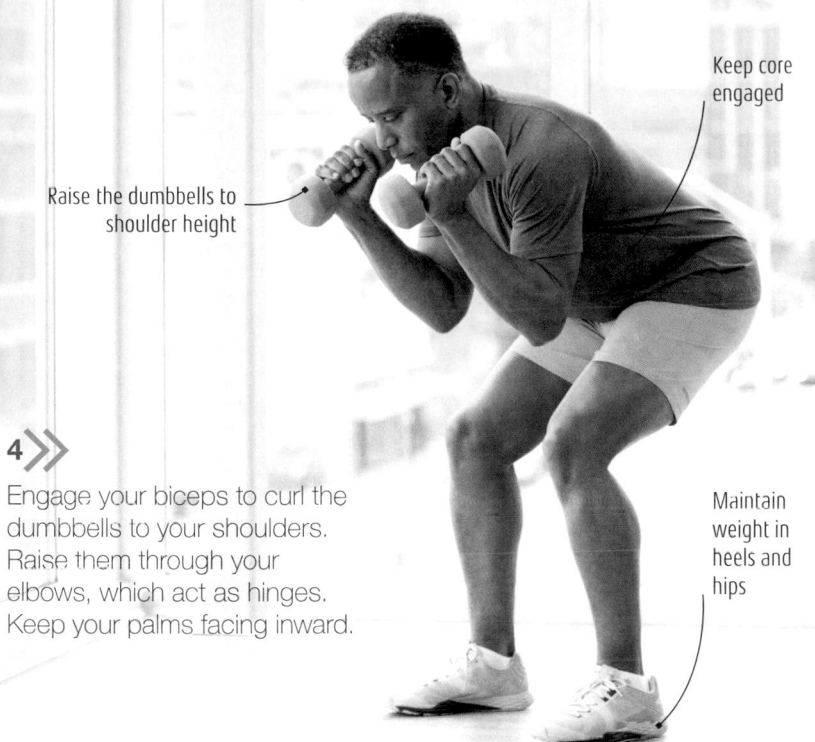

Keep core engaged

Raise the dumbbells to shoulder height

Maintain weight in heels and hips

4 »

Engage your biceps to curl the dumbbells to your shoulders. Raise them through your elbows, which act as hinges. Keep your palms facing inward.

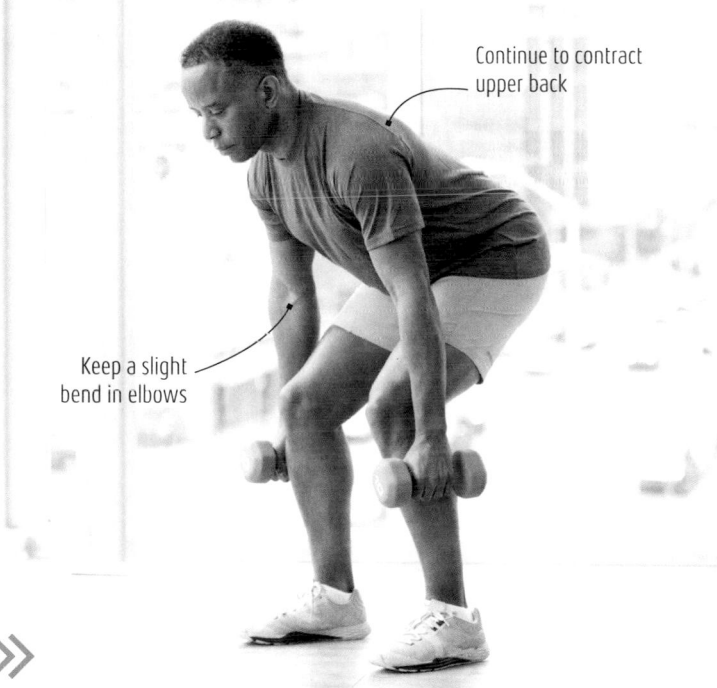

Continue to contract upper back

Keep a slight bend in elbows

5 »

In a controlled manner, extend your elbows and lower the dumbbells to the starting position. Repeat the sequence for the time given in your workout.

/// **MAKE IT easier**

To lessen the strain on your lower back, sit on the edge of a chair while performing the exercise.

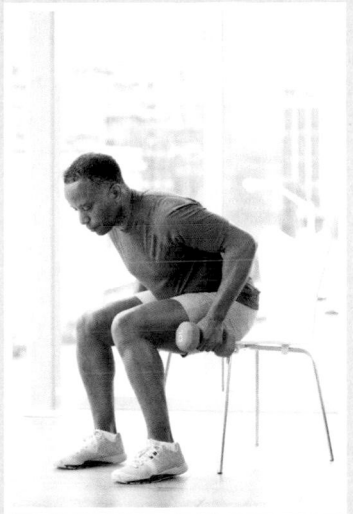

/// **MAKE IT harder**

To improve your balance, do the exercise while balanced on one leg. Bend your knees and suspend your raised foot behind you. Spend equal time balancing on each leg.

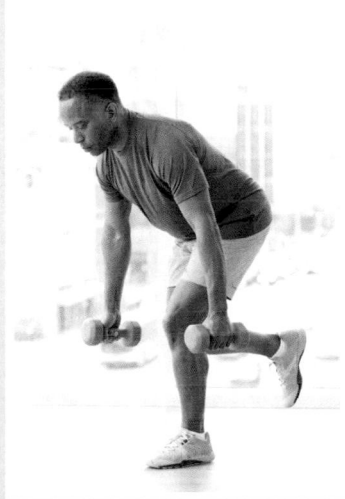

IMPROVES

/// **Posture**

/// **Strength**

/// Mobility

WHAT YOU NEED
Wall

Wall angel

Proper posture requires back strength and chest flexibility. Many daily activities such as sitting at a desk or driving a car can weaken and tighten these muscles, but you can use this stretching exercise to reverse the effects. By elongating your chest and building your back muscles, this exercise will open a tight chest and back and help fix rounded shoulders.

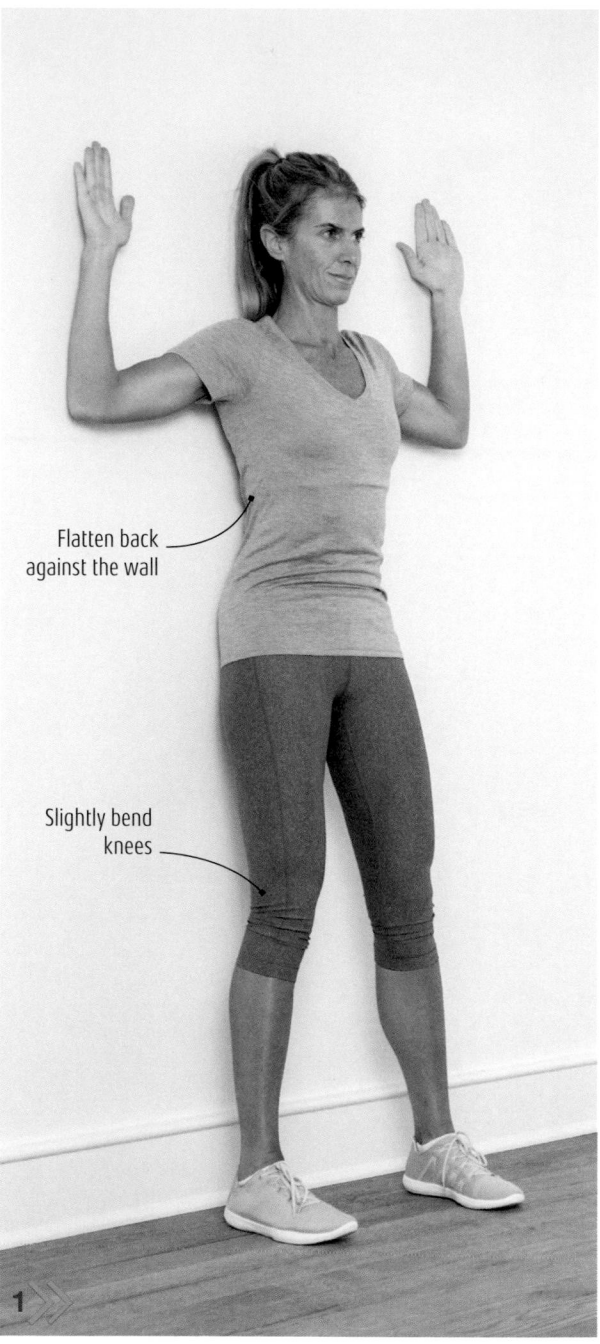

Flatten back against the wall

Slightly bend knees

1 >

Stand with your back to a wall and your feet shoulder-width apart, about 4 inches (10cm) from the wall. Rest your back and head against the wall. Raise your arms to the side, bend your elbows, and rest the backs of your arms and hands against the wall.

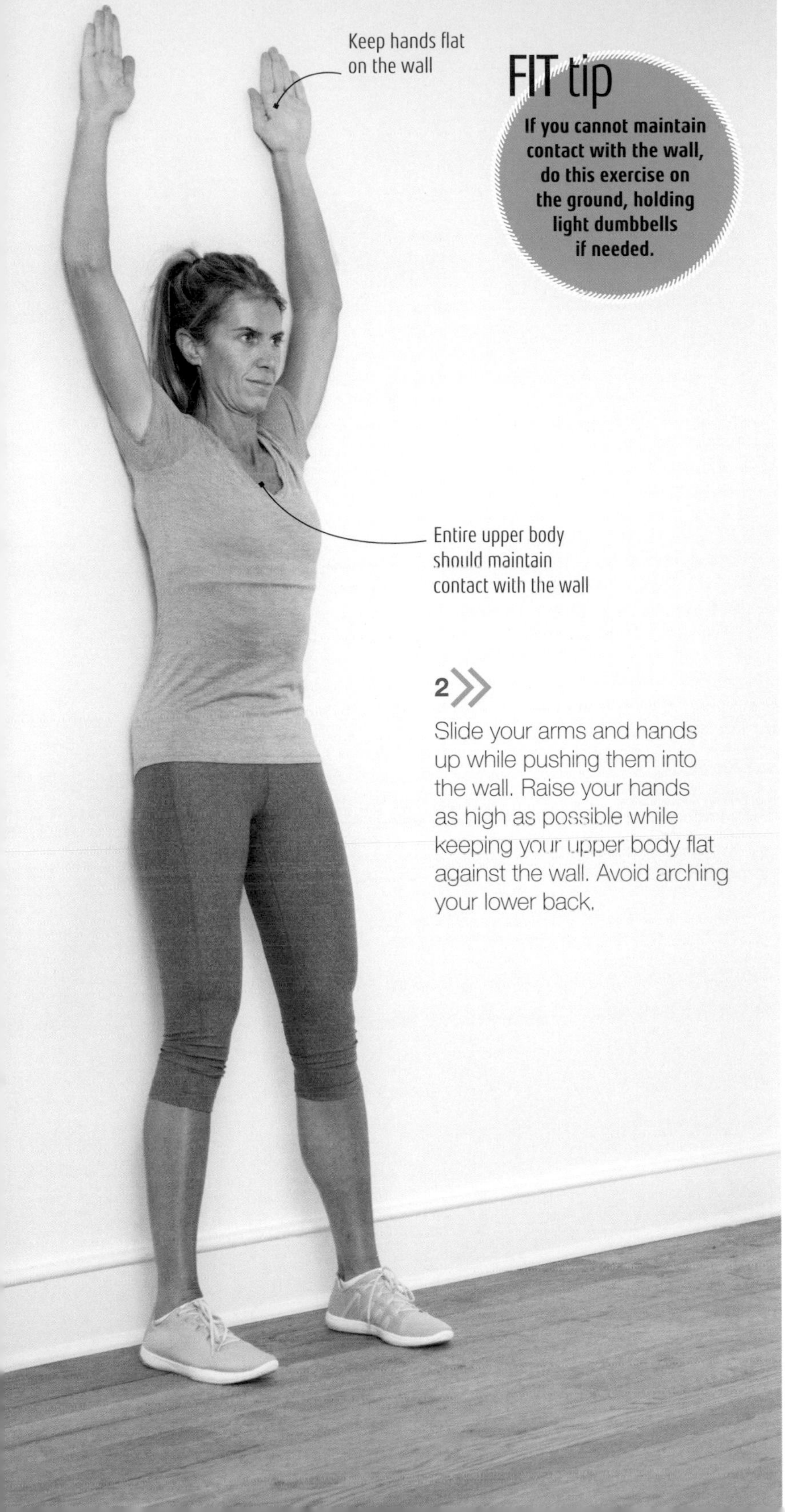

Keep hands flat on the wall

FIT tip

If you cannot maintain contact with the wall, do this exercise on the ground, holding light dumbbells if needed.

Entire upper body should maintain contact with the wall

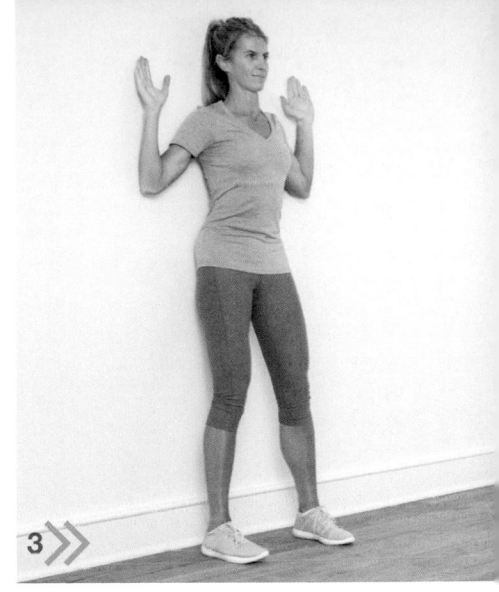

3 »

Using your back muscles, pull your arms back to the starting position. Continue to push your arms and hands into the wall, and repeat the exercise for the time given.

2 »

Slide your arms and hands up while pushing them into the wall. Raise your hands as high as possible while keeping your upper body flat against the wall. Avoid arching your lower back.

/// MAKE IT **harder**

To increase resistance to your back, add a resistance band. Hold one side of the band in each hand, place it behind your head, and pull the band apart. Maintain constant tension by pulling as you do the exercise.

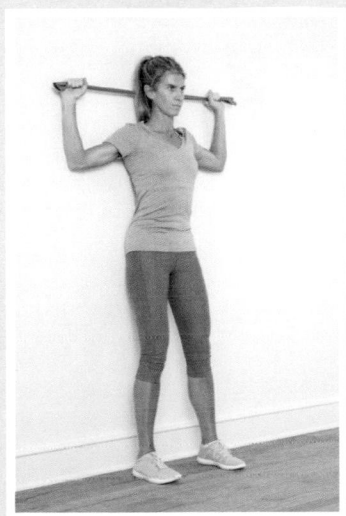

One-arm snatch

IMPROVES
//// Posture
//// Strength
//// Stability
//// Mobility

WHAT YOU NEED
Dumbbell

Your back is one of the most powerful muscle groups in your body, so it is important to train it with exercises like this snatch so that your posture is better and your full-body movements are more efficient and stable. Perform this quick power move to develop a strong upper and lower back.

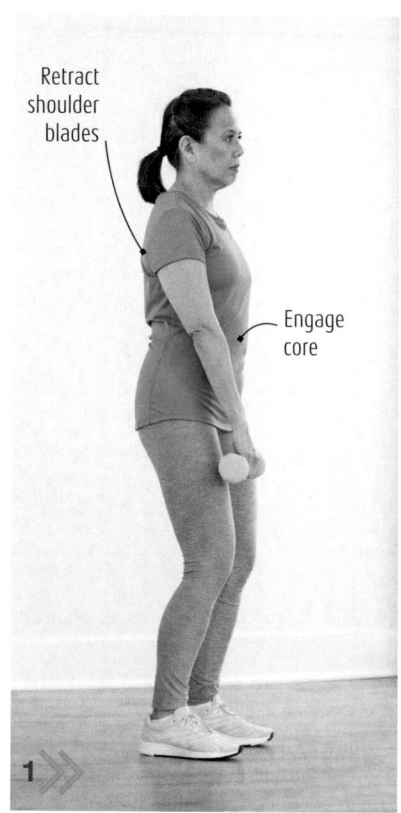

Retract shoulder blades

Engage core

1

Stand with your feet shoulder-width apart. Hold a dumbbell in your right hand, palm facing you, and let your right arm hang in front of you. Let your left arm hang at your side, and slightly bend your knees.

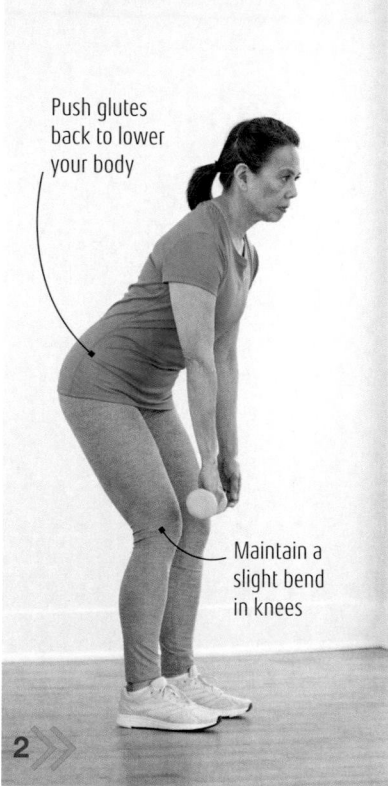

Push glutes back to lower your body

Maintain a slight bend in knees

2

Push your hips back and bend over at the waist until the dumbbell is at knee height. Keep your back straight and shoulders retracted. Let your left arm hang neutrally, keep your core engaged.

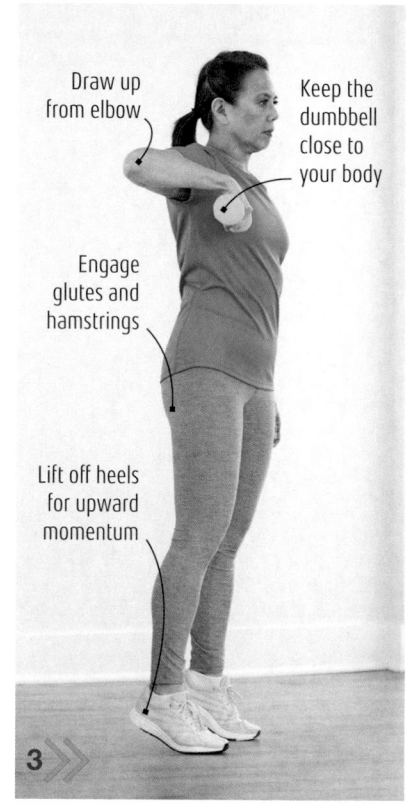

Draw up from elbow

Keep the dumbbell close to your body

Engage glutes and hamstrings

Lift off heels for upward momentum

3

In one quick motion, push your hips forward to return to an upright position, pull your right arm up from the elbow until your elbow is at shoulder height, and rise briefly onto the balls of your feet.

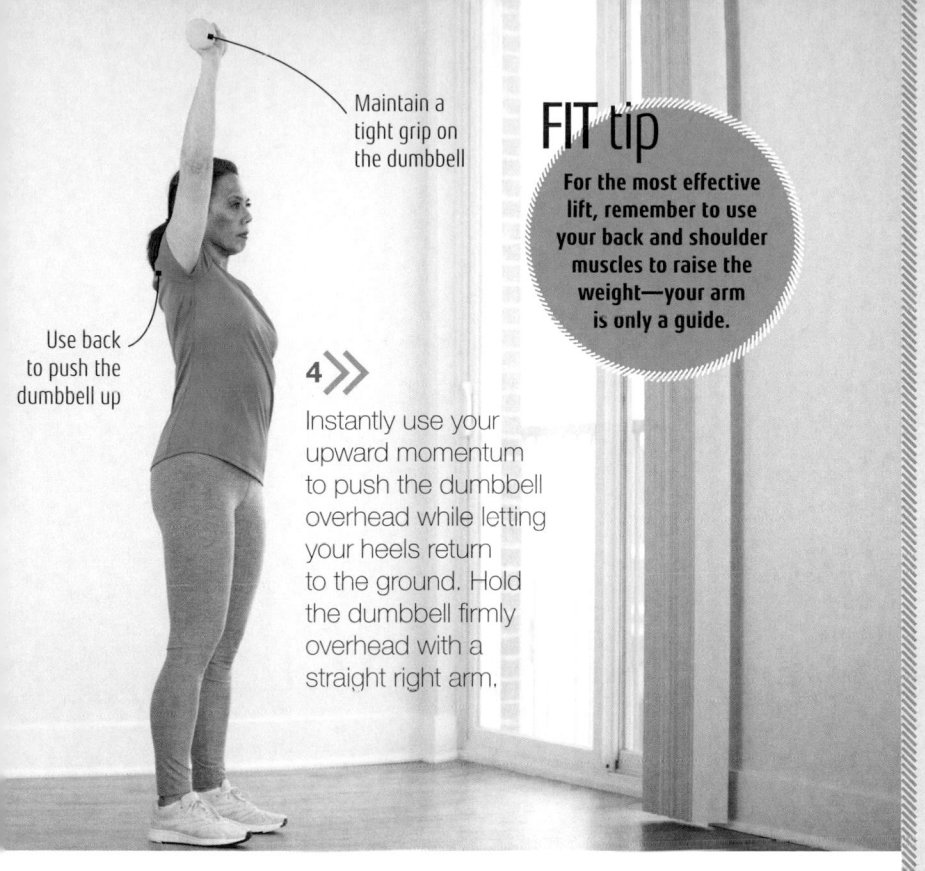

Maintain a tight grip on the dumbbell

Use back to push the dumbbell up

FIT tip

For the most effective lift, remember to use your back and shoulder muscles to raise the weight—your arm is only a guide.

4 »

Instantly use your upward momentum to push the dumbbell overhead while letting your heels return to the ground. Hold the dumbbell firmly overhead with a straight right arm.

//// MAKE IT **easier**

For a simpler movement, do steps 1–3, then lower the dumbbell in a controlled manner to the starting position without pushing the dumbbell overhead.

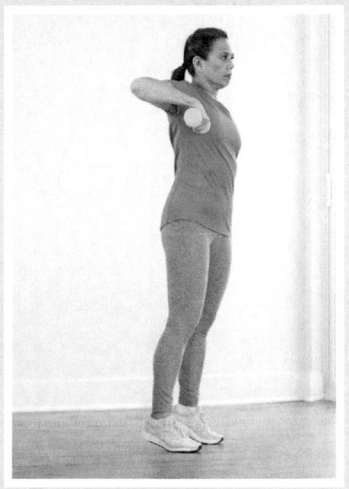

//// MAKE IT **harder**

To strengthen your legs, in step 5, sit back until your thighs are parallel to the ground. Stand back up before lowering the dumbbell.

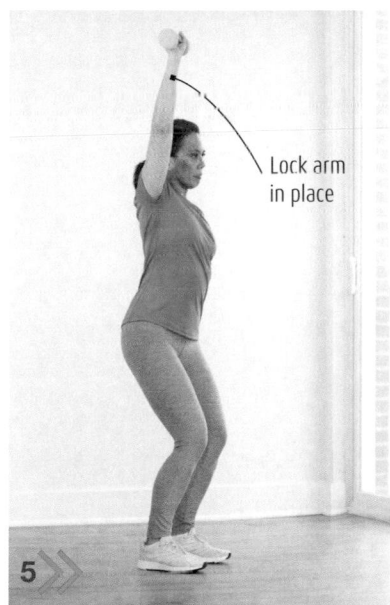

Lock arm in place

5 »

Immediately bend your knees and hips to absorb the weight of the dumbbell. Maintain a flat back and avoid hunching forward.

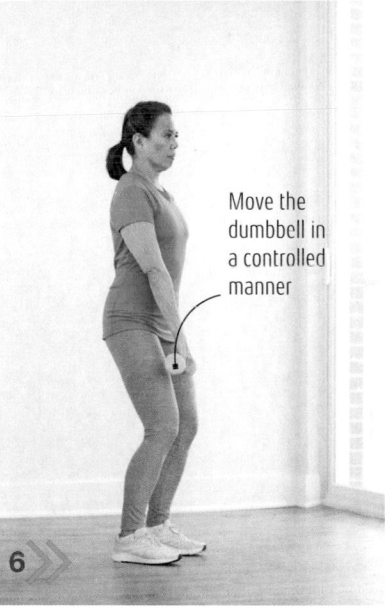

Move the dumbbell in a controlled manner

6 »

Return to the starting position. Repeat for the time given in your workout. Spend half the time on your right arm, then switch to your left arm.

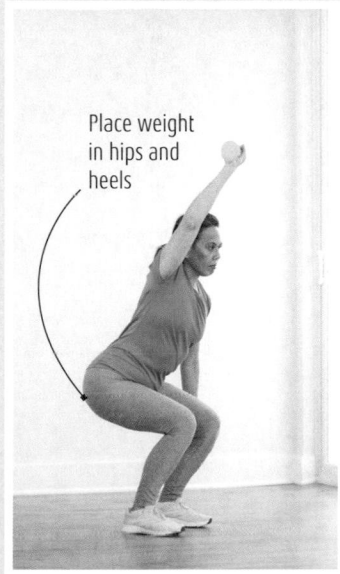

Place weight in hips and heels

Bird dog

IMPROVES
/// **Posture**
/// **Strength**
/// **Stability**
/// **Mobility**

WHAT YOU NEED
Mat

Training your abdominals but neglecting your lower back will eventually lead to poor stability and alignment. Use this yoga exercise to strengthen your core and stabilize the lower back for upper- and lower-body movements.

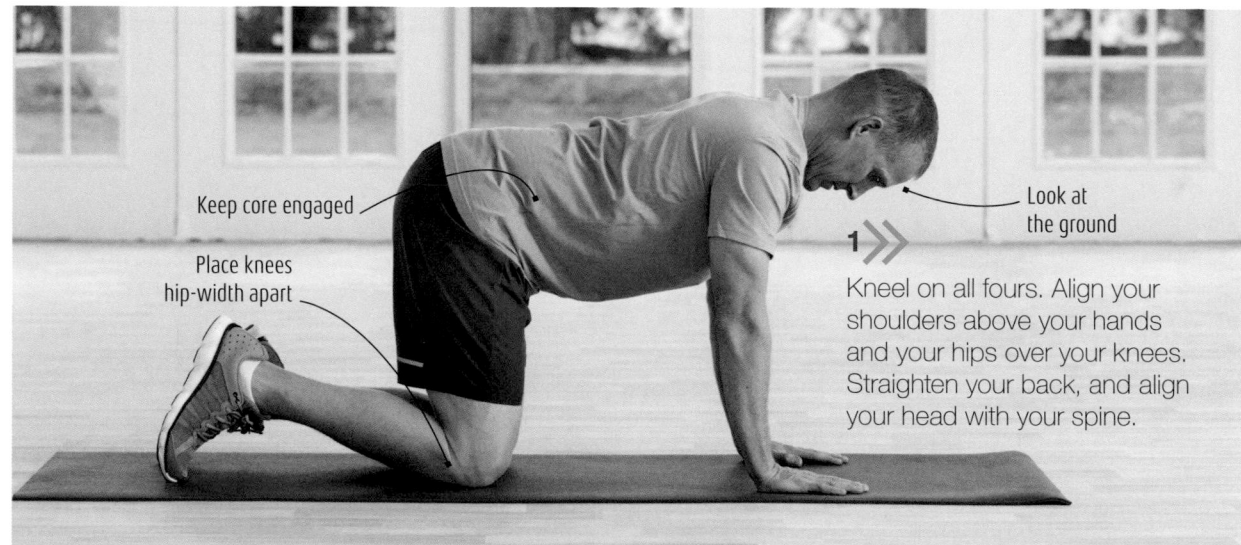

Keep core engaged

Place knees hip-width apart

Look at the ground

1

Kneel on all fours. Align your shoulders above your hands and your hips over your knees. Straighten your back, and align your head with your spine.

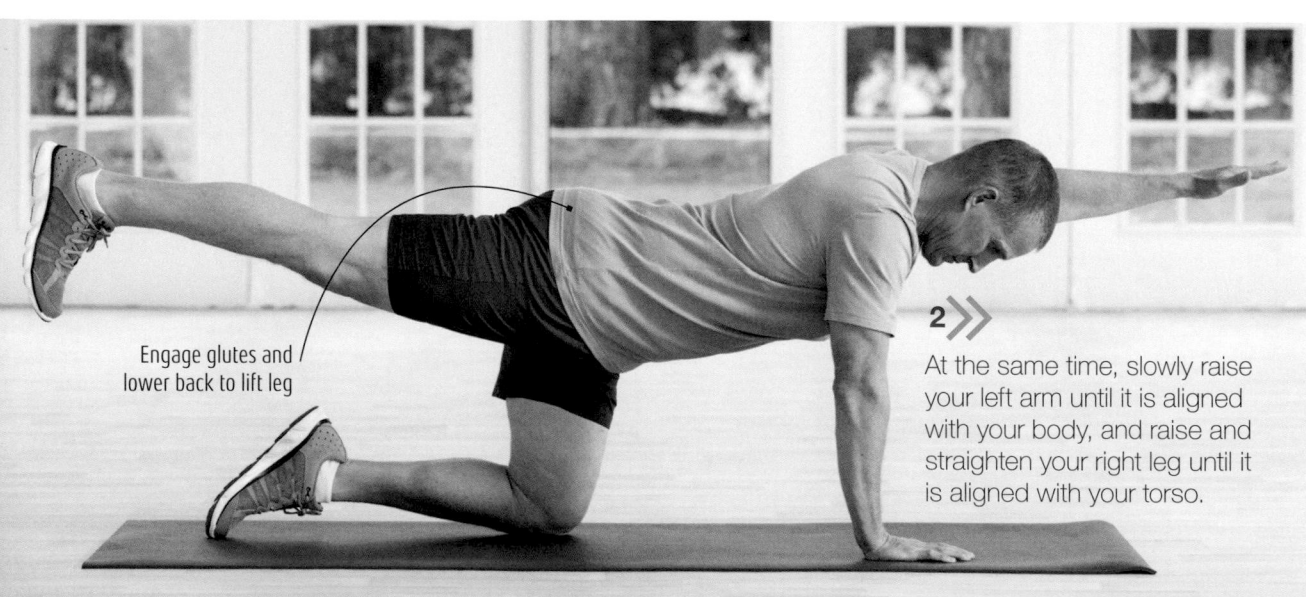

Engage glutes and lower back to lift leg

2

At the same time, slowly raise your left arm until it is aligned with your body, and raise and straighten your right leg until it is aligned with your torso.

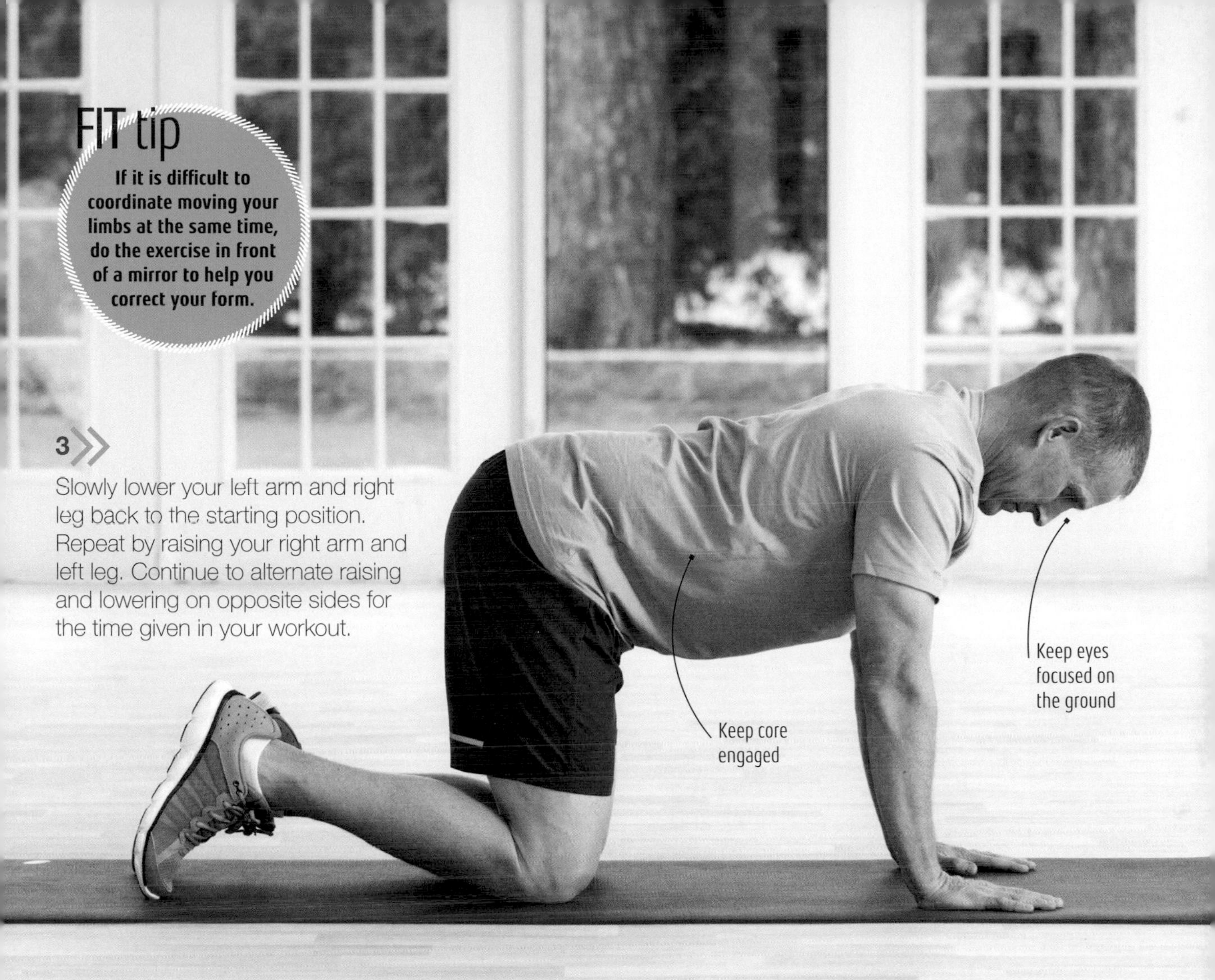

FIT tip

If it is difficult to coordinate moving your limbs at the same time, do the exercise in front of a mirror to help you correct your form.

3 »

Slowly lower your left arm and right leg back to the starting position. Repeat by raising your right arm and left leg. Continue to alternate raising and lowering on opposite sides for the time given in your workout.

Keep eyes focused on the ground

Keep core engaged

///// MAKE IT **easier**

To lessen the pressure on your lower back, in step 2, leave your hands on the ground and extend only your leg.

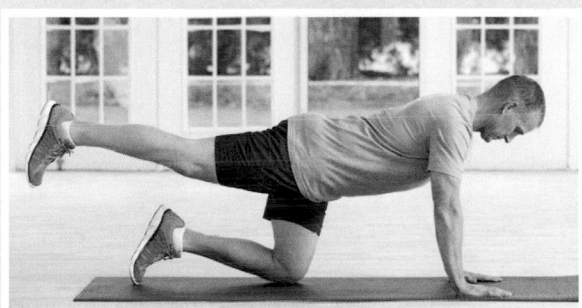

///// MAKE IT **harder**

To strengthen your abdominals, in step 3, do a crunch by pulling your elbow and knee to each other before returning to all fours.

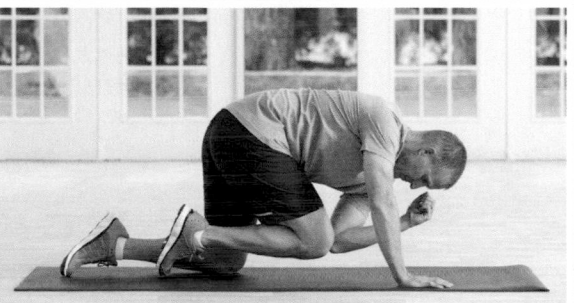

IMPROVES
▰//// Posture
▰//// Strength
▰//// Stability
▰//// Endurance

WHAT YOU NEED
Mat

High plank row

The plank is one of the best exercises for building your core strength, but it is also great for strengthening your back, glutes, and hamstrings. By combining the plank with a controlled rowing movement, this exercise develops your balance and helps improve posture.

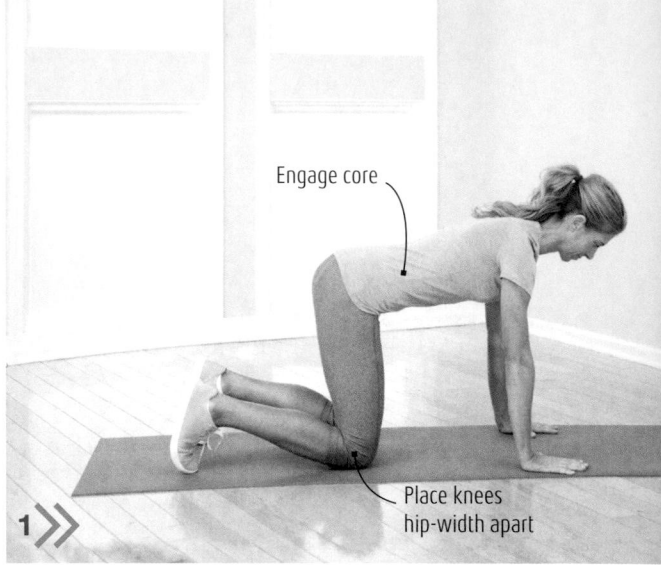

Engage core

Place knees hip-width apart

1 》

Kneel on all fours. Align your shoulders above your hands with your fingers facing forward. Straighten your back and align your head with your spine. Look at the ground and retract your shoulder blades.

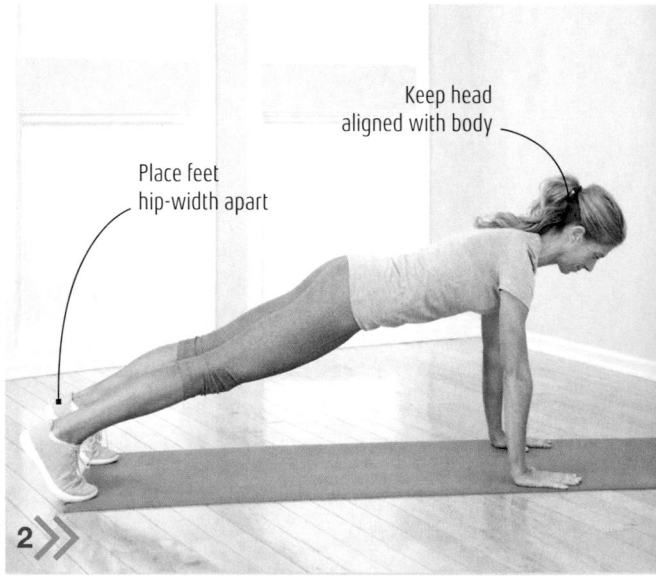

Keep head aligned with body

Place feet hip-width apart

2 》

Rise off your knees and onto the balls of your feet. Walk your feet back into a plank position to form a straight line from head to heels. Evenly distribute your weight between the balls of your feet and your hands. Do not let your hips sink down or rise up.

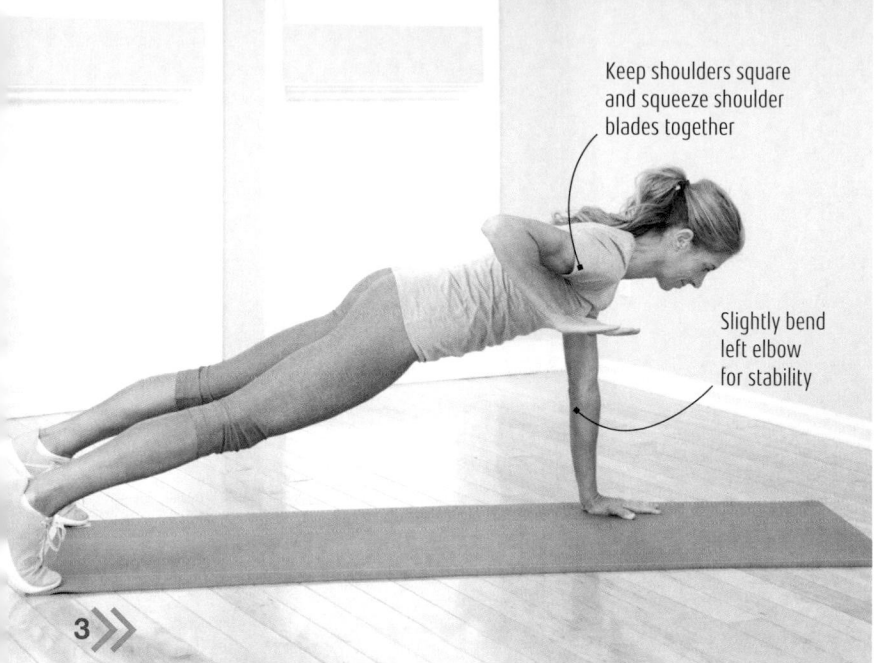

Keep shoulders square and squeeze shoulder blades together

Slightly bend left elbow for stability

3 »

In a controlled manner, pull your right arm back from your elbow, keeping your elbow close to your body and palm facing down. Contract your upper back at the top of the movement. Maintain a stable base with your left arm.

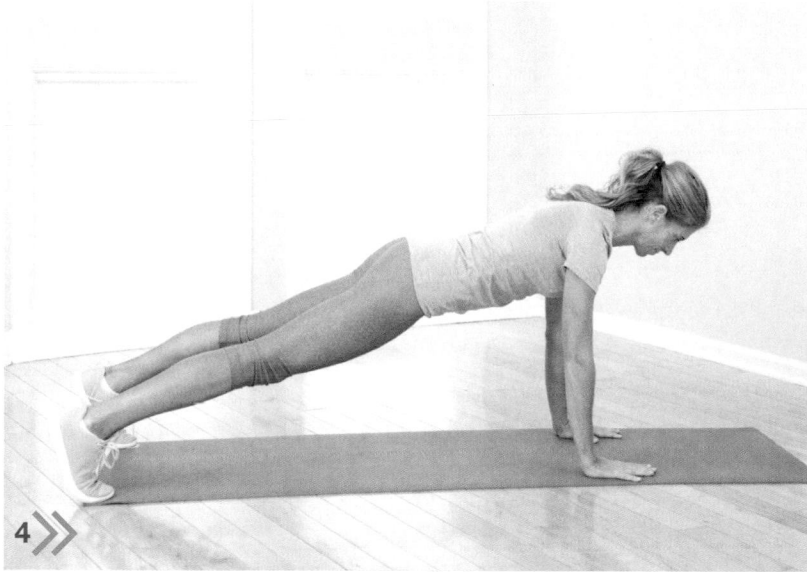

4 »

In a controlled manner, return your right arm to the starting position and redistribute your weight to both hands. Repeat the exercise with your left arm. Continue to alternate rowing with each arm for the time given in your workout.

▰/// MAKE IT **easier**

To reduce the strain on your core, remain on your knees instead of getting into a plank position. Lower your hips down until your upper body is at about a 45-degree angle to the ground.

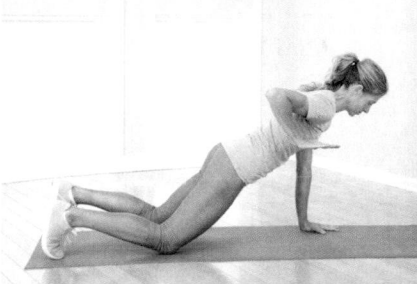

▰/// MAKE IT **harder**

To increase resistance to your back, hold a dumhhell in each hand and use the handles to support your upper body. Pull the dumbbells back from your elbow.

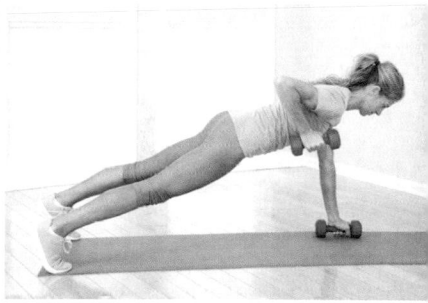

Stiff-leg deadlift and shrug

Strong muscles in the back of your body are the foundation for safe and efficient movement during daily activities. This swift, compound pulling exercise works your glutes, back muscles, and hamstrings to improve your overall stability.

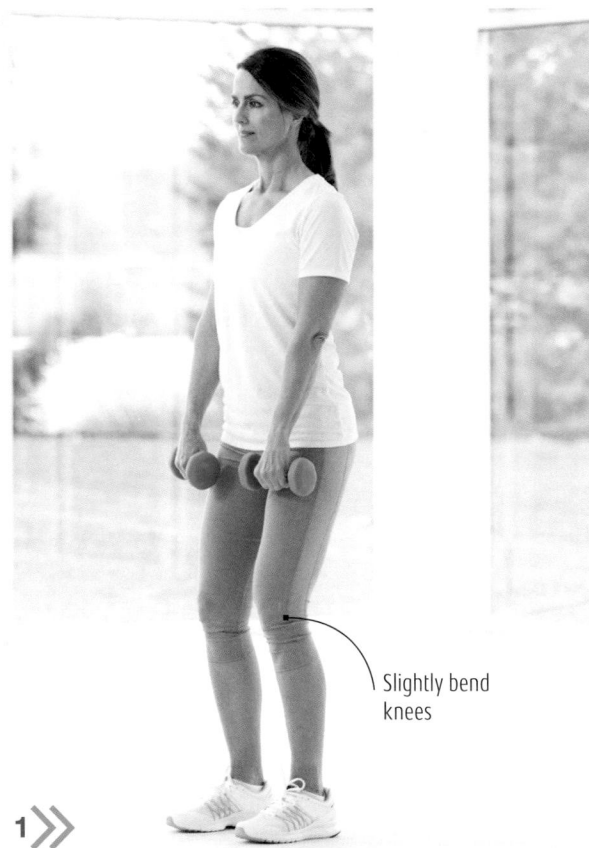

Slightly bend knees

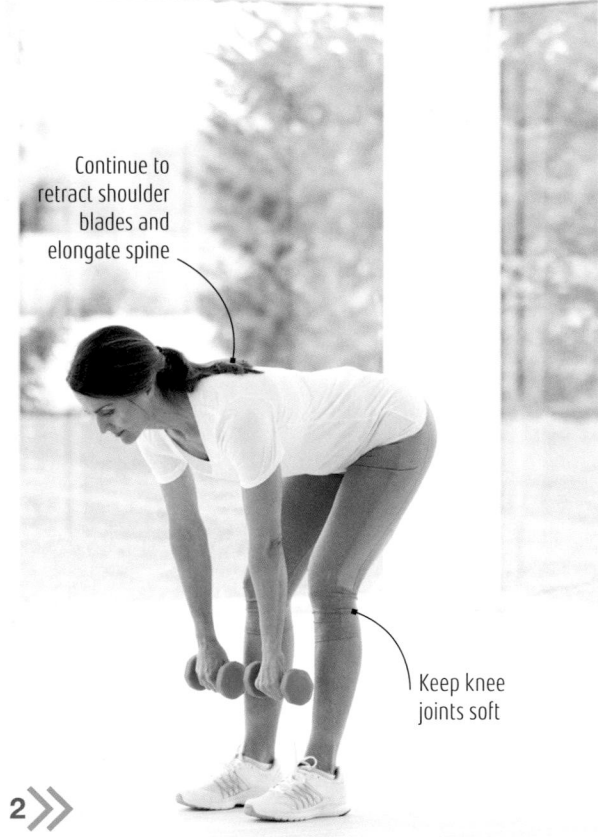

Continue to retract shoulder blades and elongate spine

Keep knee joints soft

1 >>

Stand with your feet shoulder-width apart. Hold a dumbbell in each hand, palms facing you, and let your arms hang in front of you. Engage your core and retract your shoulder blades.

2 >>

In a quick and controlled manner, push your hips back and bend at the waist until your upper body is parallel to the ground. Let your arms move downward, suspending the dumbbells above your feet.

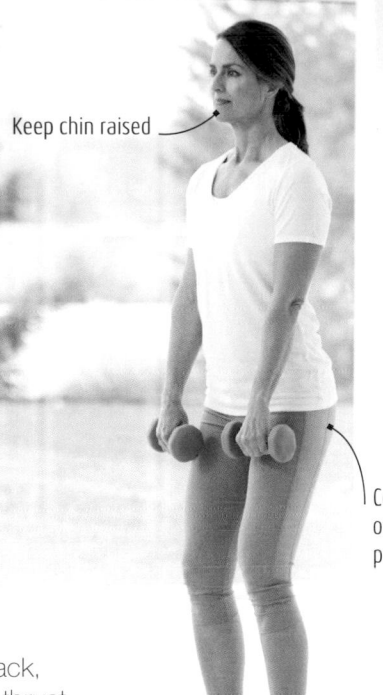

Keep chin raised

Contract glutes once in the upright position

3 »

Using your glutes, lower back, and hamstrings for power, thrust your hips forward to return to the starting position. Let your arms travel back up with your body.

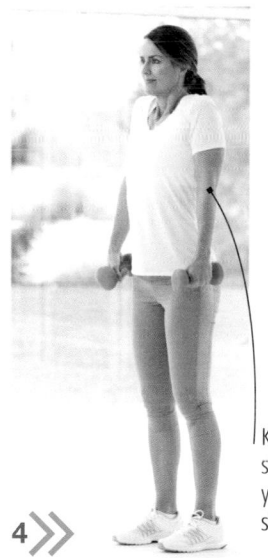

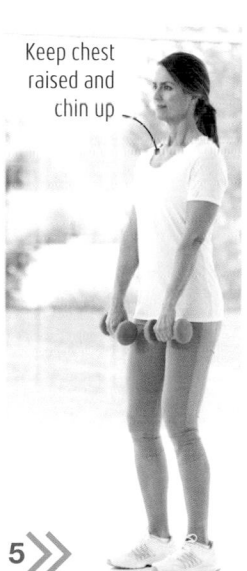

Keep chest raised and chin up

Keep arms straight as you shrug shoulders

4 »

In one motion, move the dumbbells to your sides by rotating your arms outward, and use your upper-back muscles to raise your shoulders as high as possible toward your ears.

5 »

Controlling the movement with your back, push the dumbbells down and rotate your arms to the starting position. Repeat the sequence for the time given.

/// MAKE IT **easier**

If you have limited hamstring flexibility, in step 2, push your hips back and bend at your waist until the dumbbells are at your knees.

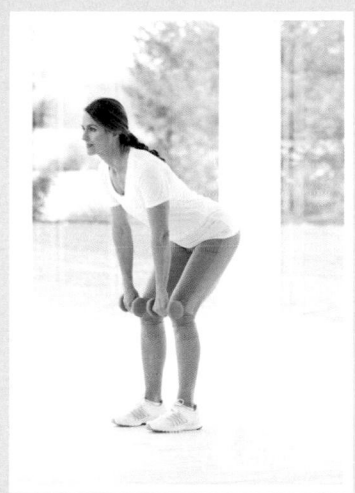

/// MAKE IT **harder**

To improve your balance, in step 2, lift your right foot off the ground and slowly kick your leg back as you bend over. Repeat the exercise by raising your left leg.

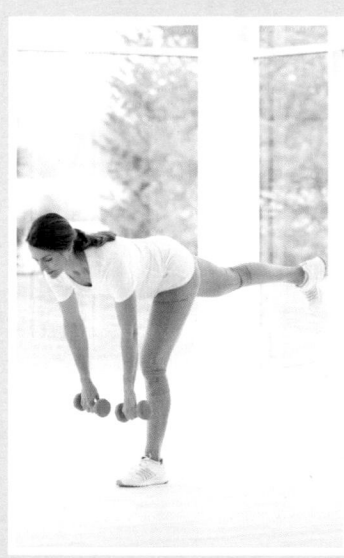

IMPROVES
/// Posture
/// Strength
/// Stability
/// Endurance

WHAT YOU NEED
Dumbbells

Seesaw row

From running to cycling, most endurance exercises are lower-body dominant, but it is important not to neglect your upper body. Perform this quick and dynamic upper-body pull to add variety to your workout and improve your upper-body endurance. Because one arm is suspended in front of you while the other is pulling up, this unique exercise also recruits your core for balance.

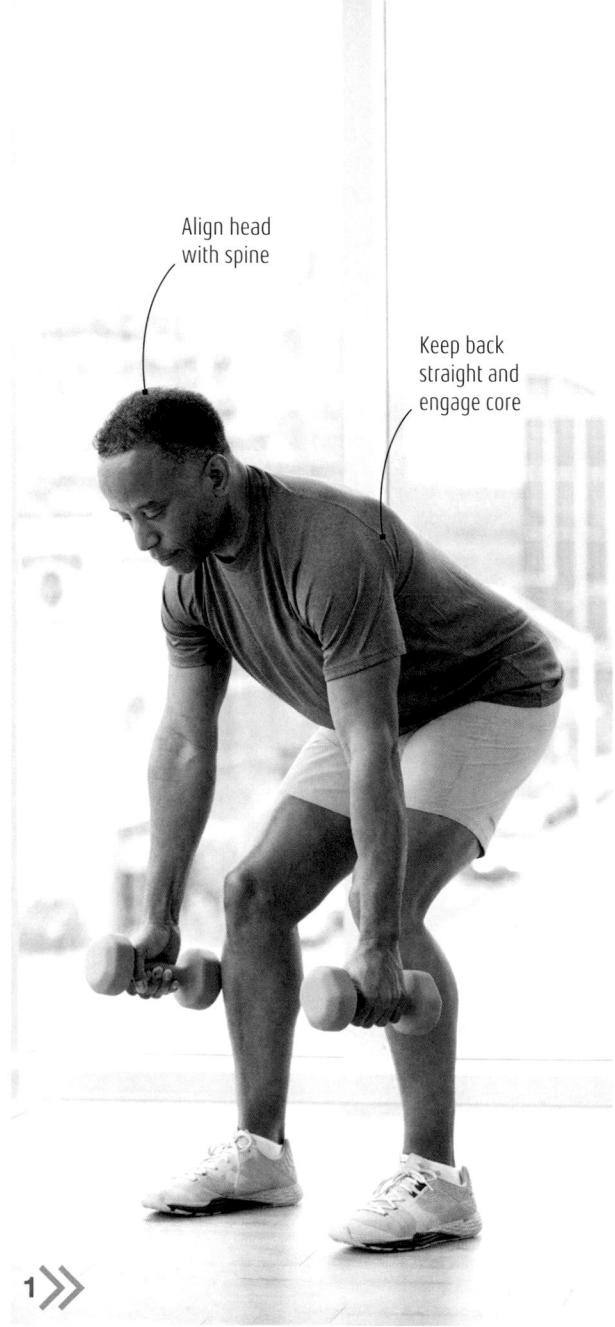

Align head with spine

Keep back straight and engage core

1 »

Stand with your feet shoulder-width apart and bend over to 45 degrees from the waist. Hold a dumbbell in each hand, palms facing each other, and let your arms hang straight down. Distribute your weight between your heels and hips.

Keep head raised

Keep shoulder blades retracted

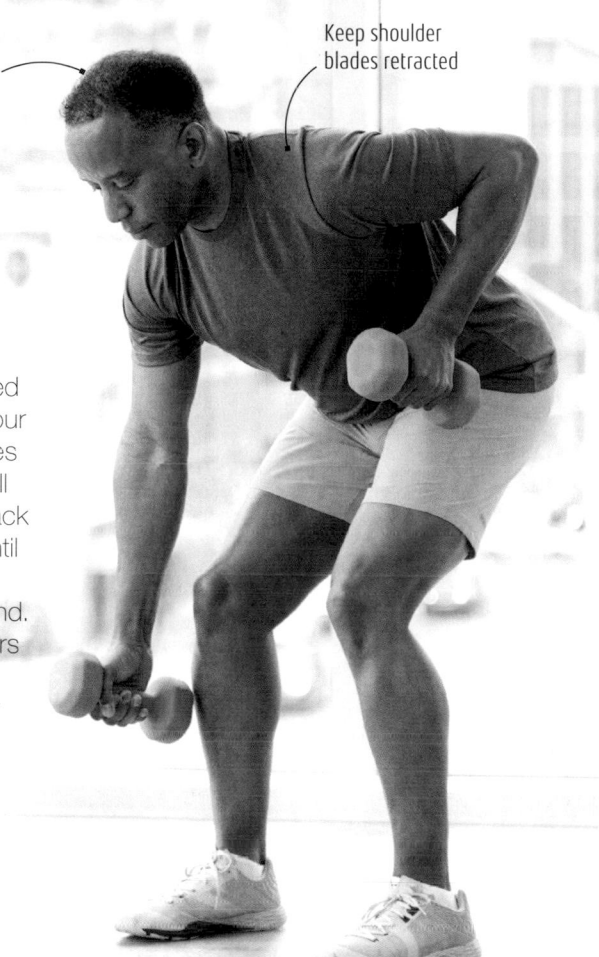

Continue to engage core

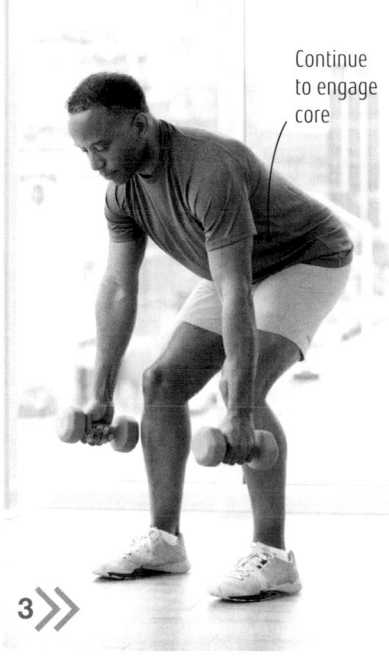

2 »

In a quick, controlled manner, engage your upper-back muscles to pull the dumbbell in your left hand back from your elbow until your upper arm is parallel to the ground. Keep your shoulders square to your feet and your left elbow tight to your body.

3 »

In a controlled manner, lower the dumbbell to the starting position, then immediately pull the dumbbell in your right hand back from your elbow. Continue to alternate rowing with each arm for the time given in your workout.

///// MAKE IT **easier**

If it is difficult to maintain balance, sit on the edge of a chair while performing the exercise.

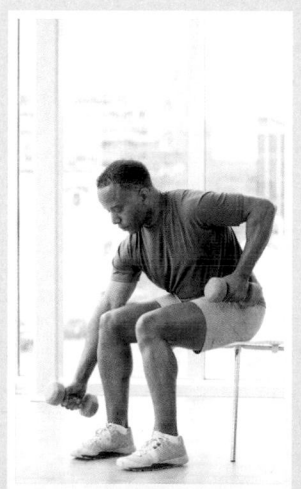

///// MAKE IT **harder**

To work your abdominals, in step 2, while you are pulling, use your core to twist your body toward the dumbbell.

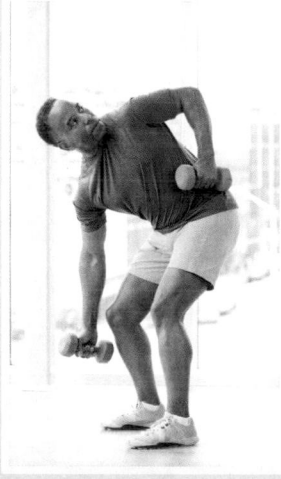

IMPROVES
■/// **Strength**
■/// **Stability**

WHAT YOU NEED
Dumbbell

Curl from one leg

Nearly every movement you make employs your balance system, recruiting the processes needed to send sensory information from your brain to your muscles. Use this quick and controlled curl to promote healthy body awareness as well as strengthen your biceps.

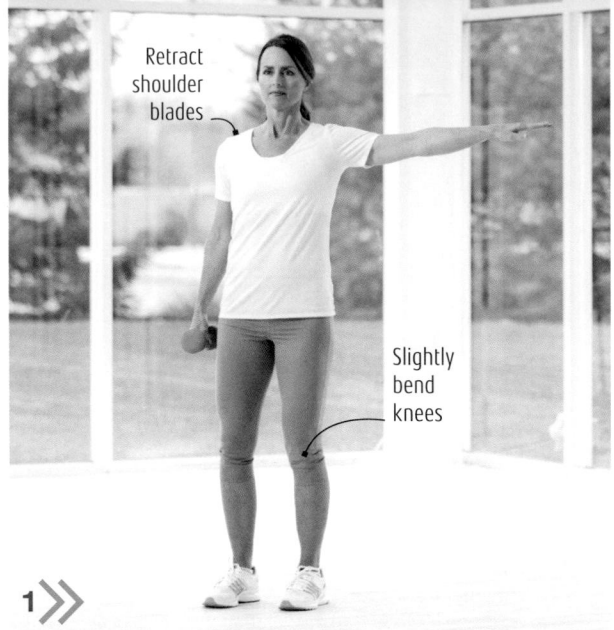

Retract shoulder blades

Slightly bend knees

1 »

Stand with your feet shoulder-width apart. Hold a dumbbell in your right hand and let your right arm hang at your side. Extend your left arm out to your side, palm facing the ground. Engage your core.

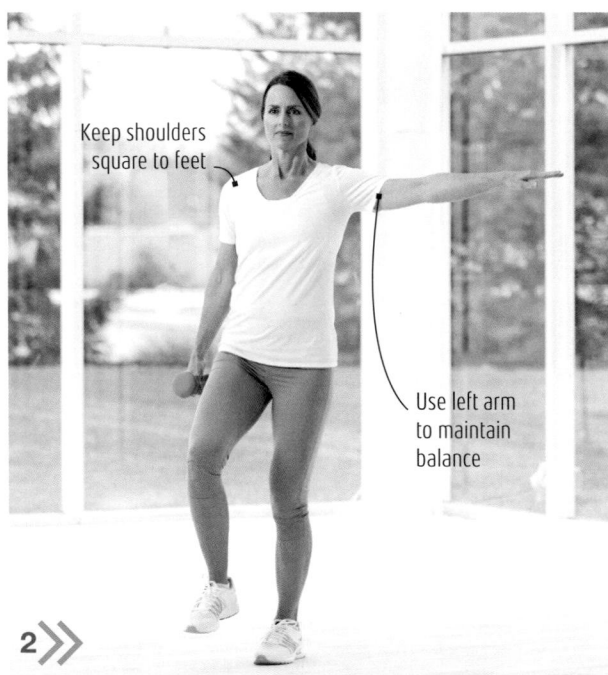

Keep shoulders square to feet

Use left arm to maintain balance

2 »

Raise your right knee until your right foot is about 5 inches (13cm) from the ground, and transfer your weight to your left heel and your hips.

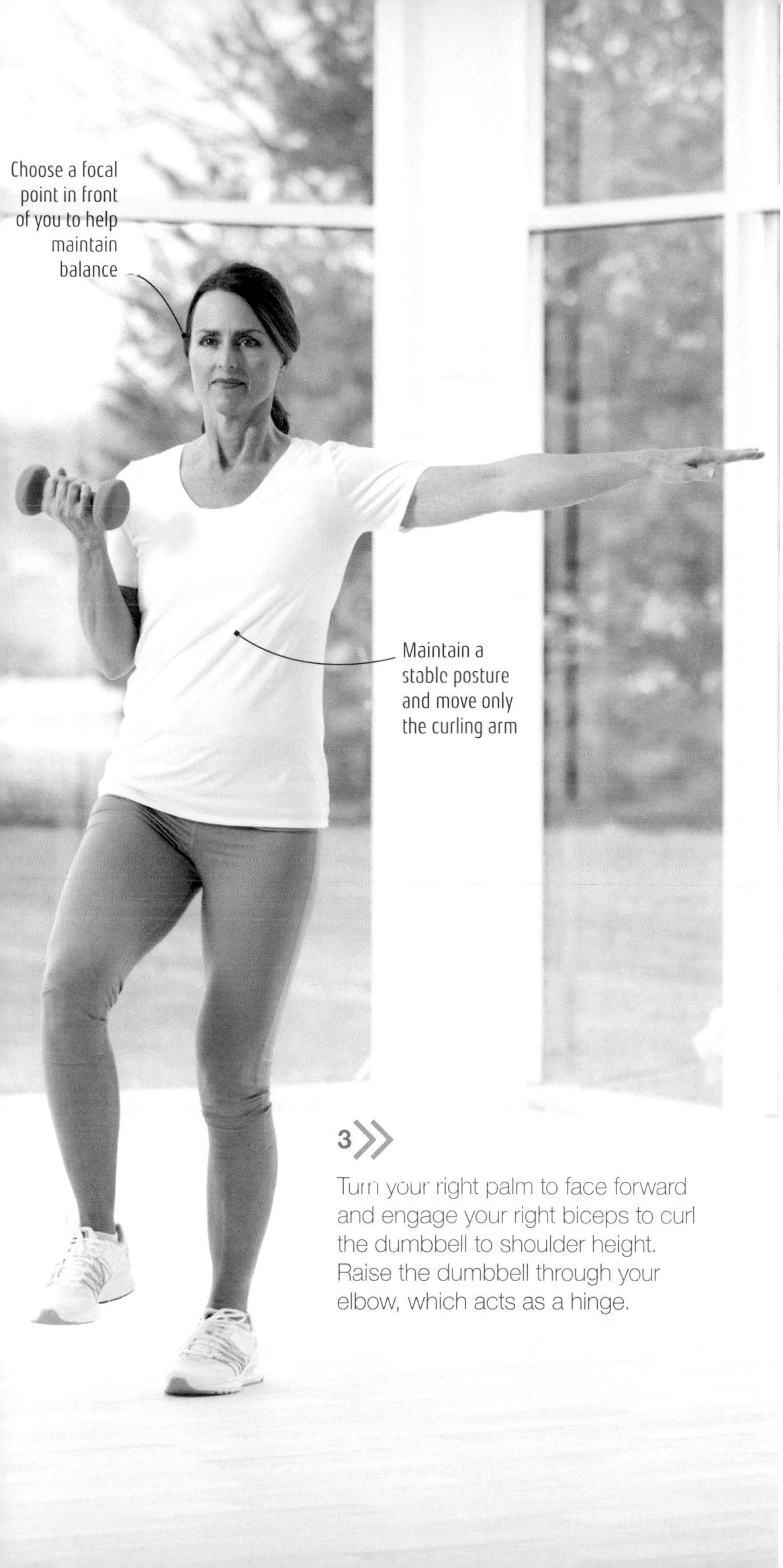

Choose a focal point in front of you to help maintain balance

Maintain a stable posture and move only the curling arm

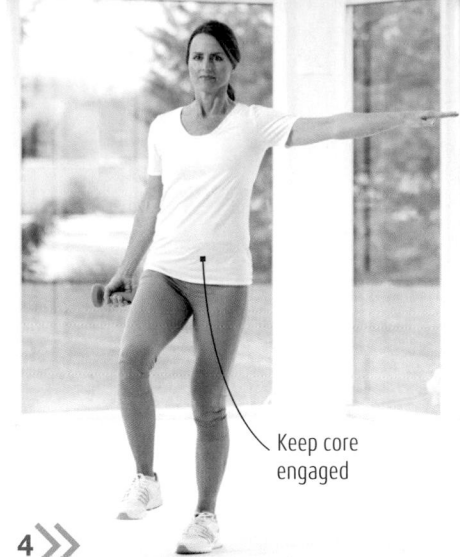

Keep core engaged

4 »

In a quick, controlled manner, lower the dumbbell straight down. Without lowering your right foot, repeat the curl. Spend half the given time curling with your right arm, then reverse your stance and curl with your left arm.

3 »

Turn your right palm to face forward and engage your right biceps to curl the dumbbell to shoulder height. Raise the dumbbell through your elbow, which acts as a hinge.

///// MAKE IT easier

For additional support, rest your extended hand on a chair or wall. Use the support when needed, but try not to rely on it too much.

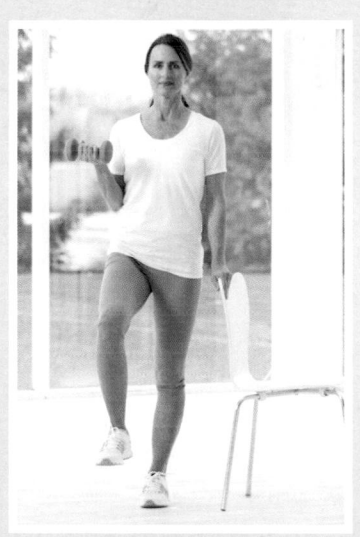

Standing elbow to knee

A firm core protects and stabilizes your spine, but it requires more than just crunches to strengthen these muscles. Do this exercise swiftly to increase your rotational ability and build your abdominals so your spine is secure and your torso remains effortlessly upright.

IMPROVES
- /// **Strength**
- /// **Stability**
- /// Mobility
- /// **Endurance**

WHAT YOU NEED
No equipment needed

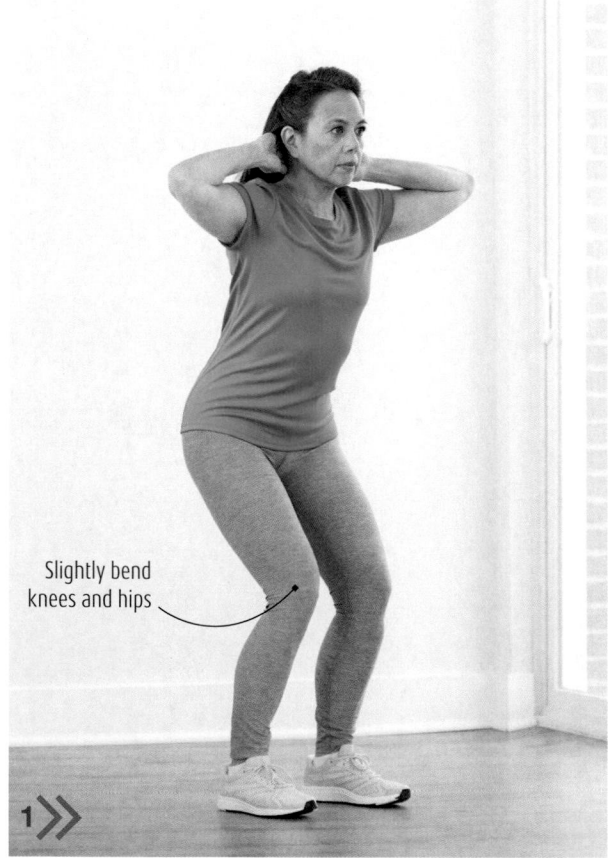

Slightly bend knees and hips

1 »

Stand with your feet shoulder-width apart. Place your hands on the back of your head and point your elbows out to your sides. Engage your core, retract your shoulder blades, and raise your chin.

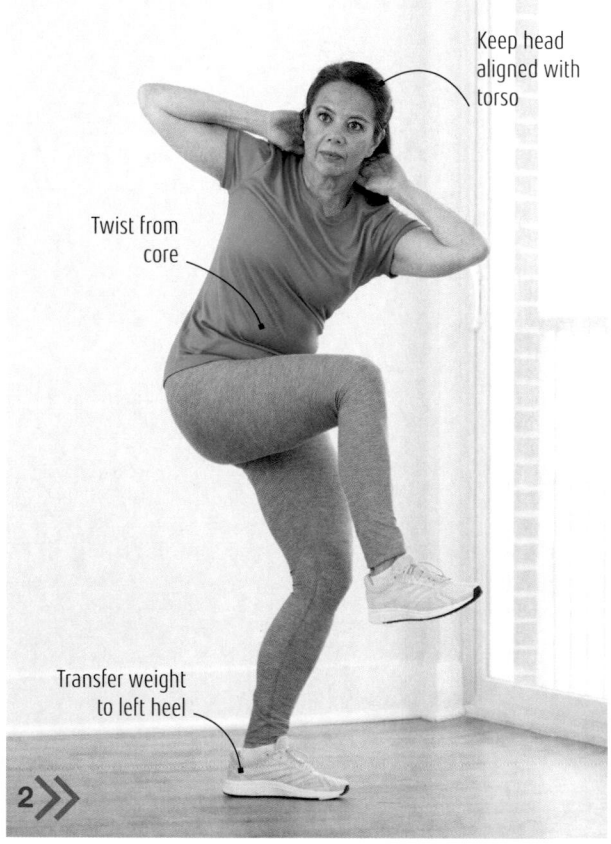

Keep head aligned with torso

Twist from core

Transfer weight to left heel

2 »

Transfer your weight to your left heel, raise your right knee and pull it toward the center of your body, and bring your left elbow toward your right knee by rotating your core. Maintain a bend in your left knee.

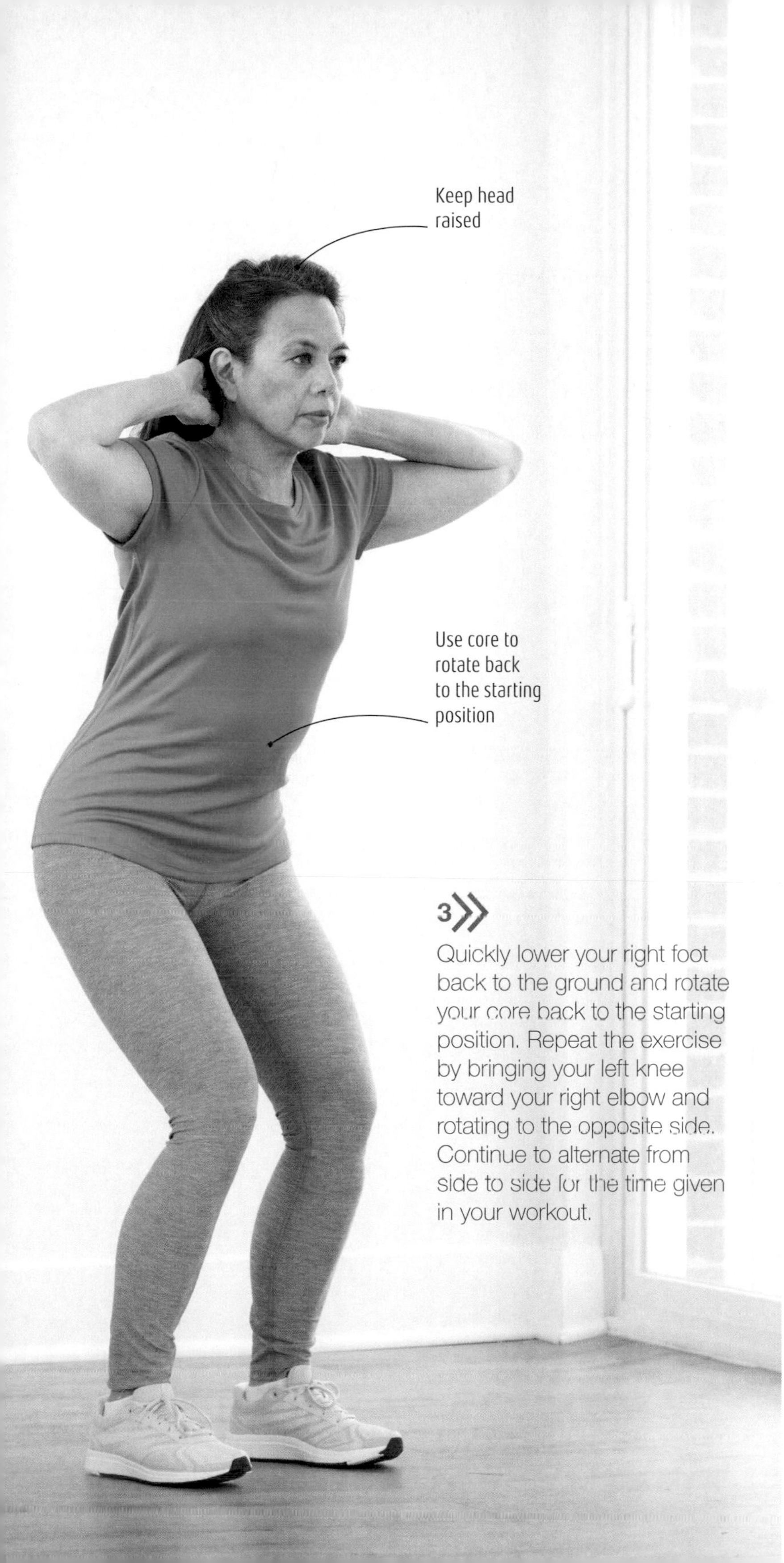

Keep head raised

Use core to rotate back to the starting position

3 »

Quickly lower your right foot back to the ground and rotate your core back to the starting position. Repeat the exercise by bringing your left knee toward your right elbow and rotating to the opposite side. Continue to alternate from side to side for the time given in your workout.

/// MAKE IT **easier**

If it is difficult to maintain balance, extend your arms out to your sides rather than placing them behind your head. Rotate your arms and core on a horizontal plane.

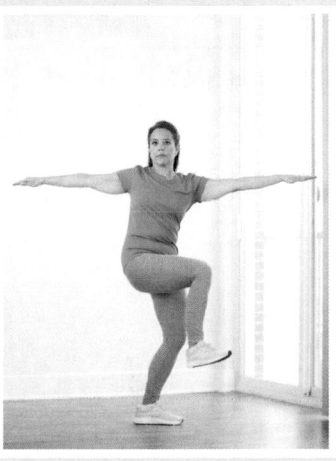

/// MAKE IT **harder**

To develop power in your legs, in step 2, jump up off the balls of your feet as you bring your knee toward your elbow. In step 3, land softly on the balls of your feet.

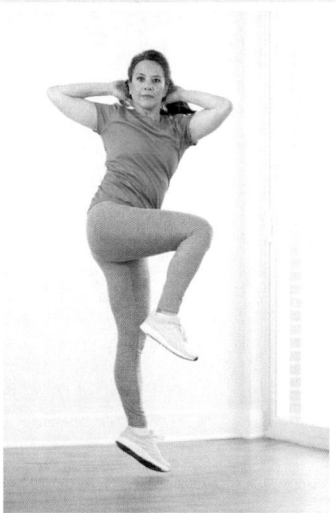

Split stance runners

Whether you are running half marathons or taking walks around the neighborhood, strong upper-body movement will immensely improve your body's efficiency. Vigorously perform this drill to practice proper walking mechanics and strengthen your upper-body muscles.

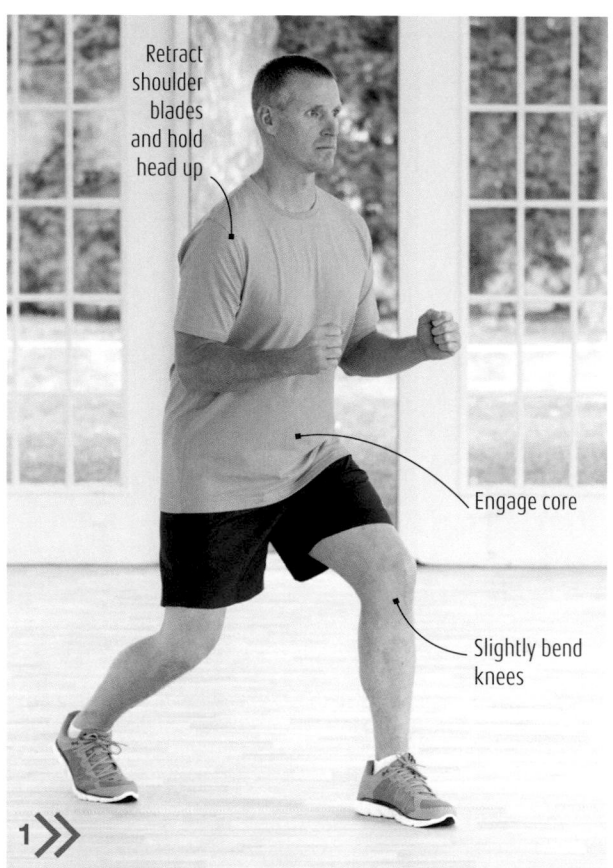

Retract shoulder blades and hold head up

Engage core

Slightly bend knees

1 »

Stand with your feet shoulder-width apart. Step your right leg back into a staggered stance and rise up onto the ball of your right foot. Bend both elbows to 90 degrees, position your forearms in front of you, and hold your hands in loose fists.

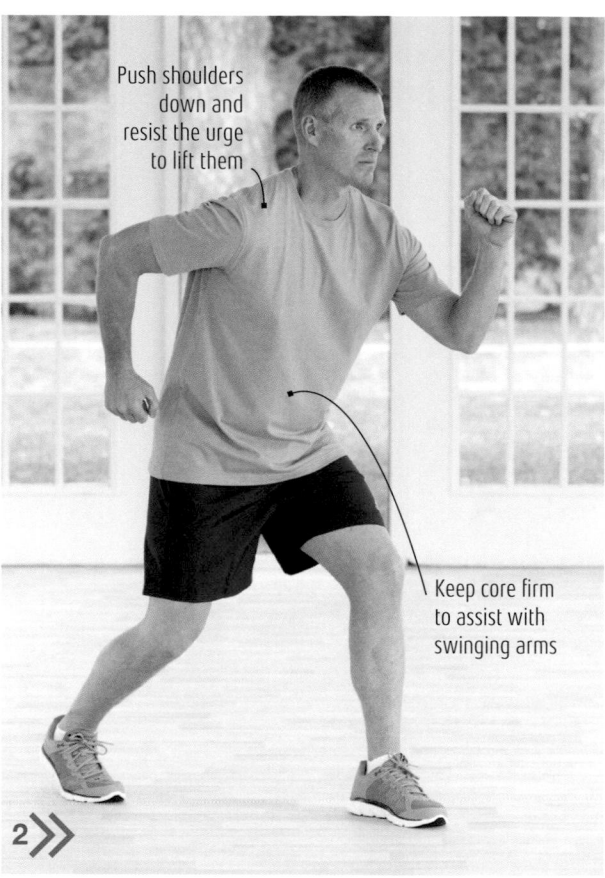

Push shoulders down and resist the urge to lift them

Keep core firm to assist with swinging arms

2 »

Using your shoulder muscles, swing your right arm back until your right hand is just behind your body, and swing your left arm forward until your left hand is at chin height. Maintain a 90-degree bend in both elbows and keep your elbows close to your body.

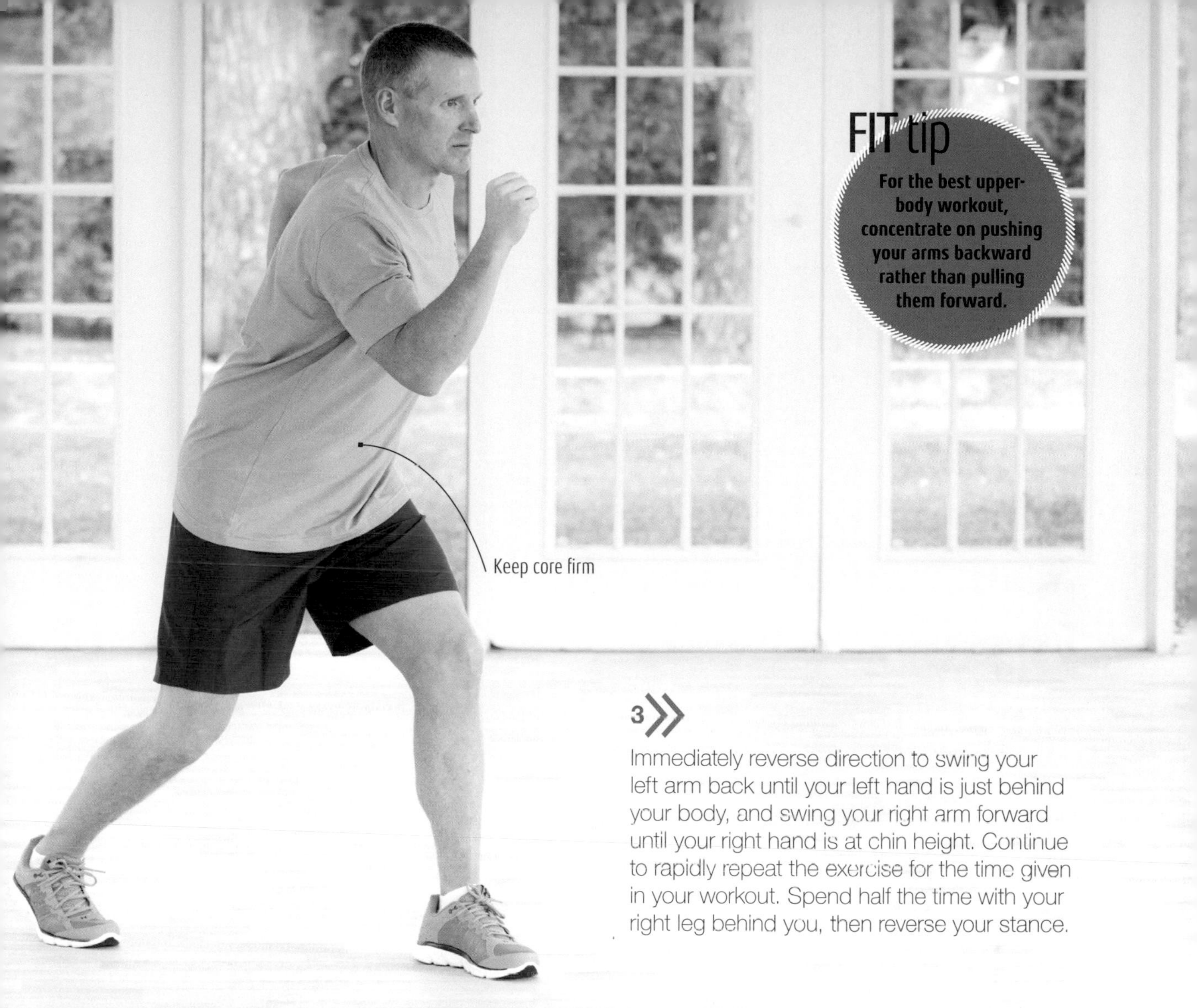

FIT tip

For the best upper-body workout, concentrate on pushing your arms backward rather than pulling them forward.

Keep core firm

3 »

Immediately reverse direction to swing your left arm back until your left hand is just behind your body, and swing your right arm forward until your right hand is at chin height. Continue to rapidly repeat the exercise for the time given in your workout. Spend half the time with your right leg behind you, then reverse your stance.

▰/// MAKE IT **easier**

If it is difficult to maintain balance, stand with your feet shoulder-width apart rather than in the staggered stance.

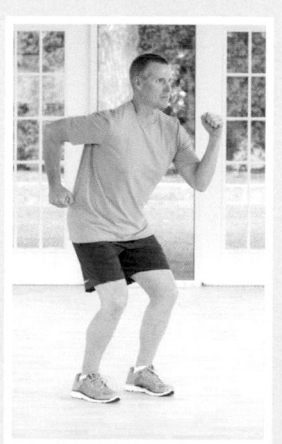

▰/// MAKE IT **harder**

To increase resistance to your shoulders, hold a dumbbell in each hand as you swing your arms.

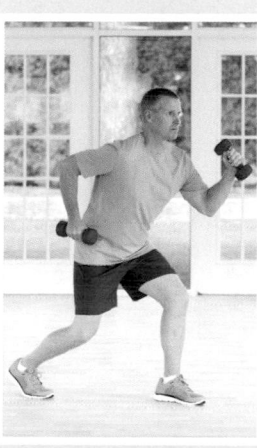

Wood chop

Rotational movements require you to activate smaller stabilizing muscles such as the hip flexors, which are not typically worked by other exercises. This fast-paced squat awakens those muscles to improve your balance.

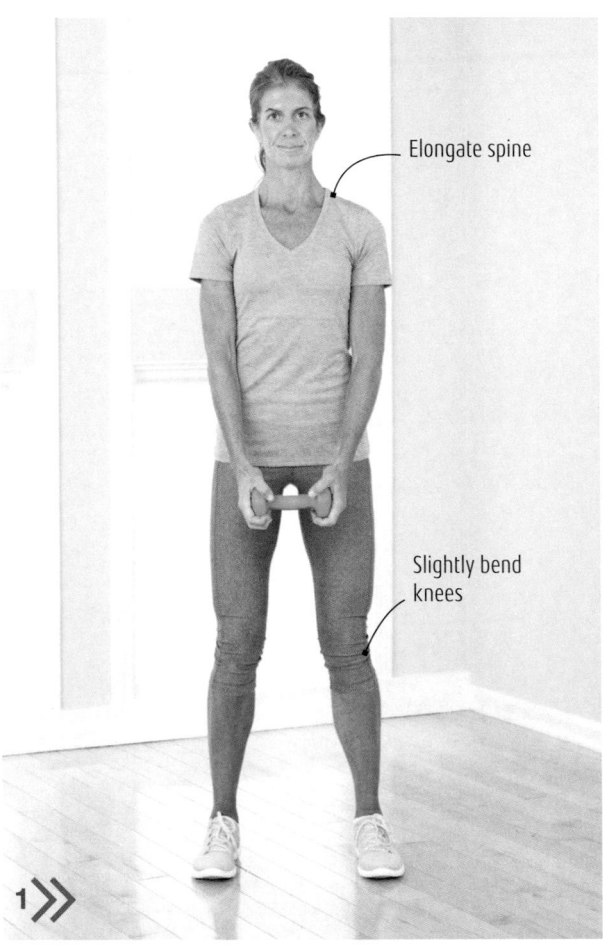

Elongate spine

Slightly bend knees

1 》》

Stand with your feet shoulder-width apart. Hold the ends of a dumbbell with both hands, and let your arms hang straight down in front of you. Engage your core and retract your shoulder blades.

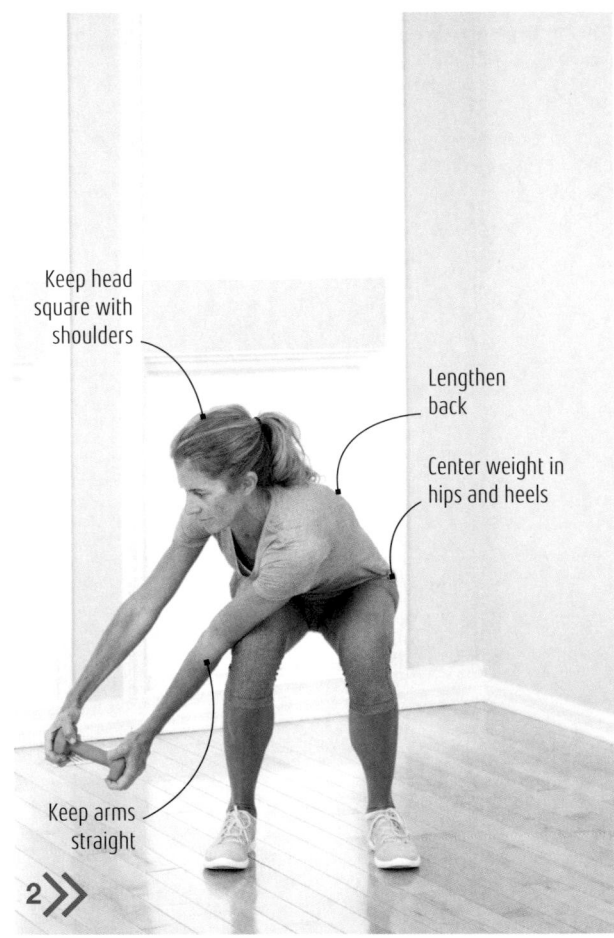

Keep head square with shoulders

Lengthen back

Center weight in hips and heels

Keep arms straight

2 》》

Push your glutes back and bend at your hips and knees to sit back into a squat until your thighs are parallel to the ground. Simultaneously rotate your core to bring the dumbbell to the outside of your right leg.

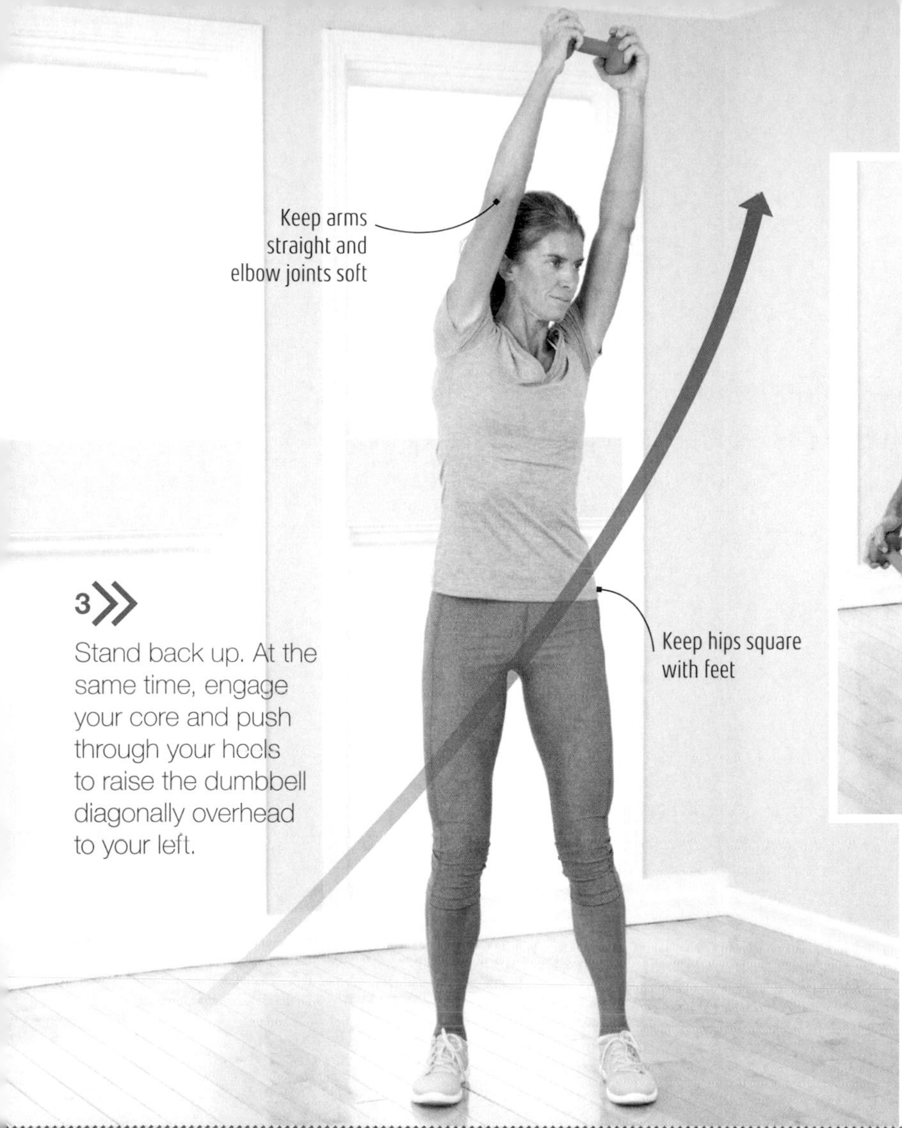

Keep arms straight and elbow joints soft

Continue to lengthen spine

3 »

Stand back up. At the same time, engage your core and push through your heels to raise the dumbbell diagonally overhead to your left.

Keep hips square with feet

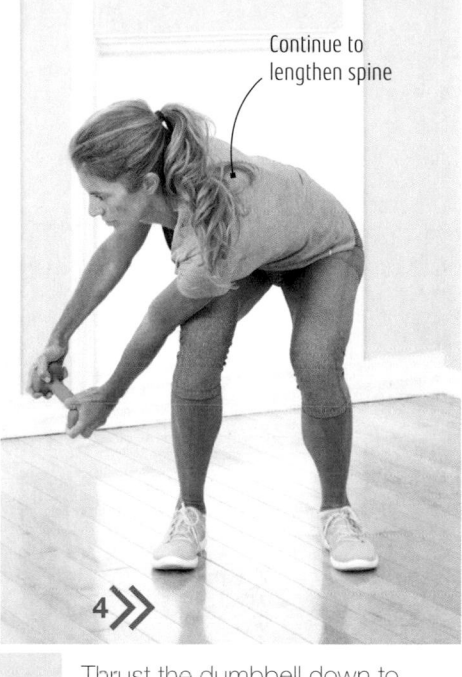

4 »

Thrust the dumbbell down to the outside of your right leg while entering into the next squat. Repeat for the time given in your workout. Spend half the time thrusting to your right, then repeat to your left.

▰▰// MAKE IT **easier**

To decrease resistance to your core, do the exercise without a dumbbell. Keep your hands and arms straight, and hold them shoulder-width apart.

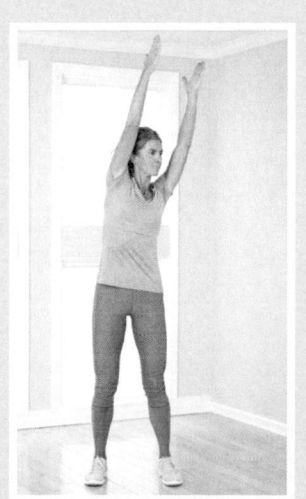

▰▰// MAKE IT **harder**

To increase resistance to your thighs, in step 1, step your right leg back into a staggered stance. In step 2, drop your back knee into a lunge rather than squatting. Remain in the staggered stance for each repetition. Reverse your stance halfway through.

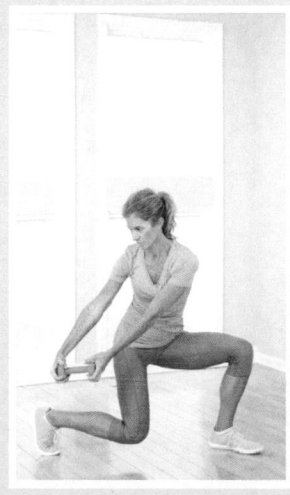

Knee chop

Training your abdominals while standing up engages more muscles and burns more calories than most ground-based exercises. Perform this standing core exercise swiftly to work your entire body, boost your endurance, burn fat, and significantly improve your posture.

IMPROVES
- Posture
- Strength
- Stability
- Mobility
- Endurance

WHAT YOU NEED
Dumbbell

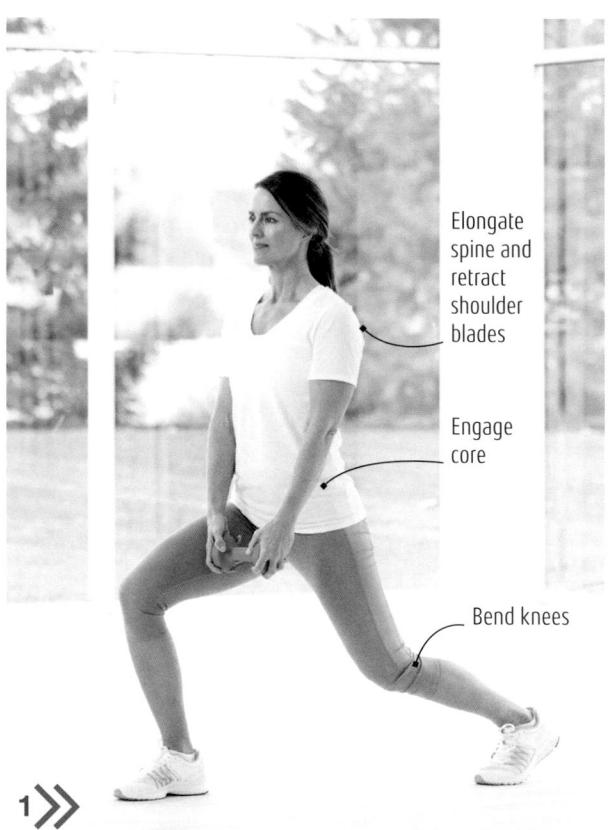

Elongate spine and retract shoulder blades

Engage core

Bend knees

1 Stand with your feet shoulder-width apart, step your left leg back into a staggered stance, and rise up onto the ball of your left foot. Hold the ends of a dumbbell with both hands, and let your arms hang straight down in front of you.

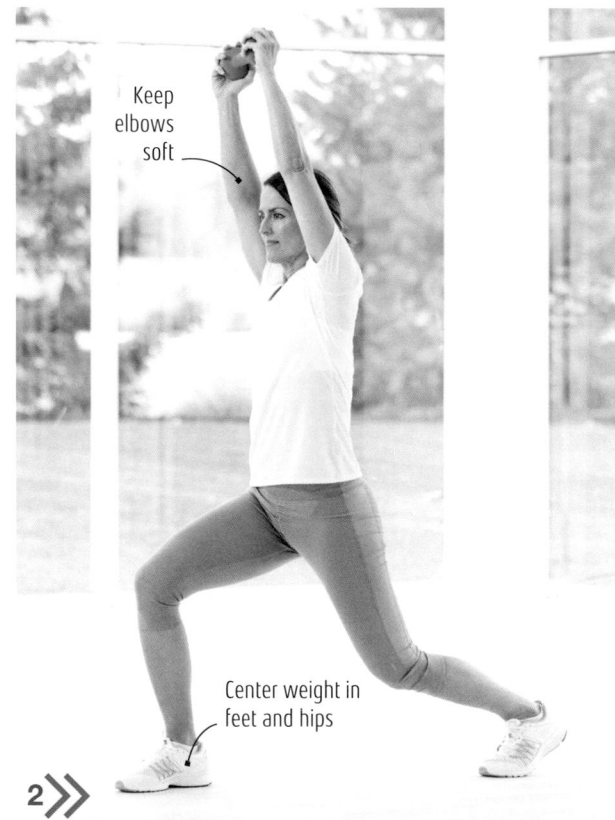

Keep elbows soft

Center weight in feet and hips

2 Keeping your arms straight, raise the dumbbell diagonally overhead to your right. Do not lock your elbow joints. Look straight ahead and maintain an upright posture. Keep your core engaged.

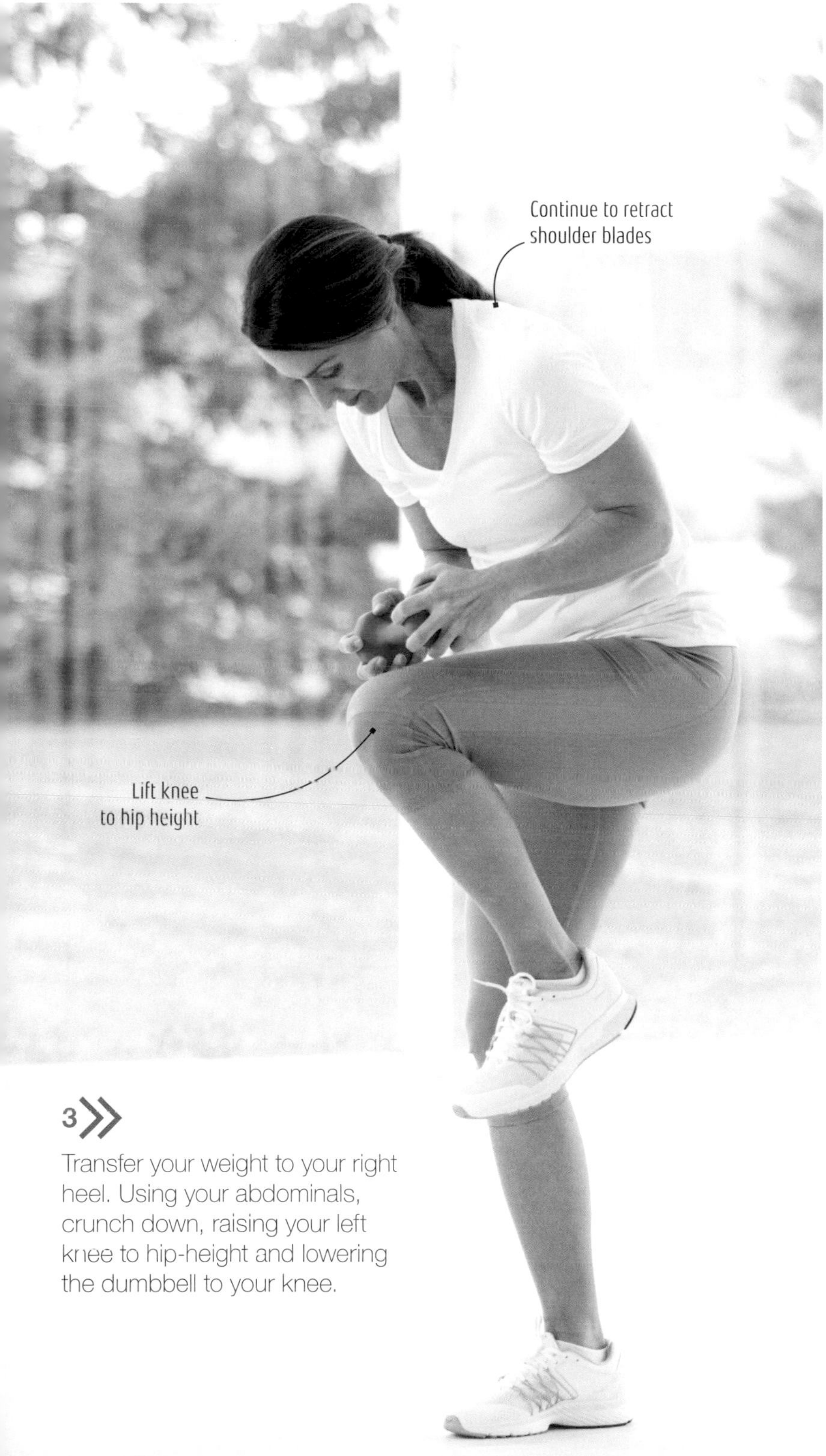

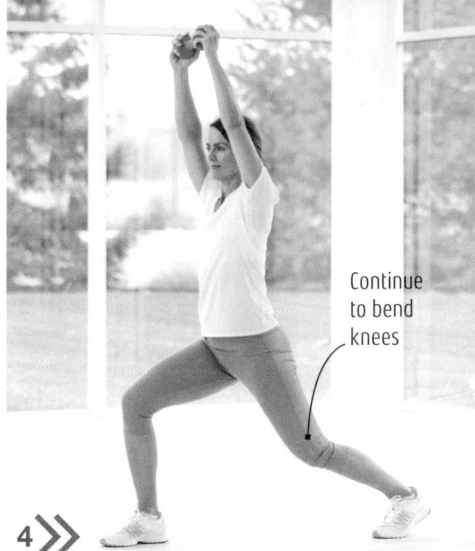

Continue to bend knees

Continue to retract shoulder blades

4 »

Return to the staggered stance, and raise the dumbbell diagonally overhead to the right. Repeat the exercise for the time given in your workout. Spend half the time raising your right leg, then switch to your left leg.

Lift knee to hip height

3 »

Transfer your weight to your right heel. Using your abdominals, crunch down, raising your left knee to hip-height and lowering the dumbbell to your knee.

▰//// MAKE IT **easier**

If it is difficult to maintain balance, do the exercise without a dumbbell, and hold your hands in fists.

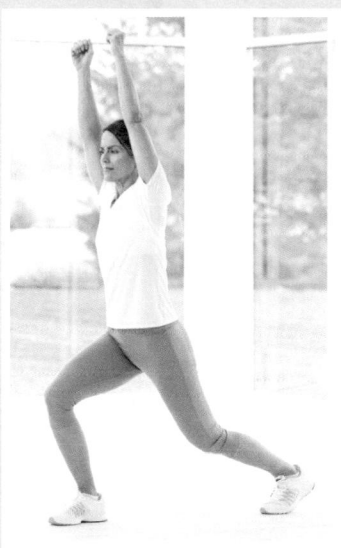

Side-to-side punch

You do not have to be a boxer to benefit from cardio boxing. This punching sequence can improve heart health, develop core strength, burn calories, and build shoulder muscles. You might also find this exercise to be a remarkable stress reliever.

IMPROVES

▰/// **Strength**

▰/// **Stability**

/// Mobility

▰/// **Endurance**

WHAT YOU NEED
Dumbbells

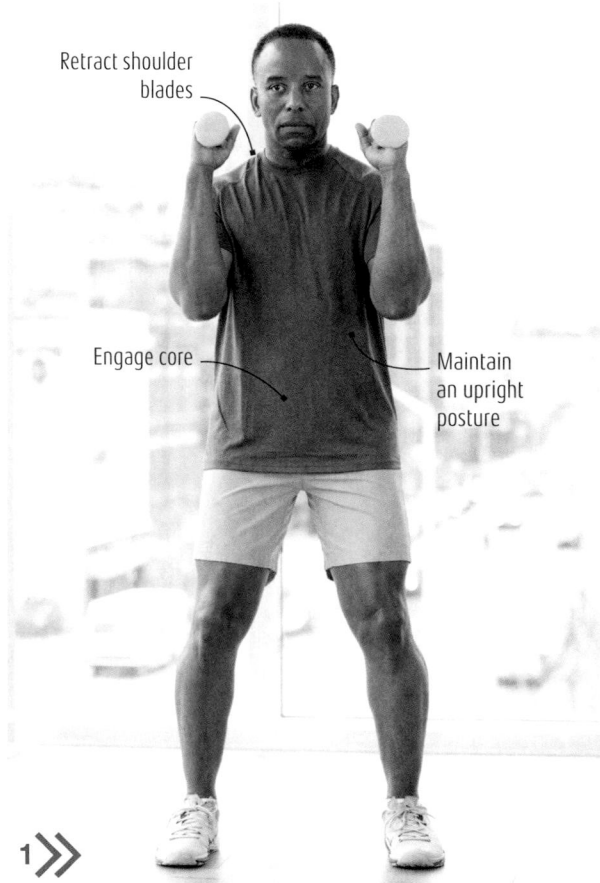

Retract shoulder blades

Engage core

Maintain an upright posture

1 》

Stand with your feet shoulder-width apart. Hold a dumbbell in each hand, raise them to chin-height with your palms facing each other, and tuck your elbows to your sides. Slightly bend your knees and hips.

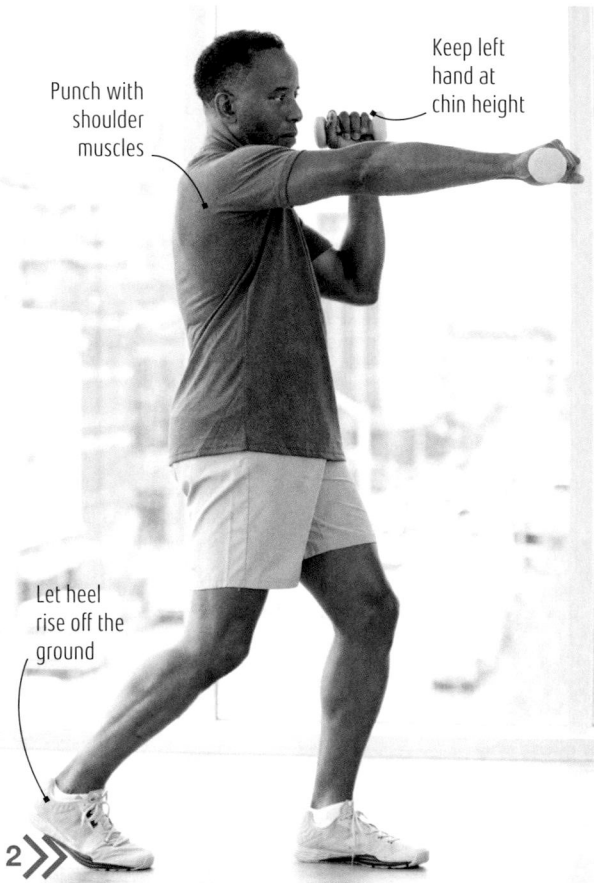

Keep left hand at chin height

Punch with shoulder muscles

Let heel rise off the ground

2 》

Engage your core and hips to rotate your body 90 degrees to the left, letting your feet rotate with you. Simultaneously punch your right arm out and rotate your arm so your palm faces the ground.

FIT tip

To protect your elbow joints from injury, always retract your punch just before reaching a full extension.

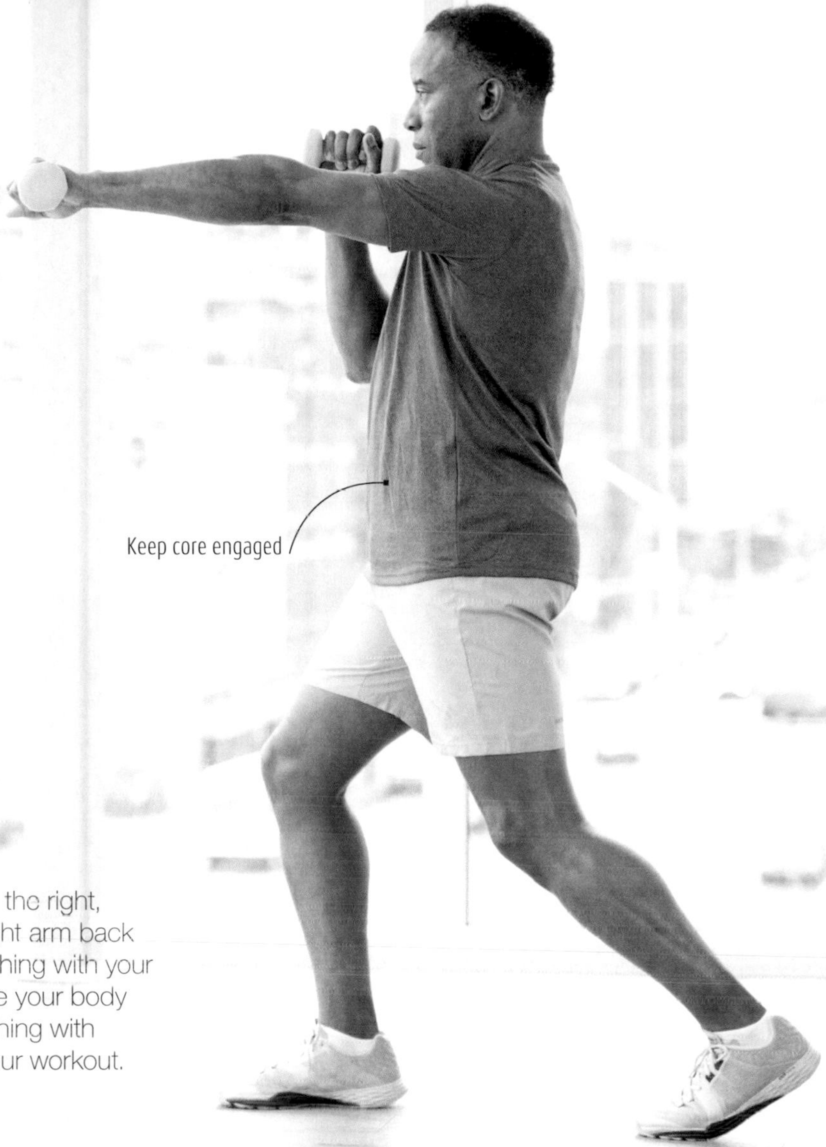

Keep core engaged

3 ≫

Powerfully rotate 180 degrees to the right, while at the same pulling your right arm back to the starting position and punching with your left arm. Continue to swiftly rotate your body 180 degrees and alternate punching with each arm for the time given in your workout.

▰/// MAKE IT **easier**

To reduce resistance to your shoulders, do the exercise without dumbbells, and hold your hands in fists.

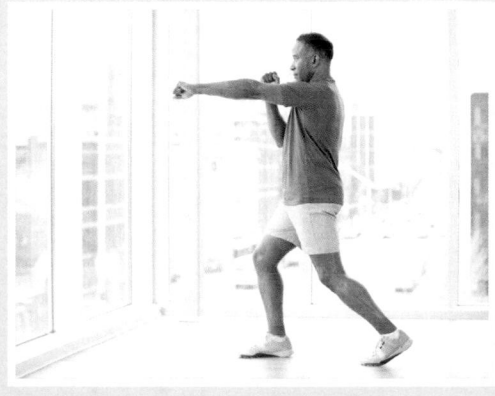

Standing twist

Spinal flexibility is just as important as muscle flexibility. A mobile spine promotes healthy posture, better enabling you to comfortably lift heavy objects or perform throwing motions. Use this swift, rotational, core-strengthening exercise to restore natural mobility to your spine, relieve chronic back pain, and reduce your chances of injury.

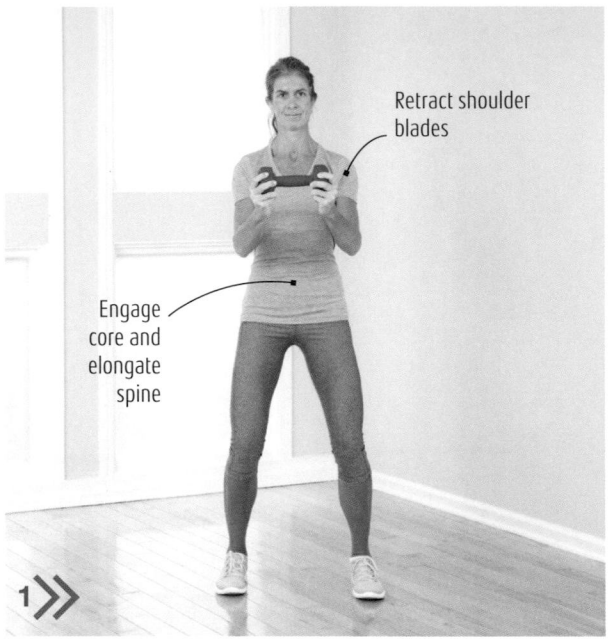

1 ≫

Stand with your feet shoulder-width apart. Hold the ends of a dumbbell with both hands, bend your elbows to 90 degrees, and raise the dumbbell to chest height. Slightly bend your knees and hips.

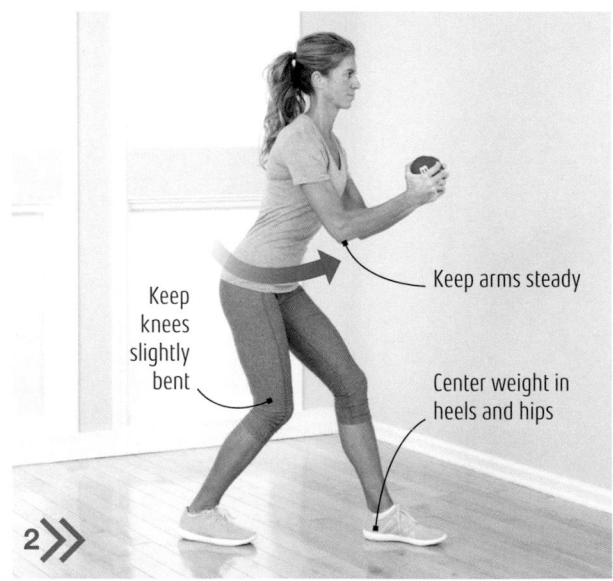

2 ≫

Using your hips and core for momentum, quickly pivot your feet and rotate your upper body 90 degrees to the left. Keep the dumbbell aligned with your chest and let your arms travel with you.

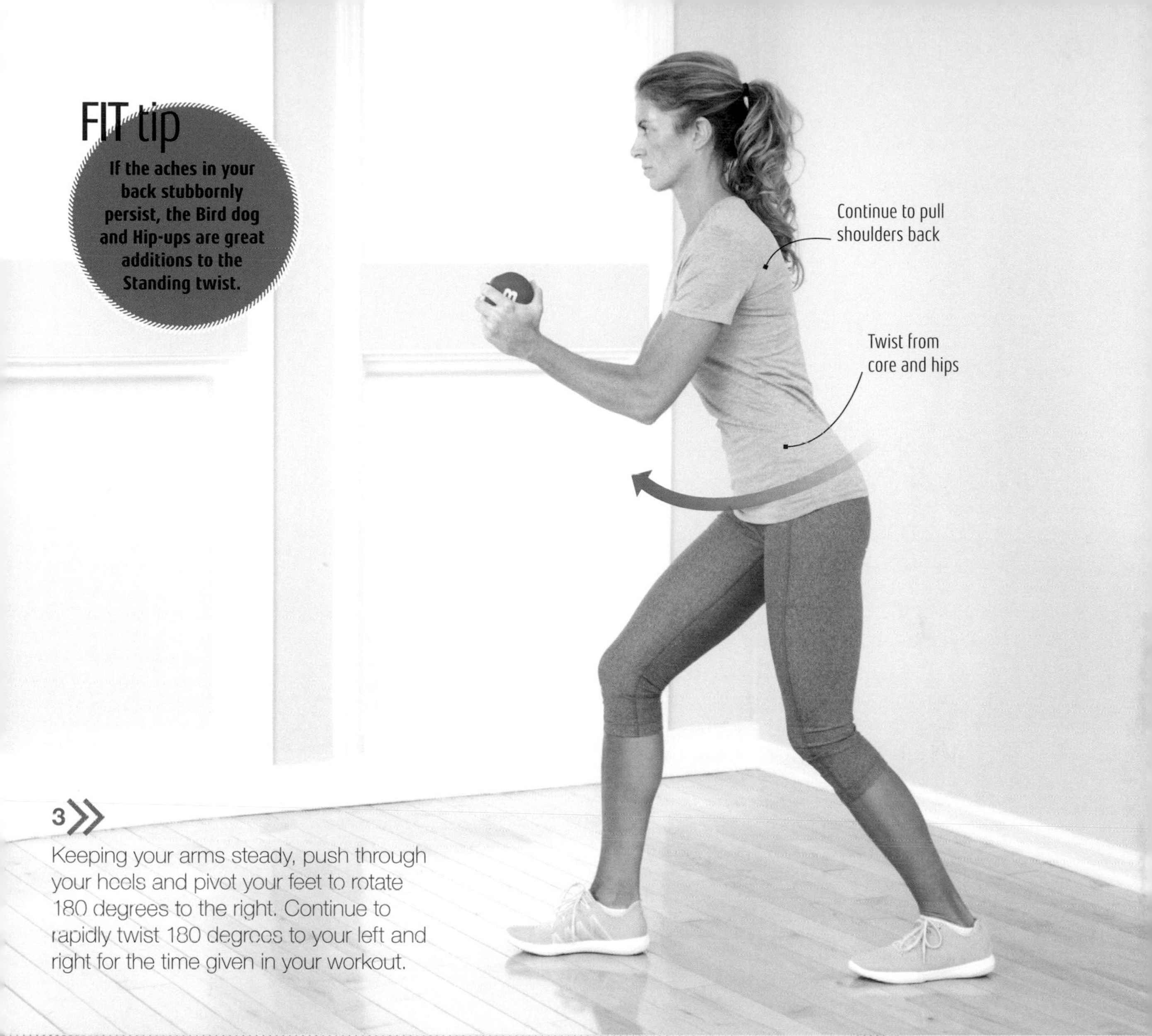

FIT tip

If the aches in your back stubbornly persist, the Bird dog and Hip-ups are great additions to the Standing twist.

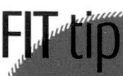

Continue to pull shoulders back

Twist from core and hips

3 »

Keeping your arms steady, push through your heels and pivot your feet to rotate 180 degrees to the right. Continue to rapidly twist 180 degrees to your left and right for the time given in your workout.

▰//// MAKE IT **easier**

If it is difficult to maintain balance, hold your arms in the same position, but do the exercise without a dumbbell.

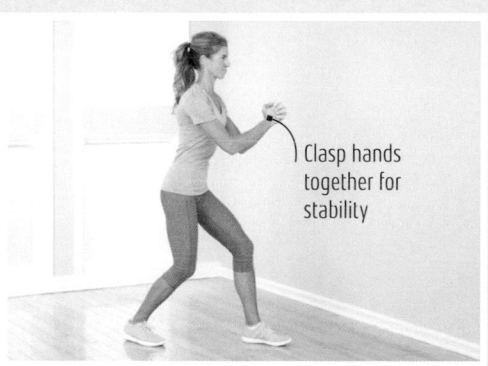

Clasp hands together for stability

Standing oblique rotation

Torso strength and mobility will stabilize your spine and make all your movements more efficient. Do this rotational exercise to strengthen your abdominals and lower back, take pressure off your spine, and help you do activities such as household cleaning or gardening more safely.

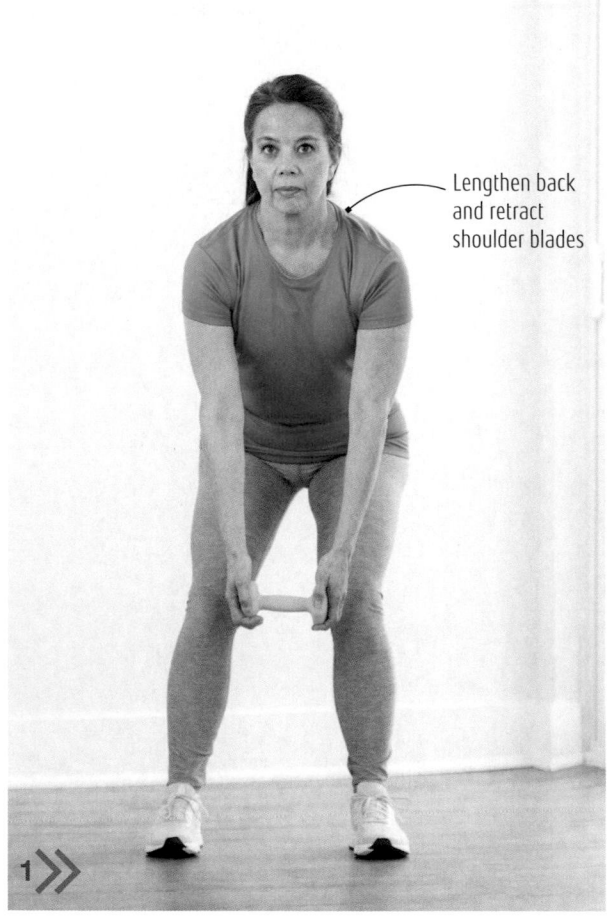

Lengthen back and retract shoulder blades

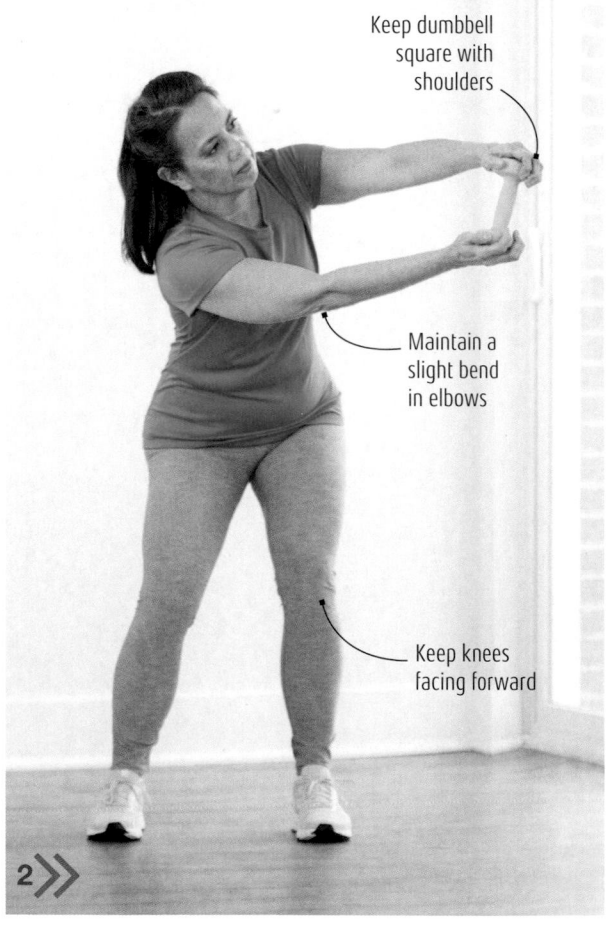

Keep dumbbell square with shoulders

Maintain a slight bend in elbows

Keep knees facing forward

1 >> Stand with your feet shoulder-width apart and bend over to 45 degrees from the hips. Hold the ends of a dumbbell with both hands and let your arms hang straight down in front of you. Slightly bend your knees.

2 >> In a quick, controlled manner, use your hips and core to rotate your torso and arms 90 degrees to the left. Move your head along with your shoulders and follow the dumbbell with your eyes.

FIT tip

If it's difficult to rotate the full 180 degrees, rotate only as much as you're comfortable and slowly increase your range.

Rotate until the dumbbell is perpendicular to the ground
Continue to draw shoulder blades together
Concentrate rotational effort in core and avoid swinging arms for momentum

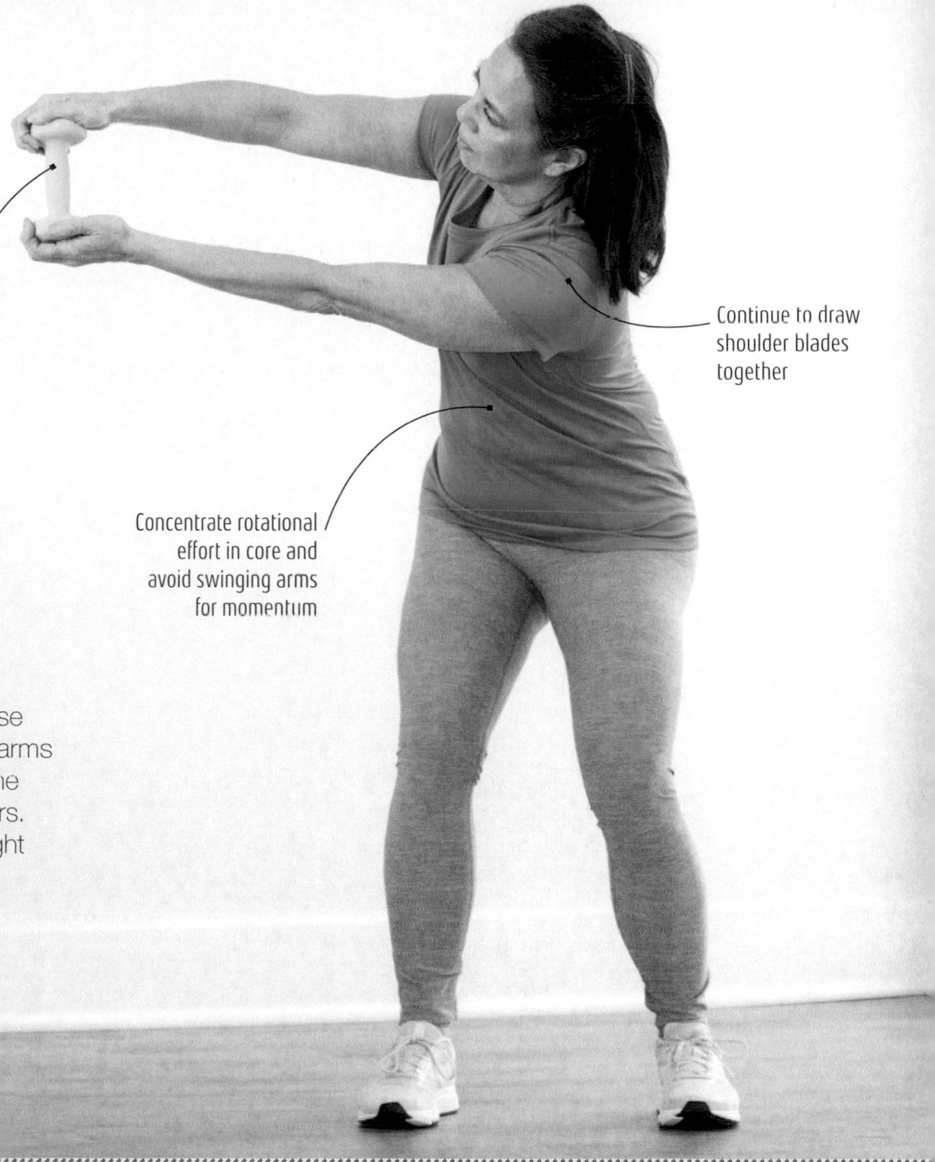

3 »

In a quick, controlled manner, reverse direction and rotate your torso and arms 180 degrees to the right, keeping the dumbbell square with your shoulders. Continue rotating to your left and right for the time given in your workout.

MAKE IT **easier**

To reduce pressure on your spine, do the exercise without a dumbbell, and hold your hands in fists.

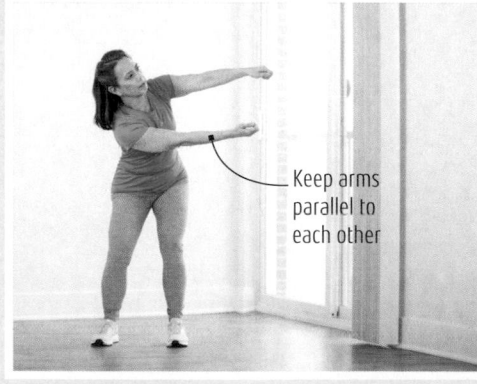

Keep arms parallel to each other

Rotational goblet squat

IMPROVES
- /// **Strength**
- /// **Stability**
- /// **Mobility**
- /// **Endurance**

WHAT YOU NEED
Dumbbell

Squatting is actually very functional—we squat naturally as babies, but many lose the ability after years of frequently sitting in unnatural positions. Perform this quick and controlled exercise to strengthen your legs and core and restore your natural ability to squat.

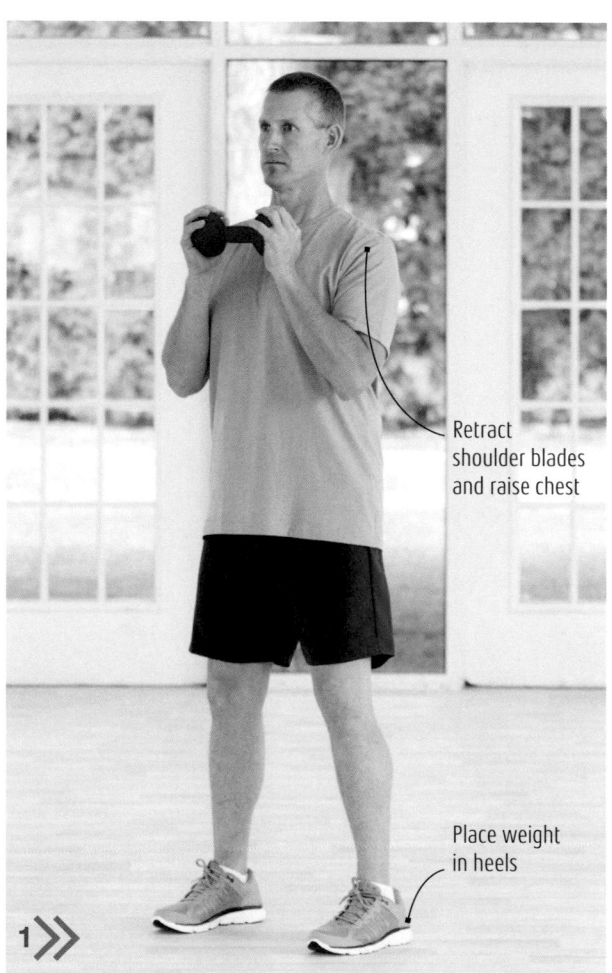

Retract shoulder blades and raise chest

Place weight in heels

1 >> Stand with your feet shoulder-width apart and hold the ends of a dumbbell with both hands. Raise the dumbbell to your chest. Engage your core.

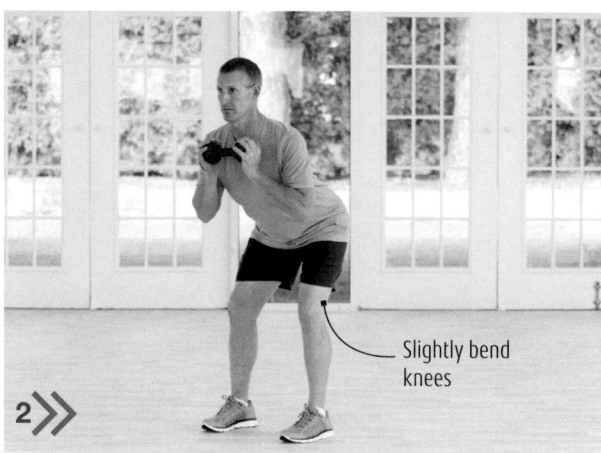

Slightly bend knees

2 >> Push your glutes back and bend at your hips. Keep your back long and straight, and keep your knees facing forward. Hold your head up.

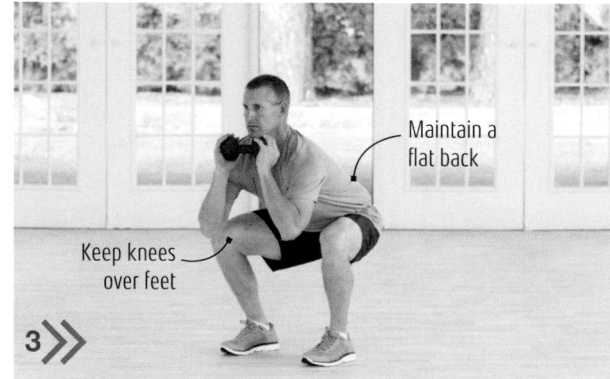

Maintain a flat back

Keep knees over feet

3 >> Without moving the dumbbell, bend your knees and sit back into a squat until your thighs are parallel to the ground. Keep your weight in your heels and hips.

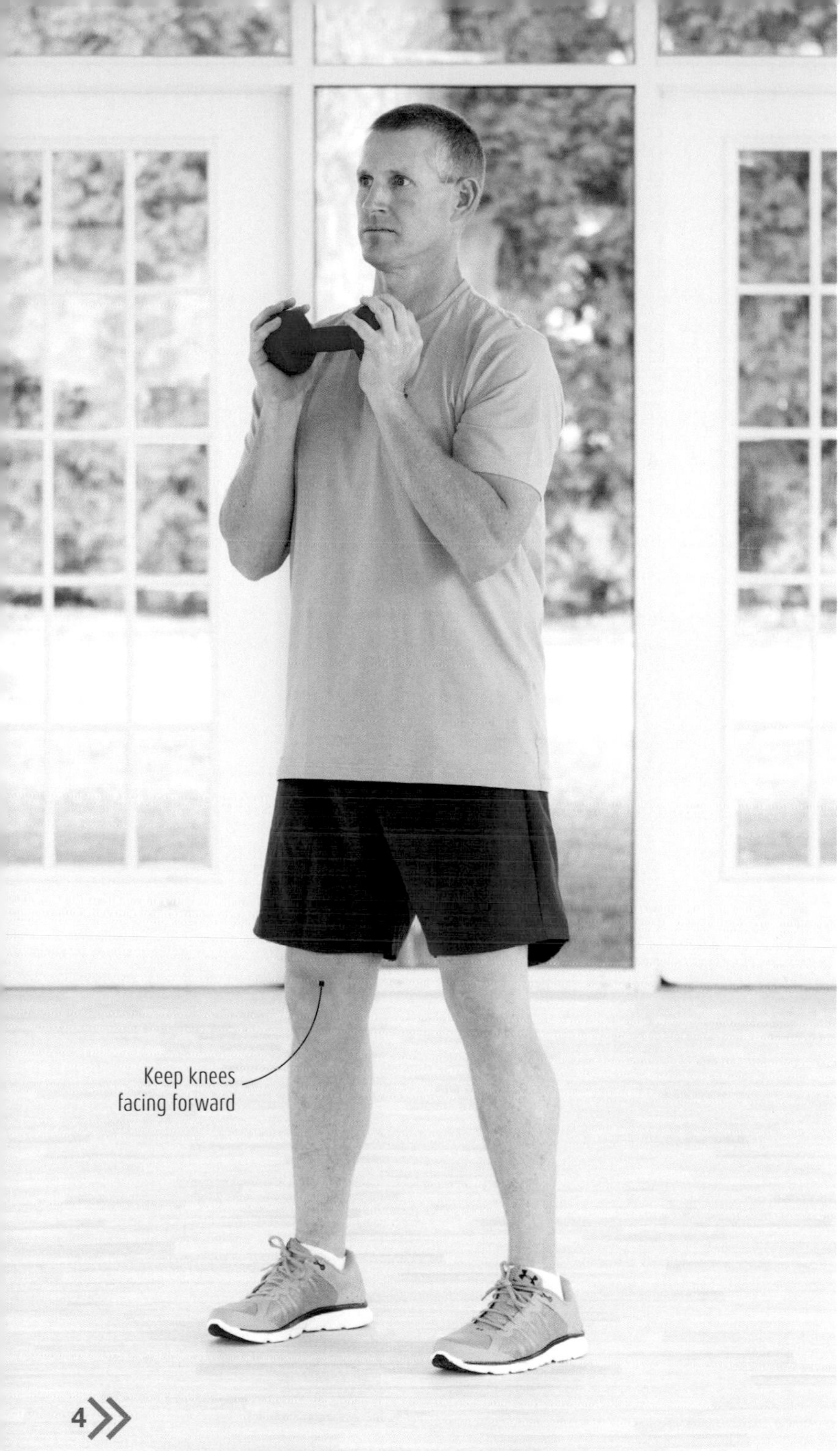

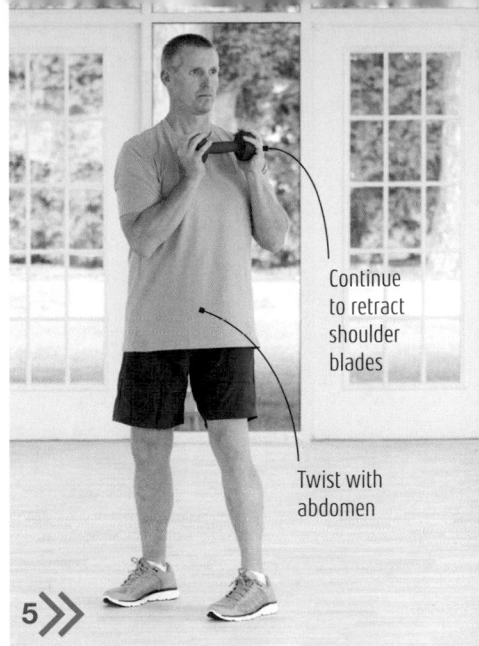

Continue to retract shoulder blades

Twist with abdomen

5 »

Using your core, rotate your torso 90 degrees to the left, letting your arms move with you. Then return to the starting position. Alternate rotating to your right and left for the time given in your workout.

Keep knees facing forward

4 »

Push through your heels and rise out of the squat until your legs are straight. Keep your head aligned with your spine and your chest raised.

///// MAKE IT **easier**

If it is difficult to maintain balance, place a chair behind you and squat until you lightly touch the chair. Do the exercise without a dumbbell, holding your hands in loose fists.

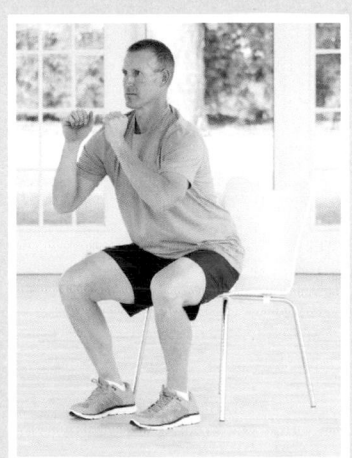

Crossover toe touch

IMPROVES
/// Posture
/// Strength
/// Stability
/// Mobility
/// Endurance

WHAT YOU NEED
No equipment needed

In order for your upper and lower body to work together harmoniously, you must train your abdominals and your lower back together. Energetically perform this exercise to work these muscles simultaneously and develop better stability and body awareness.

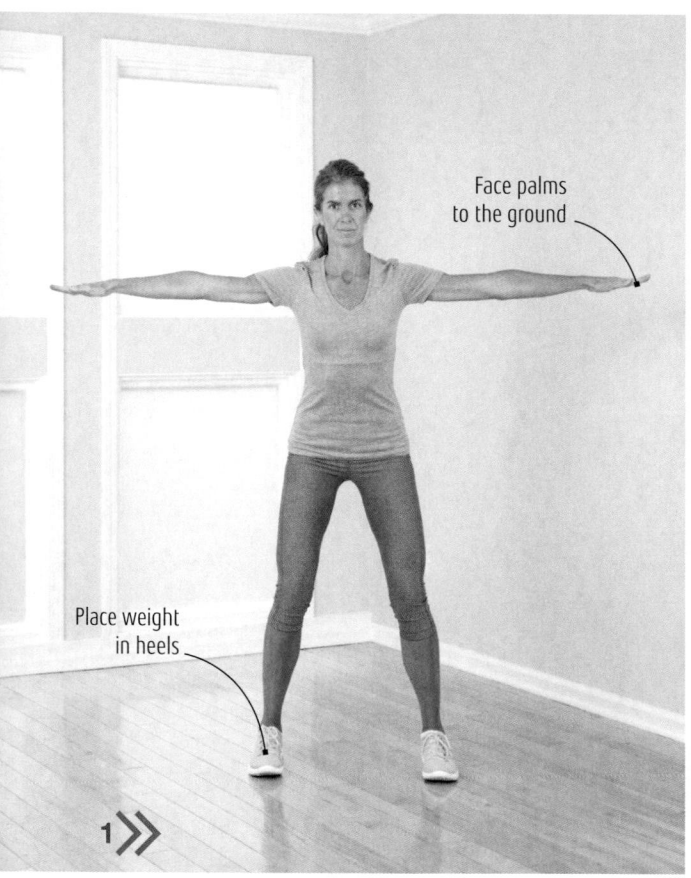

Face palms to the ground

Place weight in heels

1 >>

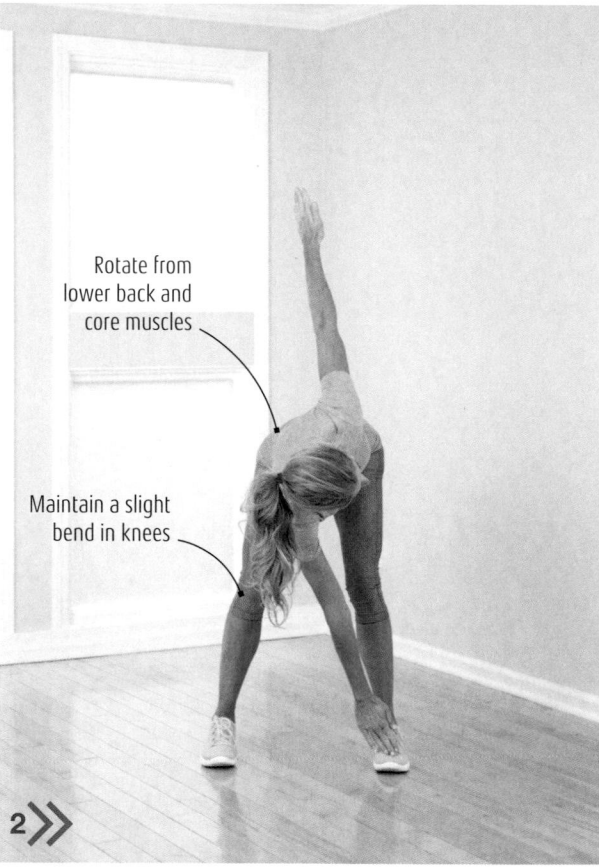

Rotate from lower back and core muscles

Maintain a slight bend in knees

2 >>

Stand with your feet slightly wider than shoulder-width apart and extend your arms straight out to your sides, palms facing down. Retract your shoulder blades and engage your core. Slightly bend your knees and hips.

Keeping your arms straight and rotating from your core, reach your right hand down to touch your left foot by bending at your hips and pushing your glutes back. Keep your head up.

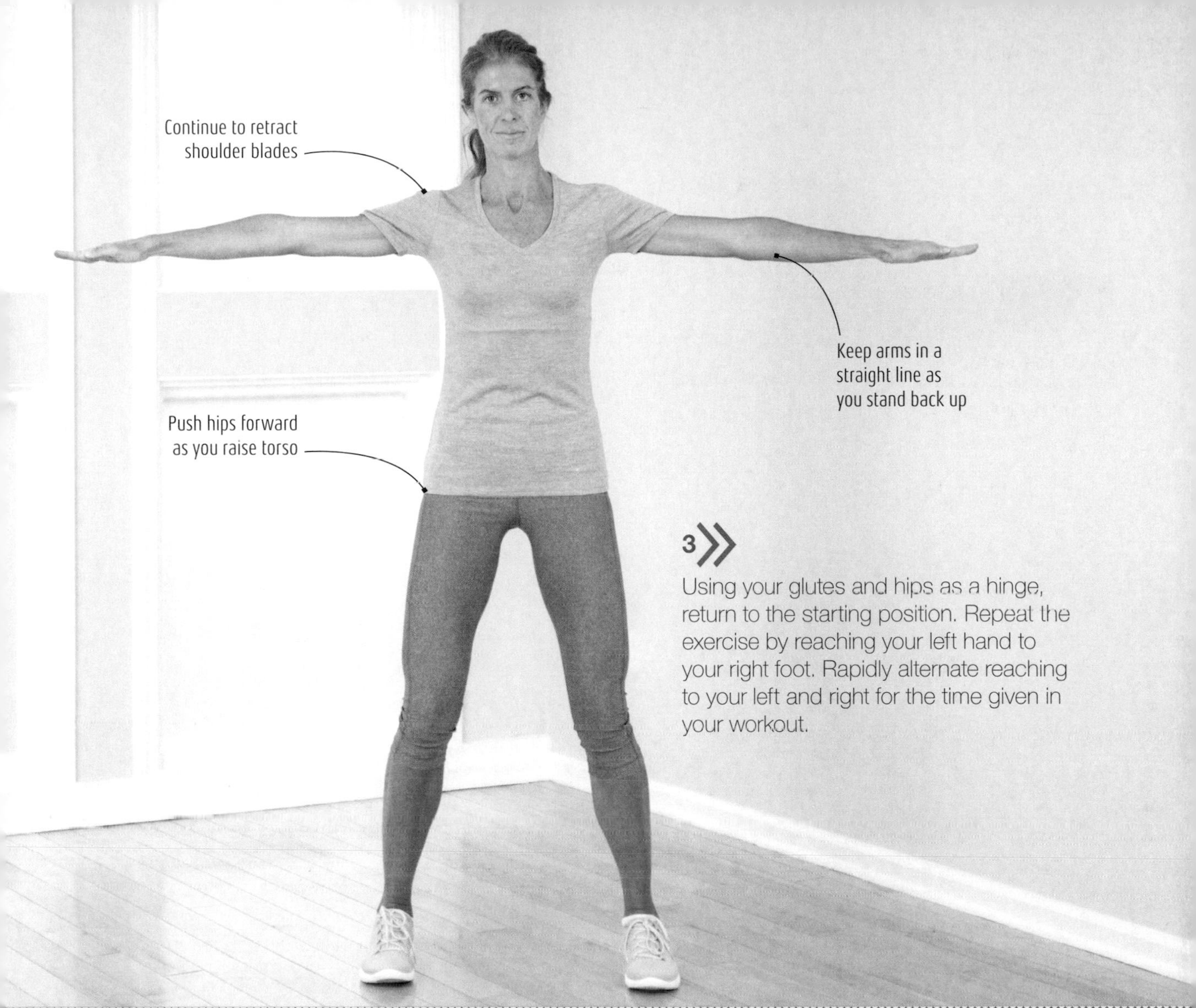

Continue to retract
shoulder blades

Keep arms in a
straight line as
you stand back up

Push hips forward
as you raise torso

3 》》

Using your glutes and hips as a hinge,
return to the starting position. Repeat the
exercise by reaching your left hand to
your right foot. Rapidly alternate reaching
to your left and right for the time given in
your workout.

///// MAKE IT **easier**

If flexibility in your hamstrings
is limited, reach to your knees
rather than your feet.

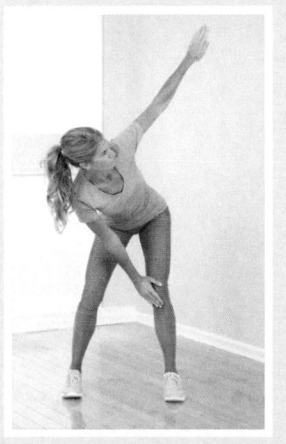

///// MAKE IT **harder**

To increase resistance to your
shoulders and core, hold a
light dumbbell in each hand.

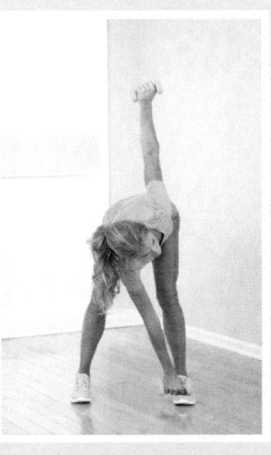

IMPROVES

//// **Posture**

//// **Strength**

//// **Stability**

//// **Mobility**

WHAT YOU NEED
Mat

High plank reach-through and fly

Planks condition your body to use your abdominals for stabilization. Plus, they are safer than crunches because they don't require you to flex your spine. Perform this rotational variation to improve your core stability and strength.

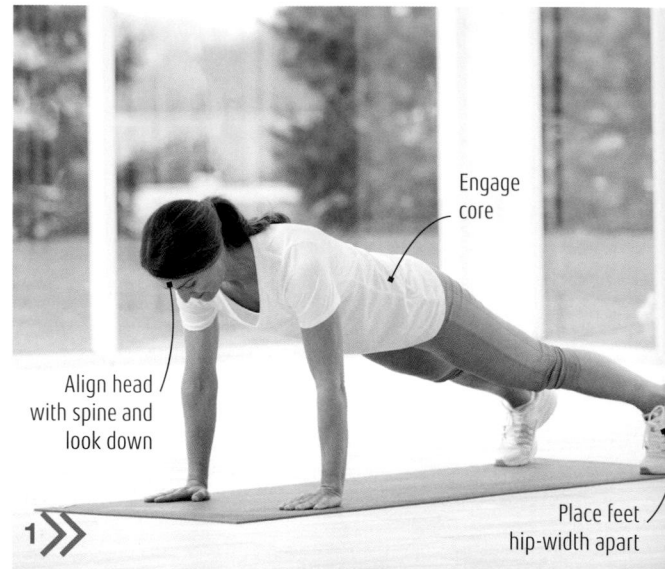

Engage core

Align head with spine and look down

Place feet hip-width apart

1 》

Kneel on all fours and align your shoulders above your hands, fingers facing forward. Rise off your knees and onto the balls of your feet, and walk your feet back into a modified plank position to form a straight line from your head to heels.

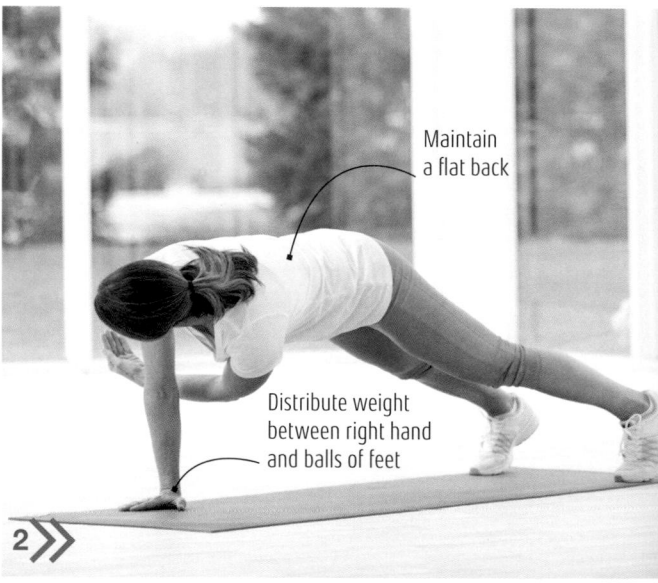

Maintain a flat back

Distribute weight between right hand and balls of feet

2 》

In a controlled manner, raise your left hand off the ground. Rotating from your core, reach your left arm under your right arm and across your body as if you are wrapping your arm around a tree trunk.

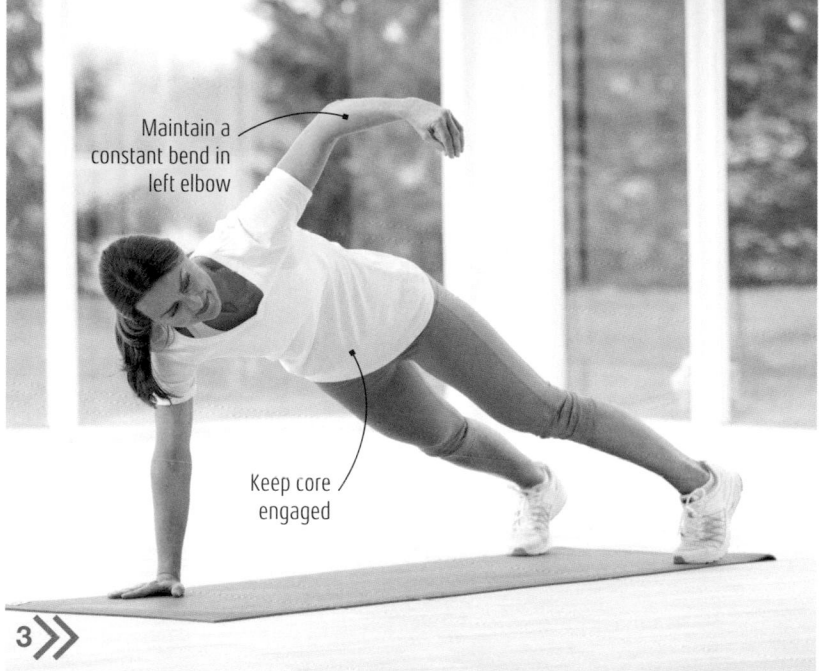

Maintain a constant bend in left elbow

Keep core engaged

3 »

Engage the muscles in your upper back and carefully pull your left arm back to open up your chest as much as possible. Contract the middle of your back at the top of the movement.

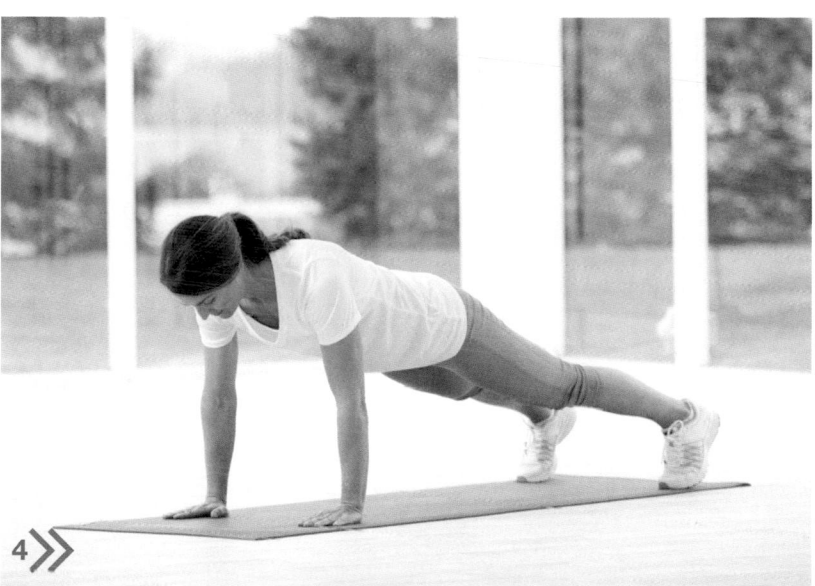

4 »

Return your left arm to the starting position and distribute your weight evenly between both hands and feet. Repeat the exercise with your right arm. Continue to alternate the exercise with each arm for the time given in your workout.

■▼/// MAKE IT **easier**

If it is difficult to maintain balance, remain on your knees instead of getting into a plank position. Lower your hips until your upper body is about 45 degrees to the ground.

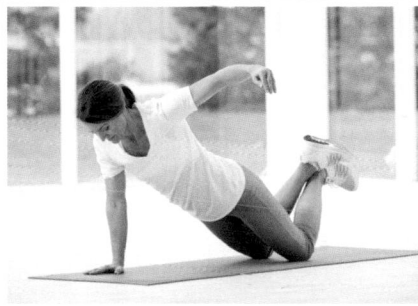

■▼/// MAKE IT **harder**

To increase resistance, hold a dumbbell in your left hand and pull it back from your elbow. Spend half the time working your left side, then repeat on your right side.

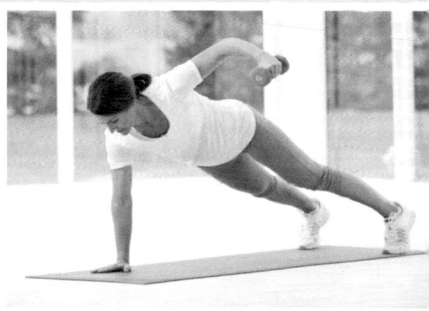

Windmill

A variety of problems can cause lower-back pain, but many back injuries are avoidable by frequently doing preventative exercises. This controlled twisting exercise can improve the strength and flexibility of your abdominals and lower-back muscles so you can stay pain- and injury-free.

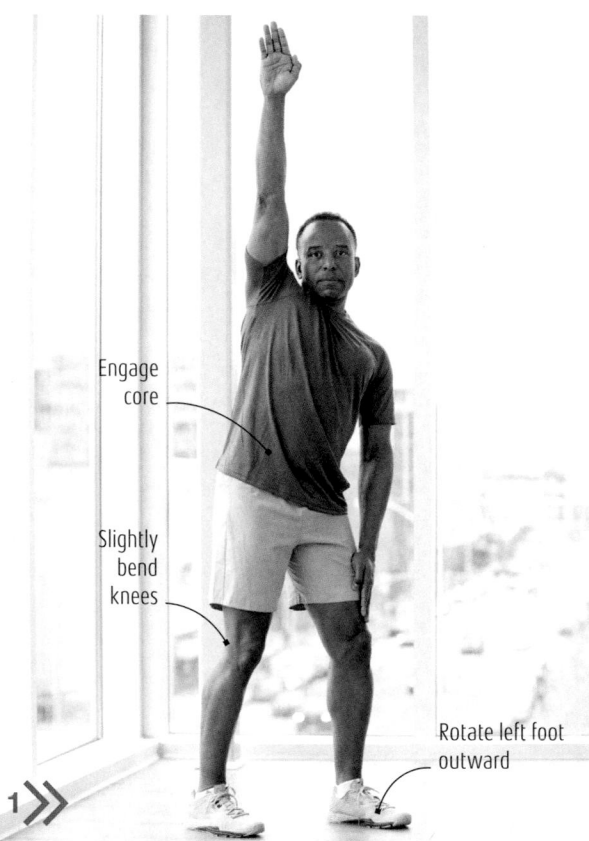

Engage core

Slightly bend knees

Rotate left foot outward

1 >> Stand with your feet slightly wider than shoulder-width apart and angle your left foot out at about 45 degrees. Fully extend your right arm straight overhead and lock your elbow. Let your left arm hang straight down.

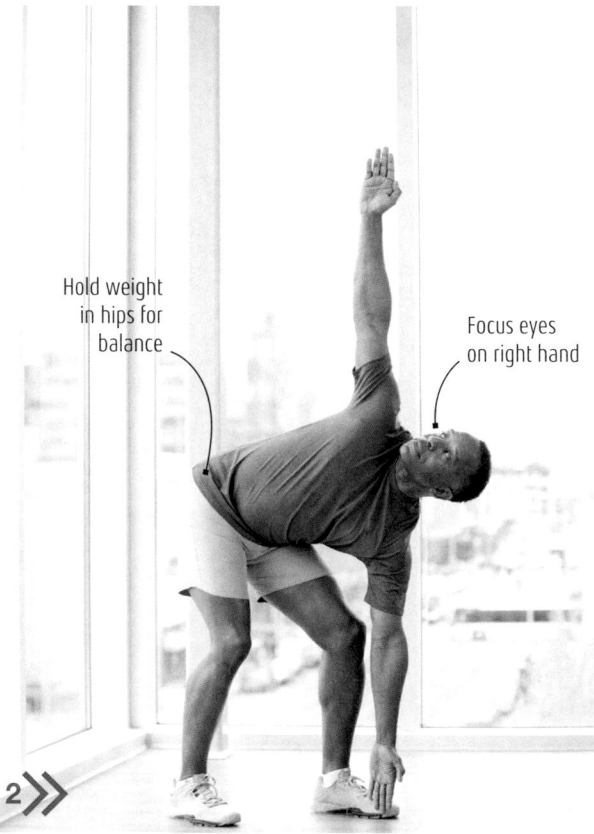

Hold weight in hips for balance

Focus eyes on right hand

2 >> Push your right hip out to your left and look up at your right hand. Keeping your back and arms straight and flexing your knees as necessary, bend to the left until your left hand touches the inside of your left foot.

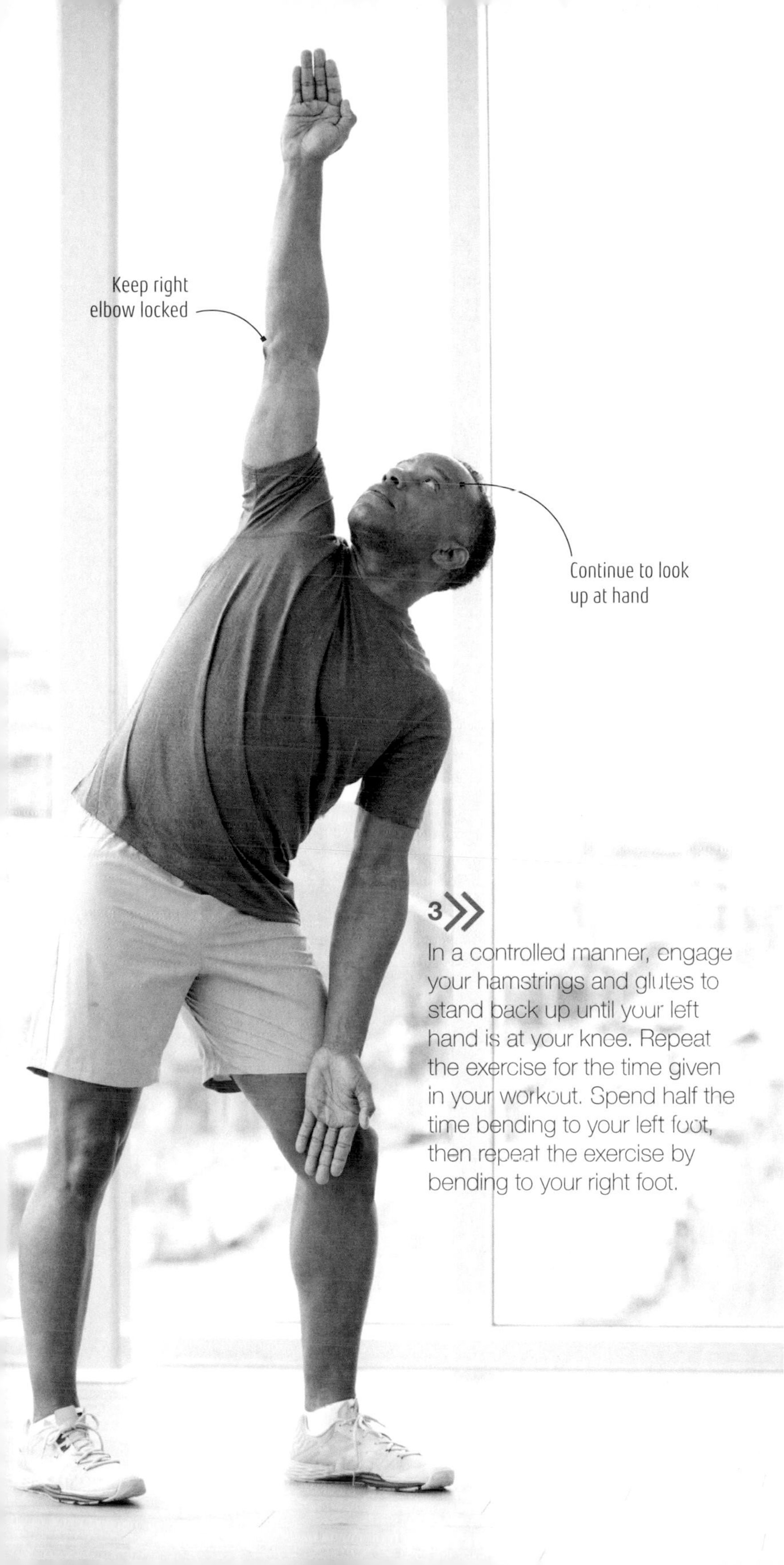

Keep right
elbow locked

Continue to look
up at hand

3 》

In a controlled manner, engage
your hamstrings and glutes to
stand back up until your left
hand is at your knee. Repeat
the exercise for the time given
in your workout. Spend half the
time bending to your left foot,
then repeat the exercise by
bending to your right foot.

■/// MAKE IT **easier**

If your flexibility is limited,
bend just until your hand
reaches your knee.

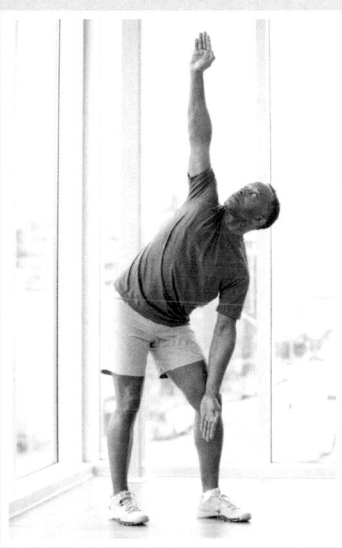

■/// MAKE IT **harder**

To increase resistance to
your shoulders and core,
hold a dumbbell in your
raised hand.

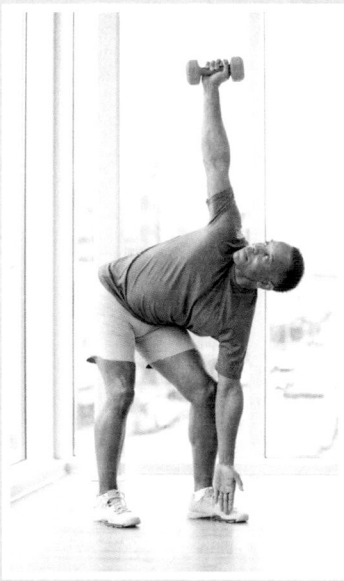

Over-the-shoulder squat

Lower-back injuries are one of the most common reasons for visits to the doctor and often occur from improperly lifting objects. Practice safe lifting and develop your lower-body strength with this weighted squat, which helps stabilize your spine and improve total-body coordination.

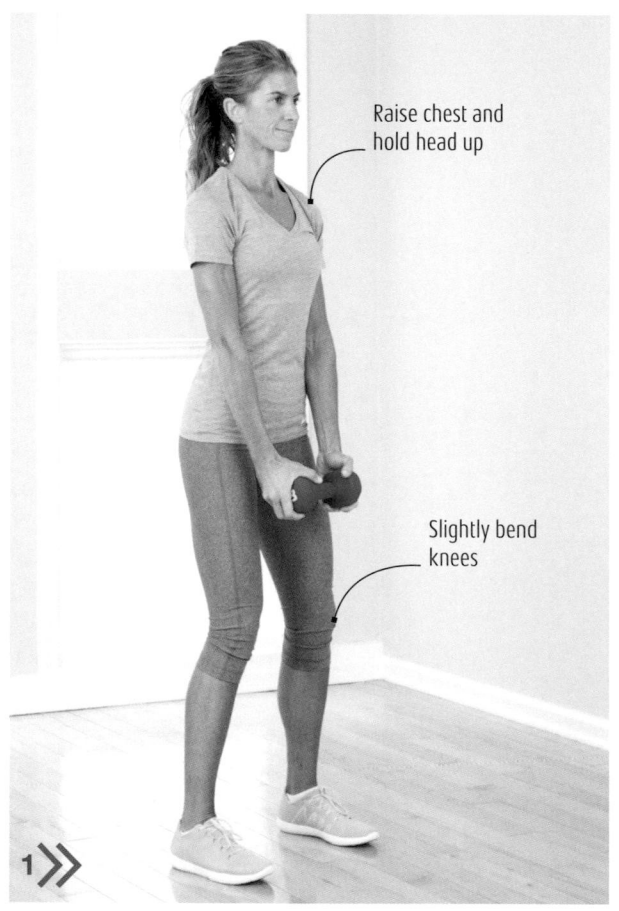

Raise chest and hold head up

Slightly bend knees

1 》》

Stand with your feet shoulder-width apart and hold the ends of a dumbbell with both hands. Let your arms hang straight down in front of you. Engage your core and retract your shoulder blades.

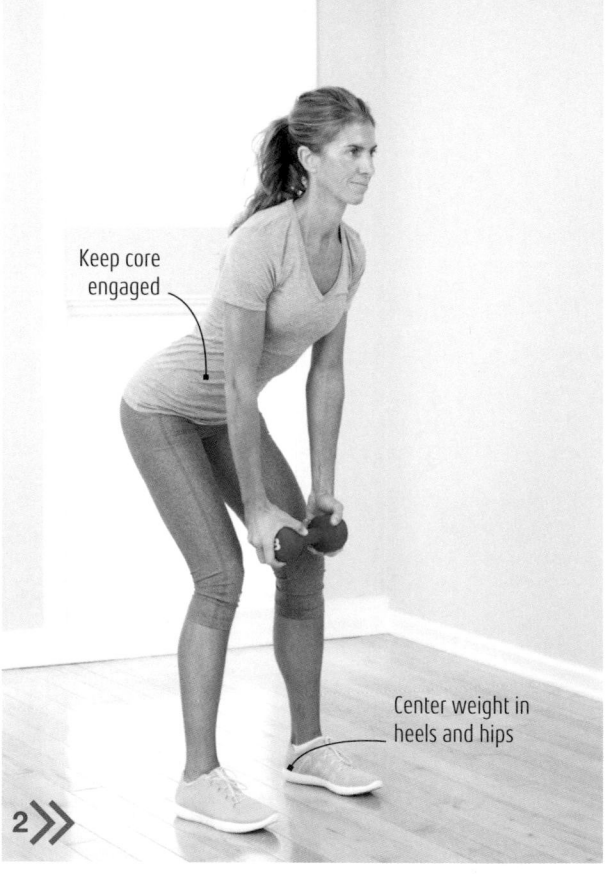

Keep core engaged

Center weight in heels and hips

2 》》

Push your glutes back and bend at your hips, letting the dumbbell move downward. Keep your back straight and your knees pointed in the same direction as your feet. Hold your head up.

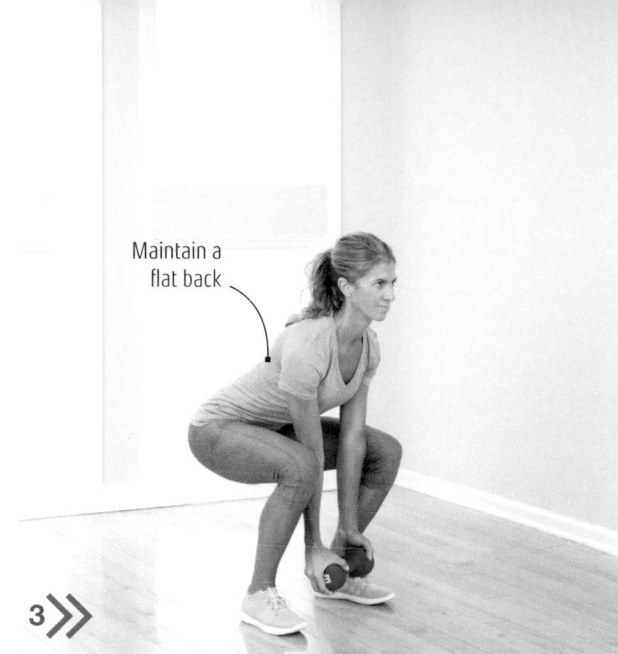

Maintain a flat back

3 »

In a quick, controlled manner, continue to bend your knees and sit back into a squat until your thighs are parallel to the ground. Let your arms hang straight down. Distribute your weight in your heels and hips.

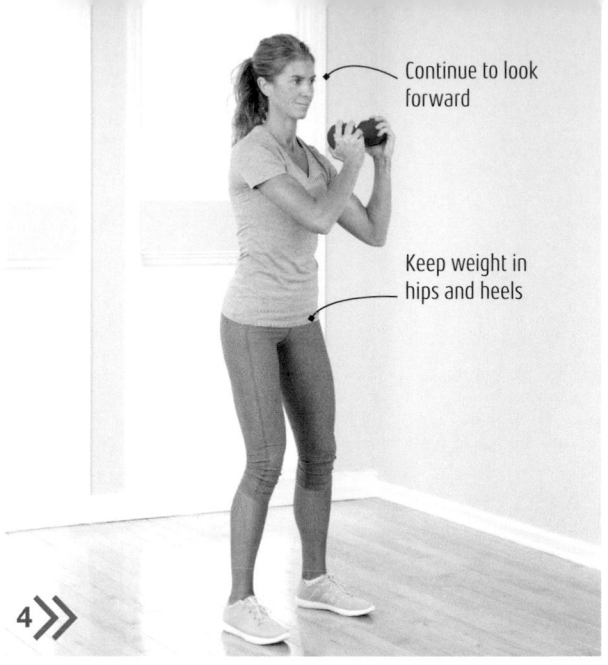

Continue to look forward

Keep weight in hips and heels

4 »

In one motion, quickly push through your heels to rise out of the squat until your legs are straight, and bend your elbows to swing the dumbbell up to your left shoulder.

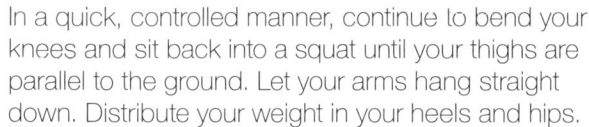

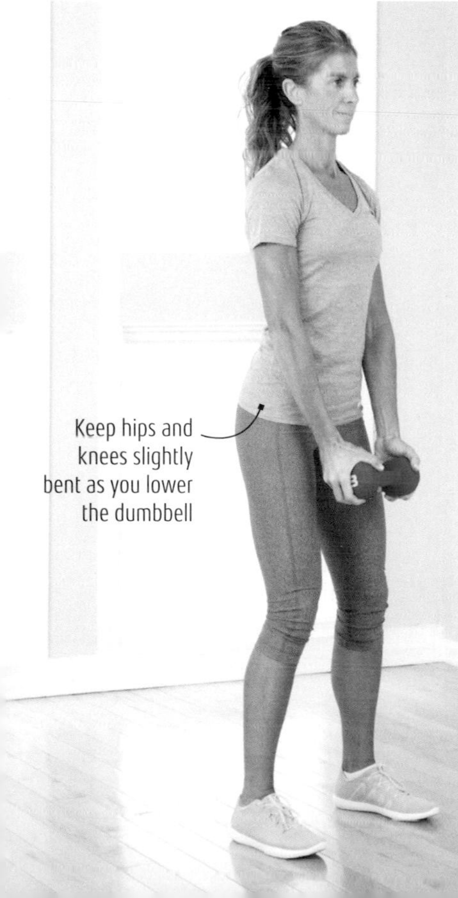

Keep hips and knees slightly bent as you lower the dumbbell

5 »

In a quick, controlled manner, return the dumbbell to the starting position and repeat the exercise by squatting then raising the dumbbell to your right shoulder. Continue to alternate the exercise to each side for the time given in your workout.

▰▰/// MAKE IT **easier**

To decrease resistance to your legs and shoulders, do the exercise without a dumbbell. Let your arms hang neutrally in front of you.

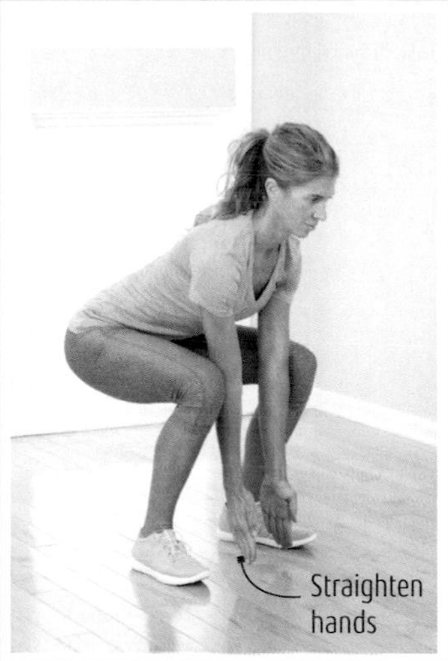

Straighten hands

Diagonal chop

IMPROVES
- ///// **Strength**
- ///// **Stability**
- ///// Mobility
- ///// **Endurance**

WHAT YOU NEED
Dumbbell

Most athletic movements involve a form of rotation, which requires your torso to generate and transfer power, but if your core is weak it can lead to poor performance or injury. Enhance your core strength, stability, and power with this energy-intensive chopping exercise.

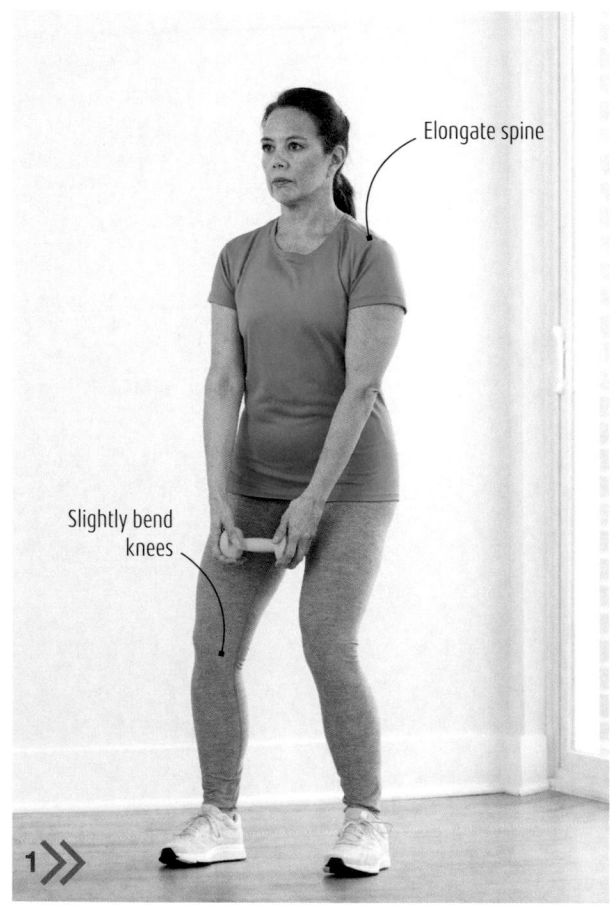

Elongate spine

Slightly bend knees

1 »

Stand with your feet shoulder-width apart. Hold the ends of a dumbbell with both hands and let your arms hang straight down in front of you. Engage your core and retract your shoulder blades.

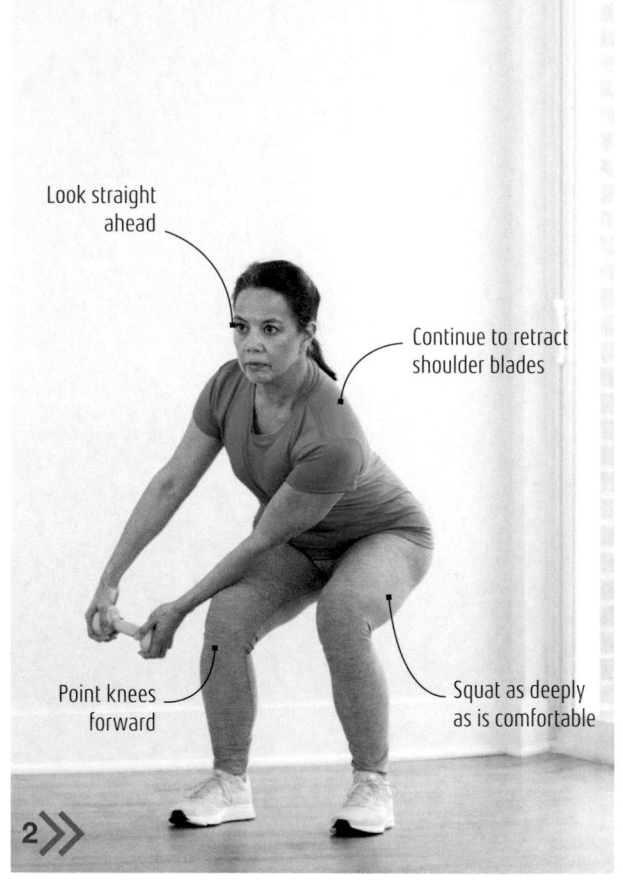

Look straight ahead

Continue to retract shoulder blades

Point knees forward

Squat as deeply as is comfortable

2 »

In one quick, controlled motion, push your glutes back and bend at your hips to sit back into a squat while rotating your core to lower the dumbbell to the outside of your right leg.

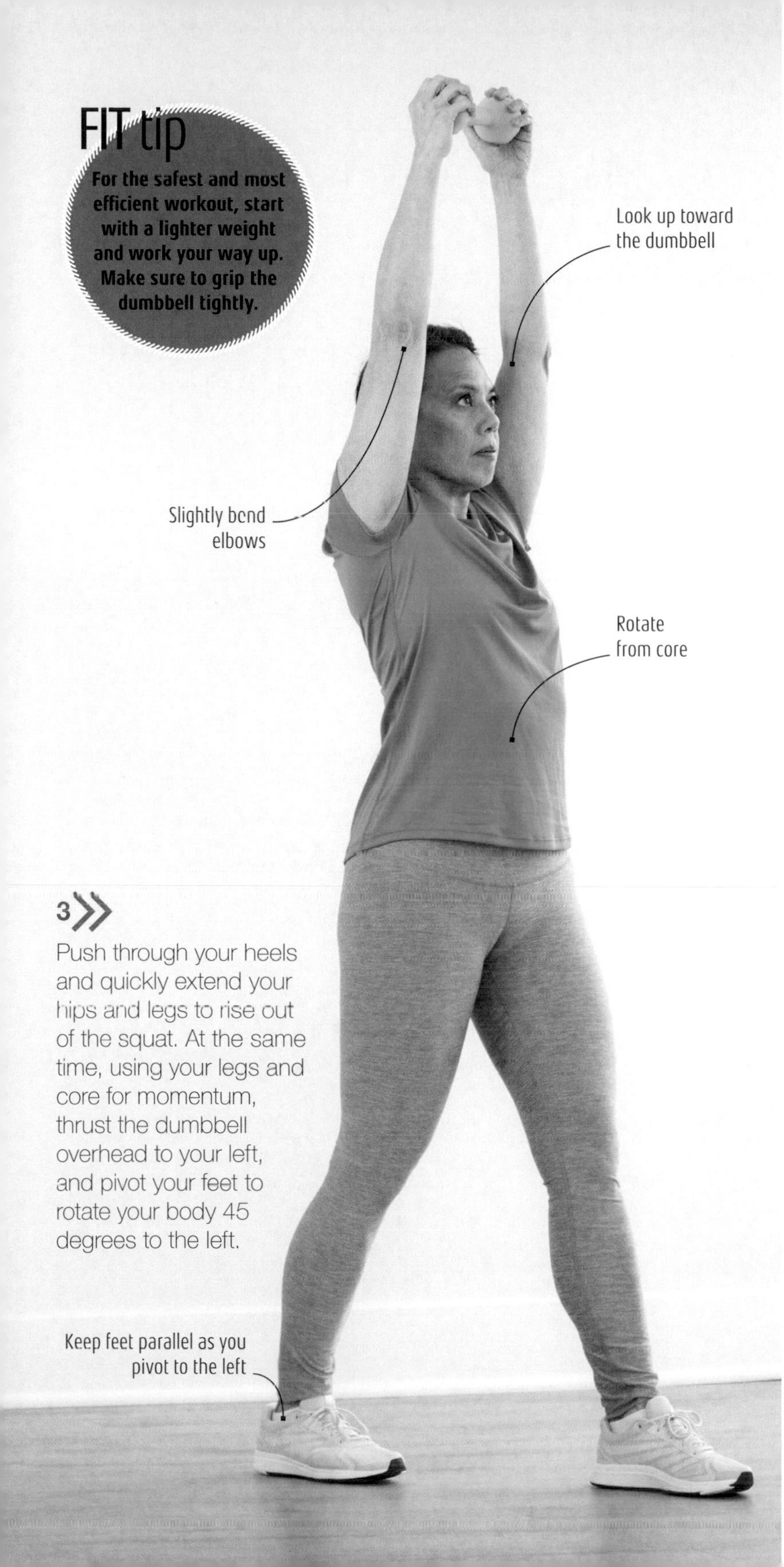

Look up toward the dumbbell
Slightly bend elbows
Rotate from core
Keep feet parallel as you pivot to the left

FIT tip

For the safest and most efficient workout, start with a lighter weight and work your way up. Make sure to grip the dumbbell tightly.

3 »

Push through your heels and quickly extend your hips and legs to rise out of the squat. At the same time, using your legs and core for momentum, thrust the dumbbell overhead to your left, and pivot your feet to rotate your body 45 degrees to the left.

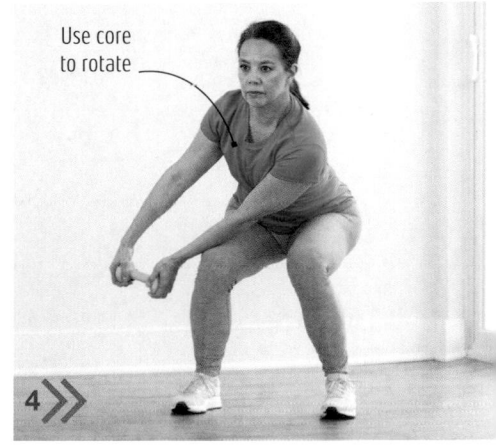

Use core to rotate

4 »

In a quick, controlled manner, enter into the next squat, pivot your feet to the starting position, and return the dumbbell to the outside of your right leg. Repeat for the time given. Spend half the time rotating to your left, then repeat to your right.

MAKE IT **easier**

To decrease the resistance to your legs, shoulders, and core, do the exercise without a dumbbell. Hold your hands in loose fists.

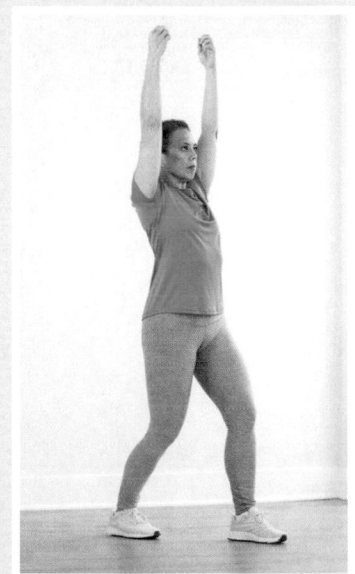

Suitcase squat

IMPROVES
- ▰/// **Strength**
- ▰/// **Stability**
- /// **Mobility**
- ▰/// **Endurance**

WHAT YOU NEED
Dumbbell

A lack of upper-leg strength can cause you to use your back muscles instead of your leg muscles for lifting heavy objects, which can lead to back injury. Perform this squat at a quick, controlled tempo to strengthen your quads and hamstrings, preparing you to safely lift anything from a suitcase to a child.

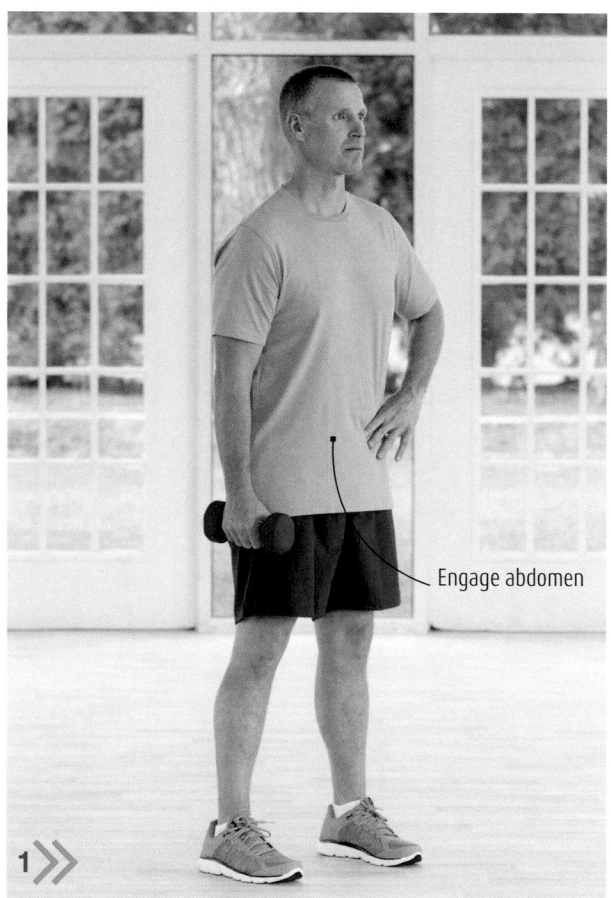

Engage abdomen

1 ≫

Stand with your feet shoulder-width apart. Hold a dumbbell in your right hand and let your right arm hang at your side. Place your left hand on your hip. Raise your head and retract your shoulder blades.

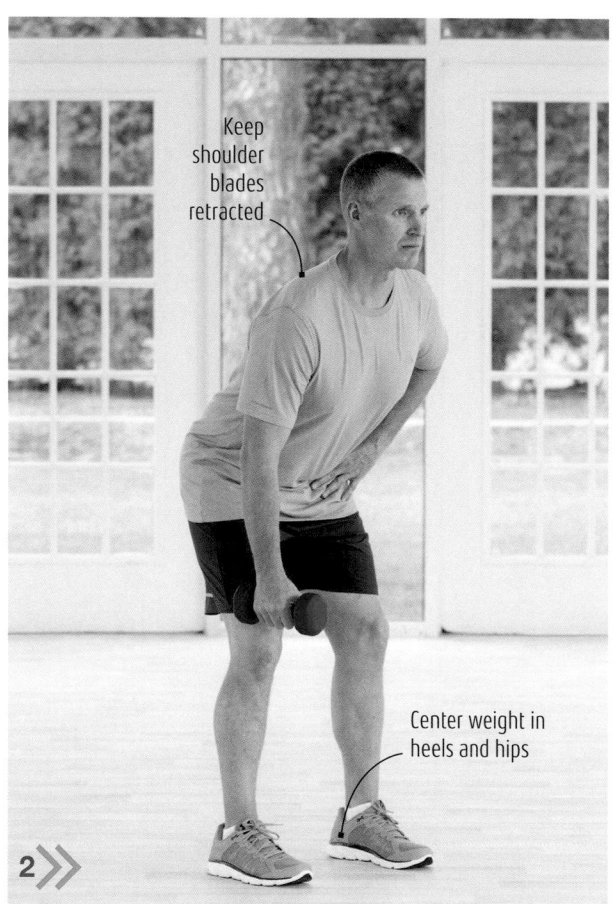

Keep shoulder blades retracted

Center weight in heels and hips

2 ≫

Push your glutes back and bend at your hips, letting the dumbbell move downward. Keep your back straight and keep your knees facing forward. Hold your head up.

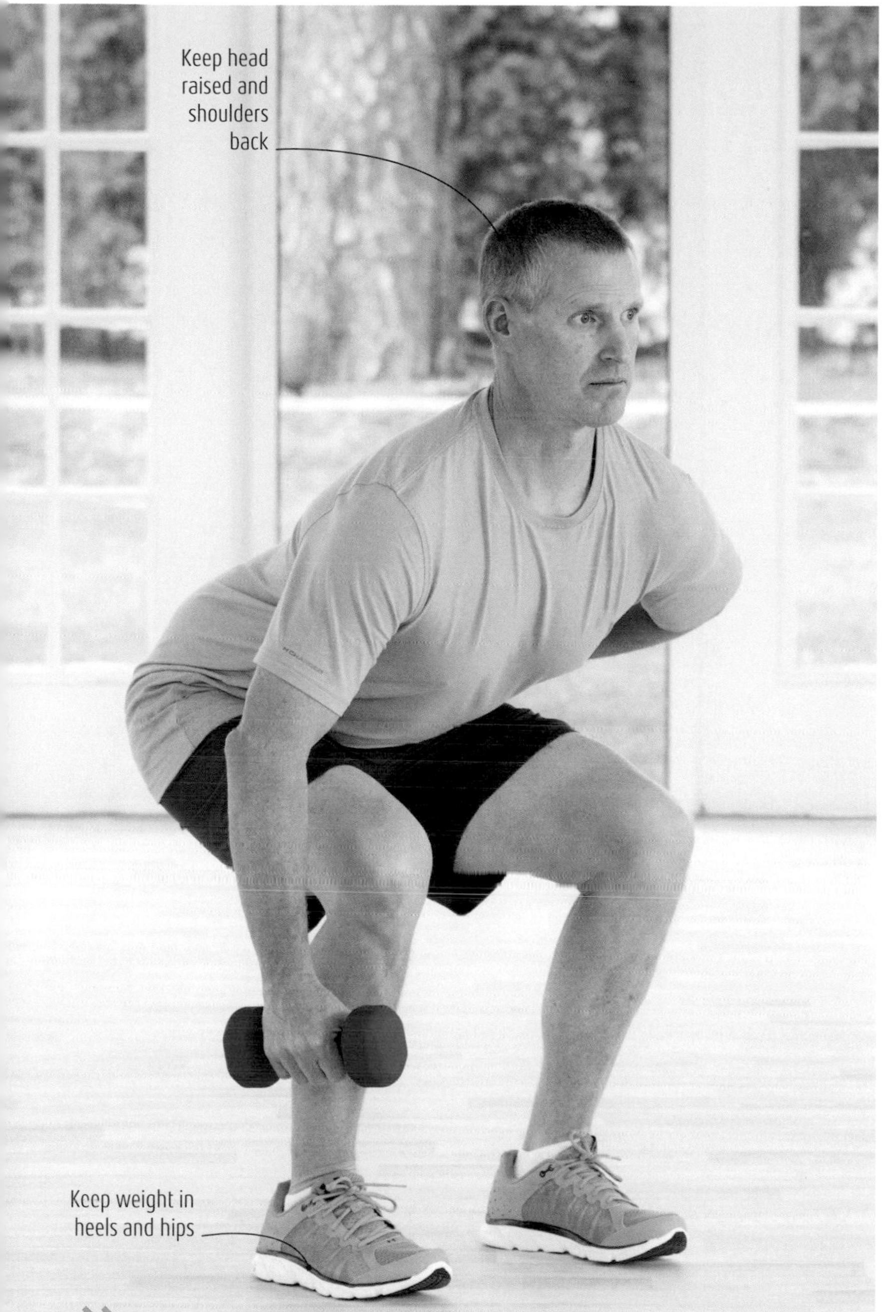

Keep head raised and shoulders back

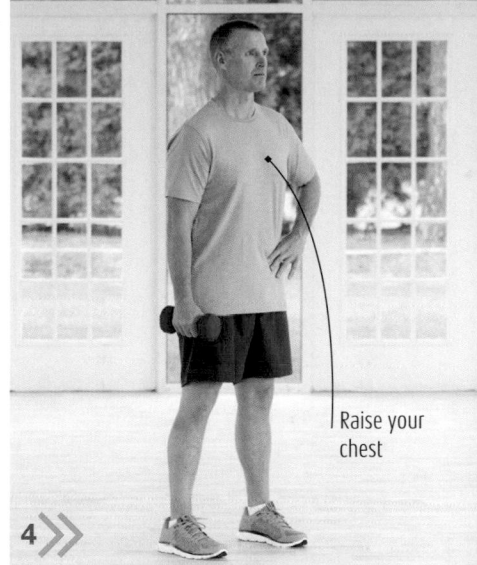

Raise your chest

4 »

Push through your heels and rise out of the squat. Repeat for the time given in your workout. Spend half the time with the dumbbell in your right hand, then switch to your left hand.

Keep weight in heels and hips

3 »

In a quick, controlled manner, continue to bend your knees and hips and sit back into a squat until your thighs are parallel to the ground. Let your right arm hang straight down.

///// MAKE IT **easier**

If it is difficult to balance, place a chair behind you and squat until your glutes lightly touch the chair.

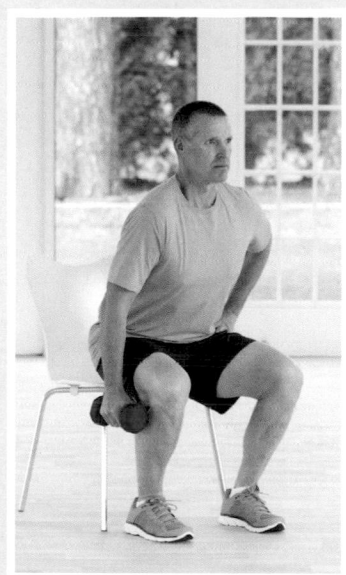

Walking reaching lunge

Your nervous system controls your movements, so it is important to train it for complex actions like bending down and reaching. Perform this exercise to build a strong mind-body connection in addition to improving your total-body strength and stability.

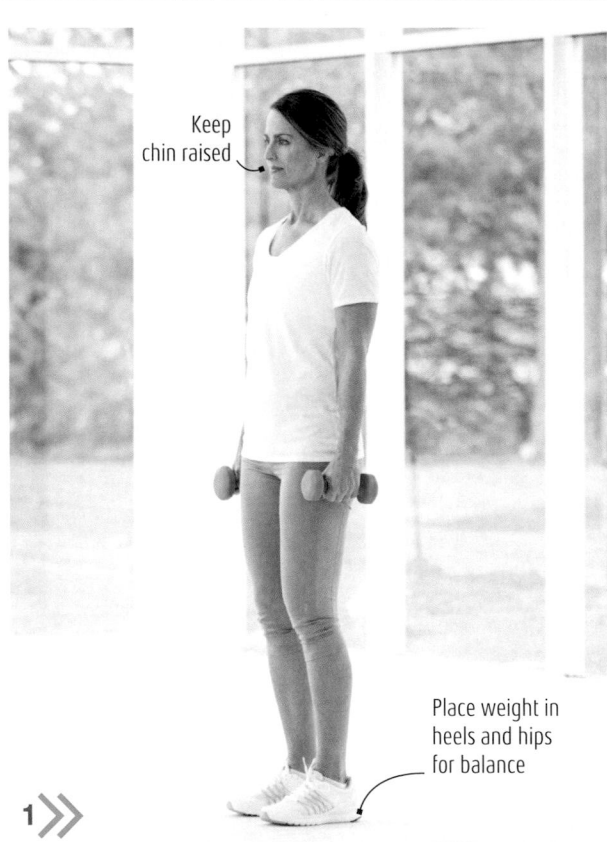

Keep chin raised

Place weight in heels and hips for balance

1 》》

Stand with your feet shoulder-width apart. Hold a dumbbell in each hand, palms facing inward, and let your arms hang at your sides. Engage your core and retract your shoulder blades.

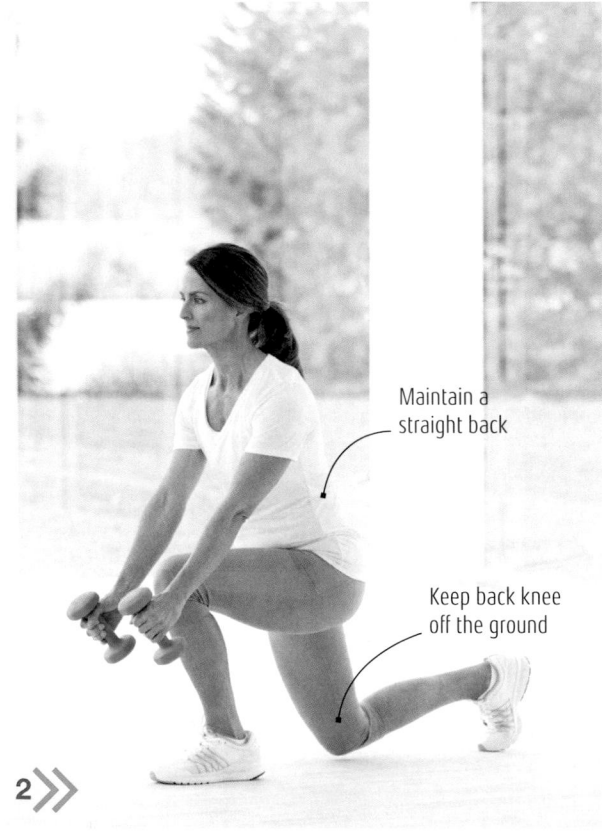

Maintain a straight back

Keep back knee off the ground

2 》》

In one quick, controlled motion, take a long step forward with your left leg, drop your right knee down until both knees are bent to 90 degrees, and extend the dumbbells down, past your left knee.

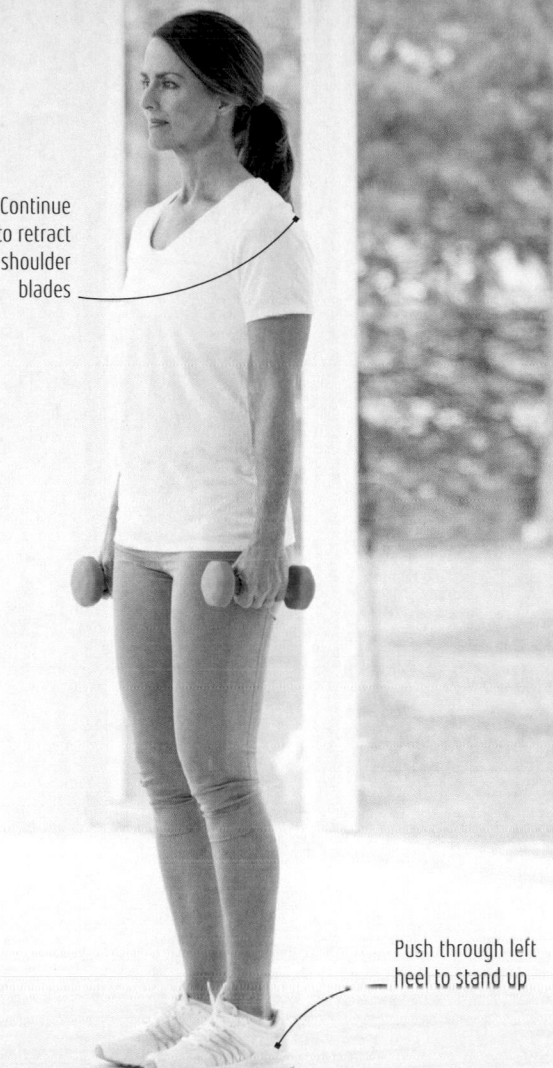

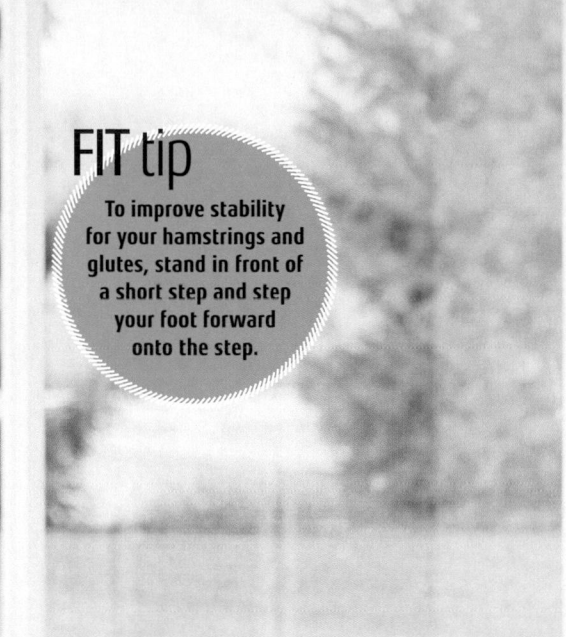

FIT tip

To improve stability for your hamstrings and glutes, stand in front of a short step and step your foot forward onto the step.

Continue to retract shoulder blades

Push through left heel to stand up

3 »

Quickly engage both legs to return to the starting position, while pulling the dumbbells back to your sides. Repeat the lunge by stepping forward with your right leg. Continue to alternate lunging on each side for the time given in your workout.

//// **MAKE IT easier**

To decrease the load on your legs, in step 1, step your right leg back into a staggered stance. In step 2, drop your right knee straight down into a lunge. Remain in the staggered stance for each repetition. Reverse your stance halfway through.

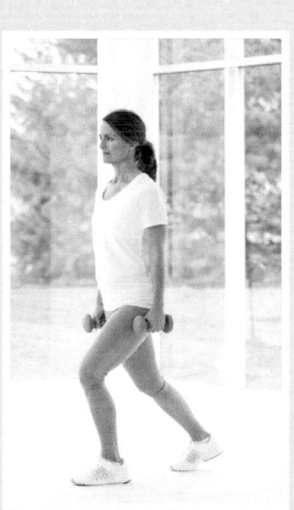

//// **MAKE IT harder**

To strengthen your arms, in step 3, after rising out of the lunge, engage your biceps to curl the dumbbells to shoulder height, then lower them again before doing the next lunge.

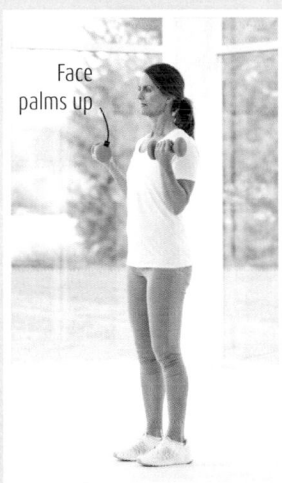

Face palms up

IMPROVES
//// **Posture**
■■// **Strength**
■// **Stability**
//// **Mobility**
■// **Endurance**

WHAT YOU NEED
Dumbbell

Reverse lunge with twist

Everyday activities like walking, hiking, and climbing stairs require a unique combination of strength and stability. Perform this dynamic exercise to strengthen your legs and prepare your body to functionally tackle activities that demand lower-body stability.

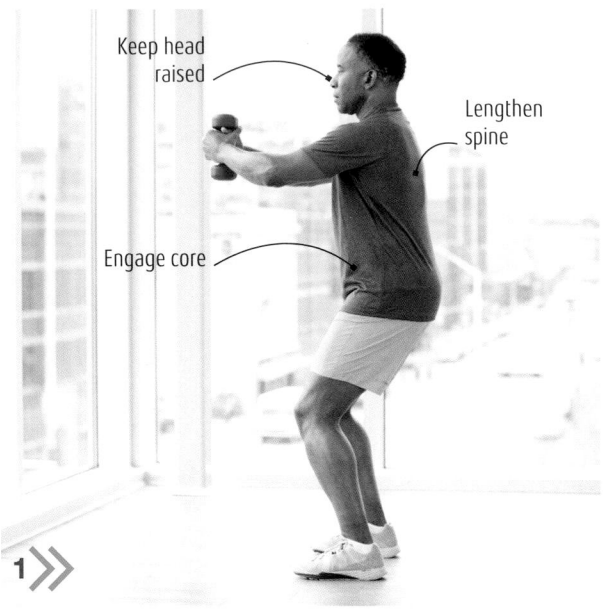

Keep head raised

Lengthen spine

Engage core

1 》》

Stand with your feet shoulder-width apart. Hold a dumbbell with both hands. Raise the dumbbell to chest height and slightly bend your elbows out to your sides. Retract your shoulder blades.

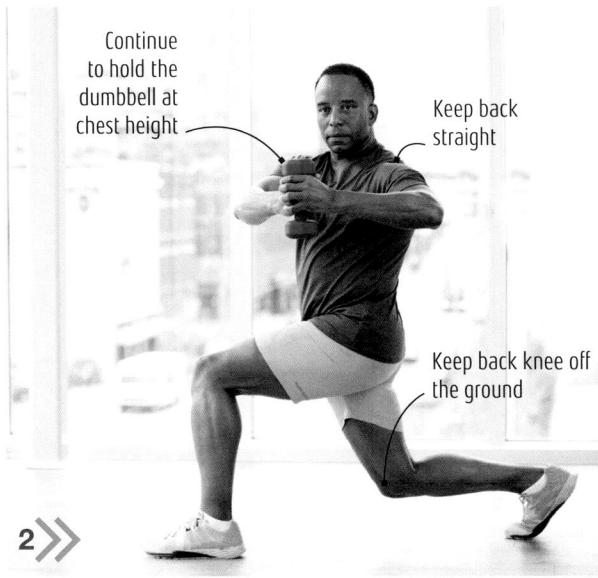

Continue to hold the dumbbell at chest height

Keep back straight

Keep back knee off the ground

2 》》

In a controlled manner, step your right leg back and drop your right knee down until both knees are bent to 90 degrees. Simultaneously engage your core to rotate your upper body 90 degrees to the left.

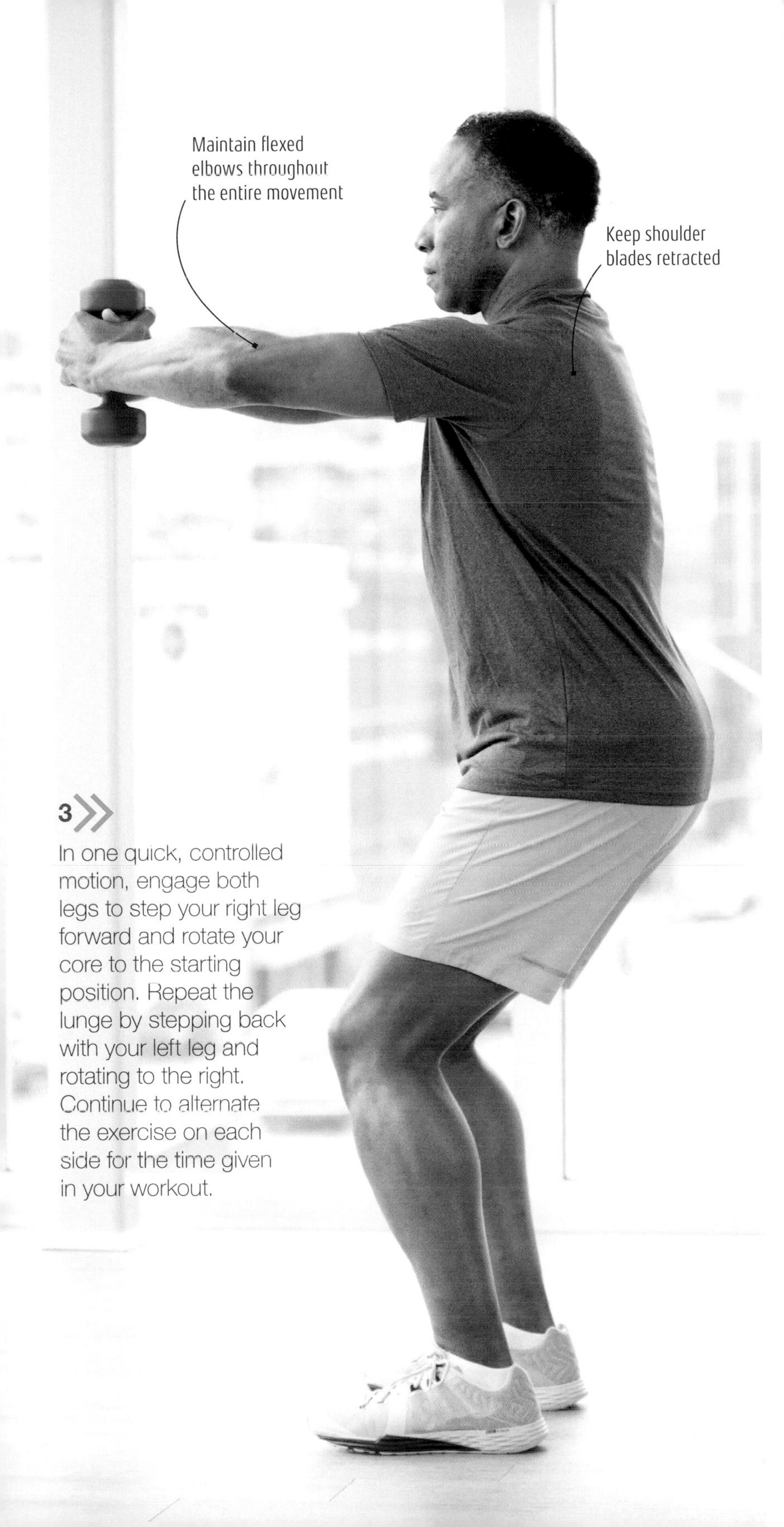

Maintain flexed elbows throughout the entire movement

Keep shoulder blades retracted

3 »

In one quick, controlled motion, engage both legs to step your right leg forward and rotate your core to the starting position. Repeat the lunge by stepping back with your left leg and rotating to the right. Continue to alternate the exercise on each side for the time given in your workout.

//// MAKE IT **easier**

To decrease resistance to your legs, in step 1, step your left leg back into a staggered stance. In step 2, drop your left knee straight down into a lunge. Remain in the staggered stance for each repetition. Reverse your stance halfway through.

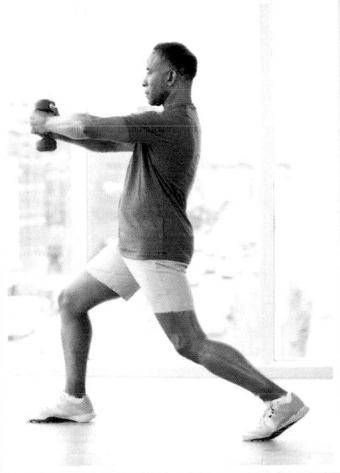

Posterior swing

This exercise strengthens your glutes, lower back, and hamstrings, doing wonders to counteract the negative effects of prolonged sitting. Use this powerful swinging movement to improve your posture and become more upright, open, and extended.

IMPROVES
//// **Posture**
//// **Strength**
//// **Stability**
//// Mobility
//// **Endurance**

WHAT YOU NEED
Dumbbell

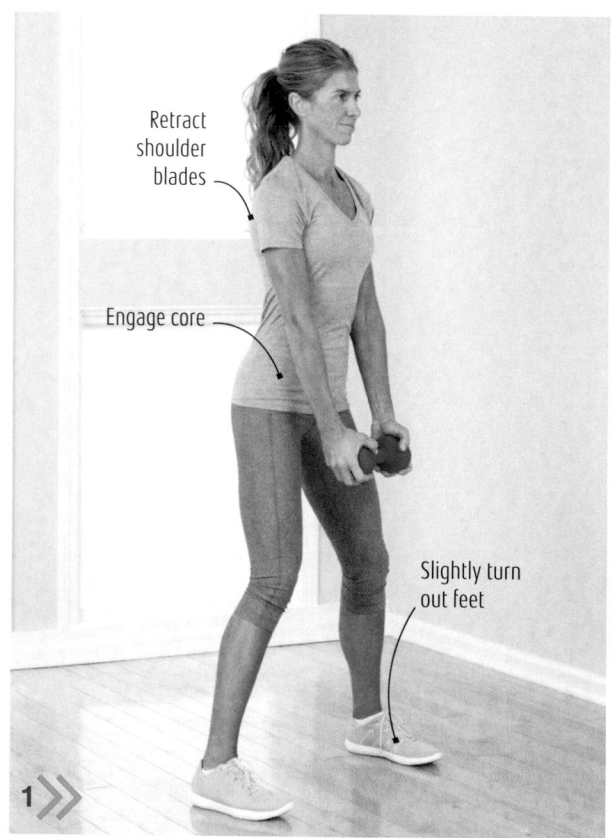

Retract shoulder blades

Engage core

Slightly turn out feet

1 >>

Stand with your feet slightly wider than shoulder-width apart. Firmly hold the ends of a dumbbell with both hands and let your arms hang straight down in front of you. Slightly bend your knees and hips.

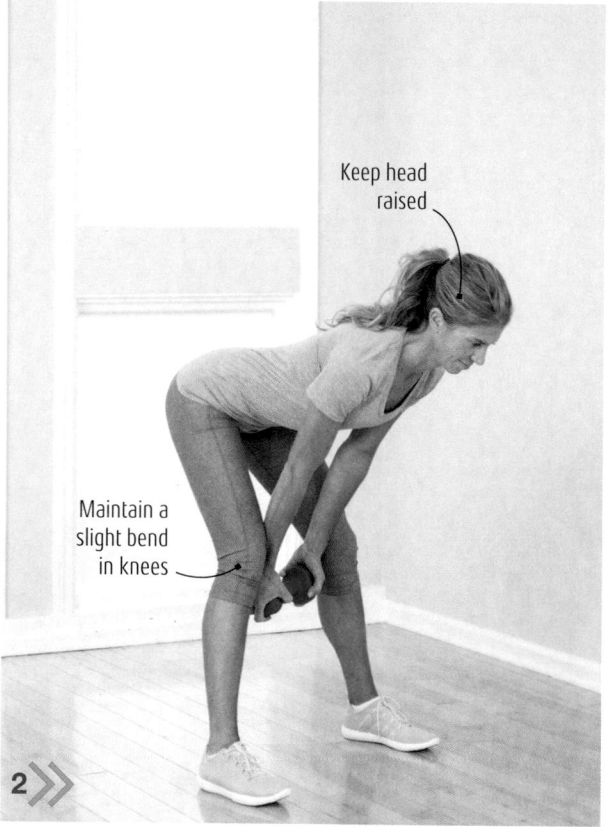

Keep head raised

Maintain a slight bend in knees

2 >>

Keeping your arms straight, quickly push your hips back, bend at the waist, and swing the dumbbell between your legs. Keep your back straight and avoid hunching forward.

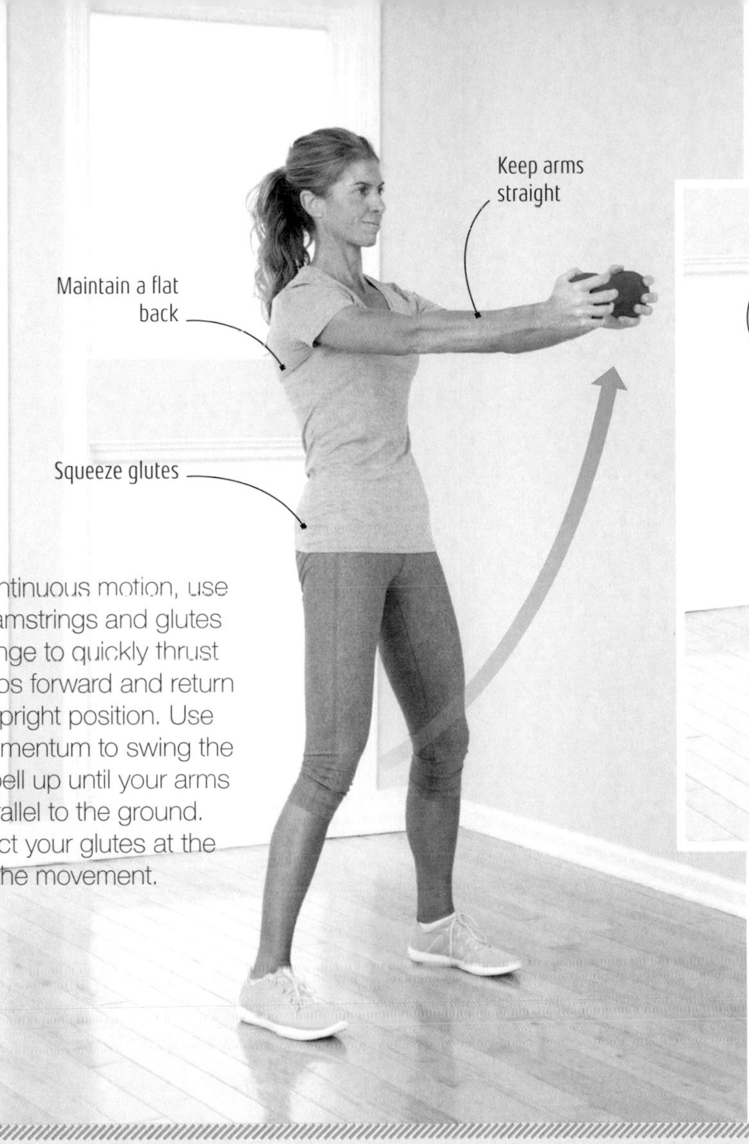

Keep arms straight

Maintain a flat back

Squeeze glutes

3 »

In a continuous motion, use your hamstrings and glutes as a hinge to quickly thrust your hips forward and return to an upright position. Use the momentum to swing the dumbbell up until your arms are parallel to the ground. Contract your glutes at the top of the movement.

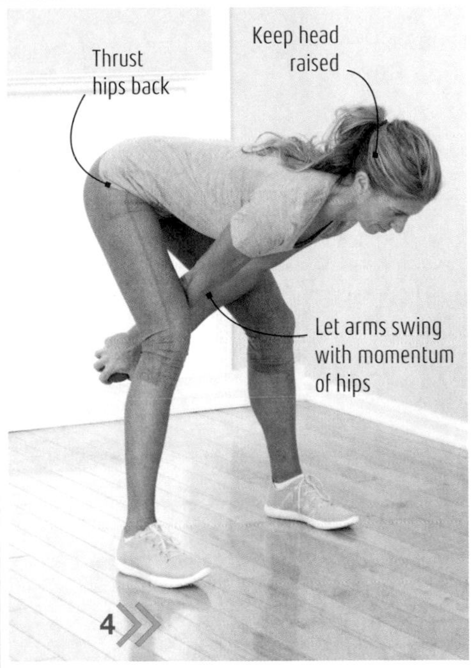

Thrust hips back

Keep head raised

Let arms swing with momentum of hips

4 »

Immediately thrust your hips back and swing the dumbbell between your legs for the next repetition. Continue to repeat the exercise swiftly for the time given in your workout.

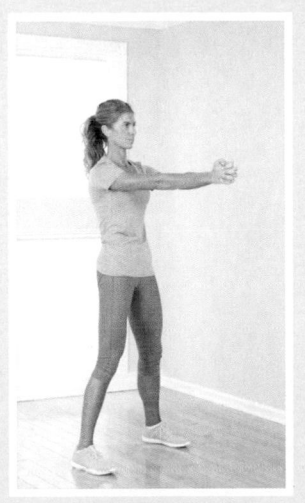

▨/// MAKE IT **easier**

To reduce resistance to your back, do the exercise without a dumbbell. Instead, lock your fingers together to make a fist.

▨/// MAKE IT **harder**

To increase resistance to your shoulders and upper back, in step 3, swing the dumbbell straight overhead.

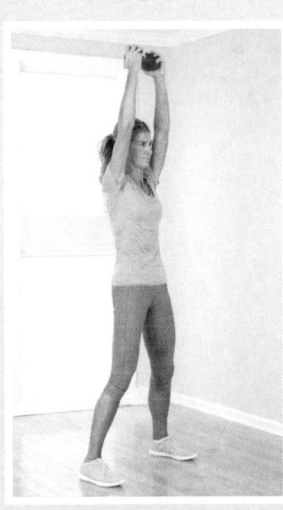

IMPROVES
//// Posture
//// Strength
//// Stability
//// Mobility

WHAT YOU NEED
Dumbbells

Good morning

Your glutes are the largest and most powerful muscle group in the body. Strong glutes can improve posture; alleviate lower back, hip, and knee pain; and even reduce bone density loss. Use this controlled power movement to strengthen these essential lower-body muscles.

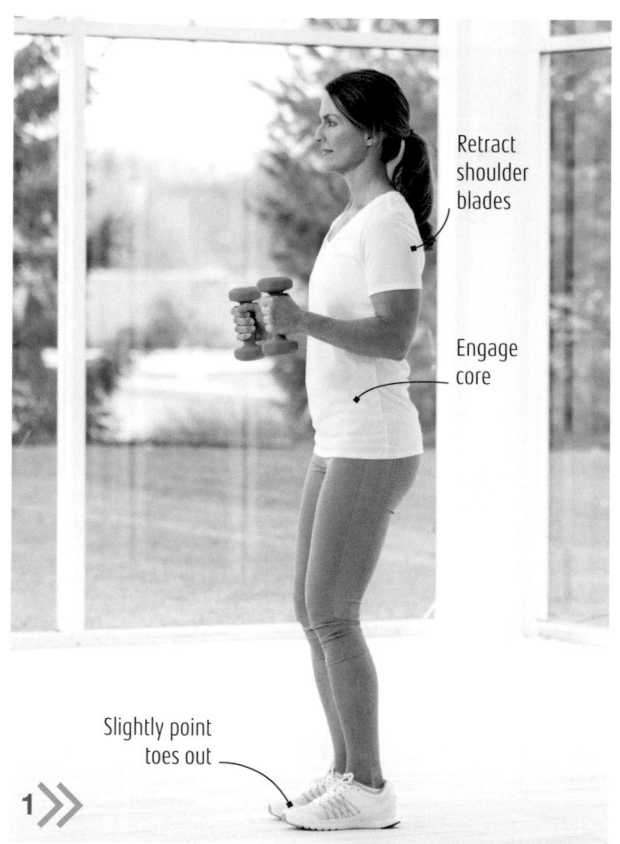

Retract shoulder blades

Engage core

Slightly point toes out

1 »

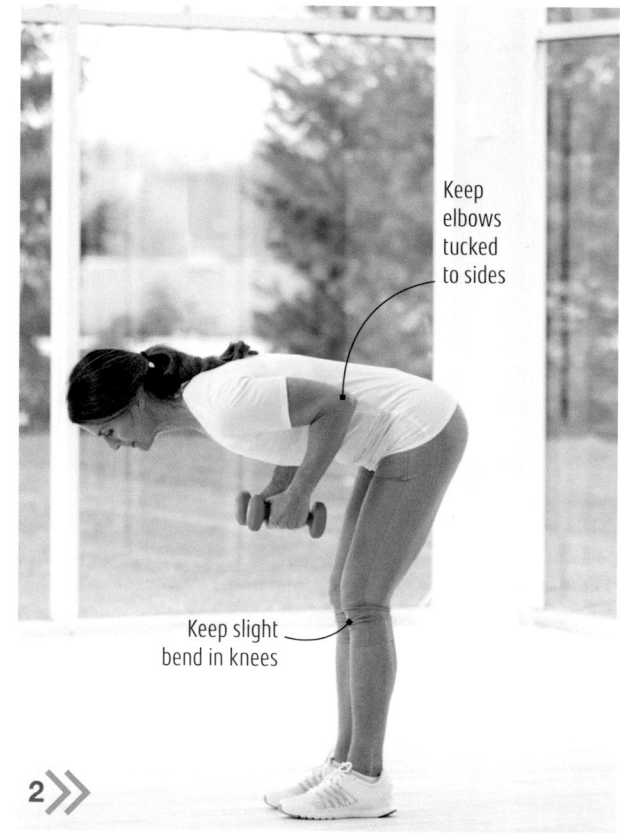

Keep elbows tucked to sides

Keep slight bend in knees

2 »

Stand with your feet shoulder-width apart. Hold a dumbbell in each hand, palms facing inward. Bend your elbows to 90 degrees, and raise the dumbbells to waist height. Slightly bend your knees and hips.

Keeping your back straight, push your hips back and bend over at the waist until your upper body is parallel to the ground. Maintain a slight bend in your knees, but avoid lowering yourself with your knees.

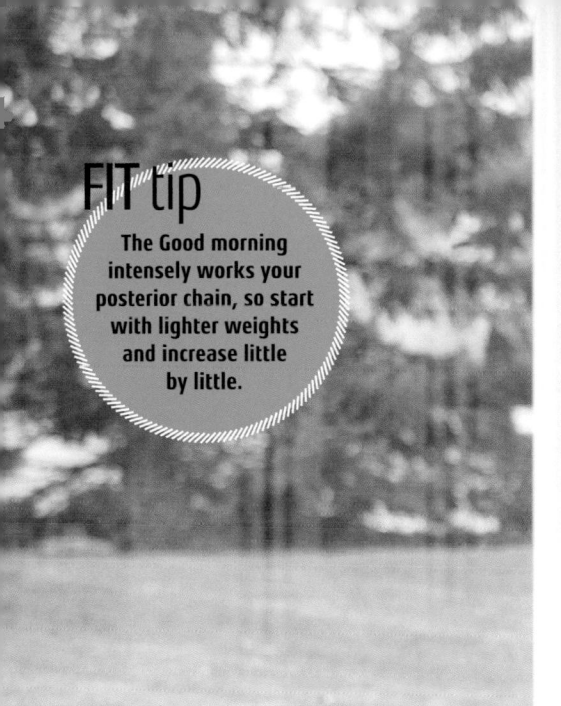

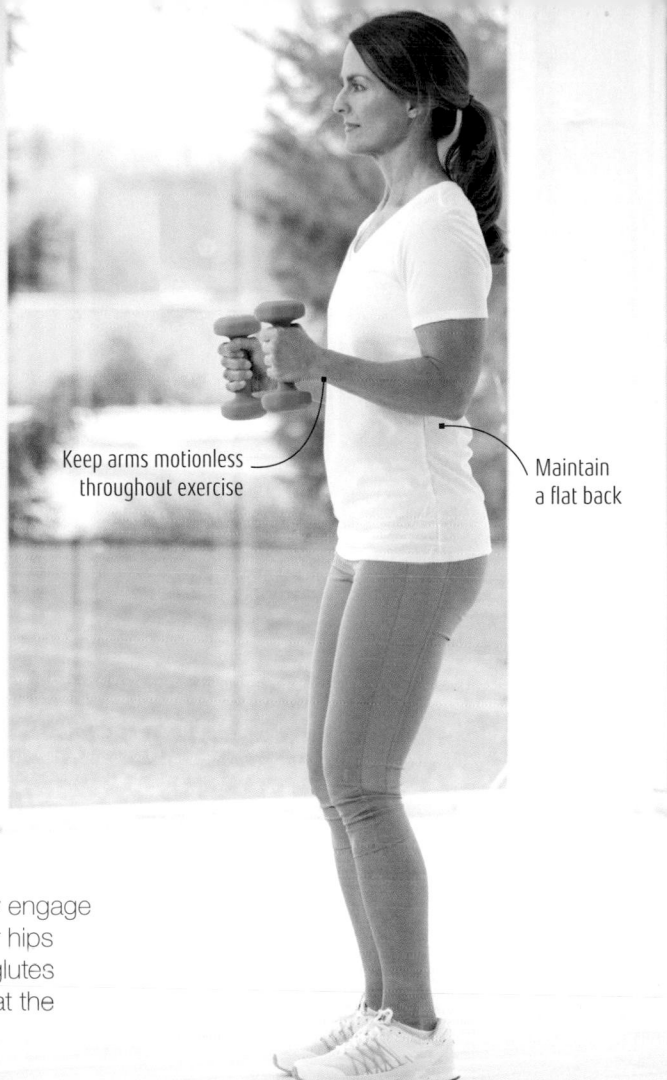

Keep arms motionless throughout exercise

Maintain a flat back

3 »

Using your hips and glutes as a hinge, quickly engage your hamstrings and lower back to thrust your hips forward to an upright position. Contract your glutes at the top of the movement. Continue to repeat the exercise for the time given in your workout.

///// MAKE IT **easier**

If it is difficult to maintain balance, do the exercise without weights. Place your hands behind your head and extend your elbows out to the sides.

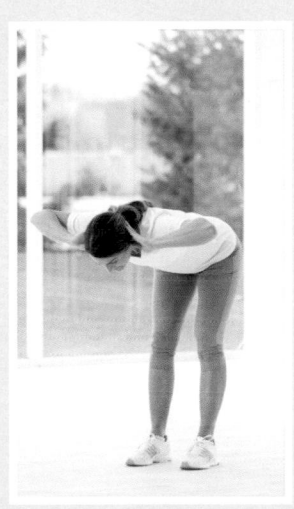

///// MAKE IT **harder**

To strengthen your upper back, after step 2, extend your arms straight down to lower the dumbbells. Then engage your upper-back muscles to pull the dumbbells back from your elbows before continuing to step 3.

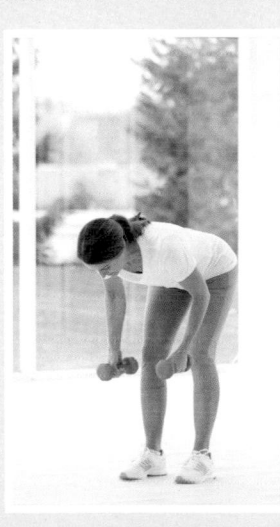

IMPROVES
▰/// Posture
▰/// **Strength**
▰/// **Stability**
▰/// Mobility
▰/// **Endurance**

WHAT YOU NEED
Dumbbells

Sumo deadlift and upright row

The deadlift is a full-body move that strengthens nearly every muscle in your body. Incorporating it with the wide stance enables you to more easily lift heavy objects. Perform this exercise to prevent or rehabilitate lifting injuries.

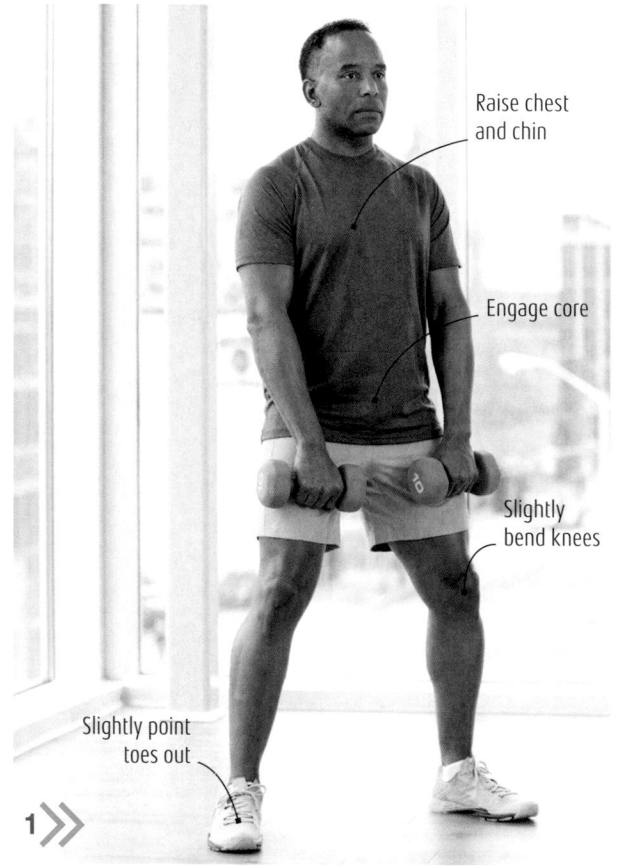

Raise chest and chin

Engage core

Slightly bend knees

Slightly point toes out

1 ≫ Stand with your feet wider than shoulder-width apart. Hold a dumbbell in each hand, and let your arms hang in front of your body, palms facing your thighs. Engage your core and retract your shoulder blades.

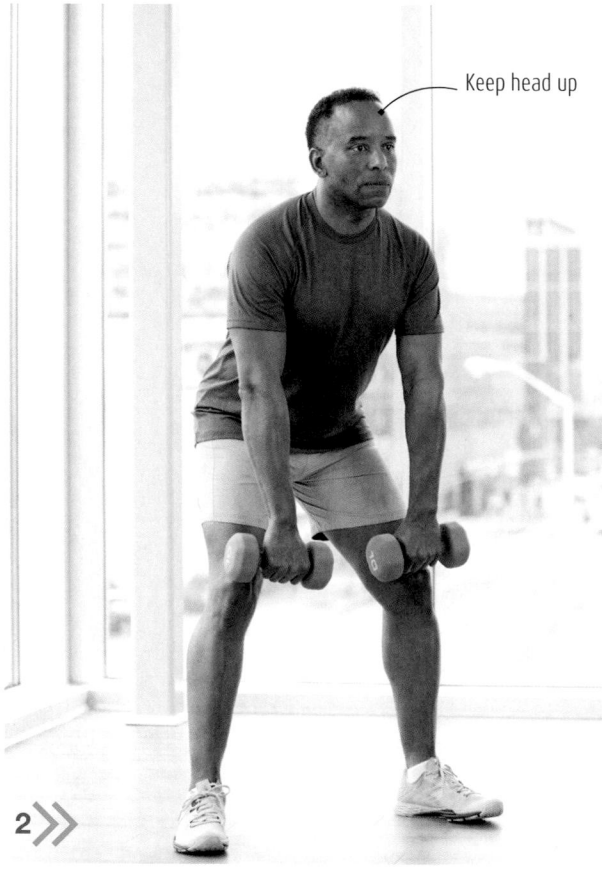

Keep head up

2 ≫ Push your glutes back and bend at your hips, letting the dumbbells move downward. Keep your back straight and hold your head up. Continue to retract your shoulder blades.

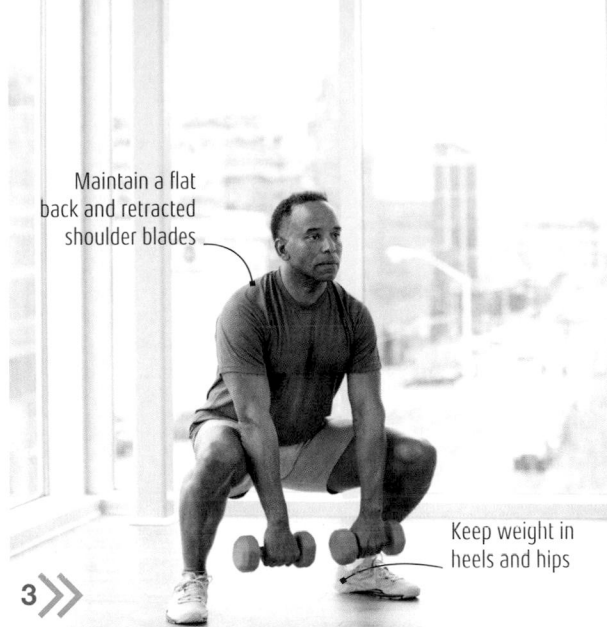

Maintain a flat back and retracted shoulder blades

Keep weight in heels and hips

3 »

In a quick, controlled manner, continue to bend your knees and sit back into a squat until your thighs are parallel to the ground. Let the dumbbells hang straight down between your legs.

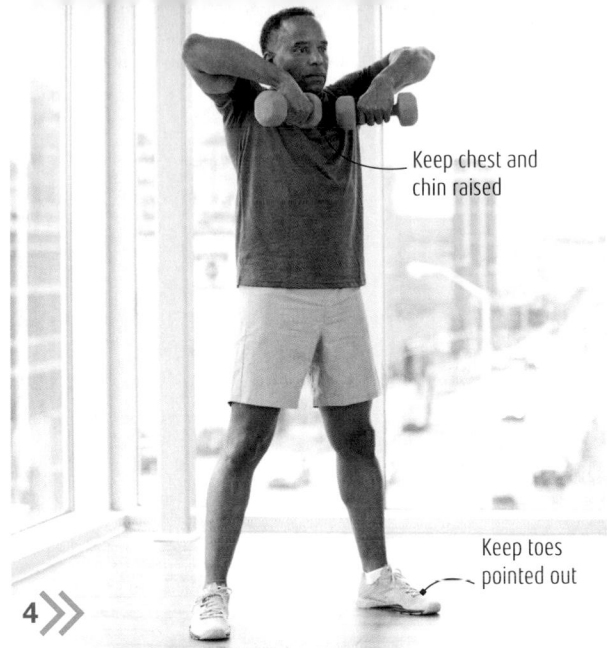

Keep chest and chin raised

Keep toes pointed out

4 »

In one swift motion, push through your heels and rise out of the squat until your legs are straight, and pull the dumbbells straight up until they are at chest height. Keep your core engaged.

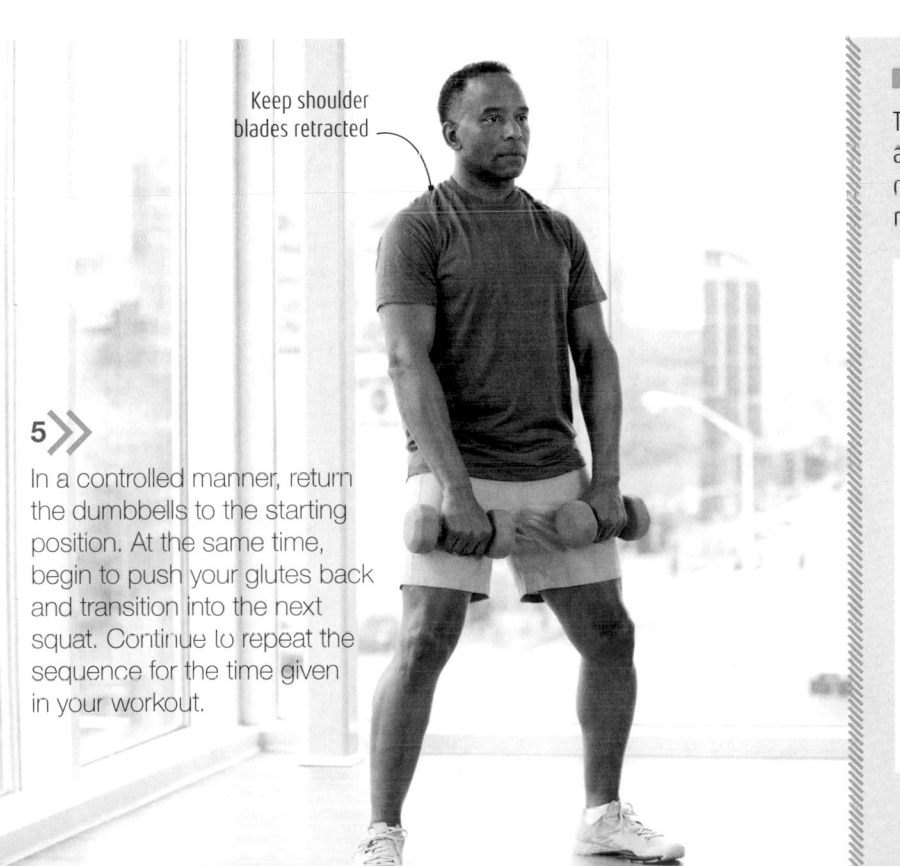

Keep shoulder blades retracted

5 »

In a controlled manner, return the dumbbells to the starting position. At the same time, begin to push your glutes back and transition into the next squat. Continue to repeat the sequence for the time given in your workout.

///// **MAKE IT easier**

To decrease resistance to your legs and back, do the movement without dumbbells. Let your arms hang neutrally in front of you.

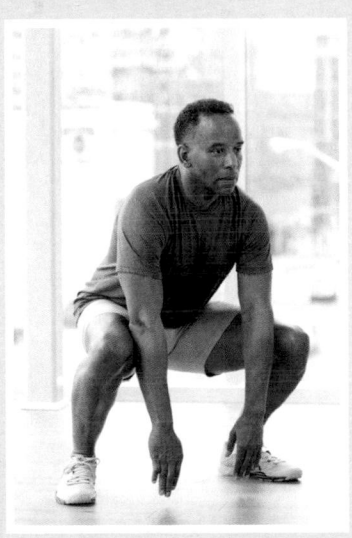

IMPROVES
▨//// Posture
▰//// Strength
▰//// Stability
▨//// Mobility

WHAT YOU NEED
Mat

Hip-ups

Your glutes can become weak and stiff when you don't use them often. Perform this powerful and controlled exercise to awaken your glutes and hip muscles and to improve your core and lower-body strength. This exercise will help you more safely execute common movements, such as standing up from a seated position.

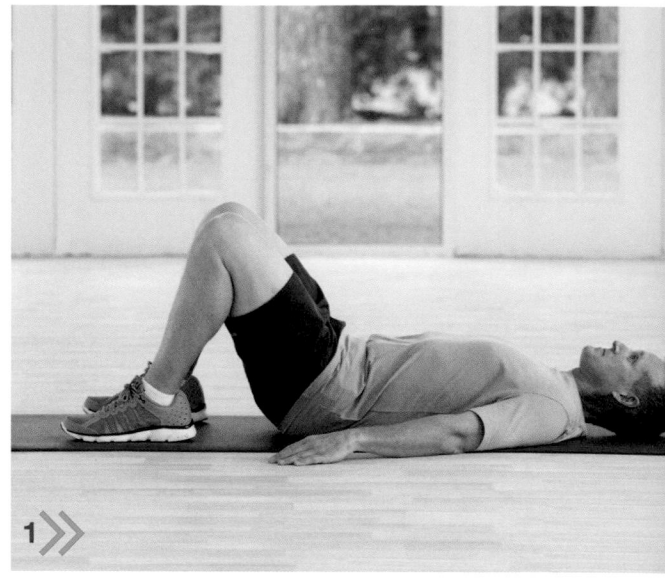

1 »

Lie on your back, bend your knees, and plant your feet flat on the ground, hip-width apart. Raise your chin and relax your arms by your sides, palms facing down.

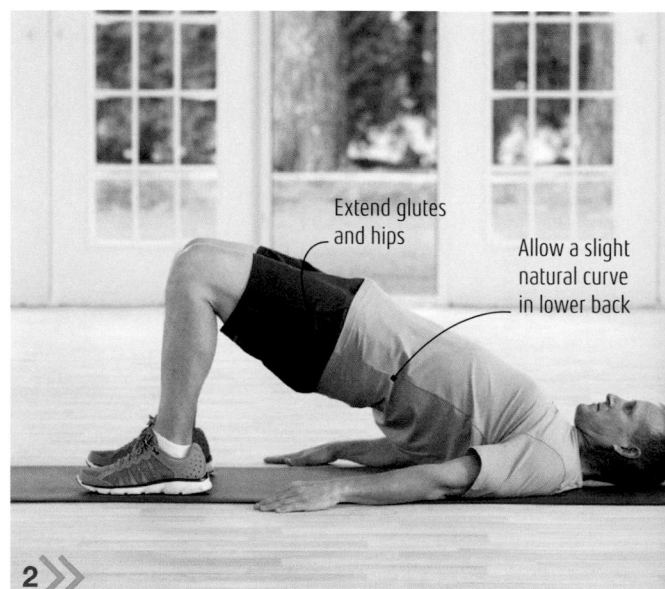

Extend glutes and hips

Allow a slight natural curve in lower back

2 »

Forcefully push your heels into the ground and raise your hips until you form a straight line from your knees to your shoulders. Contract your glutes and abdominals at the top of the movement.

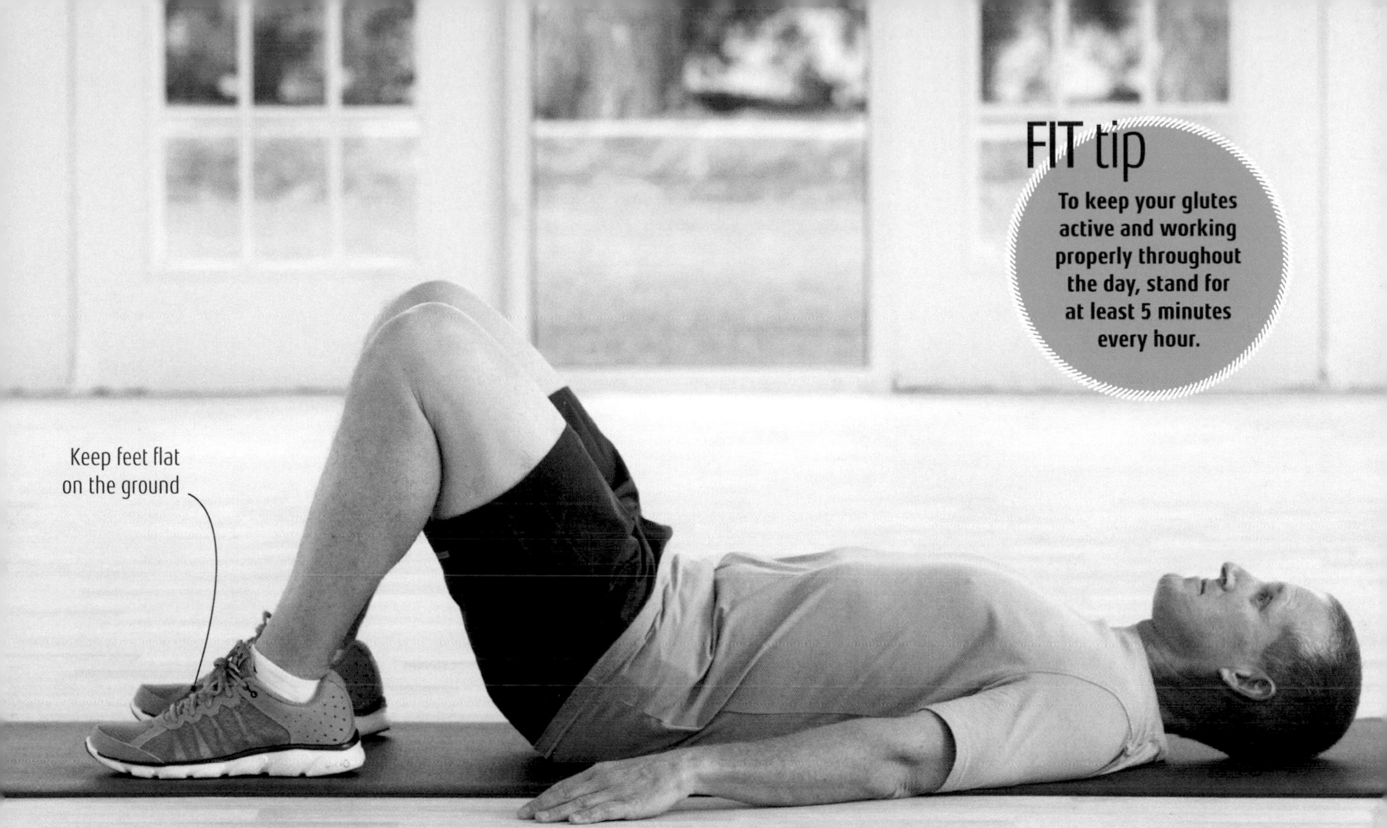

Keep feet flat on the ground

FIT tip

To keep your glutes active and working properly throughout the day, stand for at least 5 minutes every hour.

3

Using your glutes and abdominals for control, take three seconds to lower your hips to the ground. Continue to repeat the exercise for the time given in your workout.

MAKE IT **harder**

To increase resistance to your glutes, in step 2, raise one leg straight up until perpendicular to the ground. Push through your opposite heel to raise your hips. Then continue to step 3 while leaving your leg extended. Halfway through the given time, switch your legs.

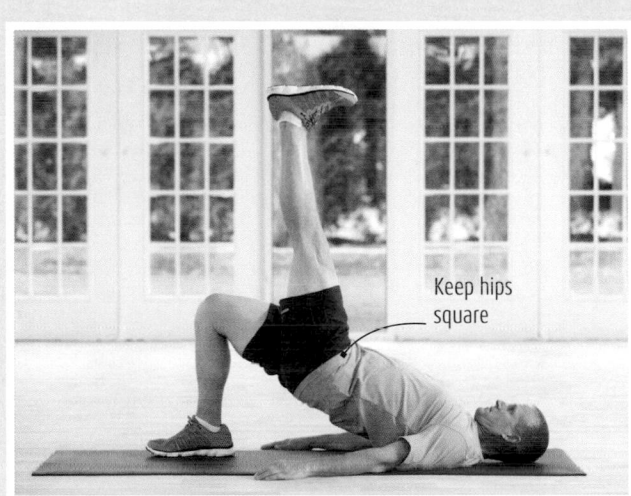

Keep hips square

Earthquakes

IMPROVES
/// **Strength**
/// **Stability**
/// **Mobility**
/// **Endurance**

WHAT YOU NEED
Dumbbell

Many activities, such as digging with a shovel, hammering, or pressing the lid down on a container, require you to generate downward power. Perform this total-body exercise swiftly to help you generate core strength for executing movements in a downward direction.

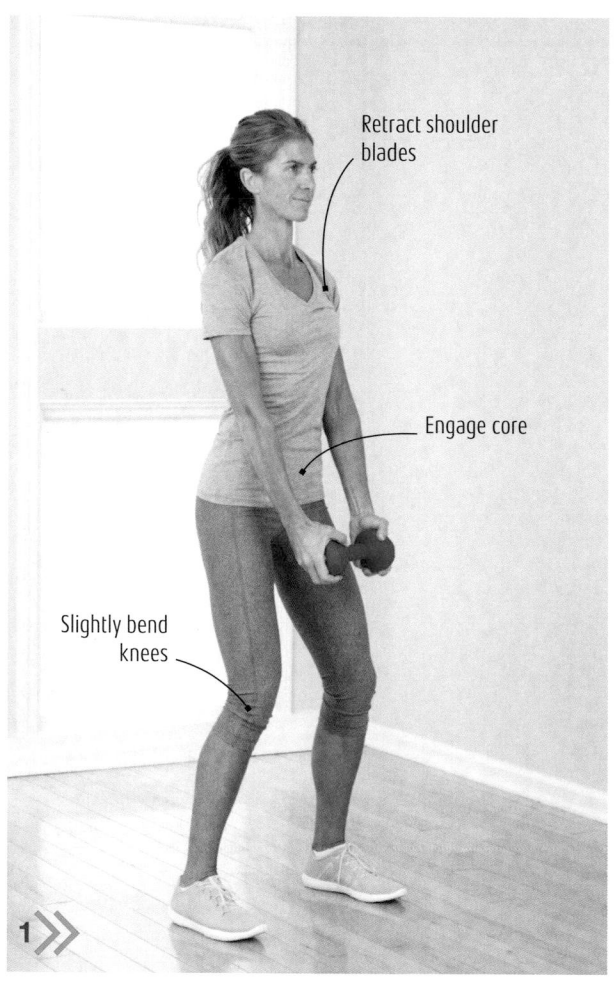

Retract shoulder blades

Engage core

Slightly bend knees

1 »

Stand with your feet slightly wider than shoulder-width apart. Hold the ends of a dumbbell with both hands and let your arms hang straight down in front of you.

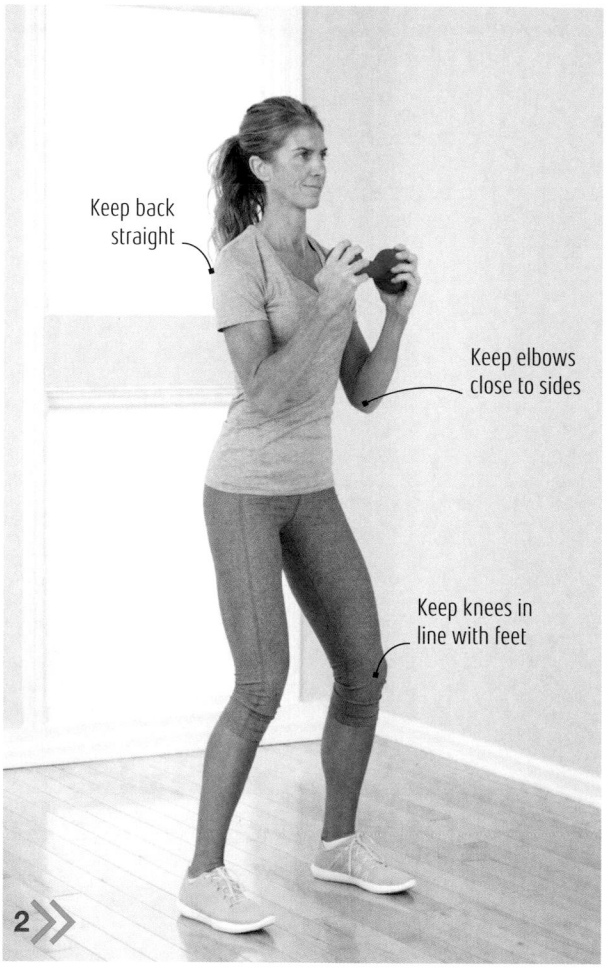

Keep back straight

Keep elbows close to sides

Keep knees in line with feet

2 »

Engage your biceps to curl the dumbbell to chest height. Raise it through your elbows, which act as hinges. Continue to retract your shoulder blades.

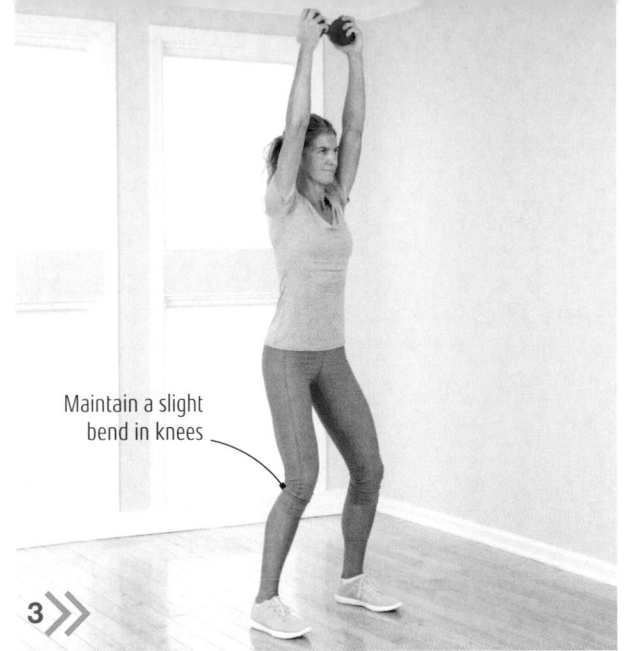

Maintain a slight bend in knees

3 »

Engage your shoulders and triceps to press the dumbbell straight up. Keep your elbows directly under the dumbbell and keep your chin raised.

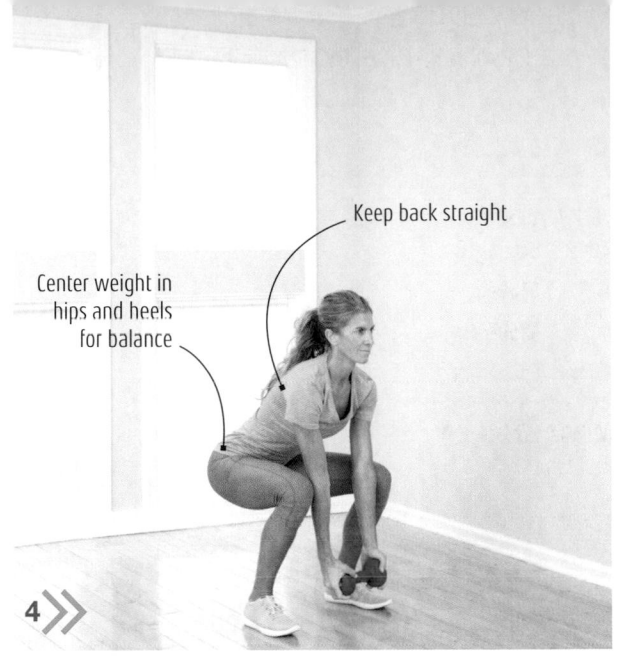

Keep back straight

Center weight in hips and heels for balance

4 »

In a continuous motion, sit your glutes back into a squat until your thighs are parallel to the ground, and powerfully thrust the dumbbell between your legs.

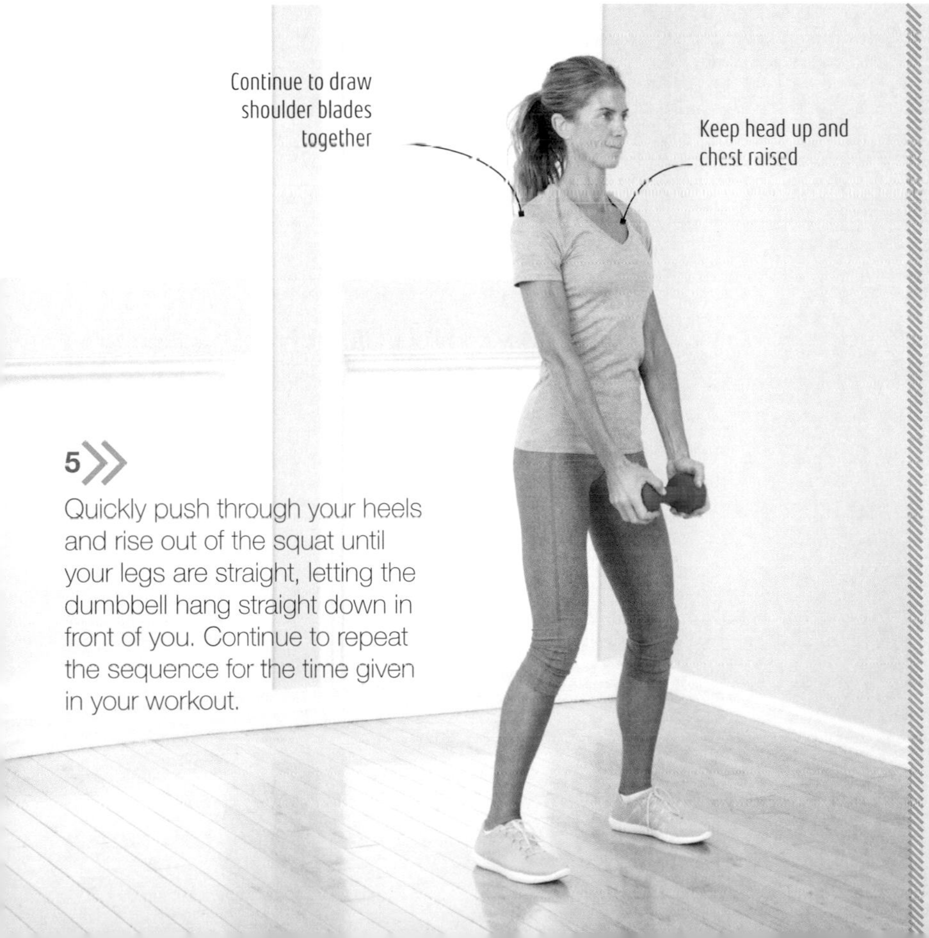

Continue to draw shoulder blades together

Keep head up and chest raised

5 »

Quickly push through your heels and rise out of the squat until your legs are straight, letting the dumbbell hang straight down in front of you. Continue to repeat the sequence for the time given in your workout.

▰▱▱ **MAKE IT easier**

If it is difficult to maintain balance, do the exercise without a dumbbell. Keep your arms parallel.

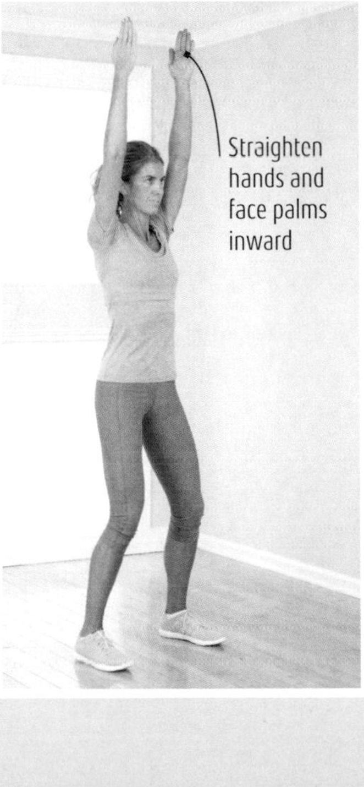

Straighten hands and face palms inward

Lateral step-ups

Many daily activities, such as climbing stairs, require your legs to work and balance independently. Build dexterity with this brisk stepping exercise that develops leg strength, improves stability, and resolves lower-body muscle imbalances.

IMPROVES
- Strength
- Stability
- Mobility
- Endurance

WHAT YOU NEED
Step

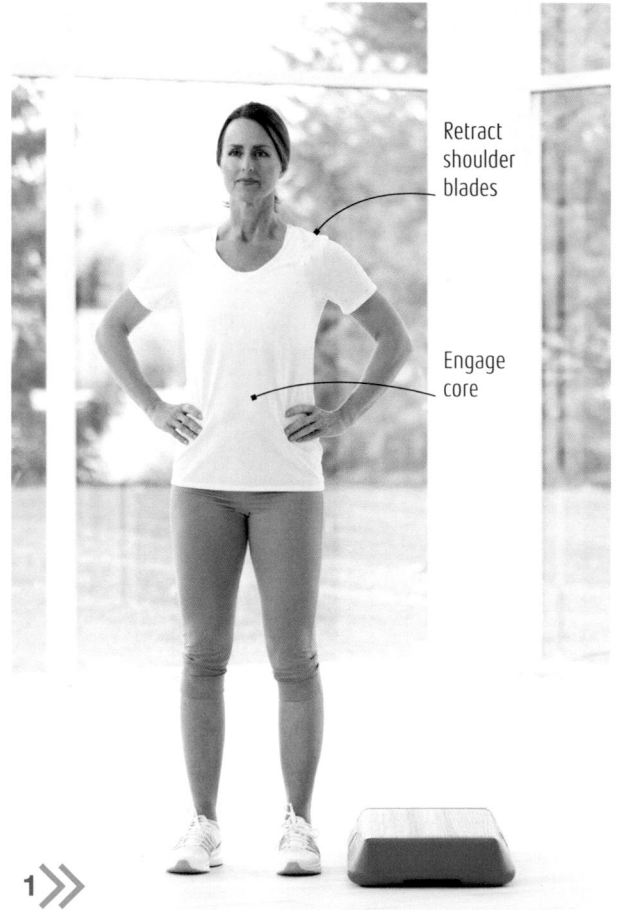

Retract shoulder blades

Engage core

1 »

Stand to the right of a step or stair with your feet shoulder-width apart. Place your hands on your hips and slightly bend your knees. Engage your core and retract your shoulder blades.

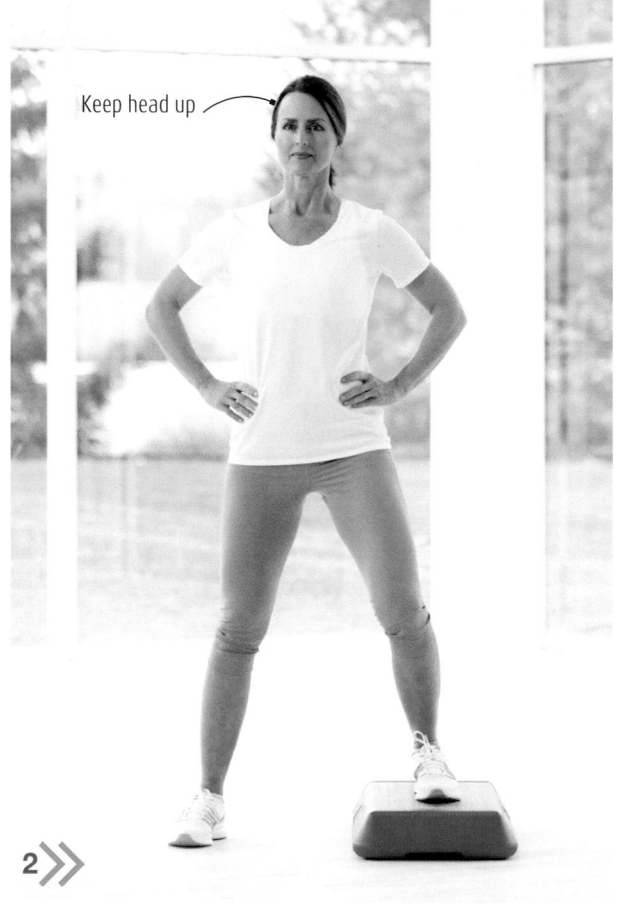

Keep head up

2 »

Lift your left leg from the knee until your left foot is about 2 inches (5cm) above the step, then place your left foot fully on the step. Keep your torso upright and your chin raised.

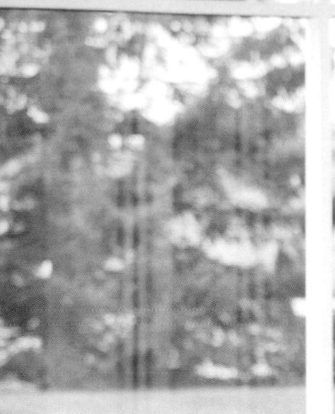
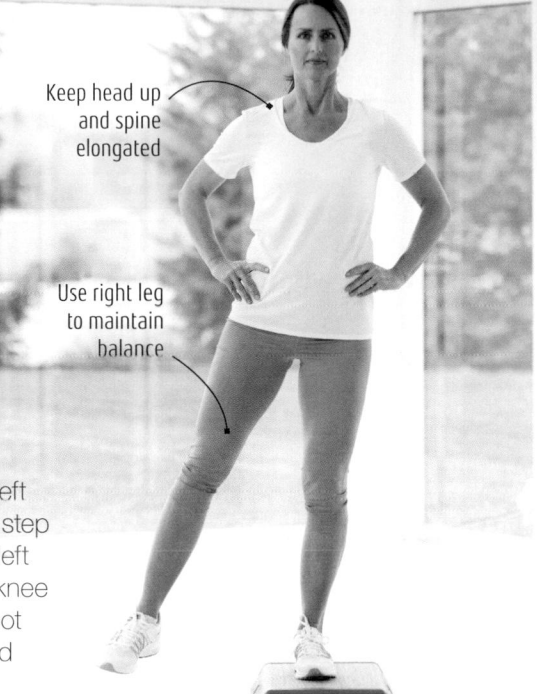

Keep head up and spine elongated

Use right leg to maintain balance

3 》》
Shift your weight to your left foot and stand up on the step by pushing through your left heel and extending your knee and hips. Let your right foot come off the ground. Hold for one second.

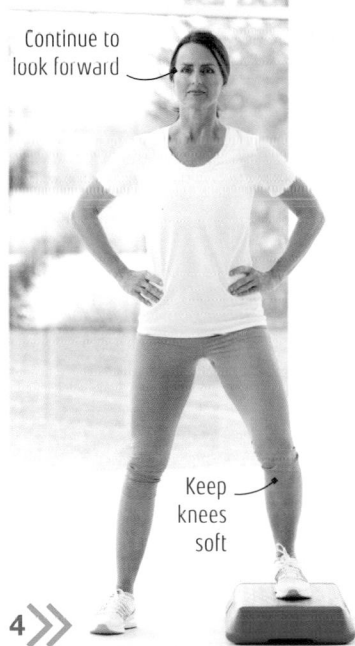

Continue to look forward

Keep knees soft

4 》》
Shift your weight back onto your right foot by lowering your right leg back to the ground. Slightly bend your knees and hips to absorb your weight.

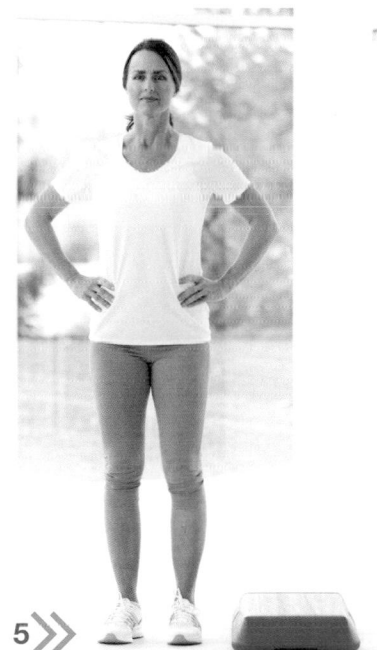

5 》》
Return your left leg to the starting position. Repeat the exercise for the time given. Spend half the time stepping onto your left foot, then repeat on the opposite side.

//// MAKE IT **easier**

If it is difficult to maintain balance, lightly rest your hand on a chair or rail for support.

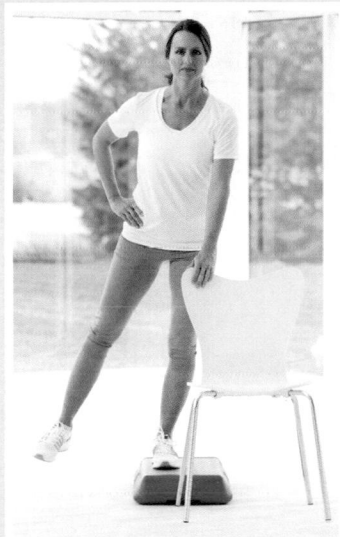

//// MAKE IT **harder**

To increase resistance to your legs, increase the height of the step.

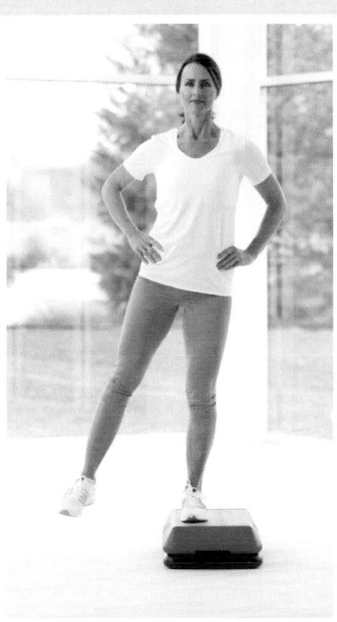

Overhead squat

Good mobility is a crucial aspect of staying fit, and it decreases your chance of injury while keeping your joints healthy. Perform this full-body squat to improve the range-of-motion of your ankles, knees, hips, back, and shoulders, while strengthening your legs.

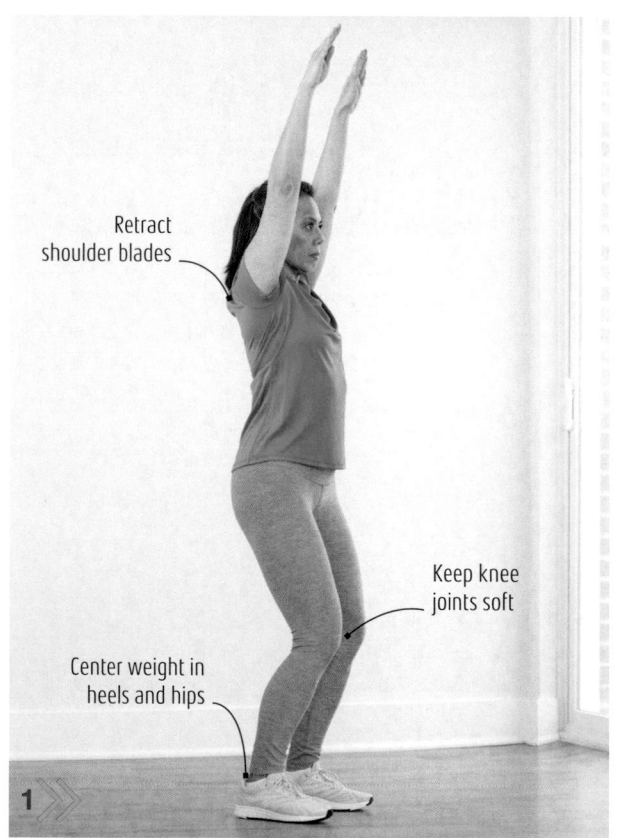

Retract shoulder blades

Keep knee joints soft

Center weight in heels and hips

1

Stand with your feet shoulder-width apart. Raise both arms straight overhead at shoulder-width, fingers together and palms facing forward. Engage your core and slightly bend your knees.

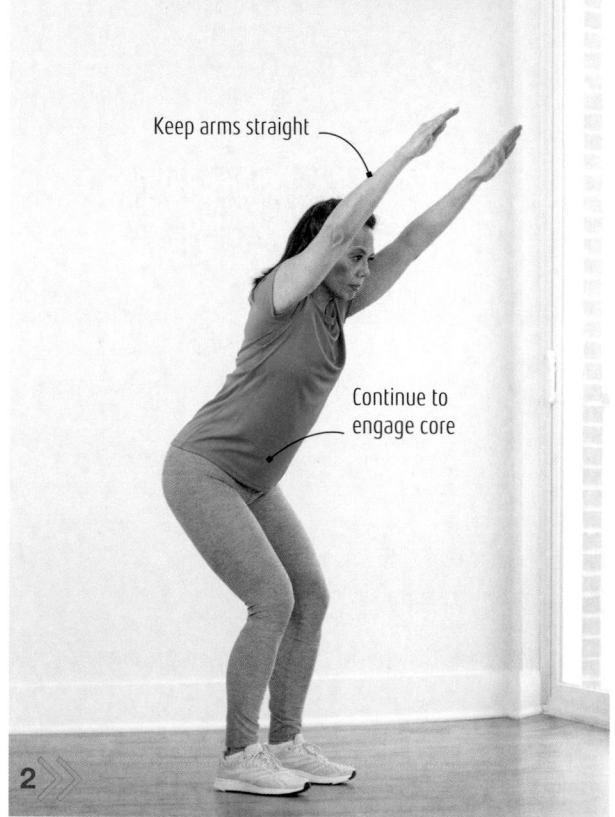

Keep arms straight

Continue to engage core

2

Push your glutes back and bend at your hips, keeping your arms aligned with your head. Keep your back straight and your toes pointed forward. Keep your head raised.

3 »

In a quick, controlled manner, bend your knees to sit back into a squat until your thighs are parallel to the ground. Keep your body as upright as possible and avoid bending forward at the waist. Distribute your weight in your hips and heels.

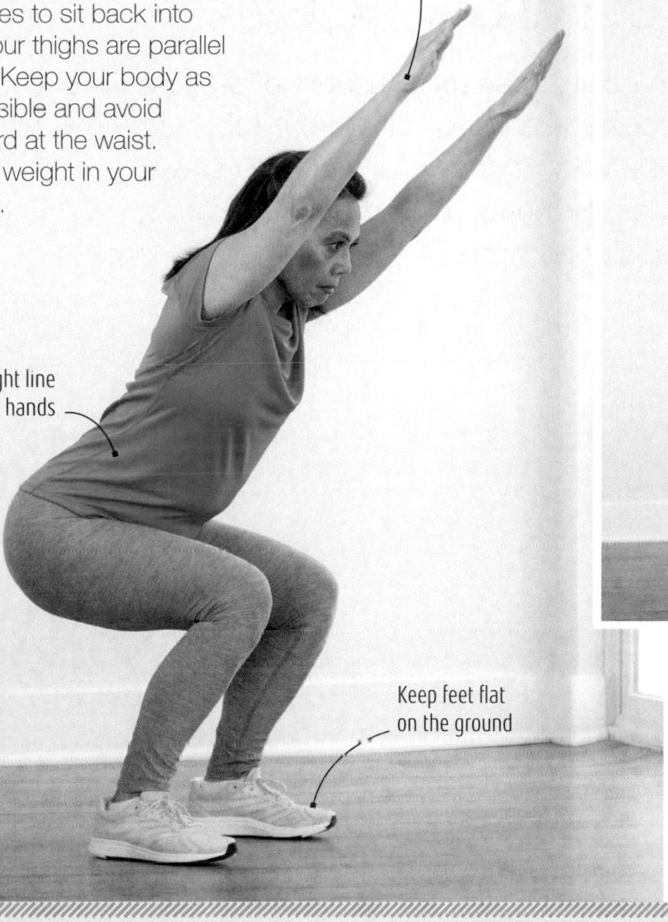

Pull arms back so they are in line with torso

Maintain a straight line from hips to hands

Keep feet flat on the ground

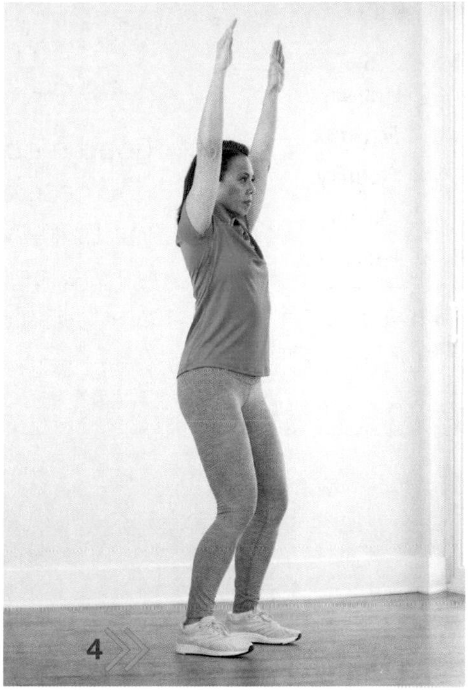

4 »

Quickly push through your heels and rise out of the squat, keeping your shoulder blades retracted and your back straight. Continue to repeat the exercise for the time given in your workout.

//// MAKE IT **easier**

If you have limited flexibility, place a folded mat under your heels to elevate them about 2 inches (5cm) while you perform the squat.

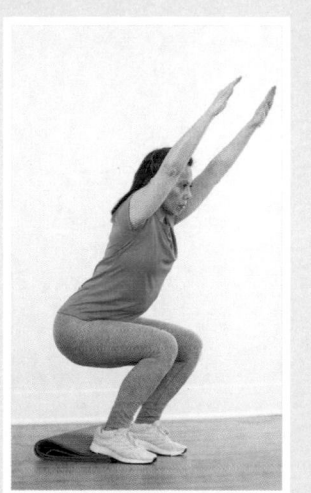

//// MAKE IT **harder**

To increase resistance to your legs, shoulders, and core, hold a dumbbell in each hand, palms facing forward.

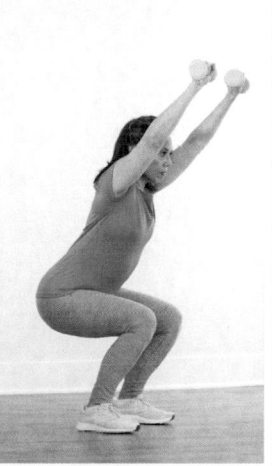

IMPROVES

//// Posture

//// Strength

//// Stability

//// Mobility

//// Endurance

WHAT YOU NEED
Dumbbells

Stationary lunge and curl

Lunges not only strengthen your legs, but they also do a remarkable job of stretching your hips. Perform this exercise for strong and flexible hip flexors, which are essential for preventing hip, knee, and lower-back pain.

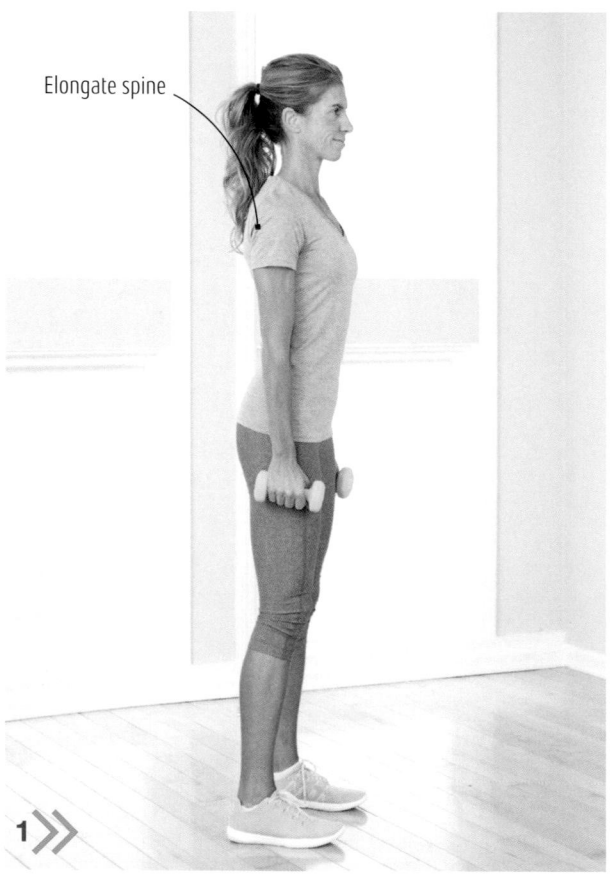

Elongate spine

1 ≫

Stand with your feet shoulder-width apart. Hold a dumbbell in each hand, palms facing inward, and let your arms hang at your sides. Engage your core and retract your shoulder blades. Raise your chin.

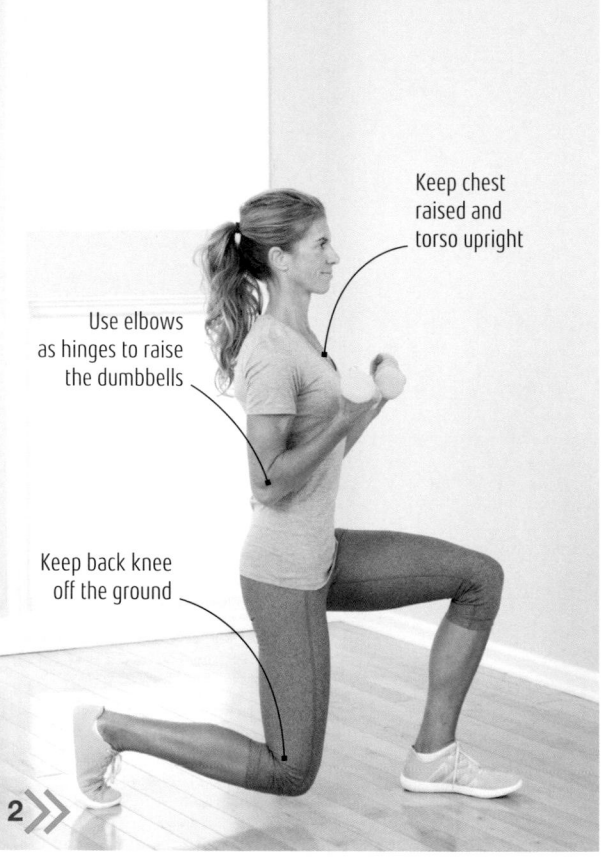

Keep chest raised and torso upright

Use elbows as hinges to raise the dumbbells

Keep back knee off the ground

2 ≫

In one quick, controlled motion, take a long step forward with your left leg, drop your right knee down until both knees are bent to 90 degrees, and curl the dumbbells to chest height, palms facing toward you.

If the strain is too great on your knees, reduce the distance you drop your back knee. Slowly increase your range of motion.

Continue to draw shoulder blades together

Rotate palms back toward body

3 »

Quickly engage both legs to return to the starting position, while using your biceps to lower the dumbbells and rotate your arms back to the starting position. Repeat the lunge by stepping forward with your right leg. Alternate lunging on each side for the time given in your workout.

//// **MAKE IT easier**

To decrease resistance to your legs, in step 1, step your right leg back into a staggered stance. In step 2, drop your right knee into a lunge. Then exit the lunge, but remain in the staggered stance. Reverse your stance halfway through.

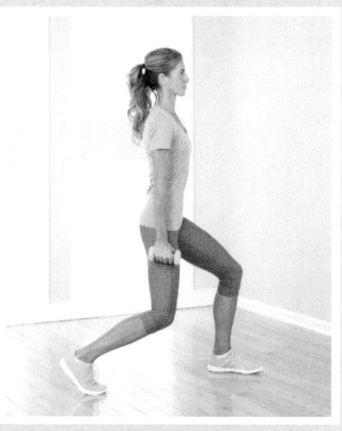

//// **MAKE IT harder**

To strengthen your shoulders, after step 2, rotate your hands 180 degrees and press the dumbbells straight overhead, then return the dumbbells to the top of the curl position. Continue to step 3.

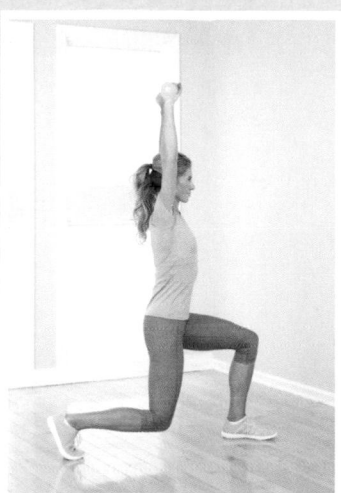

Side lunge

The human body is not only designed to move forward and backward—but also from side to side. Perform this exercise in a quick and controlled manner to strengthen your hip adductors and glutes so you can better cope with the stresses of lateral movement.

IMPROVES
- ▰/// **Strength**
- ▰/// **Stability**
- /// **Mobility**
- ▰/// **Endurance**

WHAT YOU NEED
No equipment needed

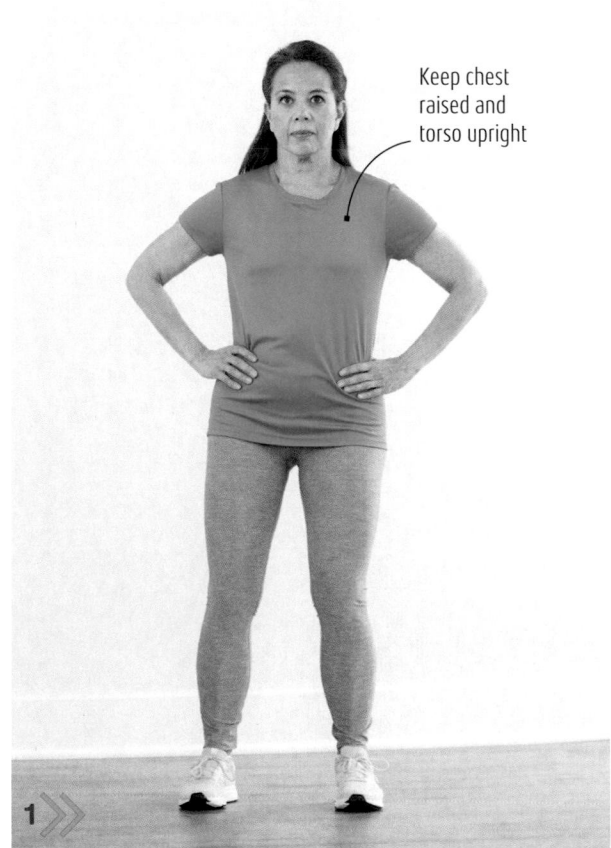

Keep chest raised and torso upright

1 Stand with your feet shoulder-width apart and place your hands on your hips. Slightly bend your knees. Engage your core and retract your shoulder blades.

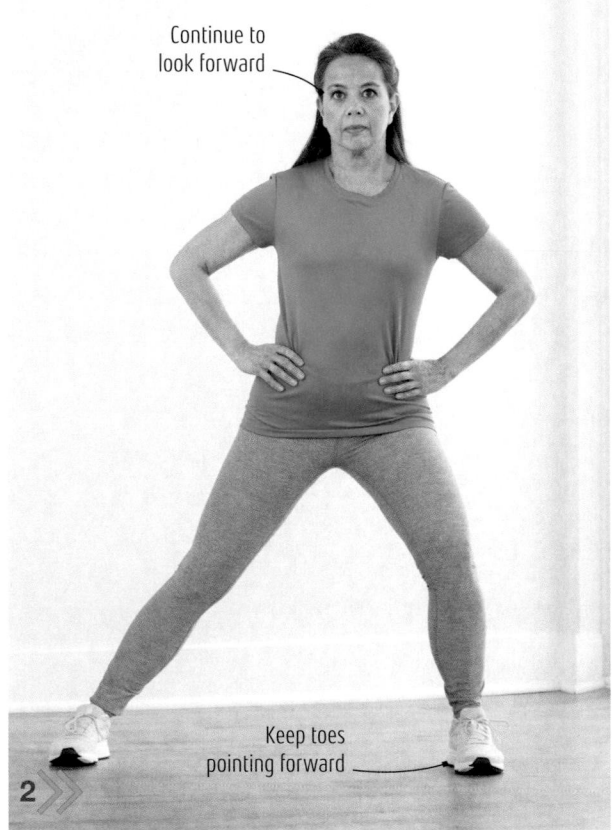

Continue to look forward

Keep toes pointing forward

2 Take a long step to the left with your left leg, landing first on the heel of your foot, and slightly bend your left knee. Keep your right leg straight.

3 »

Continue to bend your left knee, push your glutes back, and bend at the hips until your left thigh is parallel to the ground.

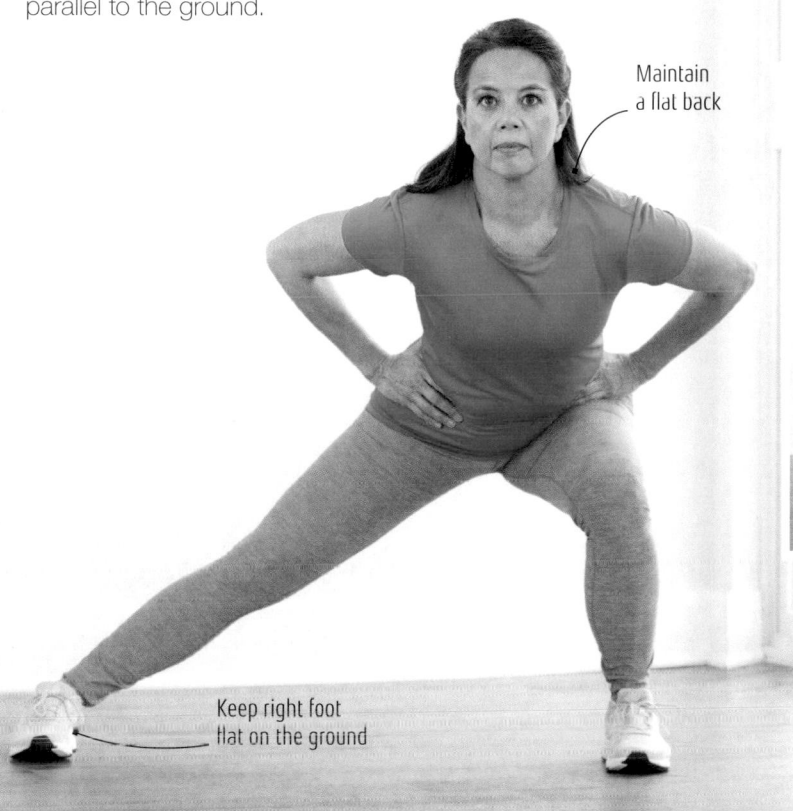

Maintain a flat back

Keep right foot flat on the ground

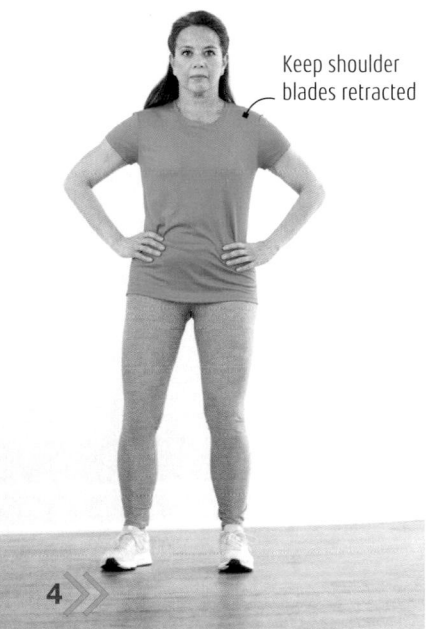

Keep shoulder blades retracted

4 »

Push through your left heel and engage your legs to return to the starting position. Repeat the exercise to your right. Alternate lunging to each side for the time given in your workout.

///// MAKE IT **easier**

To decrease the load on your legs, in step 2, take a shorter step out with your left leg. In step 3, push your glutes back until your thighs are parallel to the ground. In step 4, push through your left heel to stand up and step your leg back to the starting position. Repeat with your right leg.

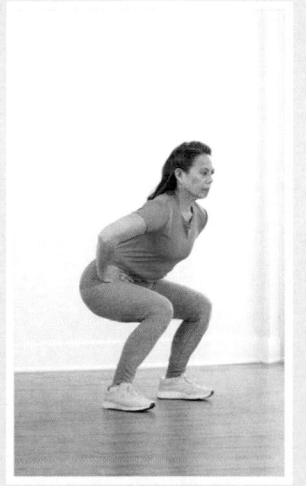

///// MAKE IT **harder**

To increase resistance to your legs, hold a dumbbell in each hand and let your arms hang straight down.

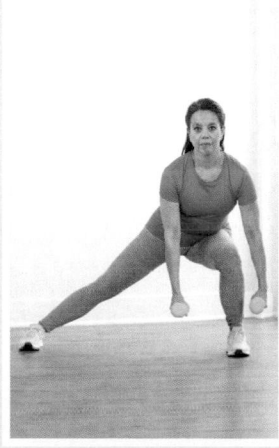

IMPROVES
/// Posture
/// Strength
/// Stability
/// Mobility
/// Endurance

WHAT YOU NEED
Dumbbells

Split squat and thruster

A principle of functional training is to choose movements that work multiple body parts together. This efficient squat and upper-body exercise uses several muscle chains at once. Perform it in a swift manner to strengthen your quadriceps, calves, glutes, lower back, hamstrings, triceps, and shoulders.

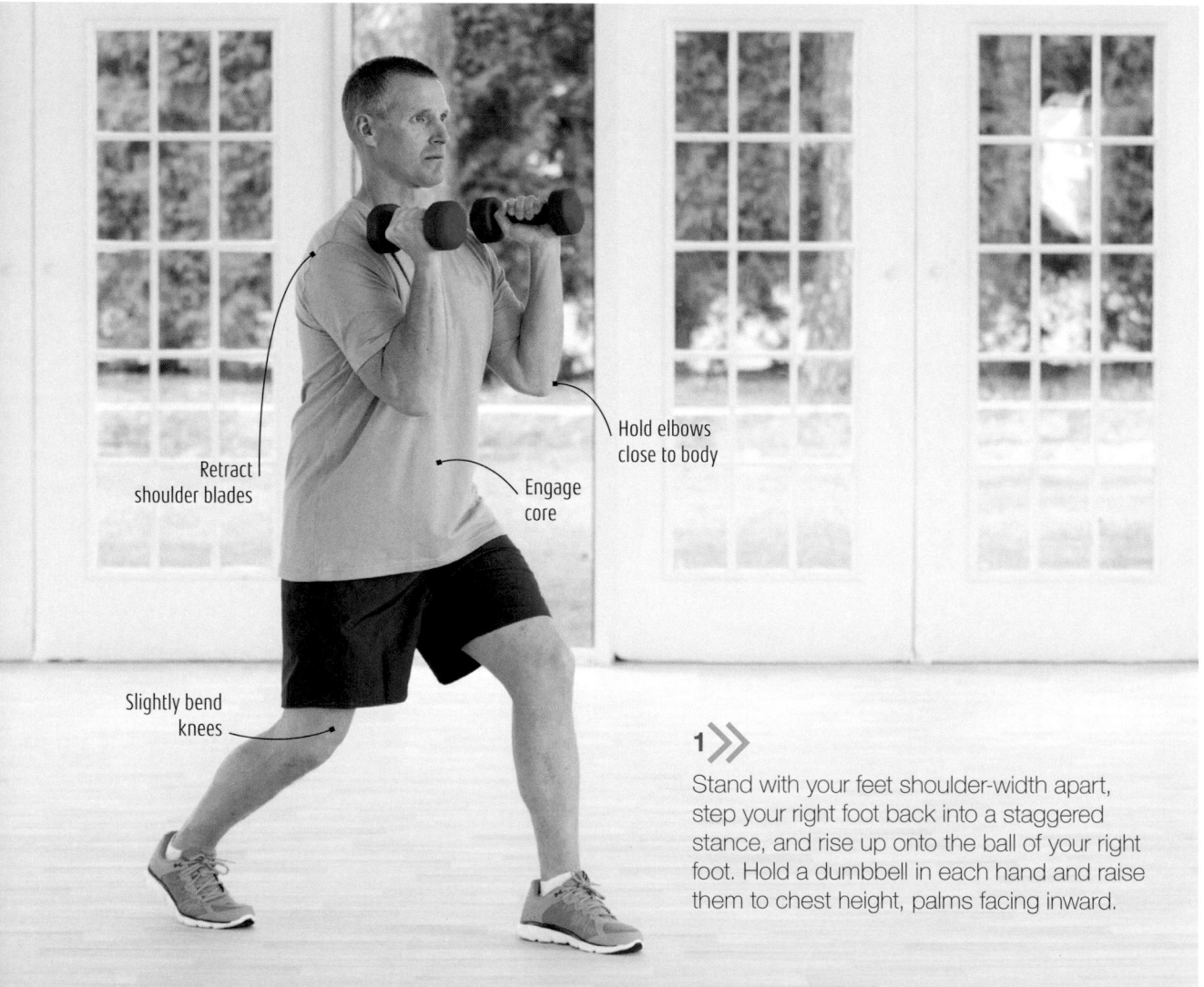

Retract
shoulder blades

Hold elbows
close to body

Engage
core

Slightly bend
knees

1 »

Stand with your feet shoulder-width apart, step your right foot back into a staggered stance, and rise up onto the ball of your right foot. Hold a dumbbell in each hand and raise them to chest height, palms facing inward.

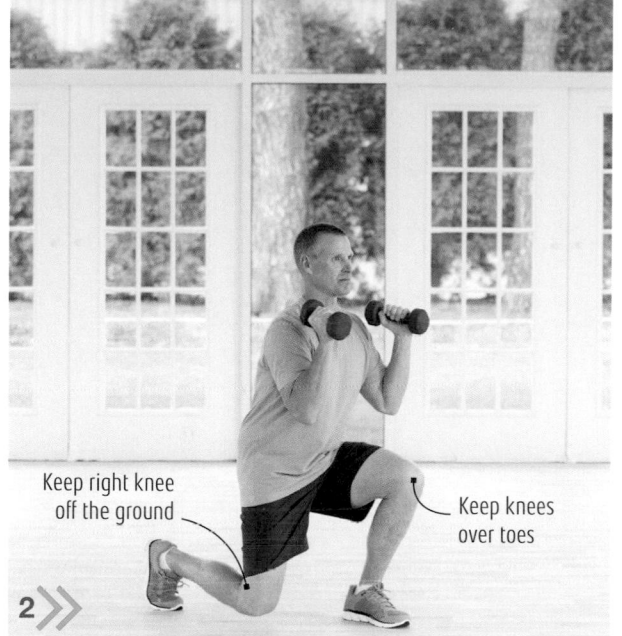

Keep right knee off the ground

Keep knees over toes

2 »

Keeping your arms in position, drop your right knee straight down until both knees are bent to 90 degrees. Keep your back straight and your head raised.

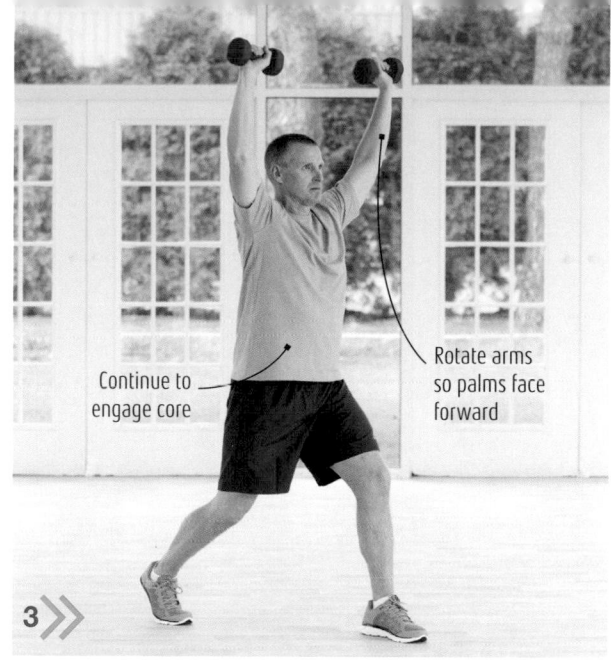

Continue to engage core

Rotate arms so palms face forward

3 »

In one swift motion, engage both legs to return to the staggered stance, rotate your arms 90 degrees forward, and press the dumbbells overhead.

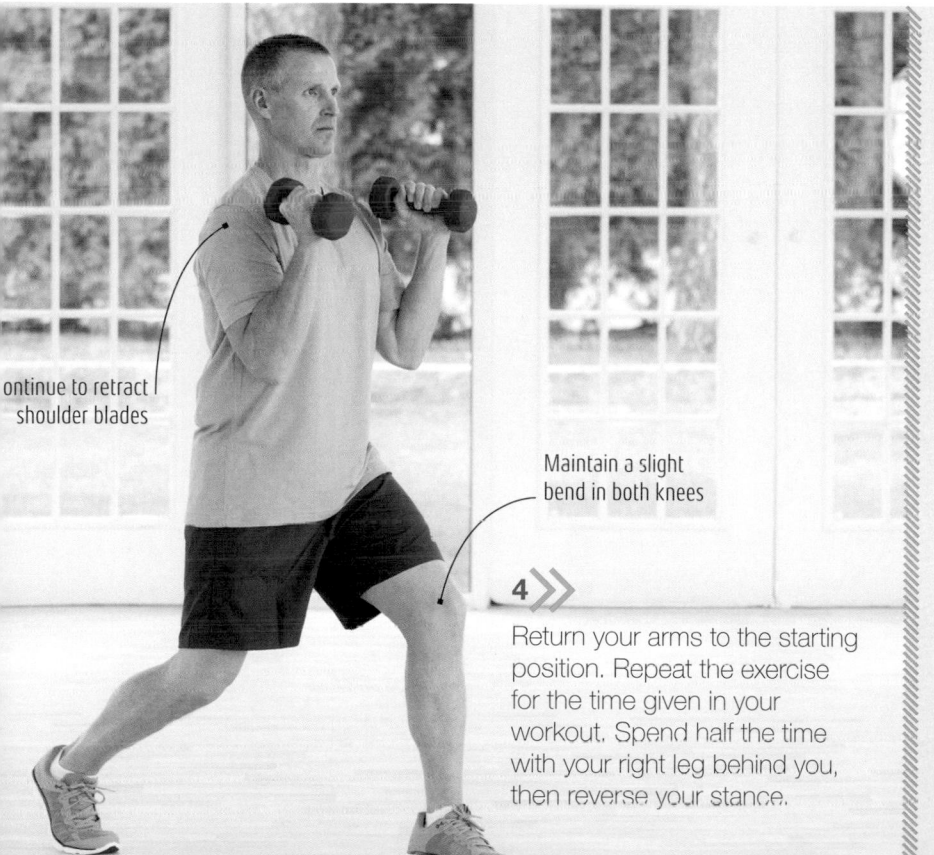

ontinue to retract shoulder blades

Maintain a slight bend in both knees

4 »

Return your arms to the starting position. Repeat the exercise for the time given in your workout. Spend half the time with your right leg behind you, then reverse your stance.

/// MAKE IT easier

If it is difficult to maintain balance, in step 1, stand with your feet shoulder-width apart. In step 2, squat until your thighs are parallel to the ground. In step 3, stand up by pushing through your heels.

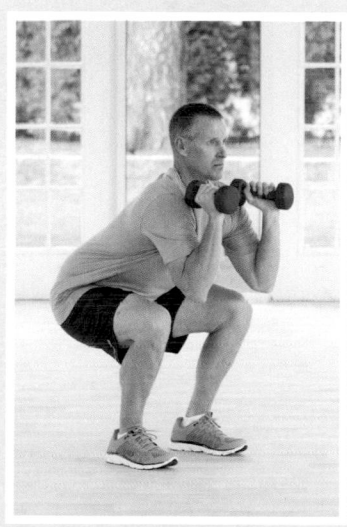

WORKOUT ROUTINES

Don't just work hard—work smart. These workout routines are purposeful collections of exercises designed to help you achieve your fitness goals. Complete the routines as required by your program to ensure that the time you spend training works your body in a safe, healthy, and balanced way.

Warm up

Dynamic stretches prepare your body for a good workout by increasing your blood flow and muscle temperature. Follow this method before every workout to improve your range of motion, activate your muscles, and prevent injury.

WHAT YOU NEED
No equipment needed

YOUR WORKOUT

- Before every workout, perform the entire sequence of warm-up exercises in order two times. Use a stopwatch to follow the work and rest intervals.
- Do not use dumbbells for any of these exercises.
- Focus on your goals and mentally prepare yourself to work hard.

THE LEVELS

ALL LEVELS

Carry out the exercise sequence
2 times

Perform each exercise for
20 seconds

Rest between each exercise for
10 seconds

Total time
5 minutes

THE EXERCISES

1	HIGH KNEE AND REACH	p.34
2	STANDING TWIST	p.108
3	POSTERIOR SWING	p.130
4	ARM PULLOVERS	p.78
5	OVERHEAD SQUAT	p.142

5-minute kick-start

Just 5 minutes of activity a day is enough to reduce your chance of heart disease by 45 percent. Use this efficient, total-body workout whenever you are running short of time and want a quick boost of energy that is good for your whole body.

WHAT YOU NEED
Dumbbells, countertop, mat

YOUR WORKOUT

- Select the level as required by your exercise program.
- Perform the entire sequence of exercises in order one time. Use a stopwatch to follow the work and rest intervals.
- If it is difficult to balance, try an easier modification or reduce the weight of your dumbbells.

THE LEVELS

LEVEL 1

Carry out the exercise sequence
1 time

Perform each exercise for
20 seconds

Rest between each exercise for
10 seconds

Total time
5 minutes

LEVEL 2

Carry out the exercise sequence
1 time

Perform each exercise for
25 seconds

Rest between each exercise for
5 seconds

Total time
5 minutes

LEVEL 3

Carry out the exercise sequence
1 time

Perform each exercise for
30 seconds

Rest between each exercise for
0 seconds

Total time
5 minutes

THE EXERCISES

1	HIGH KNEE AND REACH	p.34
2	INCLINED PUSH-UPS	p.54
3	HIP-UPS	p.136
4	FAST FEET	p.26
5	SUITCASE ROW	p.72
6	SUITCASE SQUAT	p.124
7	KNEE CHOP	p.104
8	PUSH PRESS	p.60
9	SPLIT STANCE RUNNERS	p.100
10	SUMO DEADLIFT AND UPRIGHT ROW	p.134

Cardiovascular endurance

Consistent cardiovascular exercise helps you live longer and improves your heart health and quality of life. Perform this routine vigorously to strengthen your heart, increase lung capacity, support better sleep, and improve energy levels.

WHAT YOU NEED
Dumbbells, step, chair

YOUR WORKOUT

- Select the level as required by your exercise program.
- Perform the entire sequence of exercises in order for the prescribed number of times. Use a stopwatch to follow the work and rest intervals.
- Exert maximum aerobic effort, and use the rest times between each exercise to gear up for the next drill.

THE LEVELS

LEVEL 1

Carry out the exercise sequence **2 times**

Perform each exercise for **20 seconds**

Rest between each exercise for **10 seconds**

Total time **10 minutes**

LEVEL 2

Carry out the exercise sequence **3 times**

Perform each exercise for **30 seconds**

Rest between each exercise for **10 seconds**

Total time **20 minutes**

LEVEL 3

Carry out the exercise sequence **3 times**

Perform each exercise for **35 seconds**

Rest between each exercise for **5 seconds**

Total time **20 minutes**

THE EXERCISES

1	SIDE SHUFFLE	p.30
2	SIDE-TO-SIDE PUNCH	p.106
3	STEP-UPS	p.40
4	ARM PULLOVERS	p.78
5	FAUX JUMP ROPE	p.44
6	WOOD CHOP	p.102
7	CHAIR MOUNTAIN CLIMBER	p.46
8	ONE-ARM SNATCH	p.86
9	SWITCH JUMPS	p.48
10	CURL AND ARNOLD PRESS AND REACH	p.56

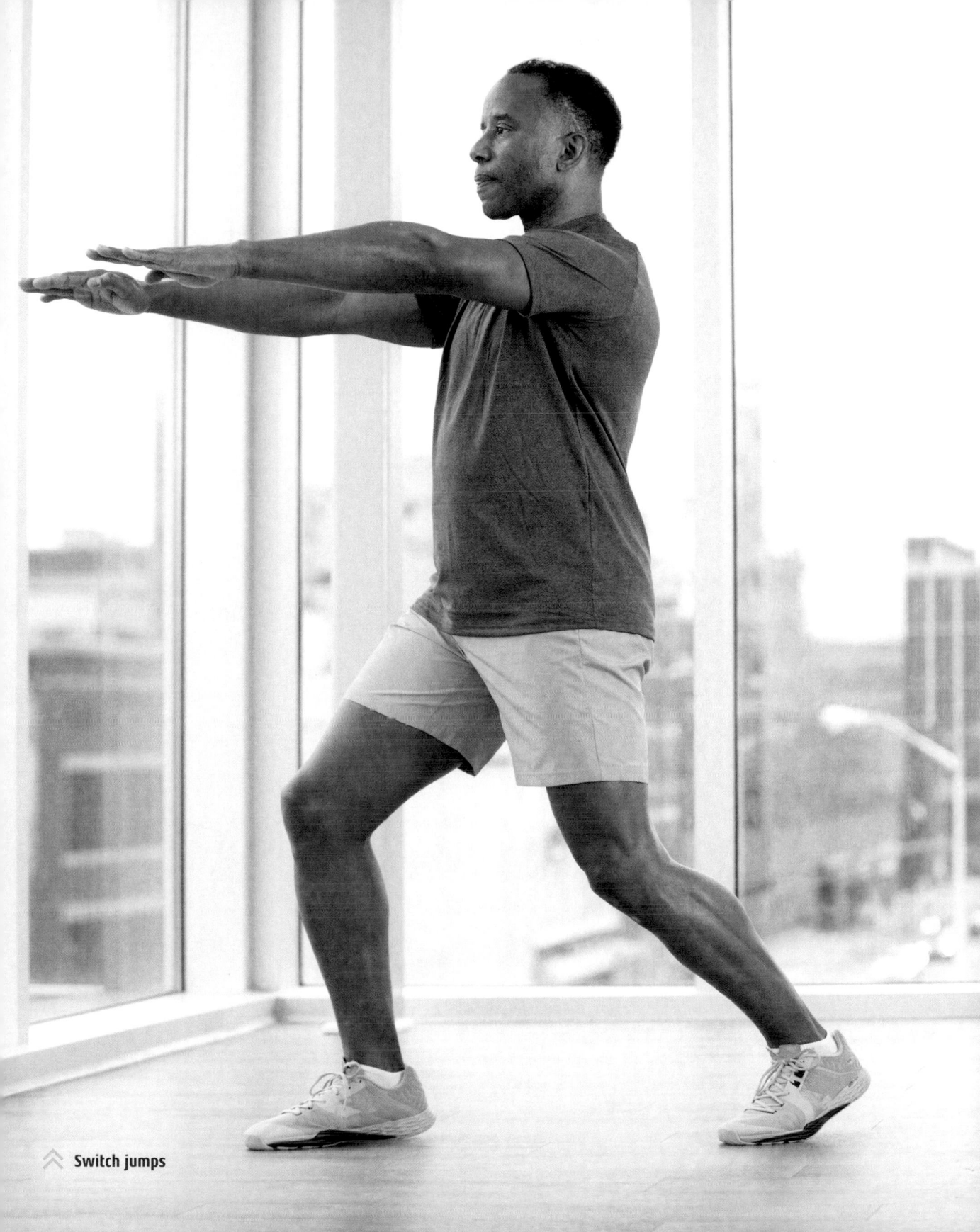

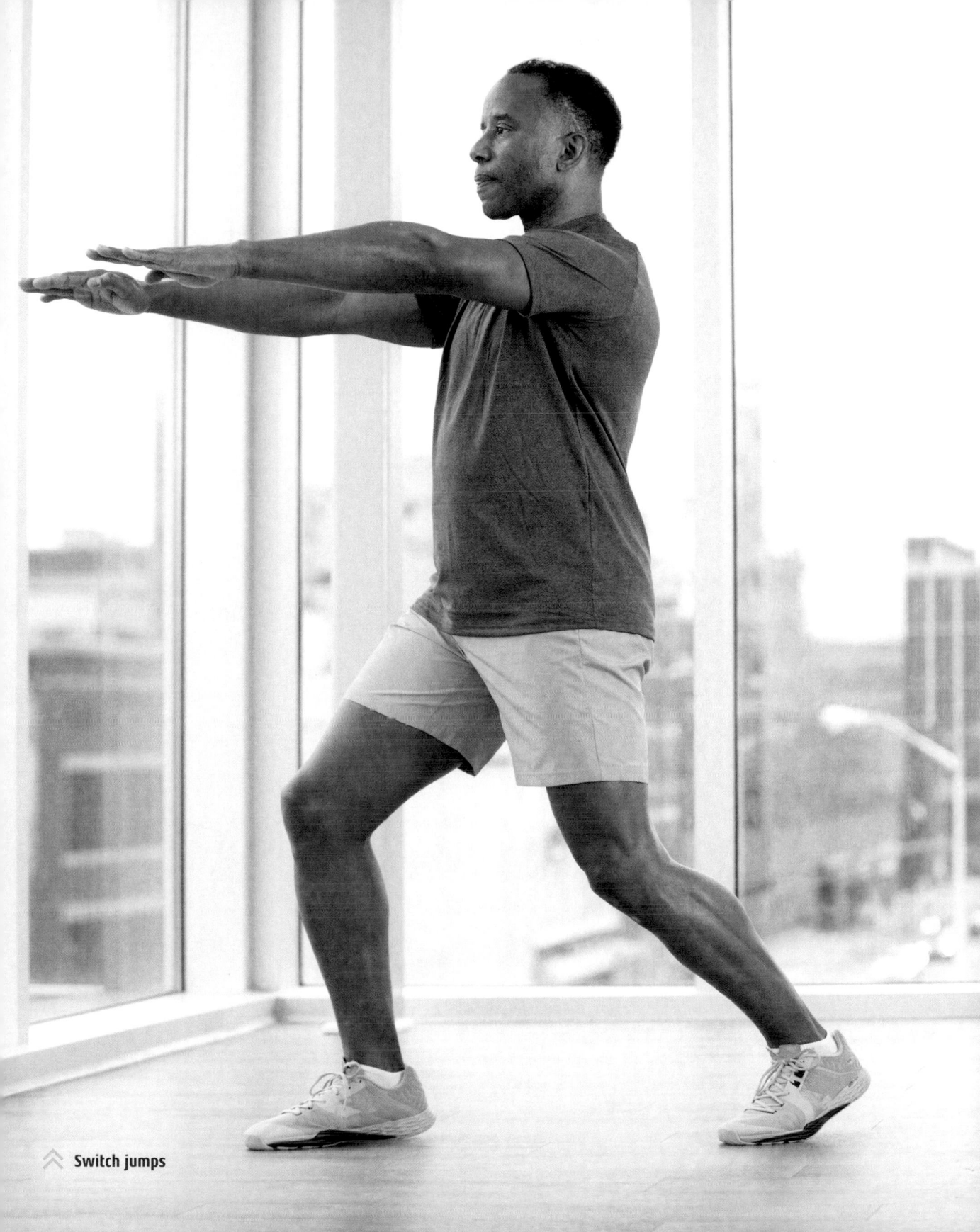Switch jumps

Beginner total body

Limited mobility does not mean you cannot exercise. If you are new to exercise, recovering from an injury, or have trouble balancing, this routine uses the seated versions of exercises to help you gain strength and improve cardiovascular endurance.

WHAT YOU NEED
Dumbbells, chair

YOUR WORKOUT
- Select the level as required by your exercise program.
- Perform the entire sequence of exercises in order two times. Use a stopwatch to follow the work and rest intervals.
- Do the seated modification for each exercise.

THE LEVELS

LEVEL 1

Carry out the exercise sequence **2 times**

Perform each exercise for **15 seconds**

Rest between each exercise for **15 seconds**

Total time **9 minutes**

LEVEL 2

Carry out the exercise sequence **2 times**

Perform each exercise for **20 seconds**

Rest between each exercise for **10 seconds**

Total time **9 minutes**

LEVEL 3

Carry out the exercise sequence **2 times**

Perform each exercise for **30 seconds**

Rest between each exercise for **10 seconds**

Total time **12 minutes**

THE EXERCISES

1	MARCH IN PLACE	p.32
2	BENT ROW AND HAMMER CURL	p.82
3	PUSH PRESS	p.60
4	FAST FEET	p.26
5	STAGGERED REVERSE FLY	p.76
6	GUNSLINGER	p.68
7	HIGH KNEE AND REACH	p.34
8	SEESAW ROW	p.94
9	ONE-ARM MILITARY PRESS	p.50

Low-intensity strength

It is never too late to start building muscle mass. Adding strength training to your program is one of the best ways to prevent or reverse bone loss and muscle atrophy. Perform these exercises to ease your way safely into resistance training.

WHAT YOU NEED
Dumbbells, countertop

YOUR WORKOUT

- Select the level as required by your exercise program.
- Perform the entire sequence of exercises in order for the prescribed number of times. Use a stopwatch to follow the work and rest intervals.
- It is okay to start without dumbbells. You can slowly increase your resistance each time you perform the routine.

THE LEVELS

LEVEL 1

Carry out the exercise sequence
2 times

Perform each exercise for
20 seconds

Rest between each exercise for
10 seconds

Total time
10 minutes

LEVEL 2

Carry out the exercise sequence
2 times

Perform each exercise for
30 seconds

Rest between each exercise for
10 seconds

Total time
13 minutes

LEVEL 3

Carry out the exercise sequence
3 times

Perform each exercise for
30 seconds

Rest between each exercise for
10 seconds

Total time
20 minutes

THE EXERCISES

#	Exercise	Page
1	ONE ARM CHEST PRESS	p.62
2	SUITCASE ROW	p.72
3	SUITCASE SQUAT	p.124
4	STANDING TWIST	p.108
5	PUSH PRESS	p.60
6	SUMO DEADLIFT AND UPRIGHT ROW	p.134
7	CURL FROM ONE LEG	p.96
8	INCLINED PUSH-UPS	p.54
9	WALKING REACHING LUNGE	p.126
10	WINDMILL	p.118

Speed and agility

Athleticism requires a combination of speed, agility, reaction time, and power. For non-athletes and weekend warriors alike, this routine will enhance athletic ability with power drills that improve footwork and boost total-body coordination.

WHAT YOU NEED
Dumbbells, chair, countertop

YOUR WORKOUT
- Select your level according to your workout program.
- Perform the entire sequence of exercises in order for the prescribed number of times. Use a stopwatch to follow the work and rest intervals.
- Begin your workout with no weights or with light dumbbells, and increase resistance as you are able.

THE LEVELS

LEVEL 1

Carry out the exercise sequence **2 times**

Perform each exercise for **15 seconds**

Rest between each exercise for **15 seconds**

Total time **10 minutes**

LEVEL 2

Carry out the exercise sequence **3 times**

Perform each exercise for **30 seconds**

Rest between each exercise for **15 seconds**

Total time **22 minutes**

LEVEL 3

Carry out the exercise sequence **3 times**

Perform each exercise for **40 seconds**

Rest between each exercise for **10 seconds**

Total time **25 minutes**

THE EXERCISES

#	Exercise	Page
1	CHAIR MOUNTAIN CLIMBER	p.46
2	SHOT-PUT PRESS	p.70
3	SIDE LUNGE	p.146
4	LAWN MOWER ROW	p.74
5	CROSS-COUNTRY SKIERS	p.42
6	INCLINED PUSH-UPS	p.54
7	SPLIT STANCE RUNNERS	p.100
8	REVERSE LUNGE WITH TWIST	p.128
9	EARTHQUAKES	p.138
10	SEESAW ROW	p.94

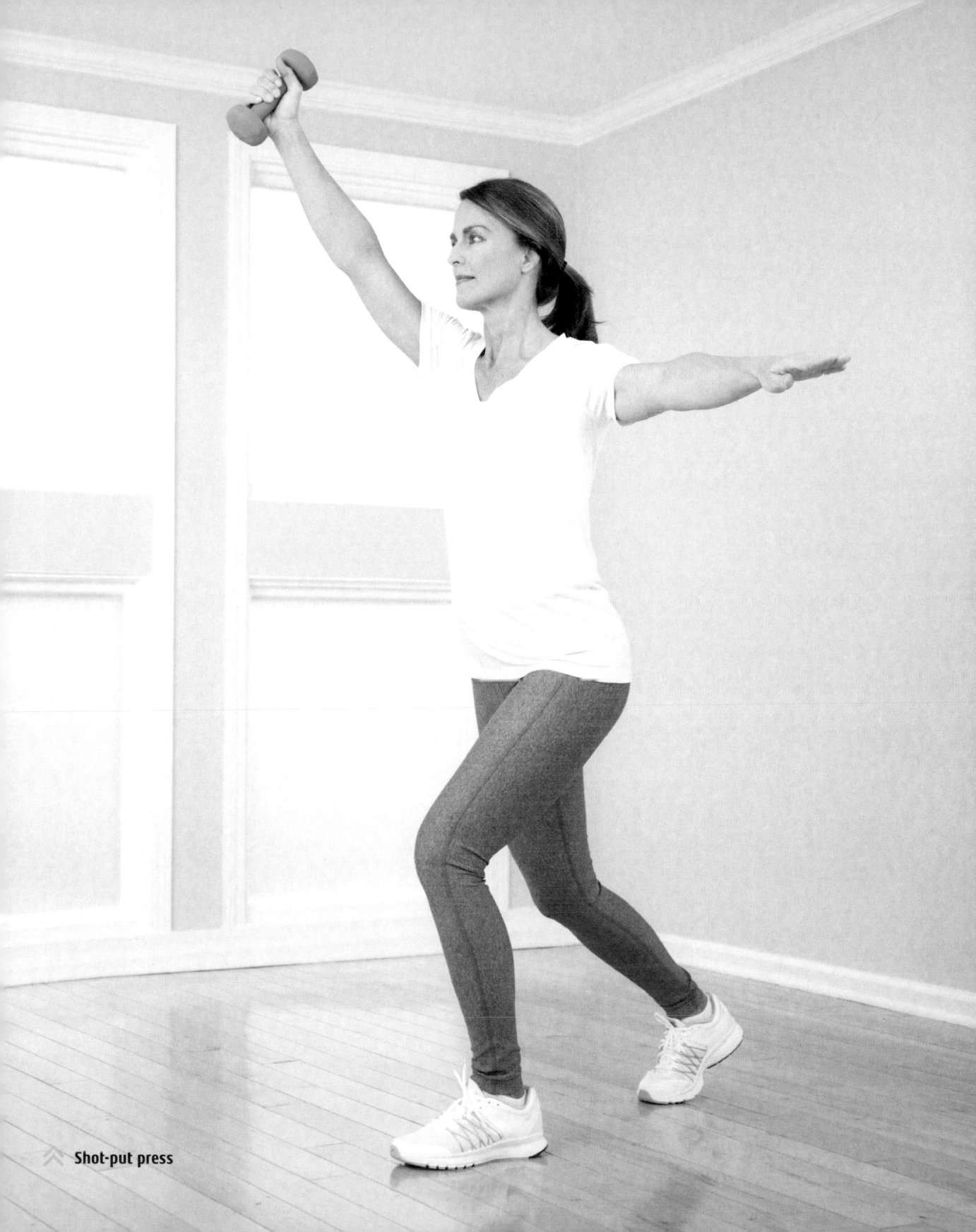

Shot-put press

Balance and stability

Control of your core and the muscles that surround your ankles, knees, hips, and shoulders is essential for good balance. Follow this routine to train those muscles, improve your posture, enhance your coordination, and boost your stability.

WHAT YOU NEED
Dumbbells, step

YOUR WORKOUT

- Select the level as required by your exercise program.
- Perform the entire sequence of exercises in order two times. Use a stopwatch to follow the work and rest intervals.
- If it is difficult to balance, try an easier modification or reduce the weight of your dumbbells.

THE LEVELS

LEVEL 1

Carry out the exercise sequence **2 times**

Perform each exercise for **15 seconds**

Rest between each exercise for **15 seconds**

Total time **10 minutes**

LEVEL 2

Carry out the exercise sequence **2 times**

Perform each exercise for **20 seconds**

Rest between each exercise for **10 seconds**

Total time **10 minutes**

LEVEL 3

Carry out the exercise sequence **2 times**

Perform each exercise for **30 seconds**

Rest between each exercise for **10 seconds**

Total time **13 minutes**

THE EXERCISES

1	HIGH KNEE AND REACH	p.34
2	CURL FROM ONE LEG	p.96
3	REVERSE LUNGE WITH TWIST	p.128
4	SUITCASE ROW	p.72
5	LATERAL STEP-UPS	p.140
6	CROSSOVER TOE TOUCH	p.114
7	ONE-LEG ARM RAISE	p.64
8	SUITCASE SQUAT	p.124
9	STANDING ELBOW TO KNEE	p.98
10	ONE-ARM MILITARY PRESS	p.50

Total-body mobility

Mobility is your body's ability to move freely without undue stress. Perform the exercises in this routine to increase the range of motion in your muscles and joints, improve your flexibility, and decrease strain on your body's systems.

WHAT YOU NEED
Dumbbells, chair, wall

YOUR WORKOUT

- Select the level as required by your exercise program.
- Perform the entire sequence of exercises in order two times. Use a stopwatch to follow the work and rest intervals.
- If any movements are painful, immediately try the modification or skip the exercise until your mobility improves.

THE LEVELS

LEVEL 1

Carry out the exercise sequence **2 times**

Perform each exercise for **15 seconds**

Rest between each exercise for **15 seconds**

Total time **10 minutes**

LEVEL 2

Carry out the exercise sequence **2 times**

Perform each exercise for **20 seconds**

Rest between each exercise for **10 seconds**

Total time **10 minutes**

LEVEL 3

Carry out the exercise sequence **2 times**

Perform each exercise for **30 seconds**

Rest between each exercise for **10 seconds**

Total time **13 minutes**

THE EXERCISES

1	GOOD MORNING	p.132
2	SIDE-TO-SIDE PUNCH	p.106
3	OVERHEAD SQUAT	p.142
4	ARM PULLOVERS	p.78
5	CHEST OPENER	p.58
6	REVERSE LUNGE WITH TWIST	p.128
7	WINDMILL	p.118
8	CHAIR DIPS	p.52
9	KNEE CHOP	p.104
10	WALL ANGEL	p.84

Cross-training

To advance your fitness level, it's necessary to keep your body alert by including variety in your workouts. This cross-training routine combines strength, aerobic, and flexibility exercises to challenge your body and help you avoid fitness plateaus.

WHAT YOU NEED
Dumbbells, mat, step

YOUR WORKOUT

- Select the level as required by your exercise program.
- Perform the entire sequence of exercises in order for the prescribed number of times. Use a stopwatch to follow the work and rest intervals.
- If you are unable to complete a round of the sequence, reduce the weight of your dumbbells or choose an easier modification.

THE LEVELS

LEVEL 1

Carry out the exercise sequence **2 times**

Perform each exercise for **15 seconds**

Rest between each exercise for **15 seconds**

Total time **10 minutes**

LEVEL 2

Carry out the exercise sequence **3 times**

Perform each exercise for **30 seconds**

Rest between each exercise for **15 seconds**

Total time **22 minutes**

LEVEL 3

Carry out the exercise sequence **3 times**

Perform each exercise for **40 seconds**

Rest between each exercise for **10 seconds**

Total time **25 minutes**

THE EXERCISES

1	HIGH PLANK ROW	p.90
2	OVER-THE-SHOULDER SQUAT	p.120
3	FARMER'S WALK	p.36
4	ONE-LEG ARM RAISE	p.64
5	POSTERIOR SWING	p.130
6	SPLIT SQUAT AND THRUSTER	p.148
7	WINDMILL	p.118
8	LATERAL STEP-UPS	p.140
9	STAGGERED REVERSE FLY	p.76
10	SIDE SHUFFLE	p.30

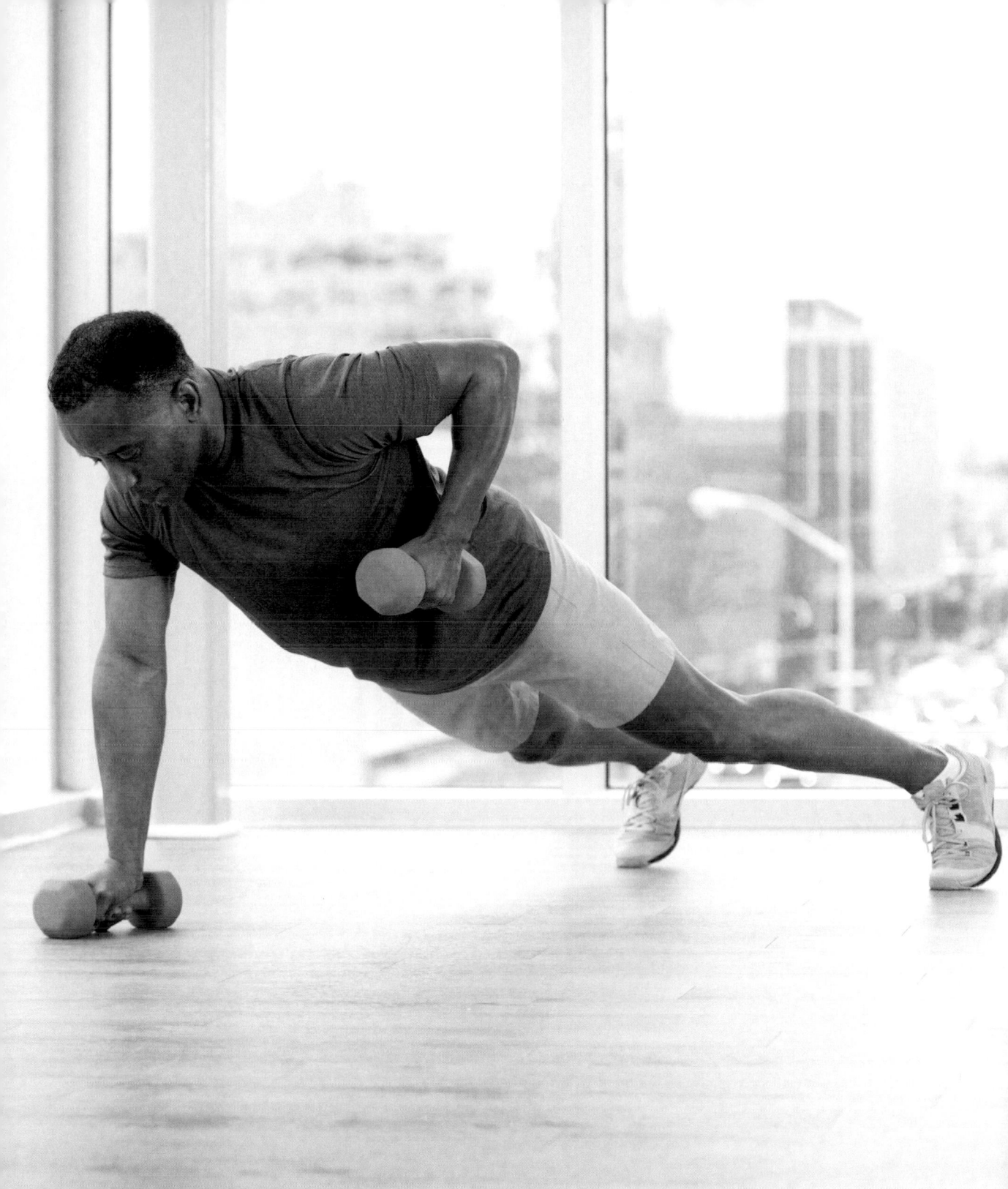

High plank row

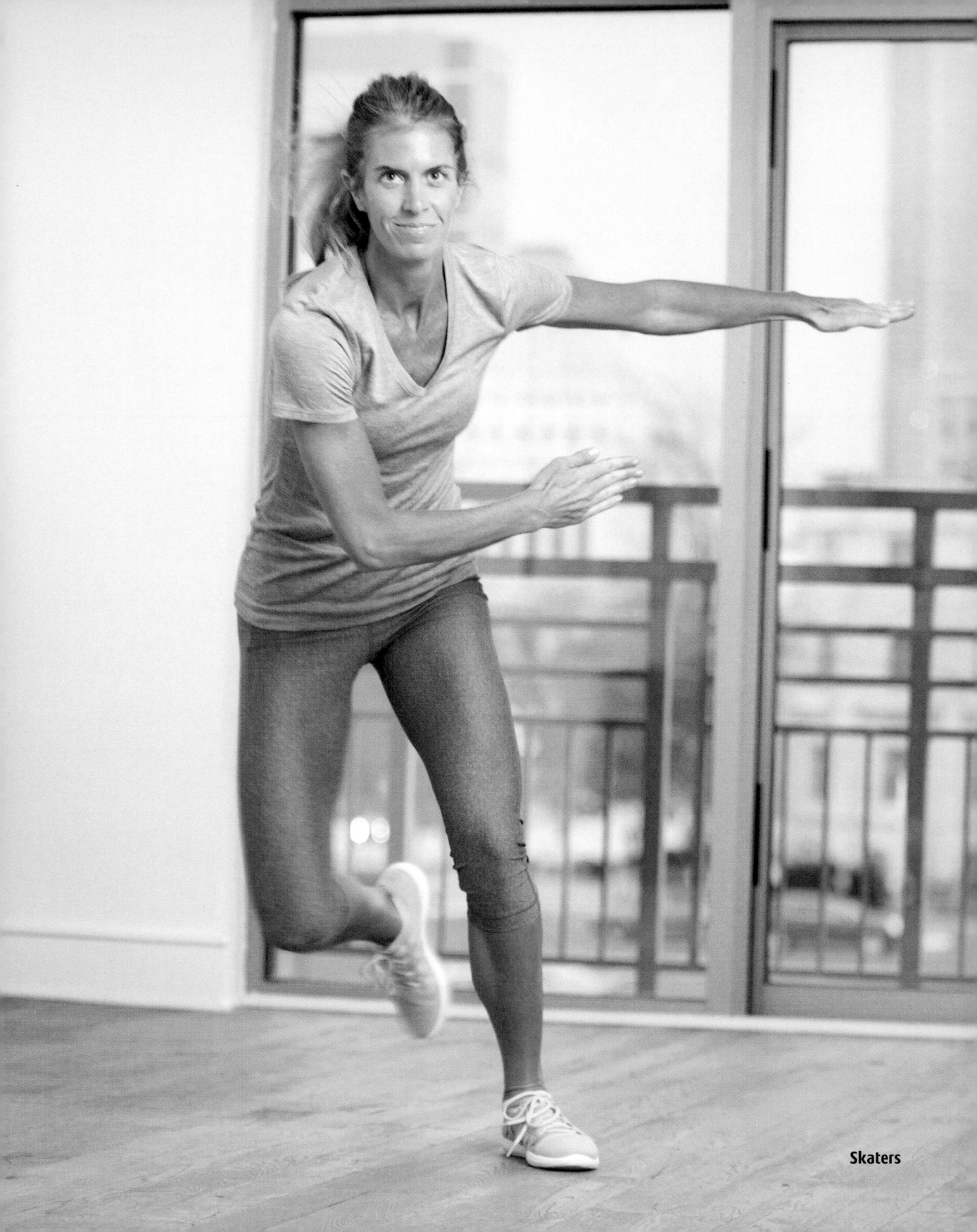

Skaters

Calorie-burning HIIT

High-intensity interval training (HIIT) is a method of exercise that alternates short bursts of intense exercise and short periods of rest. Work as hard and quickly as you can during this routine to burn a high volume of calories and fat in a short time.

WHAT YOU NEED
Dumbbells, mat, step, chair

YOUR WORKOUT

- Select the level as required by your exercise program.
- Perform the entire sequence of exercises in order for the prescribed number of times. Use a stopwatch to follow the work and rest intervals.
- Maintain a steady breathing pattern—in through your nose and out through your mouth—so you have the necessary oxygen to generate energy.

THE LEVELS

LEVEL 1

Carry out the exercise sequence **2 times**

Perform each exercise for **15 seconds**

Rest between each exercise for **15 seconds**

Total time **10 minutes**

LEVEL 2

Carry out the exercise sequence **3 times**

Perform each exercise for **30 seconds**

Rest between each exercise for **10 seconds**

Total time **20 minutes**

LEVEL 3

Carry out the exercise sequence **3 times**

Perform each exercise for **40 seconds**

Rest between each exercise for **10 seconds**

Total time **25 minutes**

THE EXERCISES

1	SUMO DEADLIFT AND UPRIGHT ROW	p.134
2	SKATERS	p.38
3	GUNSLINGER	p.68
4	HIGH PLANK REACH-THROUGH AND FLY	p.116
5	DIAGONAL CHOP	p.122
6	STEP-UPS	p.40
7	CHAIR DIPS	p.52
8	ROTATIONAL GOBLET SQUAT	p.112
9	BENT ROW AND HAMMER CURL	p.82
10	FAUX JUMP ROPE	p.44

Prehabilitation

One injury can stay with you for the rest of your life. Be proactive and use the *prehabilitation* method to help prevent injuries before they happen. These exercises will target and strengthen the areas of your body that are most susceptible to damage.

WHAT YOU NEED
Dumbbells, mat, wall, step

YOUR WORKOUT

- Select the level as required by your exercise program.
- Perform the entire sequence of exercises in order for the prescribed number of times. Use a stopwatch to follow the work and rest intervals.
- Prioritize proper technique for each exercise rather than speed, and focus on using steady, controlled movements.

THE LEVELS

LEVEL 1

Carry out the exercise sequence **1 time**

Perform each exercise for **20 seconds**

Rest between each exercise for **15 seconds**

Total time
**4 minutes
30 seconds**

LEVEL 2

Carry out the exercise sequence **2 times**

Perform each exercise for **20 seconds**

Rest between each exercise for **5 seconds**

Total time
**6 minutes
30 seconds**

LEVEL 3

Carry out the exercise sequence **2 times**

Perform each exercise for **30 seconds**

Rest between each exercise for **5 seconds**

Total time
9 minutes

THE EXERCISES

1	UPRIGHT EXTERNAL ROTATION	p.80
2	BIRD DOG	p.88
3	WALL ANGEL	p.84
4	STANDING TWIST	p.108
5	LATERAL STEP-UPS	p.140
6	CHEST OPENER	p.58
7	HIP-UPS	p.136
8	JUMPING WALL PUSH-UPS	p.66

Posture improvement

Prolonged sitting weakens your posture and wears out your muscles and joints, leading to discomfort in your neck, back, and hips. This routine strengthens those muscles so they support proper alignment and reduce the strain on your bones.

WHAT YOU NEED
Dumbbells, mat, wall

YOUR WORKOUT

- Select the level as required by your exercise program.
- Perform the entire sequence of exercises in order for the prescribed number of times. Use a stopwatch to follow the work and rest intervals.
- Remember to breathe deeply during every movement so your muscles are receptive to stretching and strengthening.

THE LEVELS

LEVEL 1

Carry out the exercise sequence **2 times**

Perform each exercise for **30 seconds**

Rest between each exercise for **15 seconds**

Total time **7 minutes**

LEVEL 2

Carry out the exercise sequence **2 times**

Perform each exercise for **30 seconds**

Rest between each exercise for **10 seconds**

Total time **6 minutes 30 seconds**

LEVEL 3

Carry out the exercise sequence **3 times**

Perform each exercise for **30 seconds**

Rest between each exercise for **10 seconds**

Total time **10 minutes**

THE EXERCISES

1	STAGGERED REVERSE FLY	p.76
2	CHEST OPENER	p.58
3	REVERSE LUNGE WITH TWIST	p.128
4	BIRD DOG	p.88
5	WALL ANGEL	p.84

Core strength

Movements such as twisting, bending, and reaching require your lower back and abdominal muscles to work together. This routine includes rotational exercises to activate those muscles, improve your flexibility, and enhance your core stability.

WHAT YOU NEED
Dumbbells

YOUR WORKOUT

- Select the level as required by your exercise program.
- Perform the entire sequence of exercises in order for the prescribed number of times. Use a stopwatch to follow the work and rest intervals.
- If any movements are too strenuous, reduce the weight of your dumbbells or try an easier modification.

THE LEVELS

LEVEL 1

Carry out the exercise sequence **1 time**

Perform each exercise for **30 seconds**

Rest between each exercise for **10 seconds**

Total time **6 minutes 30 seconds**

LEVEL 2

Carry out the exercise sequence **2 times**

Perform each exercise for **30 seconds**

Rest between each exercise for **10 seconds**

Total time **13 minutes**

LEVEL 3

Carry out the exercise sequence **3 times**

Perform each exercise for **40 seconds**

Rest between each exercise for **10 seconds**

Total time **25 minutes**

THE EXERCISES

1	STANDING ELBOW TO KNEE	p.98
2	WINDMILL	p.118
3	KNEE CHOP	p.104
4	STANDING OBLIQUE ROTATION	p.110
5	SIDE-TO-SIDE PUNCH	p.106
6	WOOD CHOP	p.102
7	CROSSOVER TOE TOUCH	p.114
8	DIAGONAL CHOP	p.122
9	STANDING TWIST	p.108
10	STANDING ELBOW TO KNEE	p.98

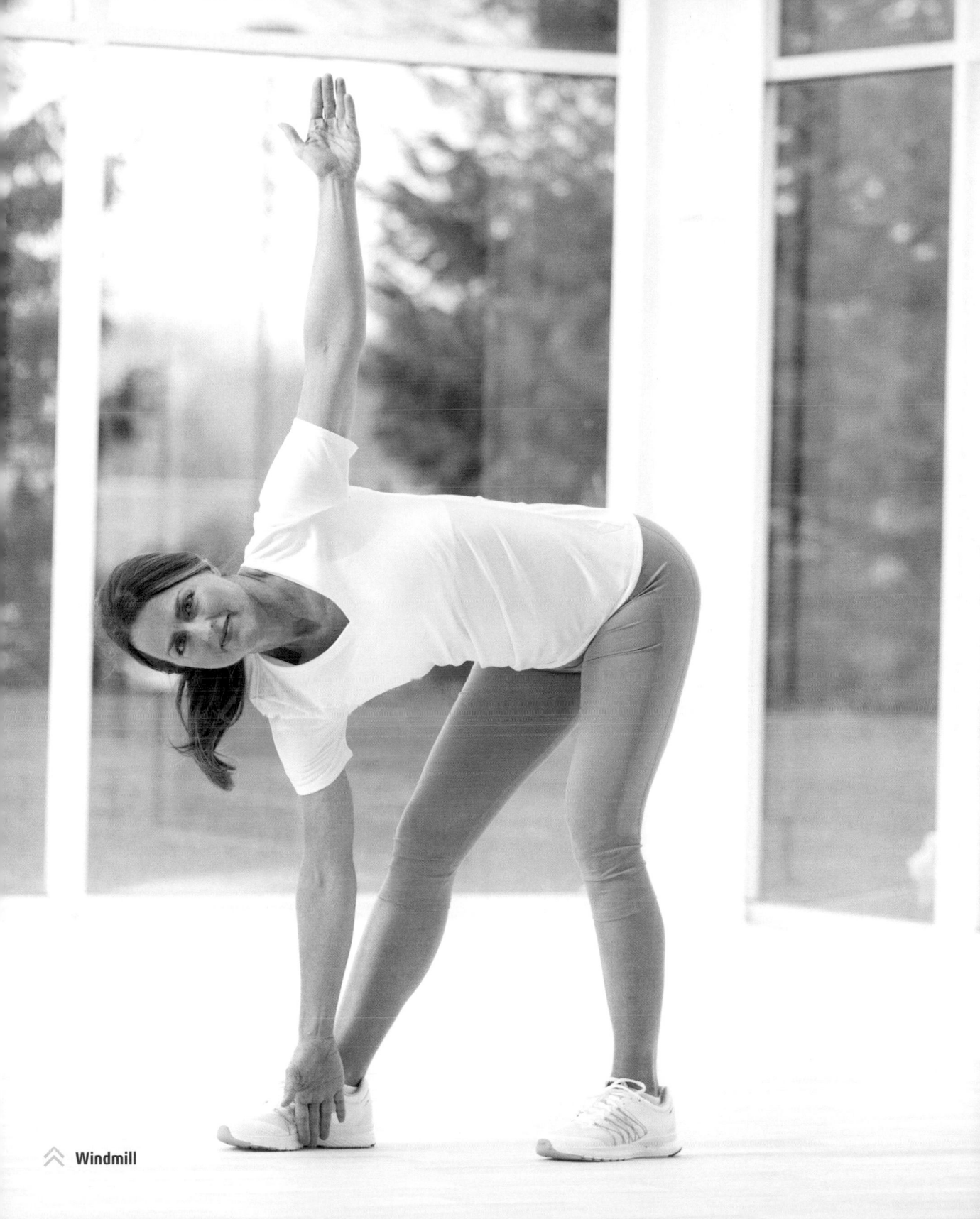

Windmill

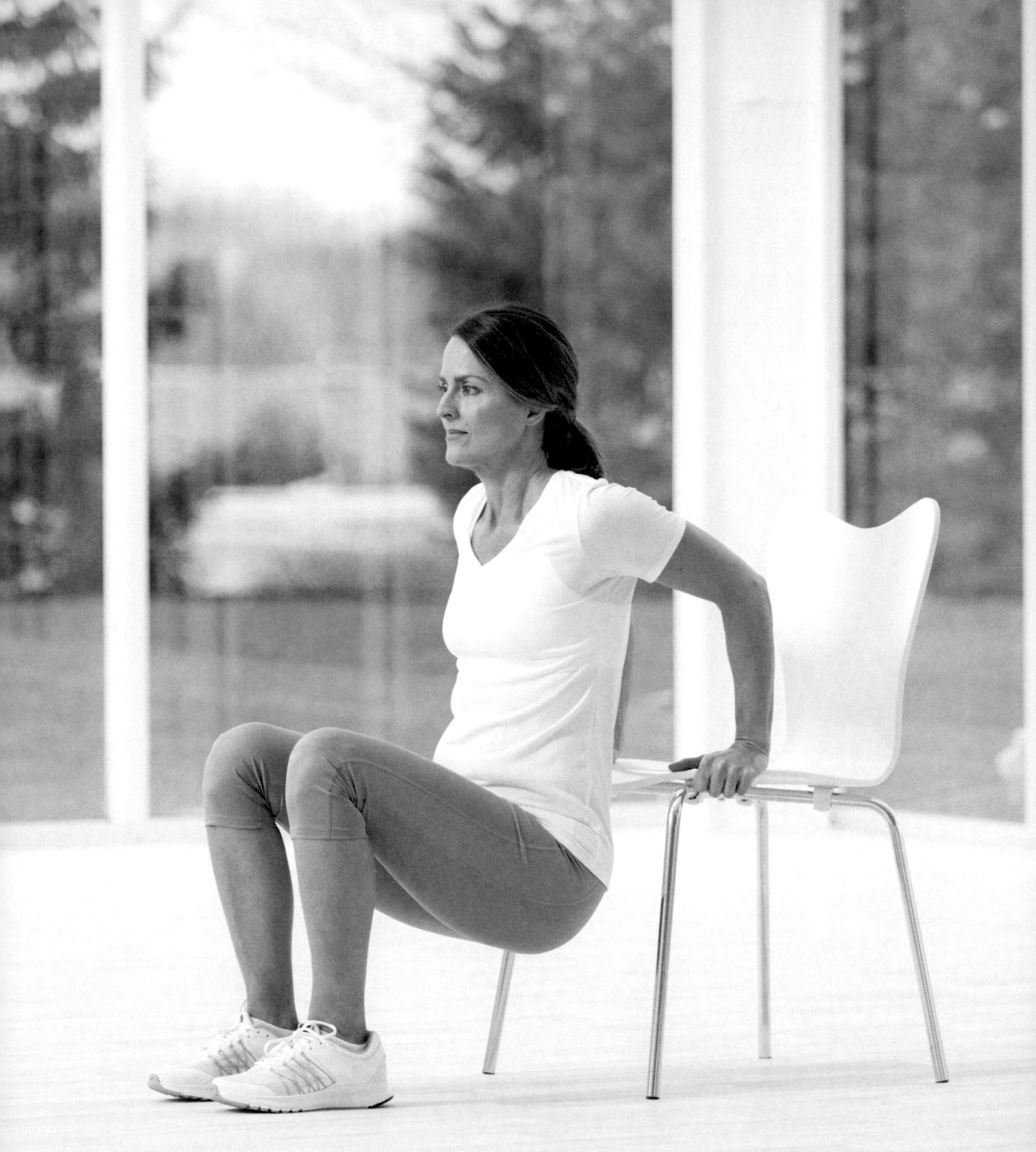

Chair dips

Total-body strength 1

Strength training tones and defines your muscles and makes your body more functional. The resistance exercises in this routine will protect your bones, aid weight loss, and build more lean muscle so your movements are safer and less strenuous.

WHAT YOU NEED
Dumbbells, chair, mat

YOUR WORKOUT

- Select the level as required by your exercise program.
- Perform the entire sequence of exercises in order for the prescribed number of times. Use a stopwatch to follow the work and rest intervals.
- Use slow, controlled movements to maximize muscle recruitment and avoid relying on momentum to move yourself or the weights.

THE LEVELS

LEVEL 1

Carry out the exercise sequence
2 times

Perform each exercise for
20 seconds

Rest between each exercise for
10 seconds

Total time
10 minutes

LEVEL 2

Carry out the exercise sequence
3 times

Perform each exercise for
30 seconds

Rest between each exercise for
15 seconds

Total time
22 minutes

LEVEL 3

Carry out the exercise sequence
3 times

Perform each exercise for
40 seconds

Rest between each exercise for
10 seconds

Total time
25 minutes

THE EXERCISES

#	Exercise	Page
1	LAWN MOWER ROW	p.74
2	CHAIR DIPS	p.52
3	STANDING OBLIQUE ROTATION	p.110
4	STIFF-LEG DEADLIFT AND SHRUG	p.92
5	CURL AND ARNOLD PRESS AND REACH	p.56
6	SIDE LUNGE	p.146
7	FARMER'S WALK	p.36
8	HIGH PLANK REACH-THROUGH AND FLY	p.116
9	GUNSLINGER	p.68
10	ROTATIONAL GOBLET SQUAT	p.112

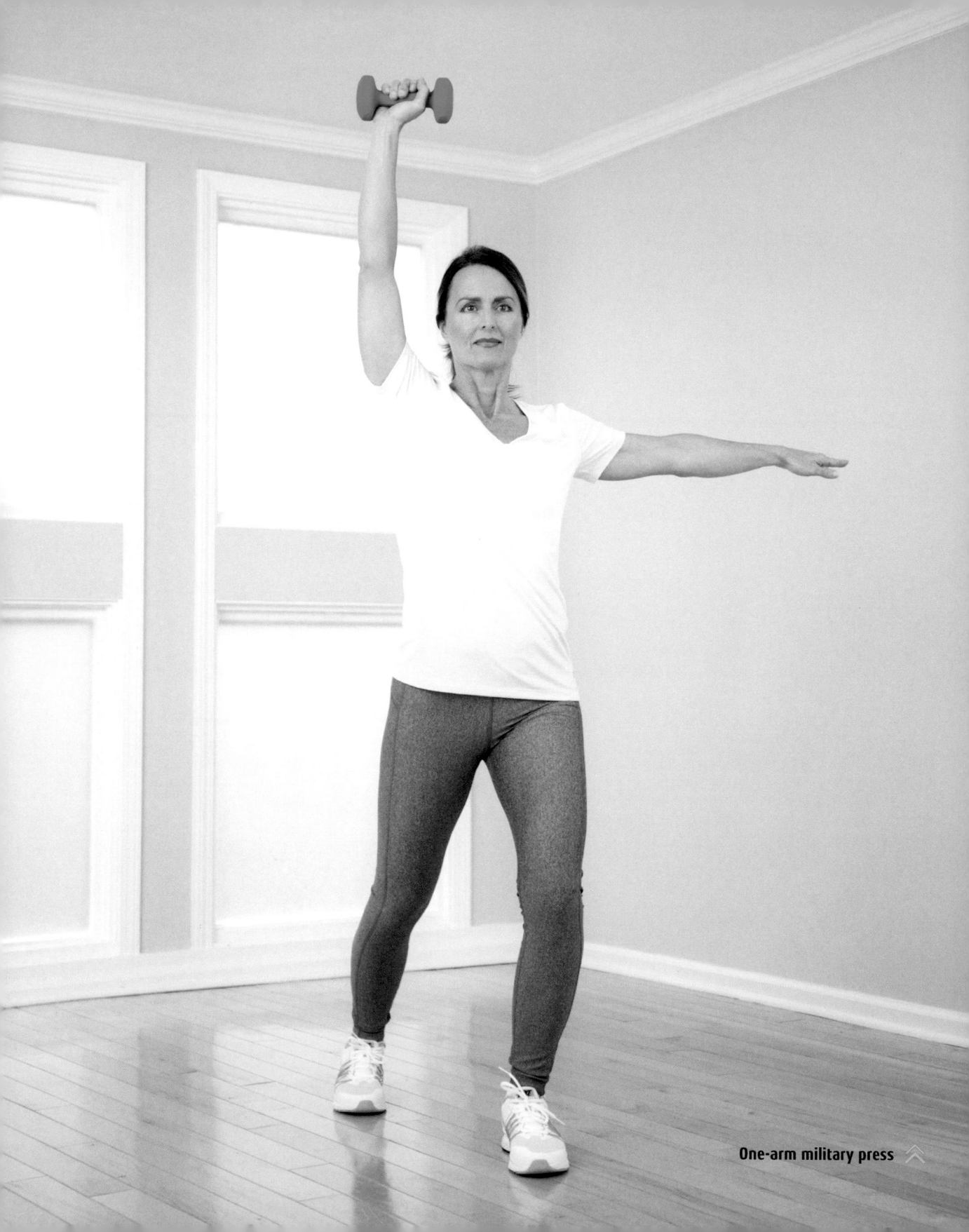

One-arm military press

Total-body strength 2

Do not underestimate the necessity of improving strength. With age, your metabolism can slow, your bones can weaken, and your posture can slump. Build muscle tissue with these exercises to offset the aging process.

WHAT YOU NEED
Dumbbells, chair

YOUR WORKOUT

- Select the level as required by your exercise program.
- Perform the entire sequence of exercises in order for the prescribed number of times. Use a stopwatch to follow the work and rest intervals.
- If you cannot maintain proper form or fully execute a movement, then reduce your resistance or don't use weights at all.

THE LEVELS

LEVEL 1

Carry out the exercise sequence
2 times

Perform each exercise for
20 seconds

Rest between each exercise for
10 seconds

Total time
10 minutes

LEVEL 2

Carry out the exercise sequence
3 times

Perform each exercise for
30 seconds

Rest between each exercise for
15 seconds

Total time
22 minutes

LEVEL 3

Carry out the exercise sequence
3 times

Perform each exercise for
40 seconds

Rest between each exercise for
10 seconds

Total time
25 minutes

THE EXERCISES

#	Exercise	Page
1	STATIONARY LUNGE AND CURL	p.144
2	STIFF-LEG DEADLIFT AND SHRUG	p.92
3	CHAIR DIPS	p.52
4	DIAGONAL CHOP	p.122
5	BENT ROW AND HAMMER CURL	p.82
6	SUITCASE SQUAT	p.124
7	ONE-ARM MILITARY PRESS	p.50
8	STAGGERED REVERSE FLY	p.76
9	REVERSE LUNGE WITH TWIST	p.128
10	STANDING ELBOW TO KNEE	p.98

Lower-back strength

The lower back is a vital link between your upper and lower body that's necessary for functional movements. Strengthen your lower back with these exercises to improve your coordination and become more physically efficient at all of your daily activities.

WHAT YOU NEED
Dumbbells, mat

YOUR WORKOUT

- Select the level as required by your exercise program.
- Perform the entire sequence of exercises in order for the prescribed number of times. Use a stopwatch to follow the work and rest intervals.
- To protect your lower back from strain, keep your core engaged and maintain a flat back for all of these exercises.

THE LEVELS

LEVEL 1

Carry out the exercise sequence
2 times

Perform each exercise for
20 seconds

Rest between each exercise for
10 seconds

Total time
5 minutes

LEVEL 2

Carry out the exercise sequence
2 times

Perform each exercise for
30 seconds

Rest between each exercise for
15 seconds

Total time
7 minutes

LEVEL 3

Carry out the exercise sequence
3 times

Perform each exercise for
40 seconds

Rest between each exercise for
10 seconds

Total time
**12 minutes
30 seconds**

THE EXERCISES

1	BIRD DOG	p.88
2	GOOD MORNING	p.132
3	HIP-UPS	p.136
4	POSTERIOR SWING	p.130
5	CROSSOVER TOE TOUCH	p.114

Upper-body strength

A well-balanced upper body is crucial for proper posture. The muscles that enable you to push and pull are often weakened, lengthened, or tightened by daily habits, so use this workout to restore muscular balance to your arms, chest, and back.

WHAT YOU NEED
Dumbbells, chair, countertop

YOUR WORKOUT

- Select the level as required by your exercise program.
- Perform the entire sequence of exercises in order for the prescribed number of times. Use a stopwatch to follow the work and rest intervals.
- For the most effective muscle recruitment, keep your focus on the muscles you are working.

THE LEVELS

LEVEL 1

Carry out the exercise sequence
2 times

Perform each exercise for
20 seconds

Rest between each exercise for
10 seconds

Total time
7 minutes

LEVEL 2

Carry out the exercise sequence
2 times

Perform each exercise for
30 seconds

Rest between each exercise for
15 seconds

Total time
10 minutes

LEVEL 3

Carry out the exercise sequence
3 times

Perform each exercise for
40 seconds

Rest between each exercise for
10 seconds

Total time
17 minutes 30 seconds

THE EXERCISES

1	ONE-ARM CHEST PRESS	p.62
2	BENT ROW AND HAMMER CURL	p.82
3	CHAIR DIPS	p.52
4	ONE-ARM SNATCH	p.86
5	CURL AND ARNOLD PRESS AND REACH	p.56
6	INCLINED PUSH-UPS	p.54
7	STAGGERED REVERSE FLY	p.76

Lower-body strength

You engage your lower body every time you squat down to pick up boxes, carry groceries, or move furniture. Perform these functional lower-body exercises to promote stability, improve strength, and prevent lower-back strains.

WHAT YOU NEED
Dumbbells, step, mat

YOUR WORKOUT

- Select the level as required by your exercise program.
- Perform the entire sequence of exercises in order for the prescribed number of times. Use a stopwatch to follow the work and rest intervals.
- For the most efficient lower-body workout, keep your core engaged and your back flat for all of these exercises.

THE LEVELS

LEVEL 1

Carry out the exercise sequence
2 times

Perform each exercise for
20 seconds

Rest between each exercise for
10 seconds

Total time
7 minutes

LEVEL 2

Carry out the exercise sequence
2 times

Perform each exercise for
30 seconds

Rest between each exercise for
15 seconds

Total time
10 minutes

LEVEL 3

Carry out the exercise sequence
3 times

Perform each exercise for
40 seconds

Rest between each exercise for
10 seconds

Total time
**17 minutes
30 seconds**

THE EXERCISES

1	LATERAL STEP-UPS	p.140
2	SUITCASE SQUAT	p.124
3	WALKING REACHING LUNGE	p.126
4	GOOD MORNING	p.132
5	REVERSE LUNGE WITH TWIST	p.128
6	HIP-UPS	p.136
7	SIDE LUNGE	p.146

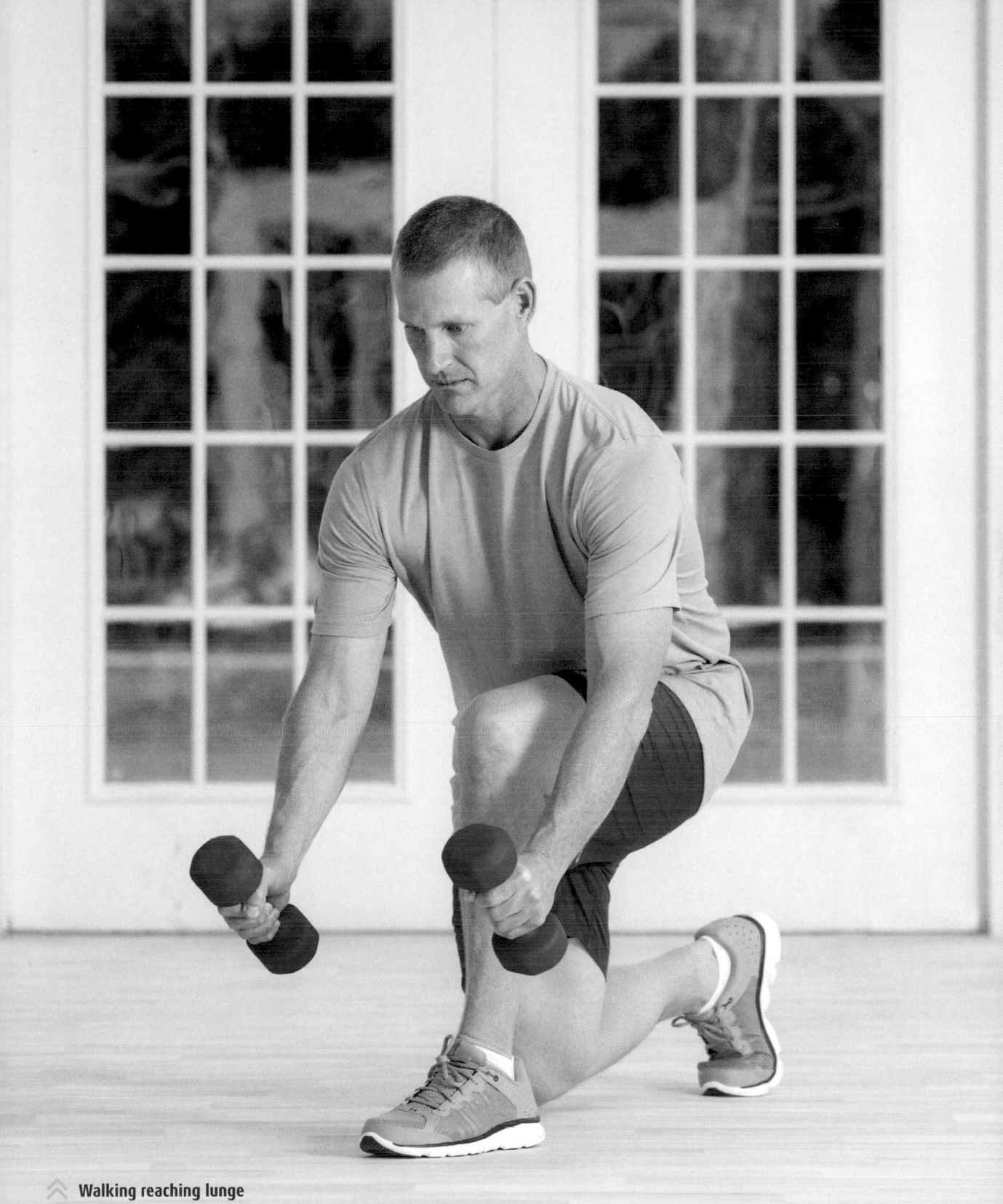

Walking reaching lunge

Low-impact aerobic

To improve your cardiovascular fitness while going easy on your joints, do this low-impact routine. This sequence of aerobic exercises places low stress on your joints while still improving your endurance and strengthening your heart.

WHAT YOU NEED
Dumbbells, wall

YOUR WORKOUT

- Select the level as required by your exercise program.
- Perform the entire sequence of exercises in order two times. Use a stopwatch to follow the work and rest intervals.
- Perform the exercises swiftly to boost your heart rate. If you can hold a conversation during your workout, push yourself a little harder.

THE LEVELS

LEVEL 1

Carry out the exercise sequence
2 times

Perform each exercise for
15 seconds

Rest between each exercise for
15 seconds

Total time
10 minutes

LEVEL 2

Carry out the exercise sequence
2 times

Perform each exercise for
20 seconds

Rest between each exercise for
10 seconds

Total time
10 minutes

LEVEL 3

Carry out the exercise sequence
2 times

Perform each exercise for
30 seconds

Rest between each exercise for
10 seconds

Total time
13 minutes

THE EXERCISES

1	FAST FEET	p.26
2	STANDING ELBOW TO KNEE	p.98
3	POSTERIOR SWING	p.130
4	JUMPING WALL PUSH-UPS	p.66
5	SIDE-TO-SIDE	p.28
6	SEESAW ROW	p.94
7	STANDING TWIST	p.108
8	PUSH PRESS	p.60
9	MARCH IN PLACE	p.32
10	EARTHQUAKES	p.138

Cool down

This quick and effective cool down helps your body smoothly transition from exercising to a resting state. Follow the routine after every workout to slowly reduce your heart rate, prevent dizziness, and resume a normal breathing pattern.

WHAT YOU NEED
Wall, mat

YOUR WORKOUT

- After every workout, perform the entire sequence of cool-down exercises in order at least once, but repeat as necessary until you reach a resting state.
- Do not use dumbbells for any of these exercises.
- Focus on gradually lowering your heart rate, and be proud of yourself for making it through the day's workout.

THE LEVELS

ALL LEVELS

Carry out the exercise sequence at least **1 time**

Perform each exercise for **20 seconds**

Rest between each exercise for **10 seconds**

Total time
**2 minutes
30 seconds**

THE EXERCISES

1	MARCH IN PLACE	p.32
2	CHEST OPENER	p.58
3	WALL ANGEL	p.84
4	UPRIGHT EXTERNAL ROTATION	p.80
5	HIP-UPS	p.136

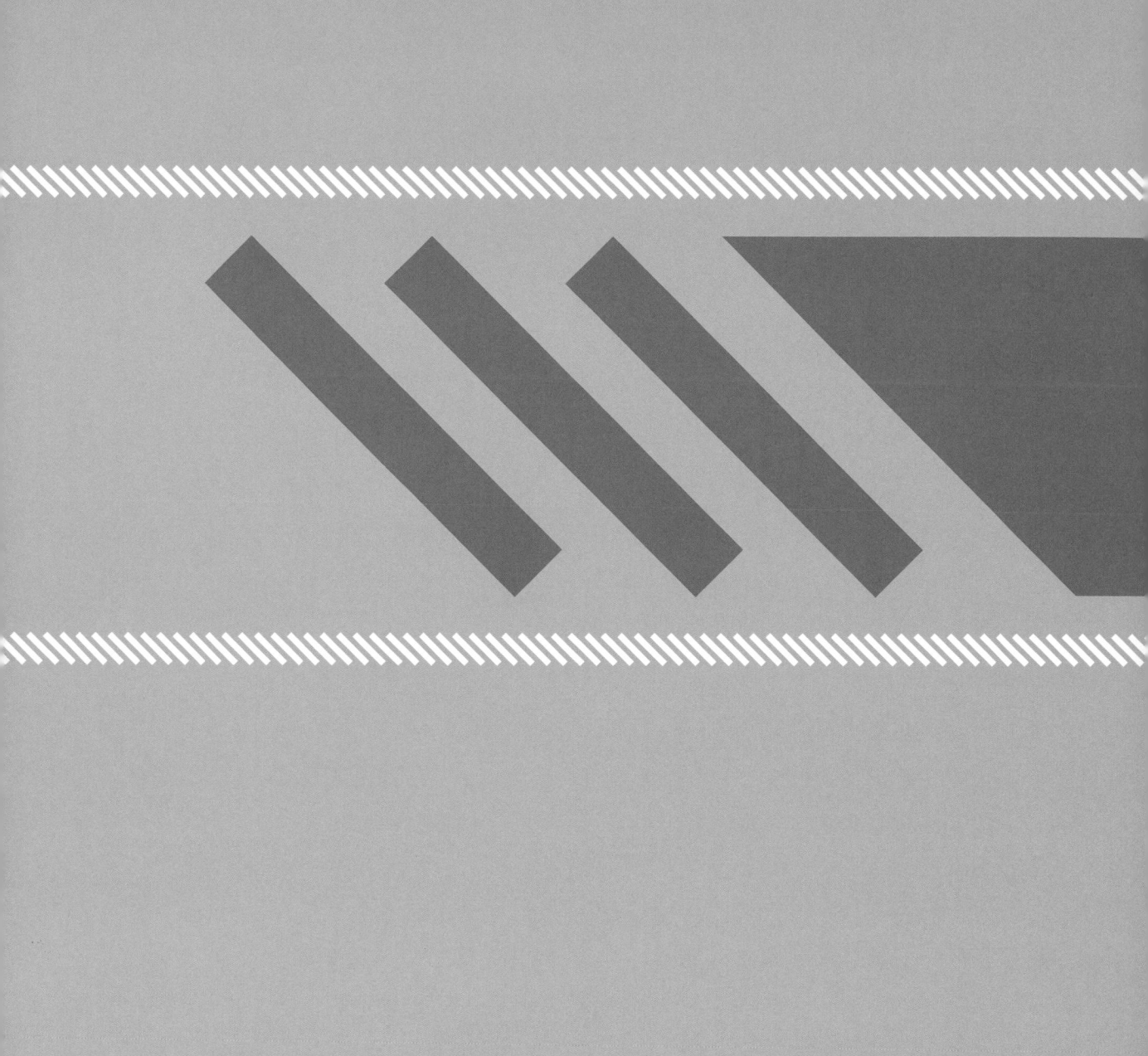

FITNESS
PROGRAMS

Regain your functional strength and mobility and create a healthy habit of exercise by following one of these 30-day fitness programs. Built from the routines in the previous chapter, each program is an easy-to-follow schedule of workouts that you can integrate into your active life.

Beginner

Every winner was once a beginner—this program is the perfect way to begin your fitness journey. Follow the schedule and notice your body becoming stronger and more mobile as you confidently attack each day.

WORK DAYS

Begin each day with the *Warm up* (p.152). After completing the day's routine(s), finish your workout with the *Cool down* (p.179).

If any week is too strenuous, repeat that week until you feel confident enough to progress. Once you complete all four weeks, re-assess your fitness level and repeat the program, or start a new program.

REST DAYS

Your body needs down time to recover, so always take two rest days per week. However, you can shift the work and rest days within each week to fit your schedule.

WEEK 1

WEEK 2

WEEK 3

WEEK 4

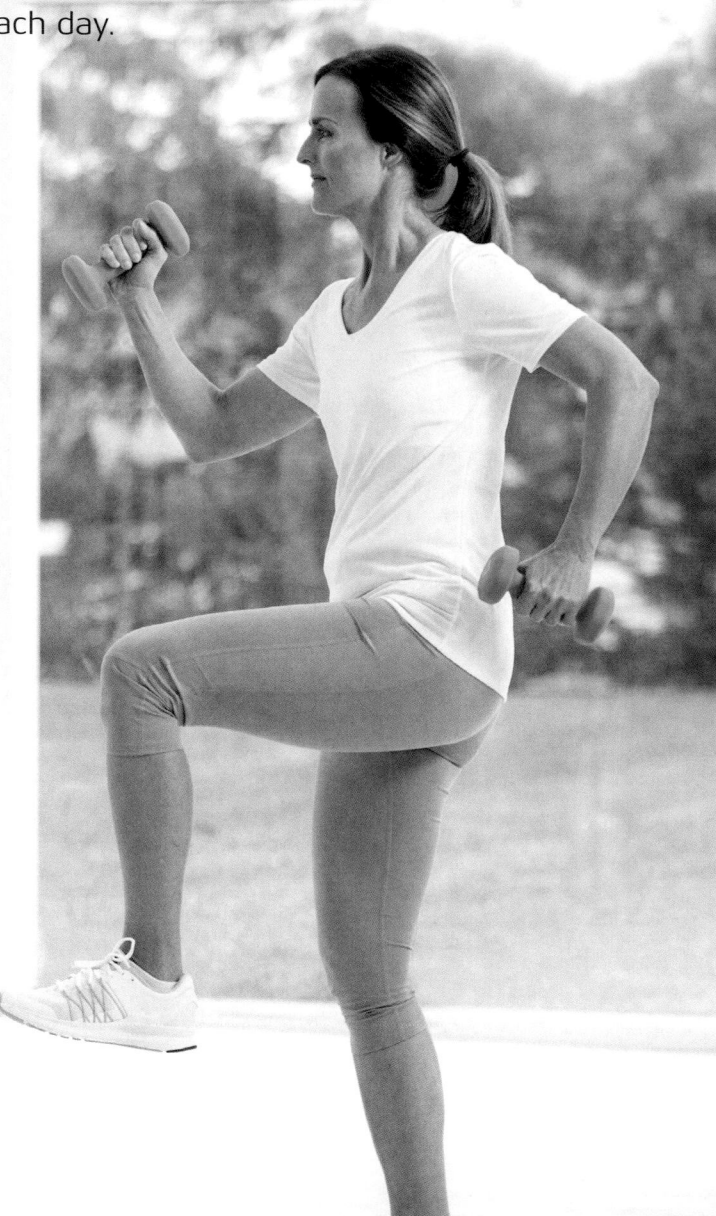

⌃ **March in place**

DAY 1	DAY 2	DAY 3	DAY 4	DAY 5	DAY 6	DAY 7
• **5-minute kick-start:** level 1 *page 153*	• **Beginner total body:** level 1 *page 156*	• **Low-intensity strength:** level 1 *page 157* • **Posture improvement:** level 1 *page 167*	• **Rest**	• **Low-impact aerobic:** level 1 *page 178*	• **Core strength:** level 1 *page 168*	• **Rest**
• **Total-body mobility:** level 1 *page 161*	• **Prehabilitation:** level 1 *page 166*	• **Beginner total body:** level 1 *page 156*	• **Rest**	• **Balance and stability:** level 1 *page 160*	• **Lower-back strength:** level 1 *page 174*	• **Rest**
• **Low-impact aerobic:** level 2 *page 178*	• **Core strength:** level 2 *page 168* • **Posture improvement:** level 1 *page 167*	• **Beginner total body:** level 2 *page 156*	• **Rest**	• **Balance and stability:** level 1 *page 160* • **Lower-back strength:** level 1 *page 174*	• **Total-body strength 2:** level 1 *page 173*	• **Rest**
• **Cardiovascular endurance:** level 1 *page 154*	• **Beginner total body:** level 2 *page 156*	• **Total-body mobility:** level 1 *page 161* • **Posture improvement:** level 1 *page 167*	• **Rest**	• **Low-impact aerobic:** level 2 *page 178*	• **Total-body strength 2:** level 2 *page 173*	• **Rest**

Intermediate

You already have a foundation of strength and stability, so break out of your comfort zone and use this program to continue growing stronger and building a lifelong habit of functional exercise.

WORK DAYS

Begin each day with the *Warm up* (p.152). After completing the day's routine(s), finish your workout with the *Cool down* (p.179).

If any week is too strenuous, repeat that week until you feel confident enough to progress. Once you complete all four weeks, re-assess your fitness level and repeat the program, or start a new program.

REST DAYS

Your body needs down time to recover, so always take two rest days per week. However, you can shift the work and rest days within each week to fit your schedule.

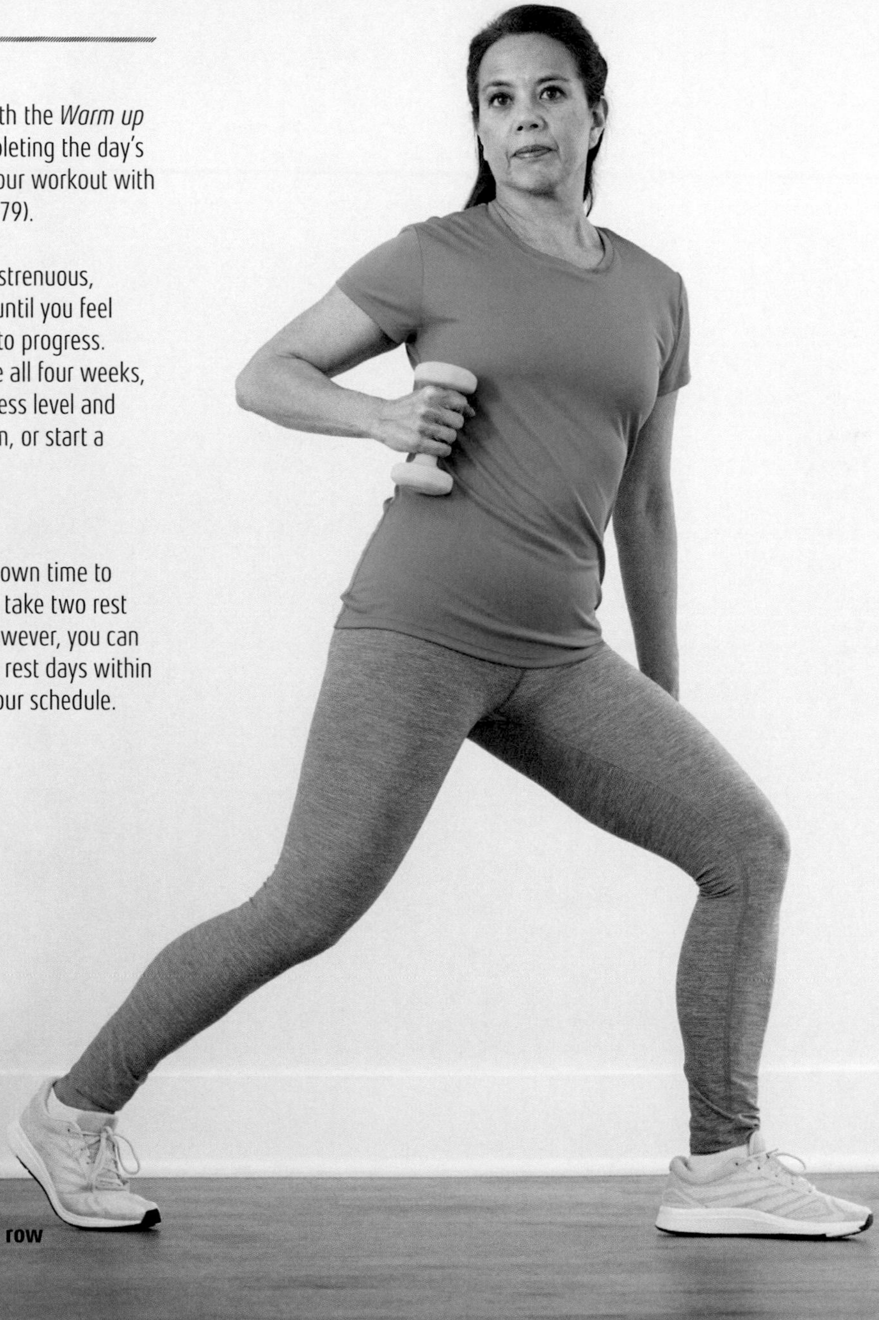

WEEK 1

WEEK 2

WEEK 3

WEEK 4

Lawn mower row

DAY 1	DAY 2	DAY 3	DAY 4	DAY 5	DAY 6	DAY 7
• **Cardiovascular endurance:** level 2 *page 154*	• **Total-body strength 1:** level 2 *page 171*	• **Core strength:** level 2 *page 168*	• **Rest**	• **Calorie-burning HIIT:** level 2 *page 165*	• **Total-body strength 2:** level 2 *page 173*	• **Rest**
• **Lower-body strength:** level 2 *page 176*	• **Upper-body strength:** level 2 *page 175*	• **Total-body mobility:** level 2 *page 161*	• **Rest**	• **Cardiovascular endurance:** level 2 *page 154*	• **Calorie-burning HIIT:** level 2 *page 165*	• **Rest**
• **Total-body strength 1:** level 2 *page 171*	• **Balance and stability:** level 2 *page 160* • **Posture improvement:** level 2 *page 167*	• **Cross-training:** level 2 *page 162*	• **Rest**	• **Prehabilitation:** level 2 *page 166* • **Low-impact aerobic:** level 2 *page 178*	• **Total-body strength 2:** level 2 *page 173*	• **Rest**
• **Speed and agility:** level 2 *page 158*	• **Total-body mobility:** level 2 *page 161*	• **Cross-training:** level 2 *page 162*	• **Rest**	• **Upper-body strength:** level 2 *page 175*	• **Lower-body strength:** level 2 *page 176*	• **Rest**

Advanced

Speed, power, strength, balance, and coordination are all necessary components of functional movement. Push yourself with this challenging program and achieve a high level of functional fitness.

WORK DAYS

Begin each day with the *Warm up* (p.152). After completing the day's routine(s), finish your workout with the *Cool down* (p.179).

If any week is too strenuous, repeat that week until you feel confident enough to progress. Once you complete all four weeks, repeat the program while increasing the weight of your dumbbells and selecting the harder modifications.

REST DAYS

Your body needs down time to recover, so always take two rest days per week. However, you can shift the work and rest days within each week to fit your schedule.

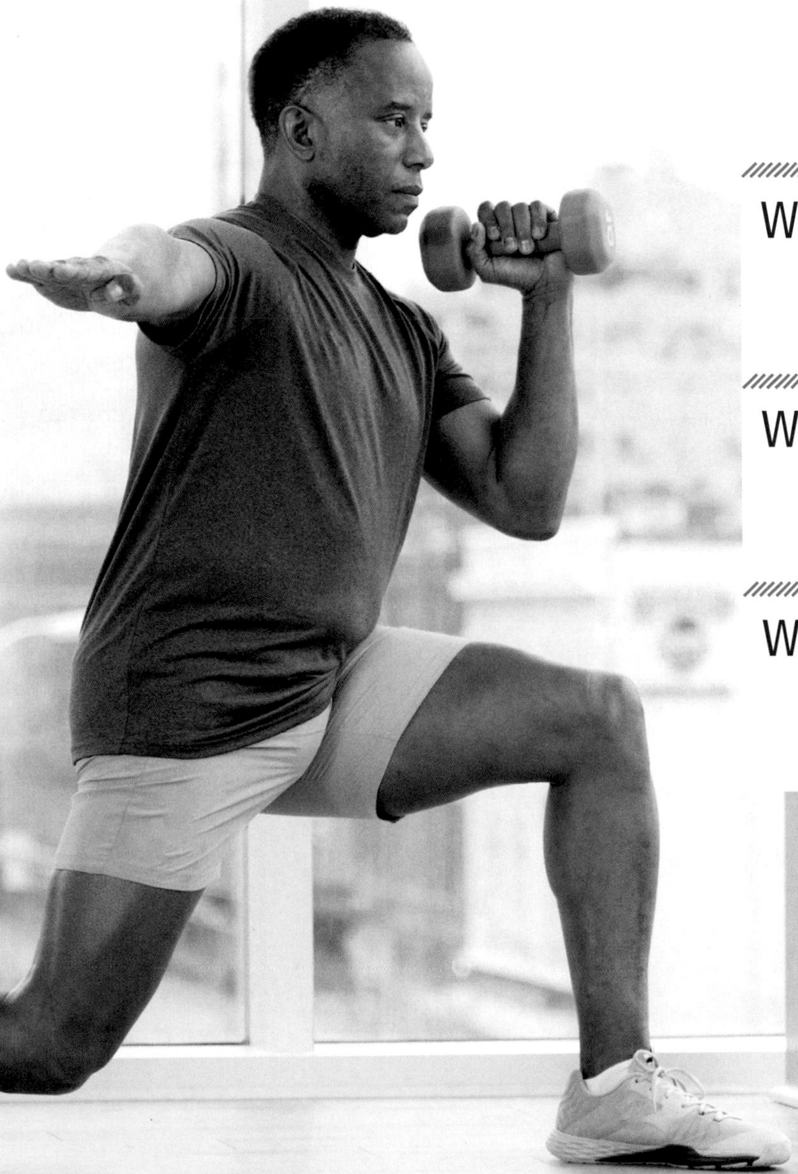

WEEK 1

WEEK 2

WEEK 3

WEEK 4

⌃ **Shot-put press**

DAY 1	DAY 2	DAY 3	DAY 4	DAY 5	DAY 6	DAY 7
• **Calorie-burning HIIT:** level 3 *page 165*	• **Total-body strength 2:** level 3 *page 173*	• **Balance and stability:** level 3 *page 160* • **Posture improvement:** level 3 *page 167*	• Rest	• **Cross-training:** level 3 *page 162*	• **Core strength:** level 3 *page 168*	• Rest
• **Total-body strength 1:** level 3 *page 171*	• **Cardiovascular endurance:** level 3 *page 154*	• **Prehabilitation:** level 3 *page 166*	• Rest	• **Lower-body strength:** level 3 *page 176*	• **Upper-body strength:** level 3 *page 175*	• Rest
• **Speed and agility:** level 3 *page 158*	• **Total-body mobility:** level 3 *page 161*	• **Total-body strength 2:** level 3 *page 173*	• Rest	• **Cross-training:** level 3 *page 162*	• **Cardiovascular endurance:** level 3 *page 154*	• Rest
• **Lower-body strength:** level 3 *page 176*	• **Upper-body strength:** level 3 *page 175*	• **Calorie-burning HIIT:** level 3 *page 165*	• Rest	• **Total-body strength 1:** level 3 *page 171*	• **Speed and agility:** level 3 *page 158*	• Rest

Index

About the author

As an ISSA-certified trainer, Joshua Kozak is a seasoned leader and motivator in the fitness industry with over 15 years of experience. Through his HASfit brand, he has helped over 60 million people all over the globe get stronger and healthier with his highly effective yet simple workouts, found on HASfit.com or YouTube. Kozak's positive motivational style has earned him many accolades, including being named one of the "Top 10 Trainers on YouTube" by Google in 2014, 2015, and 2016.

Kozak is a loving father to his daughter, Alessandra, and an adoring husband to his wife, Claudia.

Author's dedication

My dear Claudia,

You sacrifice. You support. You do all of the real work. No great woman stands behind me, because you stand beside me. Thank you for keeping me humble, making me breakfast every morning, laughing at my cheesy jokes, and listening to me while I talk your ear off. You're the greatest gift the Lord could ever give me.

Joshua

Publisher's acknowledgments

DK would like to thank the following:

Models Troy Leach, Tami Soetenga, Rachel Pfeiffer, Keith Payne, and Olga Imperial Keegan

Proofreader Laura Caddell

Indexer Celia McCoy

Bibliography

Pages 14–15
Strengthens bones J. Watkins, "Physical activity helps reduce bone loss", (extract from J. Watkins, *Structure and Function of the Musculoskeletal System, Second Edition*, Illinois, USA: Human Kinetics, 2010) Human Kinetics, http://www.humankinetics.com/excerpts/excerpts/physical-activity-helps-reduce-bone-loss; **Builds lean muscle** "Sarcopenia With Aging", WebMD Medical Reference, http://www.webmd.com/healthy-aging/guide/sarcopenia-with-aging#1; **Preserves vital joint tissues** A. Sinha, *Remedies and Cures for the Common Diseases*, New York: Page Publishing Inc., 2015; **Sharpens nervous system** "Falls Prevention Facts", National Council on Aging, https://www.ncoa.org/news/resources-for-reporters/get-the-facts/falls-prevention-facts/; **Improves heart health and blood flow** "Cardiovascular diseases (CVDs)", World Health Organization, http://www.who.int/mediacentre/factsheets/fs317/en/; **Extends life span** S.C. Moore, A.V. Patel, C.E. Matthews et al, "Leisure Time Physical Activity of Moderate to Vigorous Intensity and Mortality: A Large Pooled Cohort Analysis", *Public Library of Science* no. 9 (11), November 2012, DOI: https://doi.org/10.1371/journal.pmed.1001335; **Improves mood and confidence** A. Pietrangelo, "Depression and Mental Health by the Numbers: Facts, Statistics, and You", Healthline, http://www.healthline.com/health/depression/facts-statistics-infographic; **Increases lung function** G. Sharma and J. Goodwin, "Effect of aging on respiratory system physiology and immunology", *Clinical Interventions in Aging* no. 1 (3), September 2006, 253–260; **Boosts metabolism** G. Boston, "Basal metabolic rate changes as you age", *Washington Post*, 5 March 2013

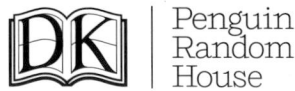

Editor Alexandra Elliott
Senior editor Brook Farling
Book designer XAB Design
Art director for photography Nigel Wright
Photographer Elese Keturah Bales
Jacket designer Steve Marsden
Associate publisher Billy Fields
Publisher Mike Sanders

First American Edition, 2017
Published in the United States by DK Publishing
6081 E. 82nd Street, Indianapolis, Indiana 46250

ISBN: 978-1-4654-6275-6

Library of Congress Catalog Number: 2017930735

Note: This publication contains the opinions and ideas of its author(s). It is intended
to provide helpful and informative material on the subject matter covered. It is sold with
the understanding that the author(s) and publisher are not engaged in rendering
professional services in the book. If the reader requires personal assistance or advice,
a competent professional should be consulted. The author(s) and publisher specifically
disclaim any responsibility for any liability, loss, or risk, personal or otherwise, which is
incurred as a consequence, directly or indirectly, of the use and application of any of
the contents of this book.

Trademarks: All terms mentioned in this book that are known to be or are suspected
of being trademarks or service marks have been appropriately capitalized. Alpha
Books, DK, and Penguin Random House LLC cannot attest to the accuracy of this
information. Use of a term in this book should not be regarded as affecting the validity
of any trademark or service mark.

DK books are available at special discounts when purchased in bulk for sales
promotions, premiums, fund-raising, or educational use. For details, contact:
DK Publishing Special Markets, 1450 Broadway, Suite 801, New York, NY 10018 USA
or SpecialSales@dk.com.

Printed and bound in Canada

All images © Dorling Kindersley Limited
For further information see: www.dkimages.com

A WORLD OF IDEAS:
SEE ALL THERE IS TO KNOW

www.dk.com

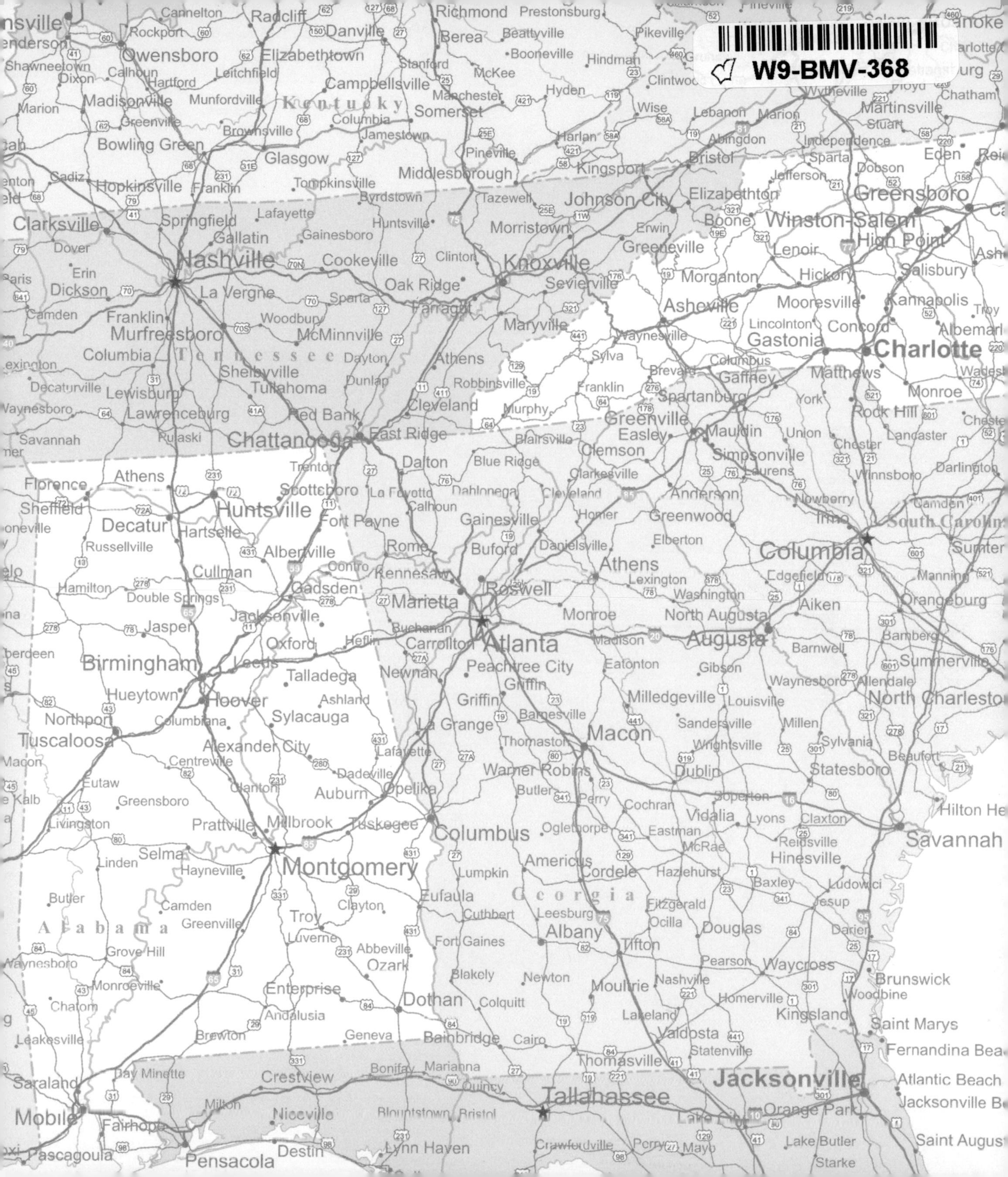
Kentucky
Tennessee
Alabama
Georgia
South Carolina
Owensboro
Elizabethtown
Danville
Richmond
Berea
Campbellsville
Somerset
Madisonville
Bowling Green
Glasgow
Hopkinsville
Middlesborough
Kingsport
Bristol
Johnson City
Clarksville
Nashville
Knoxville
Cookeville
Oak Ridge
Murfreesboro
Franklin
Columbia
Shelbyville
Tullahoma
McMinnville
Morristown
Greeneville
Sevierville
Maryville
Cleveland
Chattanooga
East Ridge
Winston-Salem
Greensboro
High Point
Hickory
Morganton
Asheville
Gastonia
Charlotte
Concord
Kannapolis
Salisbury
Rock Hill
Spartanburg
Greenville
Mauldin
Anderson
Greenwood
Columbia
Florence
Athens
Decatur
Huntsville
Gadsden
Birmingham
Hoover
Tuscaloosa
Montgomery
Dothan
Auburn
Opelika
Rome
Marietta
Roswell
Atlanta
Athens
Augusta
Aiken
Macon
Columbus
Albany
Valdosta
Savannah
Brunswick
Tallahassee
Jacksonville
Pensacola
Mobile
Orangeburg
North Charleston
Summerville
Hilton Head
Statesboro
Dublin
Warner Robins
Waycross
Thomasville
Tifton
Moultrie
La Grange
Newnan
Peachtree City
Carrollton
Cullman
Anniston
Talladega
Sylacauga
Alexander City
Selma
Prattville
Enterprise
Eufaula
Troy
Crestview
Destin
Fairhope
Saint Marys
Fernandina Beach
Atlantic Beach
Jacksonville Beach
Saint Augustine
Orange Park

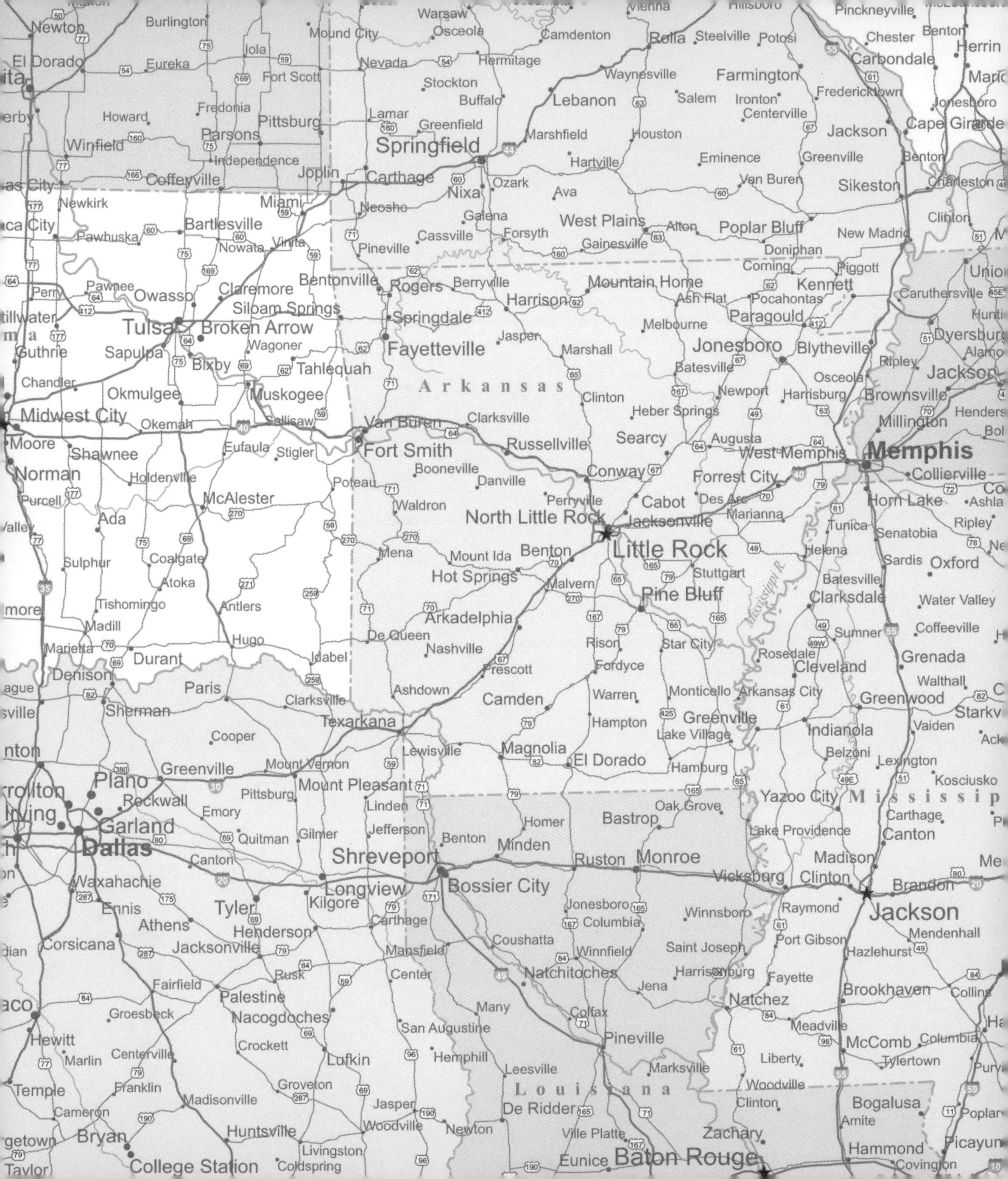

Newton
Burlington
El Dorado
Eureka
Iola
Mound City
Warsaw
Osceola
Camdenton
Rolla
Steelville
Potosi
Pinckneyville
Chester
Benton
Herrin
Carbondale
Fort Scott
Nevada
Hermitage
Waynesville
Farmington
Fredericktown
Howard
Fredonia
Stockton
Buffalo
Lebanon
Salem
Ironton
Centerville
Jonesboro
Pittsburg
Lamar
Greenfield
Marshfield
Houston
Jackson
Cape Girardeau
Winfield
Parsons
Independence
Springfield
Hartville
Eminence
Greenville
Coffeyville
Joplin
Carthage
Nixa
Ozark
Ava
Van Buren
Sikeston
Charleston
Newkirk
Miami
Neosho
Galena
West Plains
Alton
Poplar Bluff
New Madrid
Bartlesville
Pawhuska
Nowata
Vinita
Pineville
Cassville
Forsyth
Gainesville
Doniphan
Corning
Piggott
Kennett
Pawnee
Perry
Owasso
Claremore
Bentonville
Rogers
Berryville
Harrison
Mountain Home
Ash Flat
Pocahontas
Caruthersville
Siloam Springs
Springdale
Melbourne
Paragould
Tulsa
Broken Arrow
Guthrie
Sapulpa
Wagoner
Bixby
Tahlequah
Fayetteville
Jasper
Marshall
Jonesboro
Blytheville
Dyersburg
Ripley
Batesville
Osceola
Jackson
Chandler
Okmulgee
Muskogee
Arkansas
Clinton
Newport
Harrisburg
Brownsville
Heber Springs
Midwest City
Okemah
Sallisaw
Van Buren
Clarksville
Millington
Moore
Shawnee
Eufaula
Stigler
Fort Smith
Russellville
Searcy
Augusta
West Memphis
Memphis
Norman
Holdenville
Booneville
Danville
Conway
Forrest City
Collierville
Purcell
McAlester
Poteau
Waldron
Perryville
Cabot
Des Arc
Marianna
Horn Lake
Ada
North Little Rock
Jacksonville
Tunica
Ripley
Senatobia
Little Rock
Mena
Mount Ida
Benton
Helena
Sardis
Oxford
Sulphur
Coalgate
Atoka
Hot Springs
Malvern
Stuttgart
Batesville
Pine Bluff
Clarksdale
Water Valley
Tishomingo
Antlers
Arkadelphia
Mississippi R.
Madill
De Queen
Nashville
Rison
Star City
Sumner
Coffeeville
Marietta
Hugo
Idabel
Durant
Rosedale
Cleveland
Grenada
Denison
Prescott
Fordyce
Paris
Clarksville
Ashdown
Camden
Warren
Monticello
Arkansas City
Walthall
Sherman
Greenwood
Texarkana
Hampton
Greenville
Lake Village
Indianola
Vaiden
Cooper
Lewisville
Magnolia
El Dorado
Belzoni
Lexington
Greenville
Mount Vernon
Hamburg
Kosciusko
Plano
Mount Pleasant
Pittsburg
Rockwall
Linden
Oak Grove
Yazoo City
Mississippi
Irving
Emory
Garland
Homer
Bastrop
Carthage
Jefferson
Lake Providence
Canton
Quitman
Gilmer
Benton
Dallas
Minden
Shreveport
Canton
Ruston
Monroe
Vicksburg
Madison
Clinton
Waxahachie
Longview
Bossier City
Brandon
Ennis
Kilgore
Tyler
Jonesboro
Raymond
Jackson
Athens
Carthage
Winnsboro
Columbia
Henderson
Corsicana
Jacksonville
Coushatta
Port Gibson
Mendenhall
Mansfield
Winnfield
Saint Joseph
Hazlehurst
Rusk
Center
Natchitoches
Harrisonburg
Fairfield
Jena
Fayette
Palestine
Brookhaven
Natchez
Collins
Groesbeck
Nacogdoches
Many
Colfax
Meadville
Hewitt
Crockett
San Augustine
Pineville
McComb
Columbia
Marlin
Centerville
Lufkin
Hemphill
Leesville
Marksville
Liberty
Tylertown
Temple
Franklin
Groveton
Woodville
Louisiana
Madisonville
Jasper
Clinton
Bogalusa
Cameron
De Ridder
Amite
Bryan
Huntsville
Woodville
Newton
Ville Platte
Zachary
Hammond
Picayune
Livingston
College Station
Coldspring
Eunice
Baton Rouge
Covington
Taylor

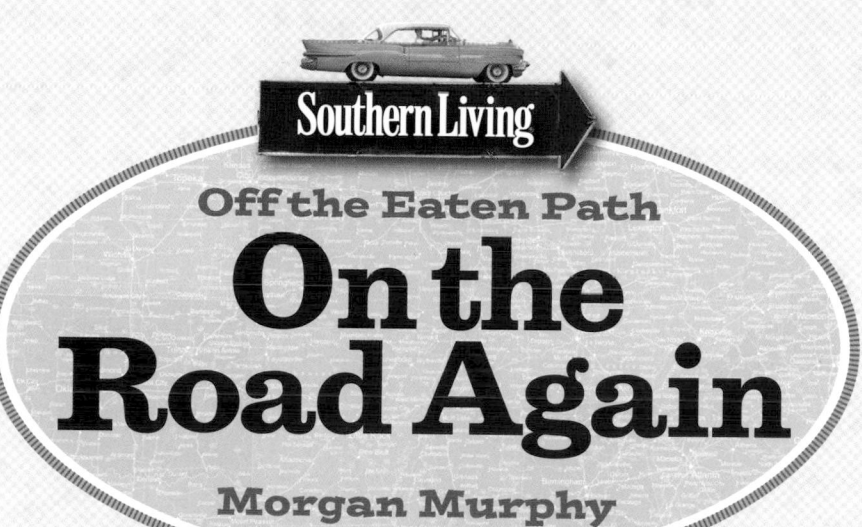

Southern Living

Off the Eaten Path
On the
Road Again

Morgan Murphy

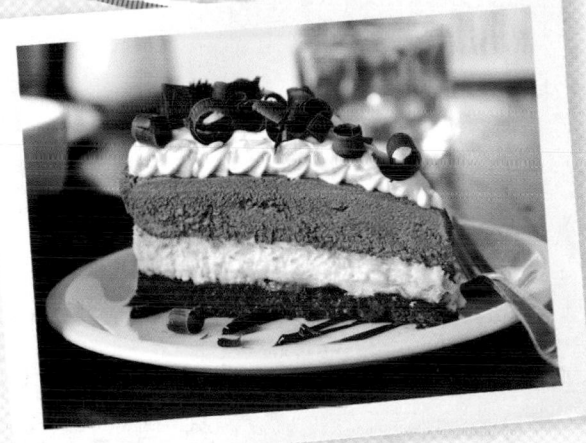

Oxmoor House®

Contents

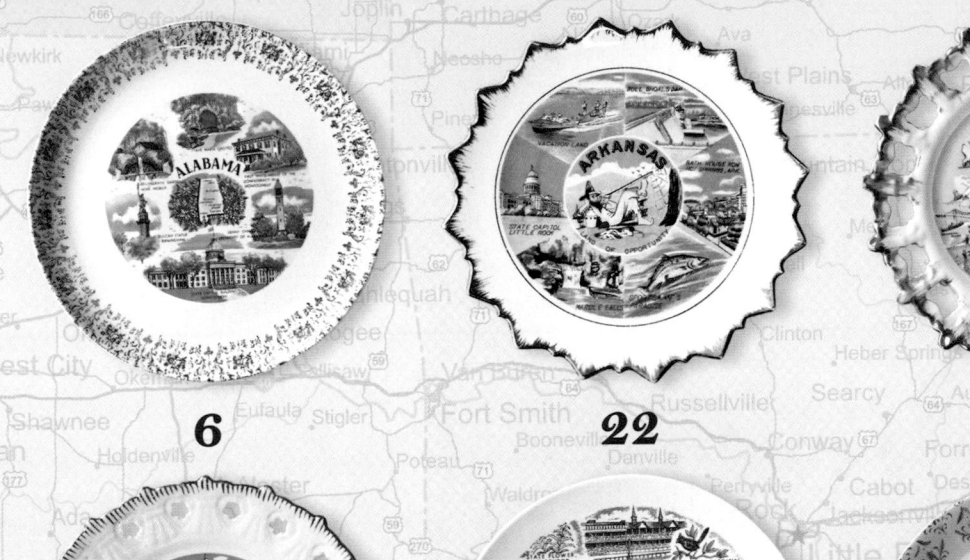
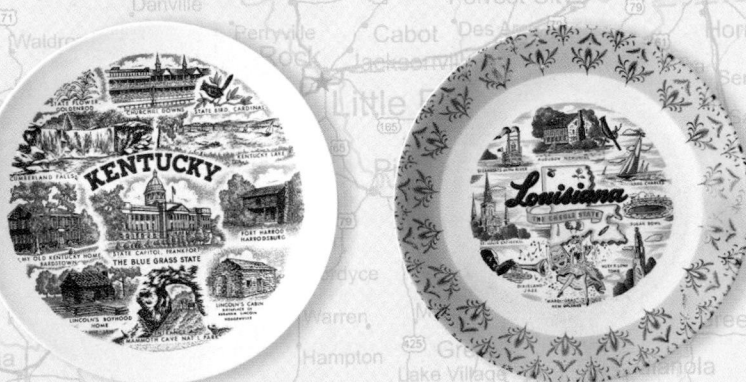
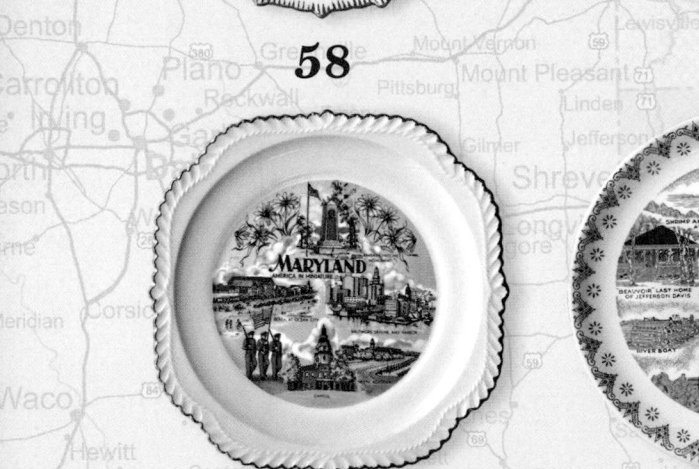
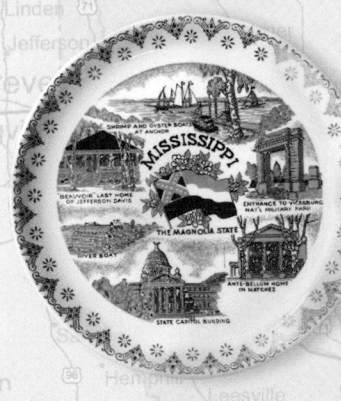
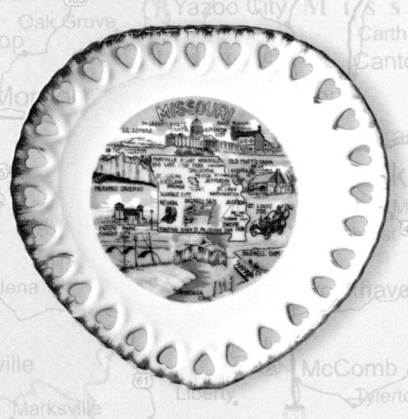

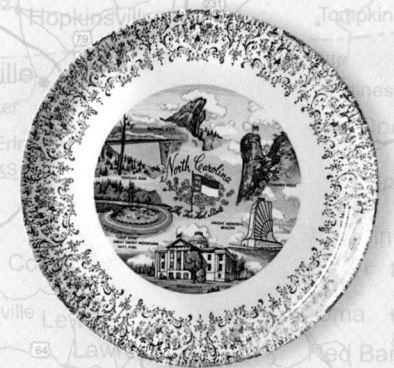

138

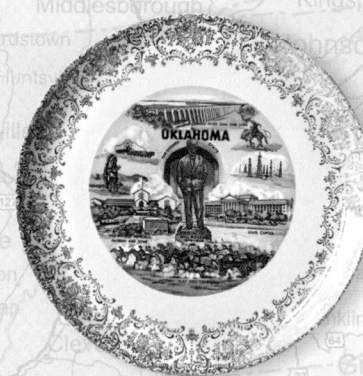

152

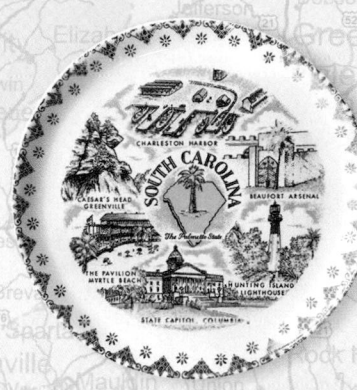

168

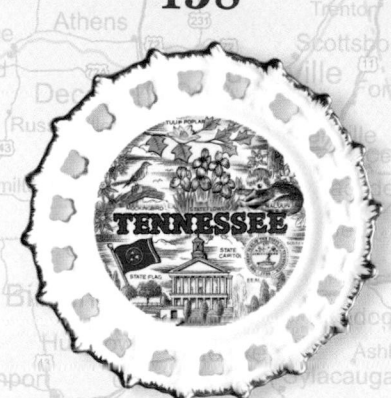

192

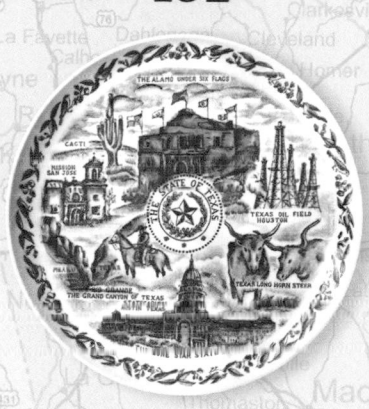

212

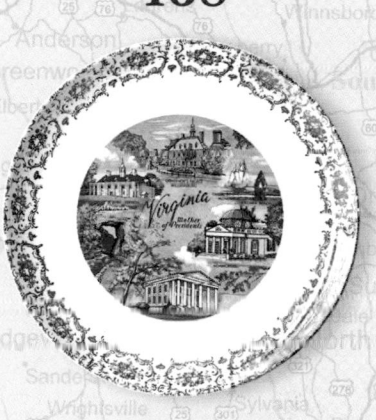

238

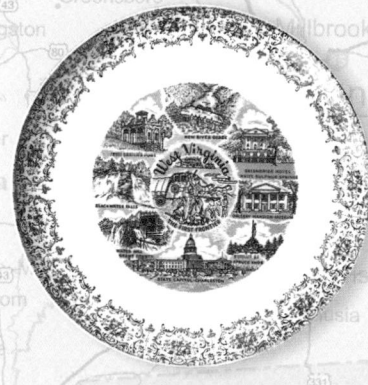

252

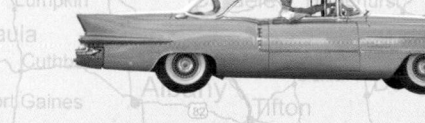

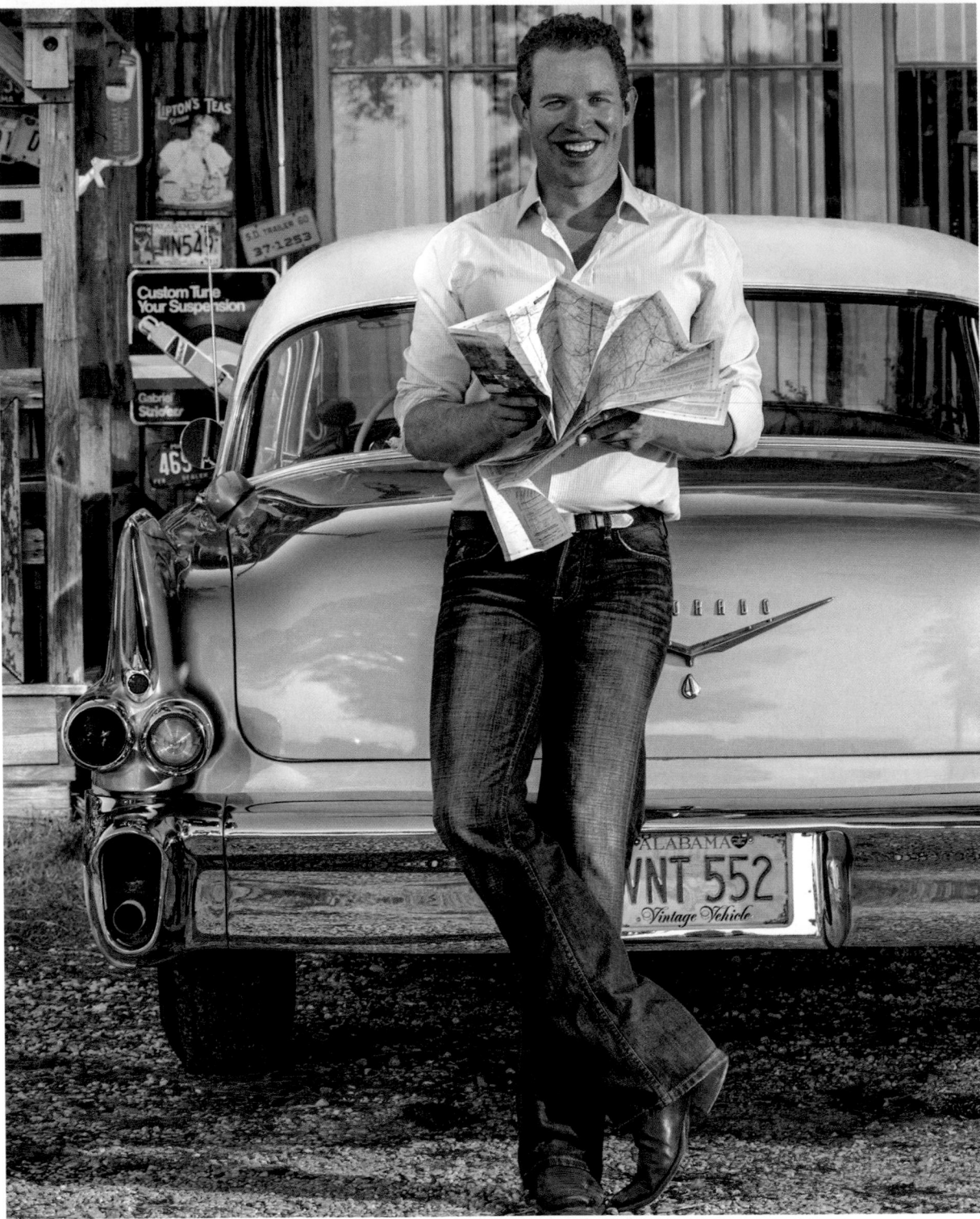

Y'all,

As much as I love searching the Internet for Kanye West memes and finding old Caddy parts on eBay, you can't Google "good restaurant" and get results that match your tastes.

The recipe-packed goodness you're holding right now required a road trip covering 60 cities, 15,000 miles, scores of restaurants, and several hundred thousand calories. I researched this book the old-fashioned way: by visiting each diner, farm, restaurant, steakhouse, and burger joint; devouring everything in sight; interviewing owners, wait staff, and customers; and cajoling the recipes from cooks and chefs.

My tastes are simple. I judge a restaurant as a stool that stands on three legs: food, service, and ambiance. To make these pages, a restaurant must be excellent in all three, and be Southern and family-owned as well.

Also, you should know that I am not a food snob. I eat just about everything from fried green tomatoes to foie gras, so that's reflected in the recipes, too. The food in *On the Road Again* is as varied as the South itself. What it is not is low calorie: If you're on a diet, put the book down and slowly back away. That said, though the dishes here are rich, you won't find artificial flavors, shortcuts, preservatives, or ingredients you can't pronounce.

Visit as many spots as I do each year and you'll see that Southern restaurants in particular anchor their communities. Dine at these places and I promise you'll make new friends. Owners such as Lisa "Sissy" Garza, who has a thing for Champagne and fried chicken at her Dallas restaurant Sissy's (page 218), can blow your diet, your wallet, and your mind with her menu. Another Lisa, Lisa Smith of Big Fatty's in Knoxville (page 202), charms customers with 50-cent happy hour, fried cornbread, and fritters crafted from pimiento cheese. If you leave and don't want to hug Lisa on your way out, you may need both a personality and taste bud transplant. When you visit these restaurants, take a pic and tag me @_morganmurphy on Twitter or Instagram.

Whether you craft these dishes in your kitchen, or map out your own Southern road trip adventure, thank you for supporting the culinary artists who make our region shine. I wish you full plates, glasses, tables, and hearts.

Eat up!

Morgan Murphy

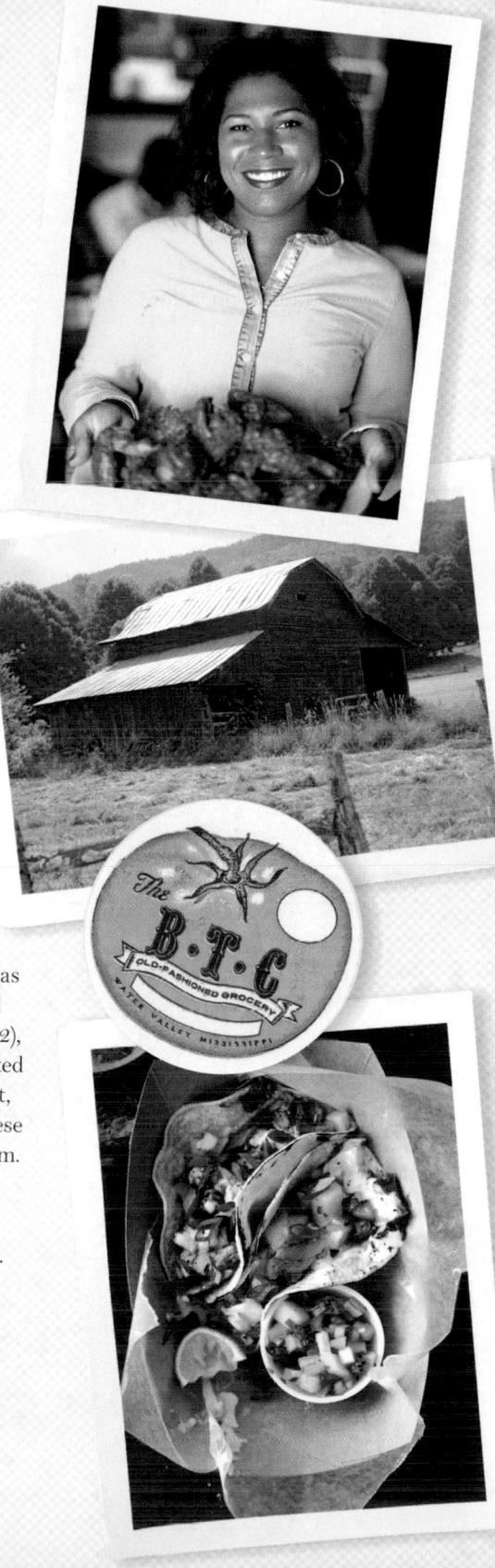

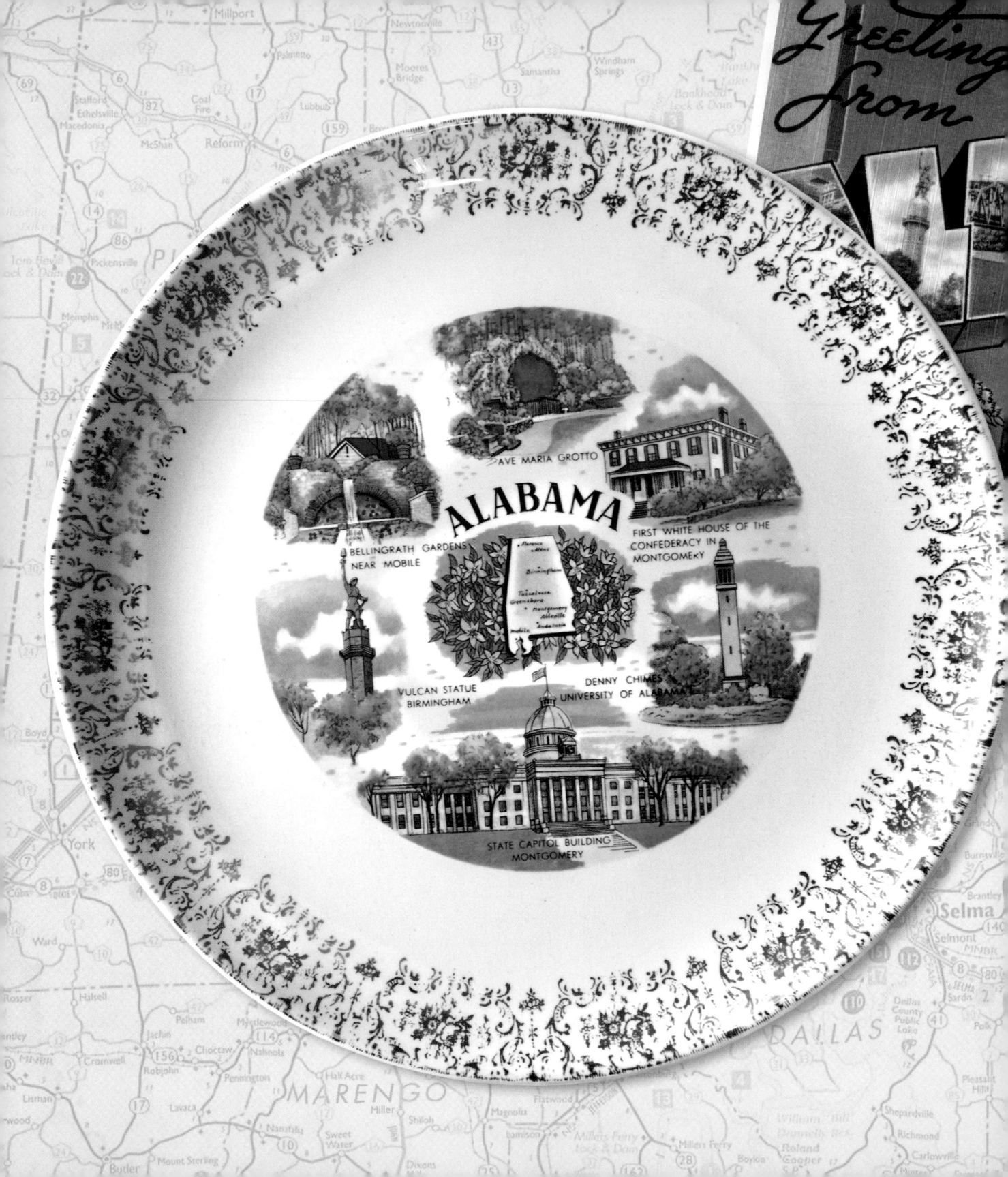

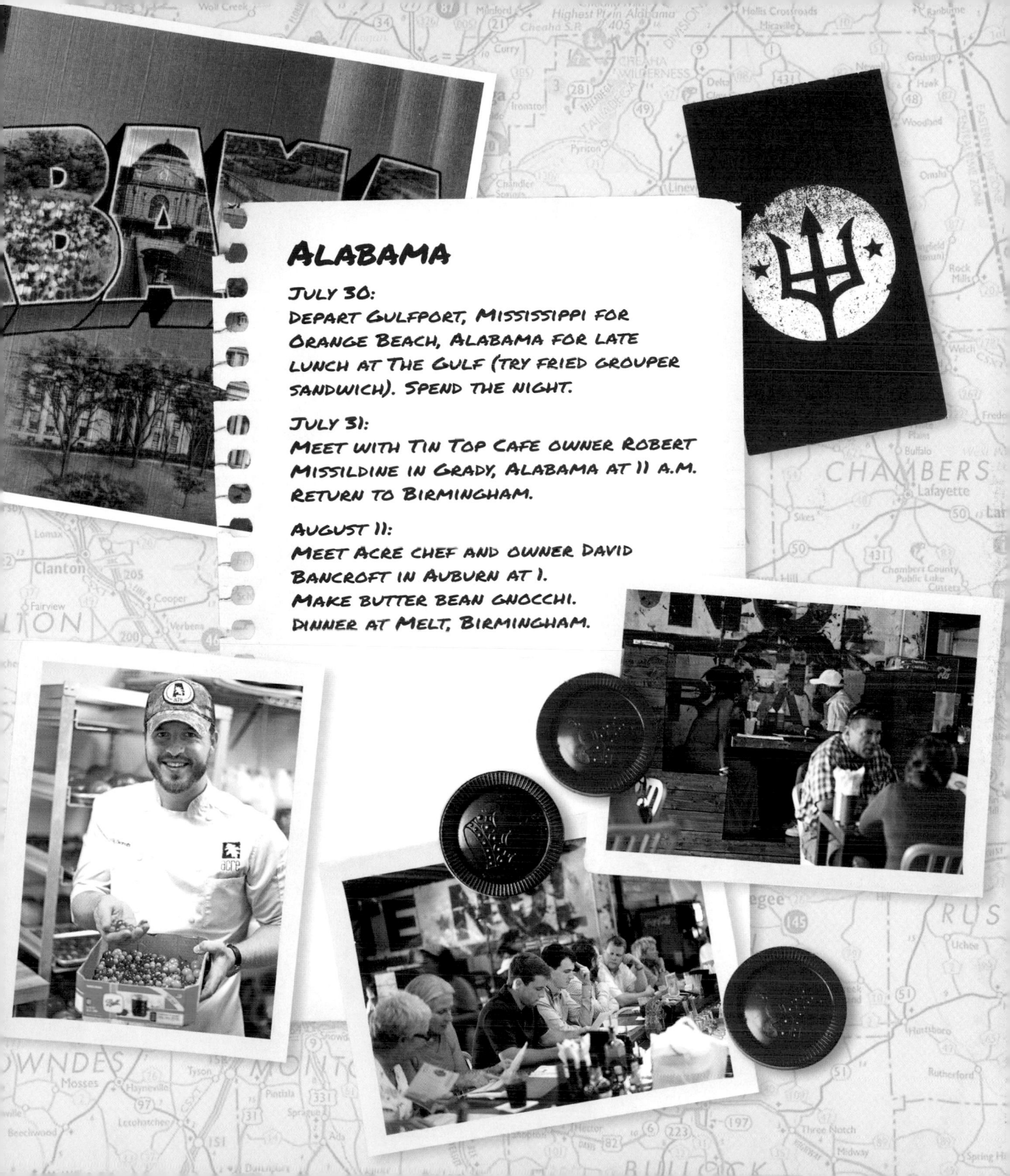

ALABAMA

July 30:
Depart Gulfport, Mississippi for Orange Beach, Alabama for late lunch at The Gulf (try fried grouper sandwich). Spend the night.

July 31:
Meet with Tin Top Cafe owner Robert Missildine in Grady, Alabama at 11 a.m. Return to Birmingham.

August 11:
Meet Acre chef and owner David Bancroft in Auburn at 1.
Make butter bean gnocchi.
Dinner at Melt, Birmingham.

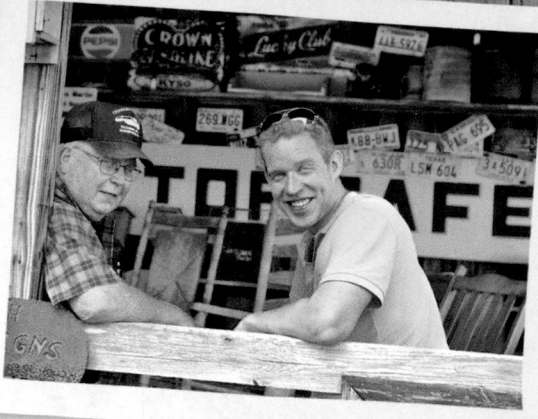

Tin Top Cafe

24319 Troy Highway
Grady, Alabama 36036
(334) 584-7518

I like to hop into my big, old Cadillac and motor down to the Tin Top Cafe in Grady, Alabama, for some country cooking like no other. Owner Robert Missildine will sit on the porch with you and swap stories about politics, fishing, and that time Kid Rock and Hank Williams Jr. sang about the Tin Top. "It's a hole in the wall, kinda small, but the people are real nice." (There's music video proof if you search for "Redneck Paradise" on YouTube.) The Tin Top's menu is traditional 'Bama meat and three, which might set you back $10 if you order sweet tea and leave a big tip. And God bless 'em; it's one of the last spots in America where you can order "orange fluff" and not be at a church revival.

Corn Salad

Nothing beats the taste of freshly shucked corn. It's that flavor, plus a good mayonnaise (preferably homemade, but Duke's if you're short on time), that is the key to Tin Top Cafe's corn salad.

3	ears bicolored fresh corn, husks removed
½	cup mayonnaise
1½	Tbsp. chopped fresh thyme
½	tsp. table salt
½	tsp. freshly ground black pepper
1½	cups diced seeded tomato
1	cup chopped green bell pepper
½	cup thinly sliced green onions

1. Cook corn in boiling salted water in a large Dutch oven 6 minutes or until tender. Drain. Let stand 20 minutes or until cool. Cut kernels into a large bowl to measure 3½ cups. Discard cobs.
2. Stir together mayonnaise and next 3 ingredients until blended. Stir mayonnaise mixture, tomato, and remaining ingredients into corn. Cover and chill 30 minutes. **Makes: 9 servings**

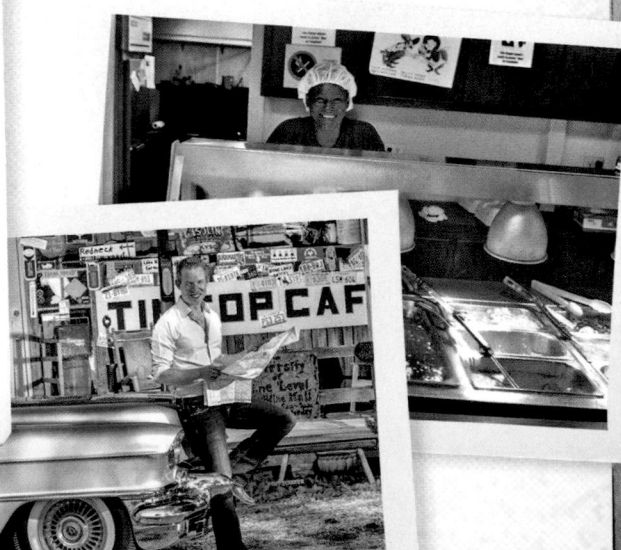

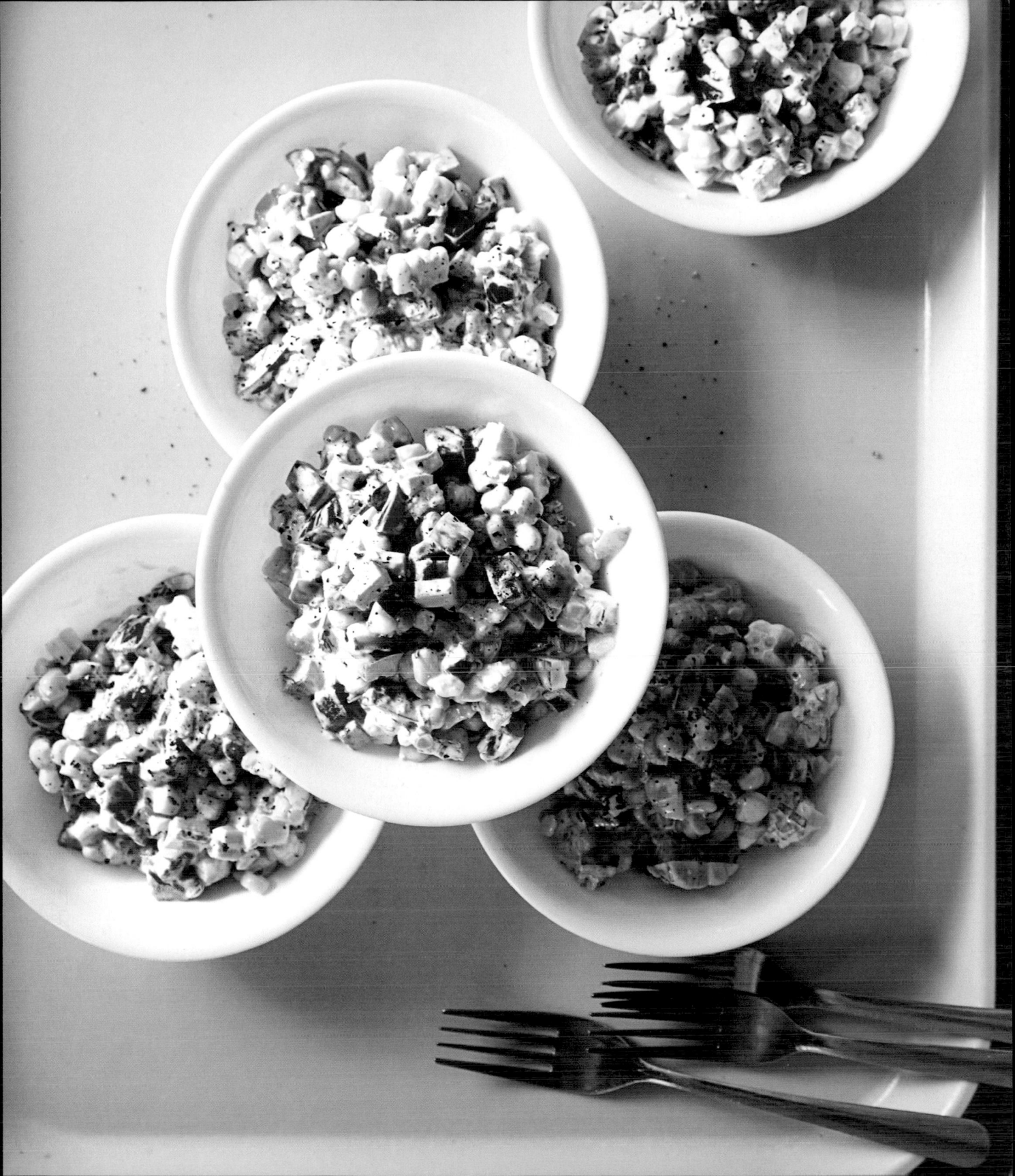

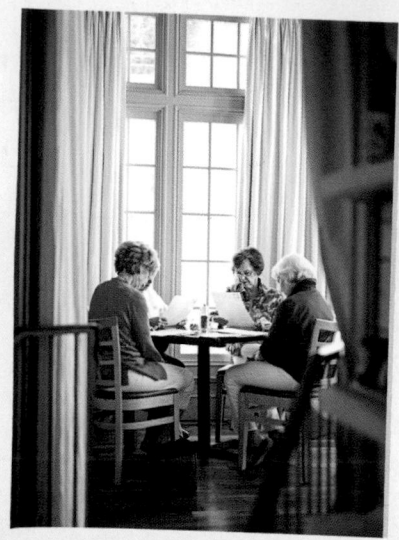

Acre

210 East Glenn Avenue
Auburn, Alabama 36830
(334) 246-3763
acreauburn.com

One of Alabama's most beautiful restaurants sits on the "Loveliest Village on the Plains." Acre, as its name suggests, encompasses an acre. Chef and owner David Bancroft built the wood-and-stone restaurant out of local, reclaimed lumber. Nearly every board has a story. "That was from my grandfather's barn in Hartford," he says. "This table came from the guy who sells me our rabbits." David is equally passionate about his Southern fare. All of his produce is local—much of it from the restaurant garden. Try his blueberry ice cream—it's a perfect balance of sweet and tart—or the fried green tomatoes with pimiento cheese and crab, and you'll taste the difference local, fresh makes.

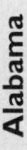
Butter Bean Gnocchi

The butter beans add a Southern twist to this Italian favorite, and makes the gnocchi slightly green (and very delicious).

1   large baking potato (about 1 lb.)
½   (16-oz.) package frozen baby lima beans
½   cup frozen English peas
1½   tsp. kosher salt
1¾   cups all-purpose flour
1   large egg, beaten
¼   cup butter
¼   cup freshly grated Parmesan cheese
2   tsp. chopped fresh thyme

1. Preheat oven to 450°. Scrub potato; pat dry. Wrap potato in aluminum foil. Bake at 450° for 1 hour or until tender when pierced with a sharp knife. Cool 20 minutes; unwrap potato, and peel. Press potato through a ricer into a bowl to measure 2 cups.
2. Cook lima beans in boiling salted water to cover 30 minutes, adding peas during last 5 minutes of cooking. Drain.
3. Process lima bean mixture in a food processor until pureed. Stir lima bean puree and salt into potato until blended.
4. Sprinkle ½ cup flour on a work surface. Place potato mixture on floured surface; make a well in center of mixture. Pour beaten egg into well; sprinkle 1 cup flour over top. Using fingers, work egg and flour into potato mixture, gently folding and gathering mixture together. Knead 10 times, adding remaining ¼ cup flour to form a smooth dough.
5. Roll dough into a 6- x 3½-inch rectangle, 1½ inches thick, on a lightly floured surface. Cut dough lengthwise into quarters; cut each quarter lengthwise into thirds. Roll each portion of dough into a 12-inch rope. Cut ropes into 1-inch pieces. (If desired, place each piece onto a lightly floured fork or gnocchi paddle, pressing

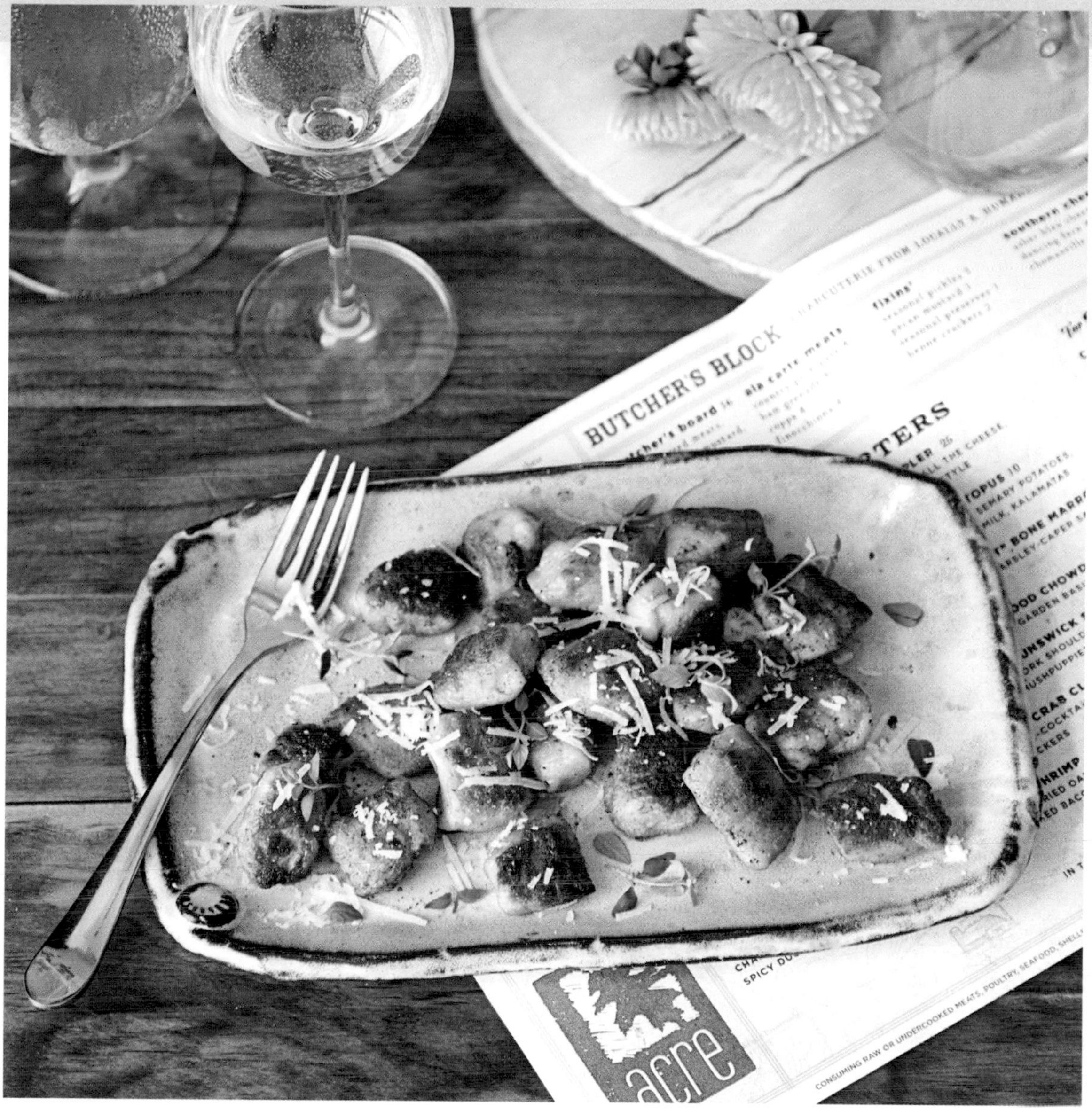

lightly to roll with thumb into a ridged dumpling.)

6. Melt butter in a large nonstick skillet over medium heat. Remove from heat.

7. Cook gnocchi in batches in boiling salted water 1 minute or until gnocchi float to surface; cook 2 more minutes. Remove gnocchi from boiling water using a slotted spoon, and place in melted butter in skillet.

8. Place skillet over medium-high heat, and cook gnocchi 4 to 5 minutes or until browned, stirring occasionally. Remove from heat, and sprinkle with cheese, thyme, and salt and pepper to taste; toss gently. Serve immediately.

Makes: 12 small or 10 large servings

Fried Green Tomatoes with Crab and Pimiento Cheese

RÉMOULADE

- 1 cup mayonnaise
- ⅓ cup Creole mustard
- 1 Tbsp. Creole seasoning
- 1½ Tbsp. fresh lemon juice
- ½ Tbsp. hot sauce
- 1 sweet-and-spicy bread and butter pickle chip, finely minced

MARINATED CRAB

- 1 lb. fresh crabmeat
- 1 tsp. lime zest
- 2 Tbsp. fresh lime juice
- 1 Tbsp. chopped fresh cilantro
- 1 Tbsp. extra virgin olive oil
- ½ tsp. kosher salt
Dash of hot sauce
- 1 jalapeño pepper, seeded and minced
- 1 garlic clove, minced

FRIED GREEN TOMATOES

Peanut oil
- 1 cup buttermilk
- 2 cups plain yellow cornmeal
- 24 (¼-inch-thick) green tomato slices
Table salt
- 2 cups homemade or store-bought pimiento cheese
- 8 fresh basil leaves

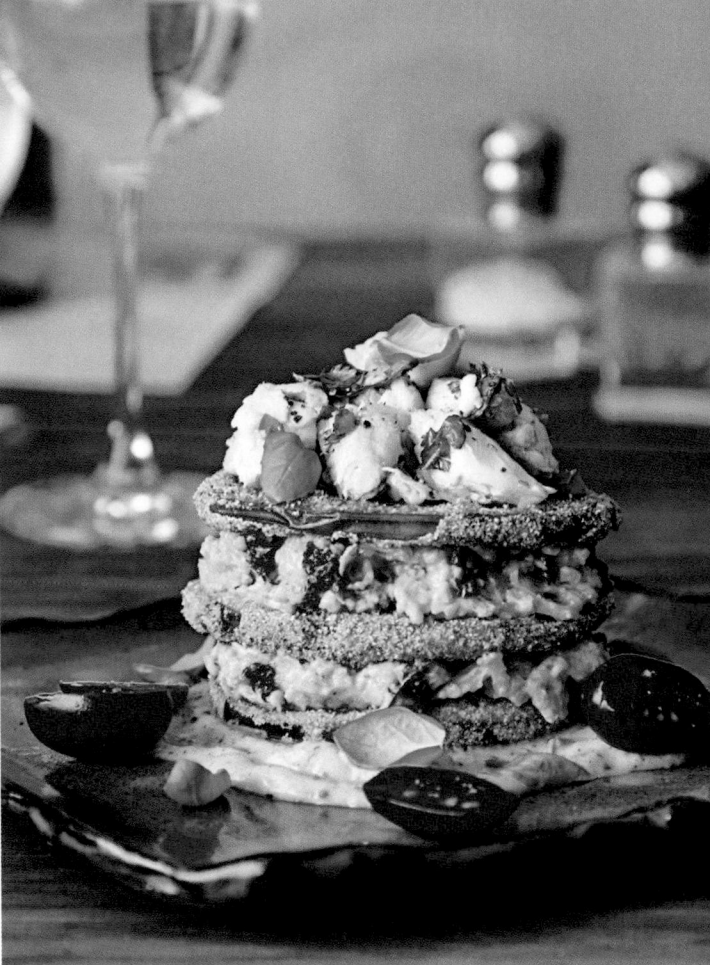

1. **Prepare Rémoulade:** Stir together all ingredients and 1 Tbsp. water in a small bowl. Cover and chill.

2. **Prepare Marinated Crab:** Pick crabmeat, removing any bits of shell. Stir together lime zest and next 7 ingredients in a large bowl. Gently fold in crabmeat. Cover and chill.

3. **Prepare Fried Green Tomatoes:** Pour peanut oil to depth of ½ inch in a large cast-iron skillet; heat to 350°. Place buttermilk in a bowl. Place cornmeal in a shallow dish. Dip tomato slices in buttermilk, shaking off excess; dredge in cornmeal. Fry tomato slices, in batches, 2 minutes or until golden brown. Drain on paper towels. Sprinkle with salt while hot.

4. Spread Rémoulade evenly on 8 plates. Place 1 tomato slice on top of Rémoulade on each plate. Top with 2 Tbsp. pimiento cheese, 1 tomato slice, 2 Tbsp. pimiento cheese, and 1 tomato slice. Top each stack with ⅓ cup Marinated Crab and 1 basil leaf. **Makes: 8 servings**

Note: We tested with Wickles Pickle Chips.

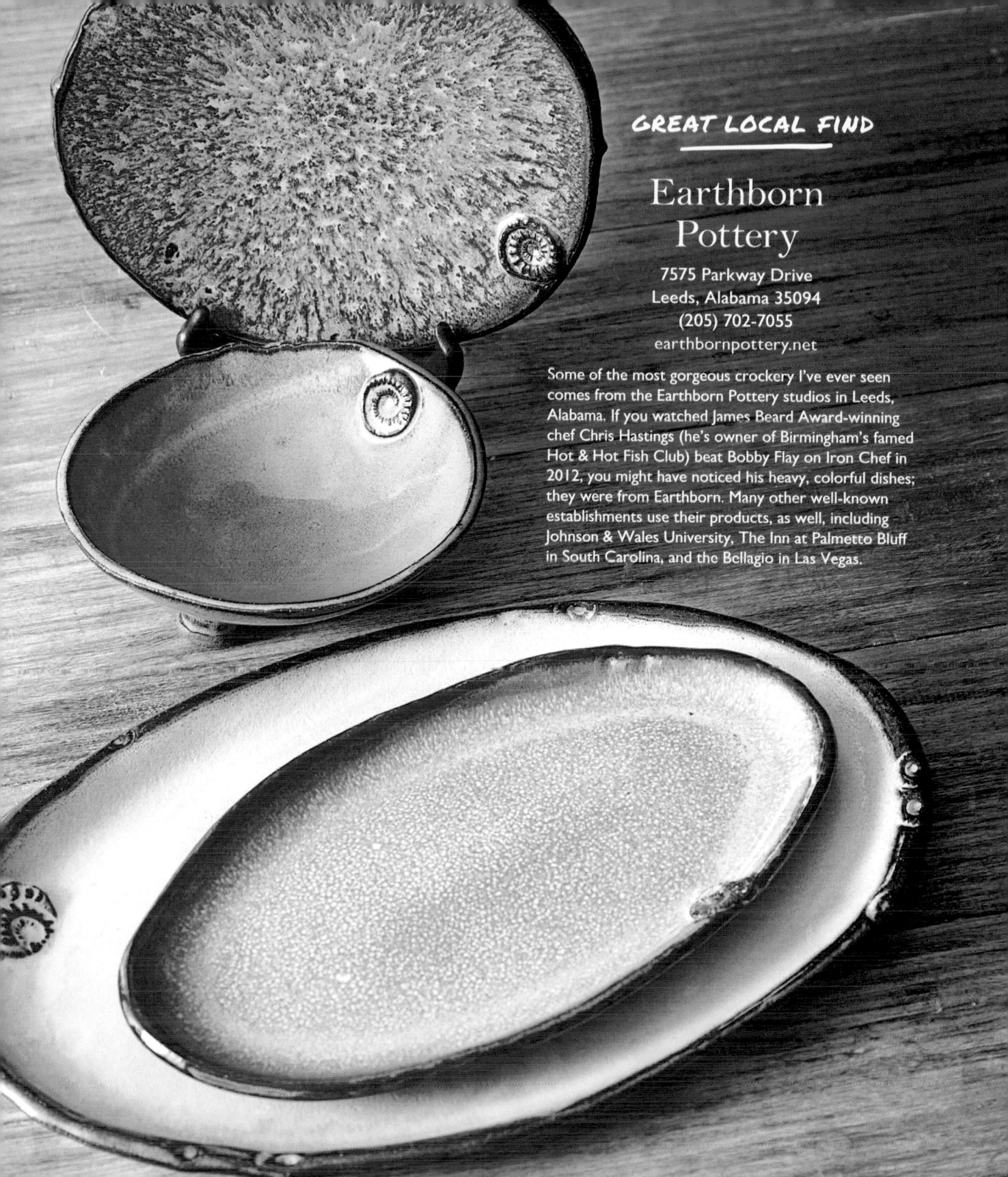

Earthborn Pottery

7575 Parkway Drive
Leeds, Alabama 35094
(205) 702-7055
earthbornpottery.net

Some of the most gorgeous crockery I've ever seen comes from the Earthborn Pottery studios in Leeds, Alabama. If you watched James Beard Award-winning chef Chris Hastings (he's owner of Birmingham's famed Hot & Hot Fish Club) beat Bobby Flay on Iron Chef in 2012, you might have noticed his heavy, colorful dishes; they were from Earthborn. Many other well-known establishments use their products, as well, including Johnson & Wales University, The Inn at Palmetto Bluff in South Carolina, and the Bellagio in Las Vegas.

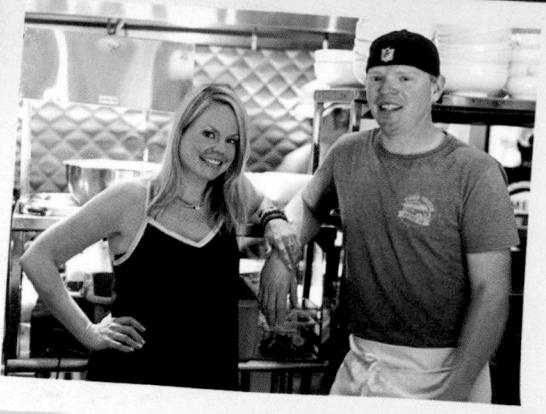

Melt Avondale

4105 4th Avenue South
Birmingham, Alabama 35222
(205) 917-5000
meltbham.com

My friend Paget Pizitz has a serious cheese problem. What started as a food truck in Birmingham (or B'ham as locals say) bloomed into a full-fledged restaurant in the Magic City's cool Avondale district. Located in a former gas station, MELT is far more than a spot to grab a grilled cheese. Fresh, local ingredients dominate the menu, and Paget will stuff you like a frequent flier's carry-on bag with delicious French fries, inventive sandwiches, and craft beer. If you leave here hungry, seek counseling. That's probably why, just a year into operation, MELT already boasts a loyal fan base of locals. Hurrah for cheese obsession!

Black 'n' Bleu

This hearty sandwich includes ingredients that simply can't fail. Both hands mandatory, bib optional.

8   oz. sirloin steak
¼   tsp. table salt
¼   tsp. freshly ground black pepper
2   (1.5-oz.) slices sourdough bread
1   Tbsp. unsalted butter, softened
2   oz. blue cheese, crumbled
⅓   cup thin vertical red onion slices
4   plum tomatoes, sliced
¼   cup baby arugula

1. Preheat grill to 350° to 400° (medium-high) heat. Sprinkle steak with salt and pepper. Grill steak, covered with grill lid, 5 to 6 minutes on each side (medium-rare). Let stand 5 minutes.
2. Spread 1 side of bread slices with butter; grill 30 seconds on each side or until toasted. Sprinkle cheese evenly on buttered sides of bread slices. Place bread, cheese side up, on grill; grill, covered, 30 seconds or until cheese melts.
3. Cut steak diagonally across the grain into thin slices. Place steak slices on 1 cheese-topped bread slice. Top with onion, tomato, arugula, and remaining bread slice, cheese side down. Cut sandwich diagonally in half, and serve immediately. Makes: 1 serving

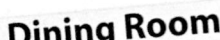

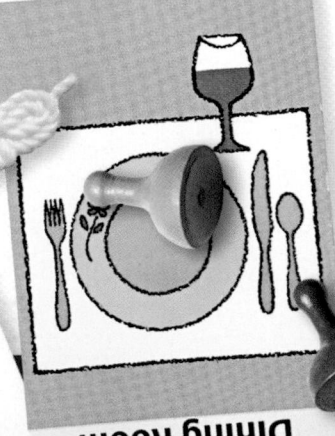

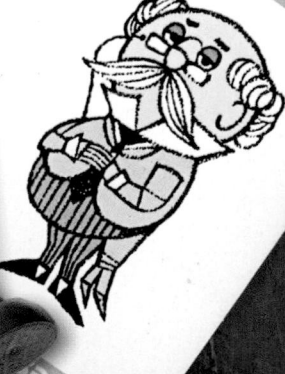

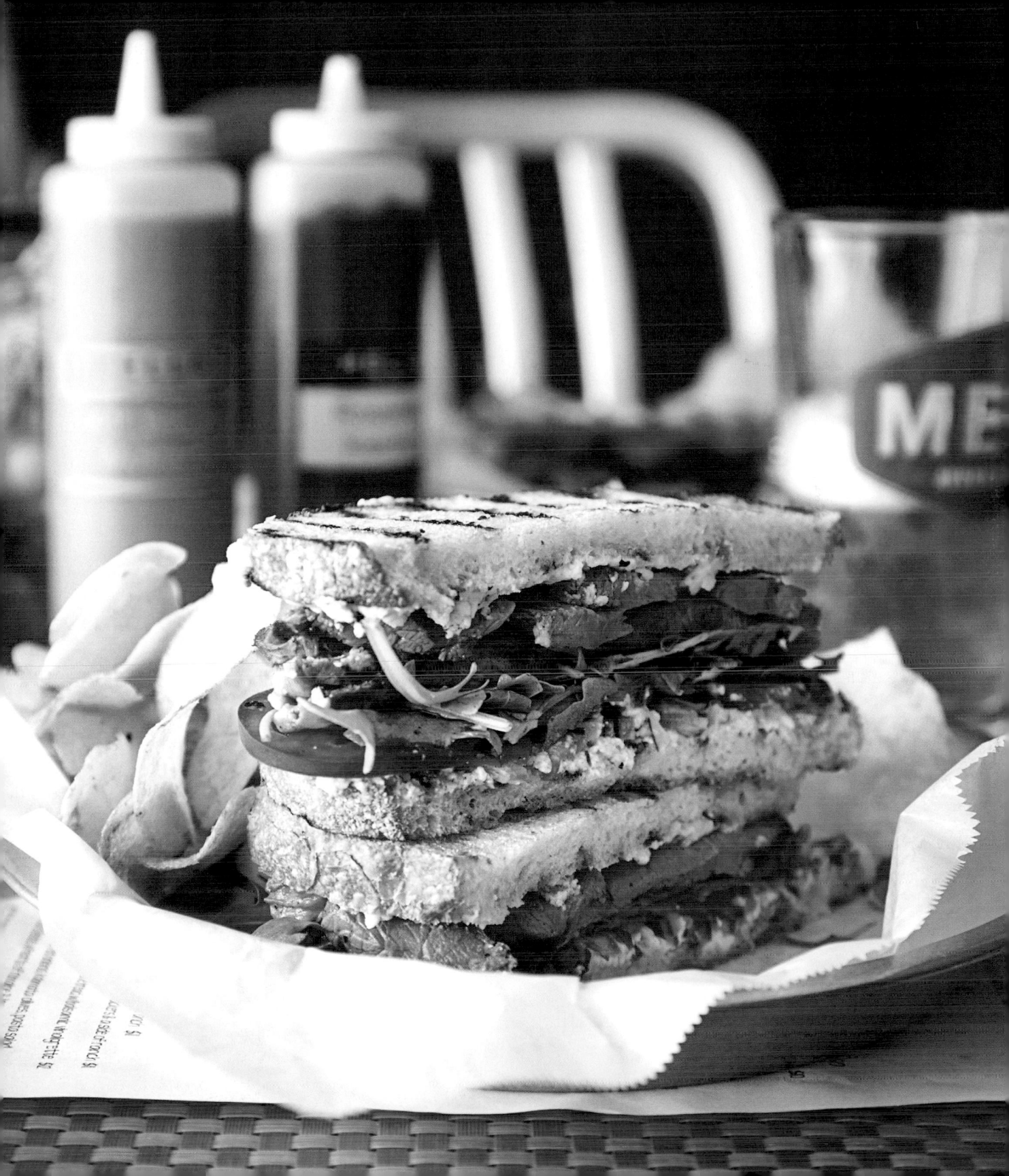

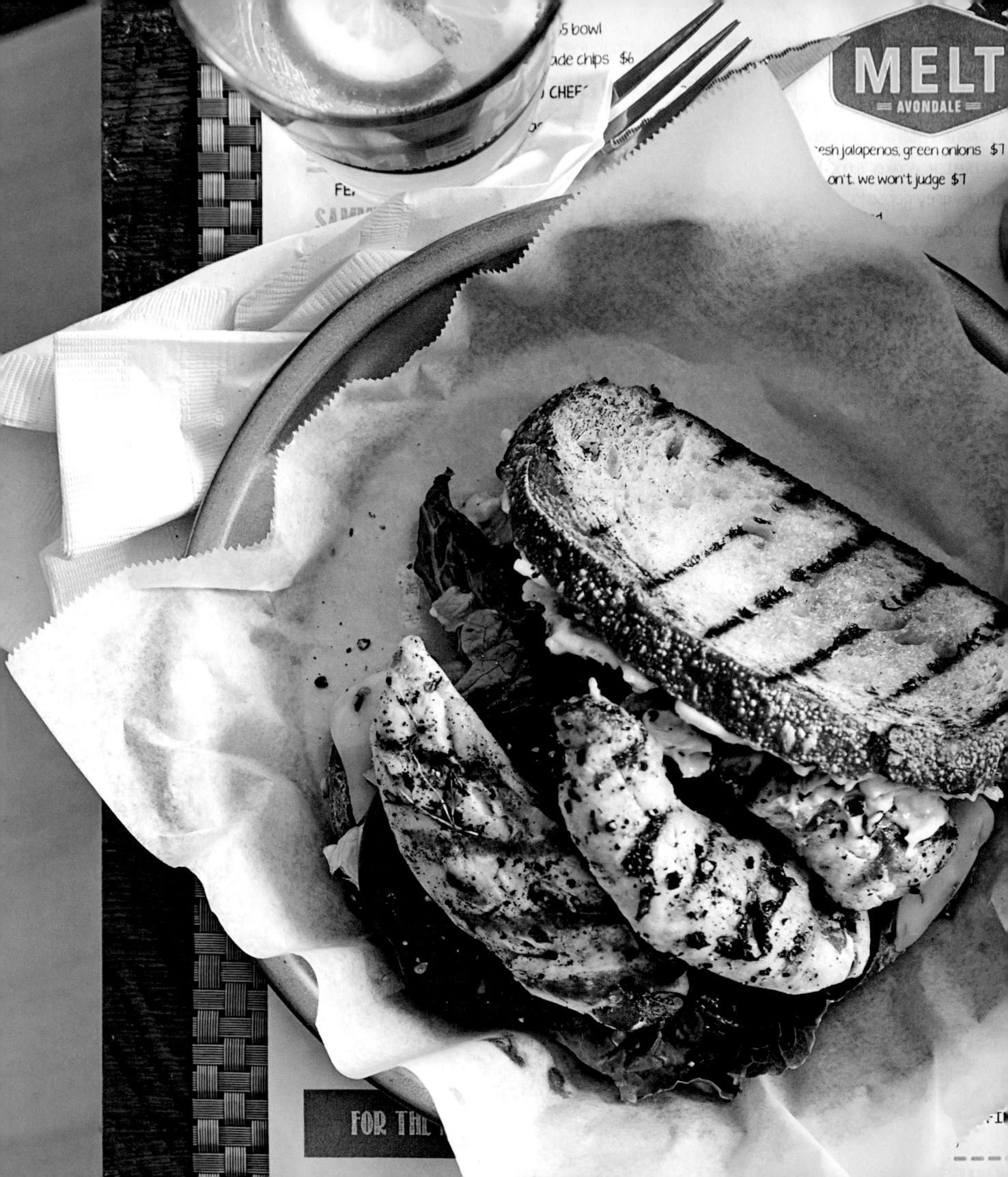

Great Caesar's Ghost

This flavorful chicken "sammich" puts a regular Caesar salad to shame. It gets quite a kick from the ghost pepper Jack cheese. For less heat, opt for classic pepper Jack instead.

CHICKEN

2	lb. boneless chicken breast tenders
½	tsp. table salt
½	tsp. freshly ground black pepper
1	cup olive oil
4	fresh thyme sprigs, coarsely chopped
2	fresh rosemary sprigs, coarsely chopped
2	fresh basil sprigs, coarsely chopped

CAESAR DRESSING

¾	cup mayonnaise
6	Tbsp. freshly grated Parmigiano Reggiano cheese
1	tsp. lemon zest
1	Tbsp. fresh lemon juice
¼	tsp. table salt
¼	tsp. freshly ground black pepper
½	tsp. chopped fresh thyme leaves
2	drained anchovy filets, minced

SANDWICHES

¼	cup unsalted butter, softened
8	(1-oz.) slices sourdough bread
4	(¾-oz.) slices ghost pepper Jack cheese
4	(¼-inch-thick) slices tomato
4	leaves romaine lettuce

1. Prepare Chicken: Sprinkle chicken with salt and pepper. Place in a large zip-top plastic freezer bag; add olive oil and herbs. Seal bag, and chill 2 hours.

2. Meanwhile, prepare Caesar Dressing: Stir together all ingredients in a medium bowl. Cover and chill.

3. Preheat broiler. Heat a cast-iron grill pan over medium-high heat. Remove chicken from herb mixture, discarding herb mixture. Cook chicken, in 2 batches, in grill pan 4 to 5 minutes on each side or until done. Keep warm.

4. Prepare Sandwiches: Spread butter on 1 side of bread slices. Place 1 cheese slice on unbuttered side of 4 bread slices. Place, buttered side down, in a large nonstick skillet. Cook over medium heat 2 minutes or until bread is golden brown. Place on a baking sheet. Place plain bread slices, buttered side down, in skillet. Cook over medium heat 2 minutes or until golden brown. Transfer, buttered side down, to baking sheet. Broil 2 minutes or until cheese melts and bread is toasted.

5. Spread 1½ to 2 Tbsp. Caesar Dressing on unbuttered side of 4 plain bread slices. Layer 1 tomato slice and 1 lettuce leaf over cheese-topped slices. Divide chicken evenly over top of lettuce. Top with remaining bread slices, dressing side down. Serve immediately. **Makes: 4 servings**

SOUNDTRACK:

"NOW THAT I'VE FOUND YOU" BY PAUL MCDONALD

"DON'T GET ABOVE YOUR RAISIN'" BY FLATT & SCRUGGS

"REDNECK PARADISE" BY KID ROCK

"OLD ALABAMA" BY BRAD PAISLEY

"UP THE HICKORY AND DOWN THE PINE" BY SHELLY COLVIN

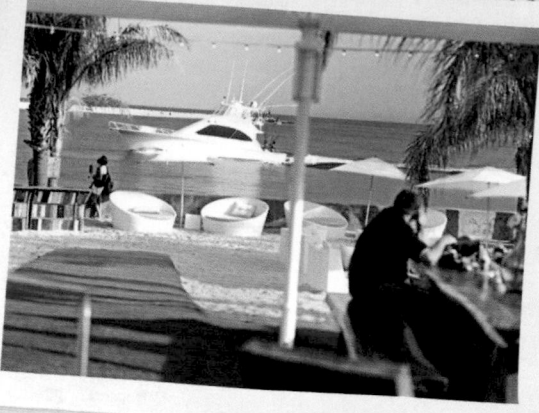

The Gulf

27500 Perdido Beach Blvd.
Orange Beach, Alabama 36561
(251) 424-1800

Seven repurposed shipping containers make up this restaurant—yes, metal shipping containers, each now painted a royal blue. Yet once you walk through the entrance, a wondrous transformation takes place: palm trees, white sand, gorgeous furniture (made from old wooden boats), and delicious food await. The name of the restaurant is The Gulf, so the majority of the ever-changing menu features fresh Gulf seafood and local farmers' produce. "The farmers drive up, lift their tailgates, and we shop," says the restaurant's consulting chef Ephraim Kadish. As beautifully designed as the space is, there's one thing it is not and that's pretentious. You'll find families (with small children) relaxing the afternoon away as they overlook the sparkling blue Perdido Pass. Ephraim describes his restaurant as fast casual—you order at the window and seat yourself. "My guess is you'll want to stay seated here for a long, long time," he says. No doubt.

Fried Grouper Sandwich with Lemon-Dill Sauce

LEMON-DILL SAUCE

6	Tbsp. sour cream
2	Tbsp. mayonnaise
1	Tbsp. chopped fresh dill
1	tsp. sugar
½	tsp. table salt
2	Tbsp. fresh lemon juice

SANDWICHES

Canola oil

4	large eggs
2	cups all-purpose flour
4	(6-oz.) grouper fillets (1 inch thick)
½	tsp. table salt
½	tsp. freshly ground black pepper
4	(3.6-oz.) brioche buns, halved horizontally
¼	cup butter, softened
8	tomato slices
1	cup shredded iceberg lettuce
4	dill pickle spears

1. Prepare Lemon-Dill Sauce: Stir together all ingredients in a small bowl. Cover and chill 1 hour.
2. Prepare Sandwiches: Pour oil to depth of 3 inches in a Dutch oven; heat to 350°. Whisk eggs in bowl until foamy. Place flour in a shallow dish.
3. Sprinkle fish on both sides with salt and pepper. Dip fish in egg; dredge in flour. Dip fish again in egg; dredge in flour, shaking off excess. Fry in hot oil 7 minutes or until crust is golden and fish flakes easily. Drain on paper towels.
4. Spread buns with butter. Cook bun halves, buttered sides down, in a large nonstick skillet 2 minutes or until toasted. Spread each bun bottom with 1½ tsp. Lemon-Dill Sauce. Place fish fillets on bun bottoms; spoon remaining Lemon-Dill Sauce evenly over fish. Top evenly with tomato slices and lettuce. Cover with bun tops, cut sides down. Serve with pickle spears. **Makes: 4 servings**

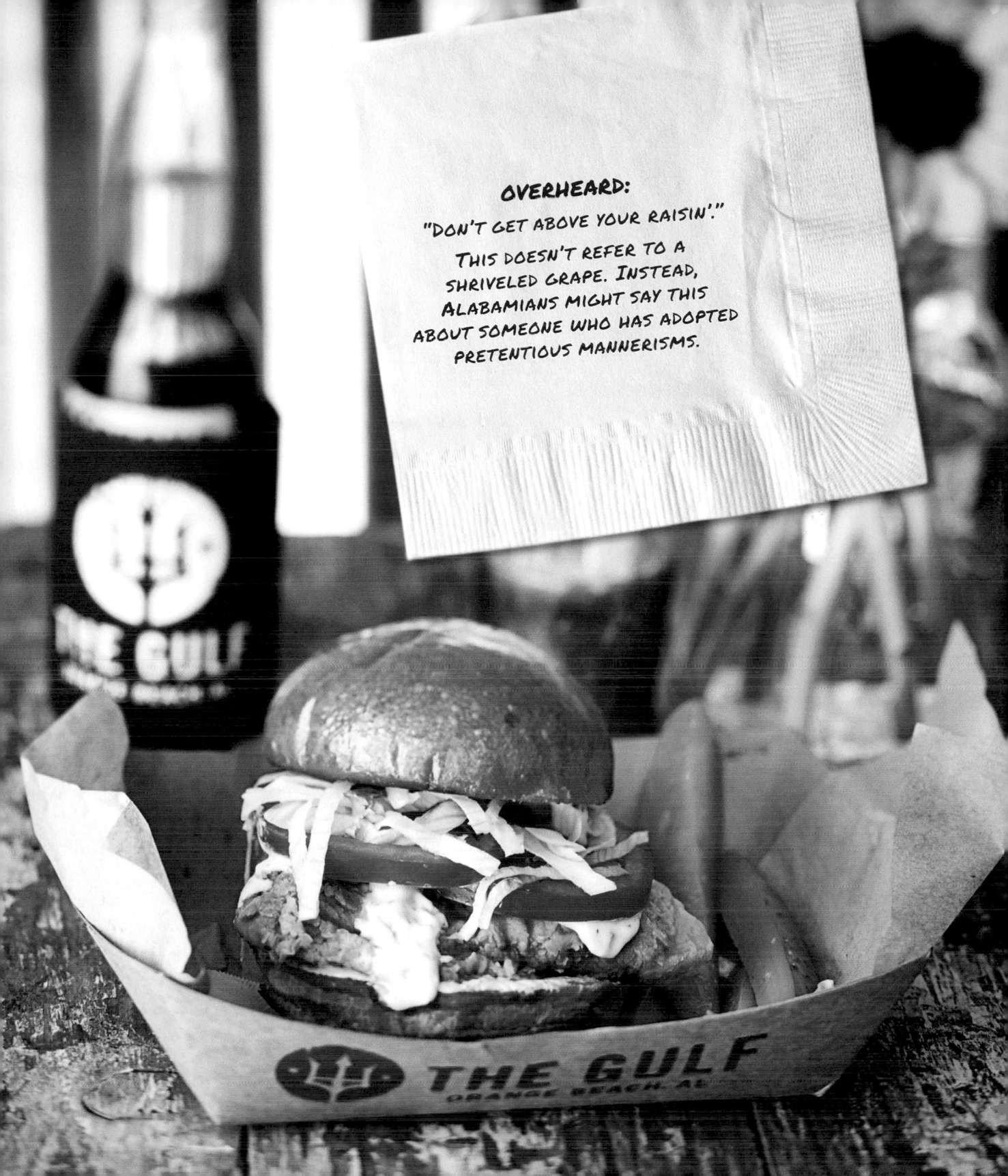

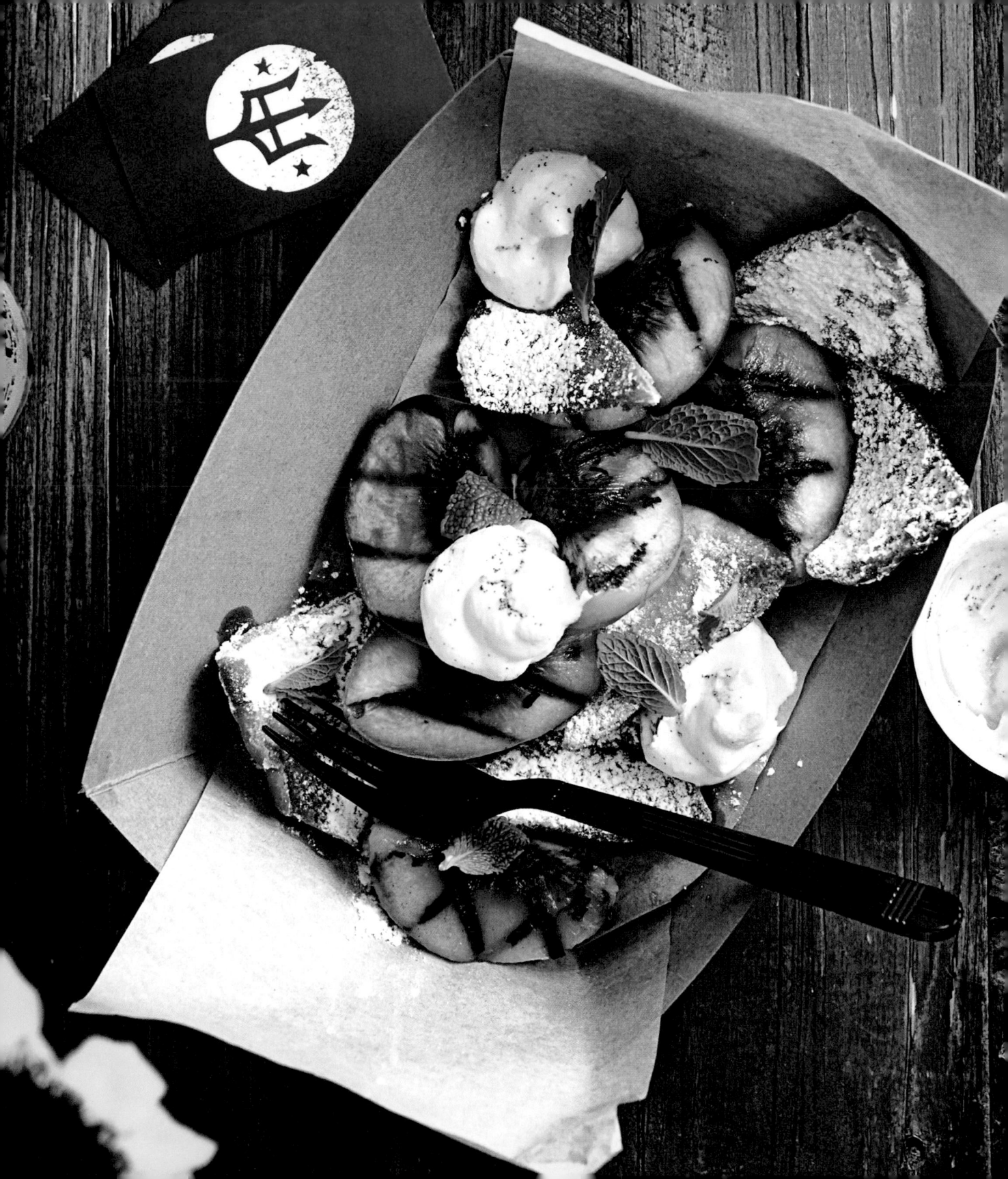

Grilled Peaches with Whipped Cream and Sweet Pita Chips

Sweet peaches are the perfect match for vanilla-infused whipped cream and powdered sugar-dusted fried pita chips.

6	large ripe peaches (about 4 lb.), pitted and quartered

Vegetable cooking spray

1	vanilla bean, halved lengthwise
1	cup heavy cream
$\frac{1}{3}$	cup plus 2 tsp. powdered sugar, divided

Canola oil

2	(6½-inch) pita rounds, each cut into 8 wedges

Garnish: fresh mint leaves

1. Preheat grill to 350° to 400° (medium-high) heat. Coat peach quarters with cooking spray, and place on grill rack. Grill, covered with grill lid, 4 minutes on each side. Transfer to a bowl; cover and let stand 15 minutes.

2. Meanwhile, scrape seeds from vanilla bean into a bowl; discard vanilla bean pod or reserve for another use. Add cream and 2 tsp. of the powdered sugar. Beat at high speed with an electric mixer until soft peaks form. Cover and chill.

3. Pour oil to depth of 1 inch in a large skillet; heat to 350°. Separate each pita wedge into 2 halves. Fry pita wedges, in 3 batches, in hot oil 2 to 3 minutes or until crisp, turning halfway through. Drain on paper towels.

4. Place remaining ⅓ cup powdered sugar in a large zip-top plastic freezer bag. Add pita wedges, a few at a time, to bag. Seal bag, and gently shake until wedges are coated.

5. Carefully remove skins from peach quarters; cut quarters into slices, and divide evenly among 8 dessert bowls. Spoon whipped cream on top of peaches. Serve with pita wedges. **Makes: 8 servings**

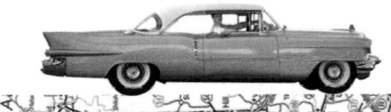

Alabama bucket list

things to see and do (besides eat) here

❶ Purchase a piece for your house at **Southern Accents Architectural Antiques** in Cullman, where you can peruse through mantels, door-knobs, and thousands of old and interesting home accessories.

❷ Catch a movie or concert and listen to "The Mighty Wurlitzer" pipe organ at Birmingham's historic **Alabama Theatre**, one of the most elaborate movie palaces in the country.

❸ Stroll through **Bellingrath Gardens** *(pictured)* in Theodore just south of Mobile, which covers approximately 900 acres along the Fowl River.

❹ Groove at the **Hangout Music Festival**, one of the largest three-day music events in the nation—which takes place every May on the beach in Gulf Shores.

❺ You can catch an IndyCar race, check out more than 1,000 vintage and modern motor-cycles (and race cars), or attend the Porsche Sport Driving School at the **Barber Motor-sports Park** near Leeds.

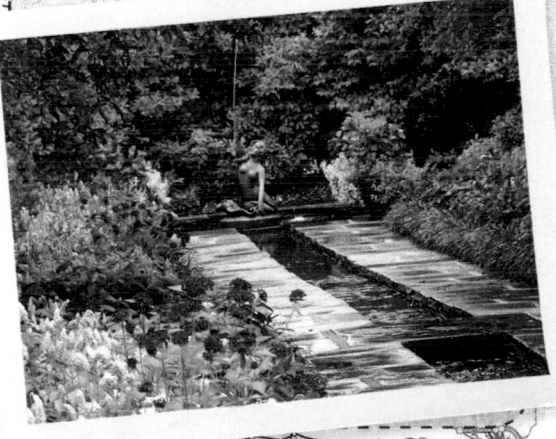

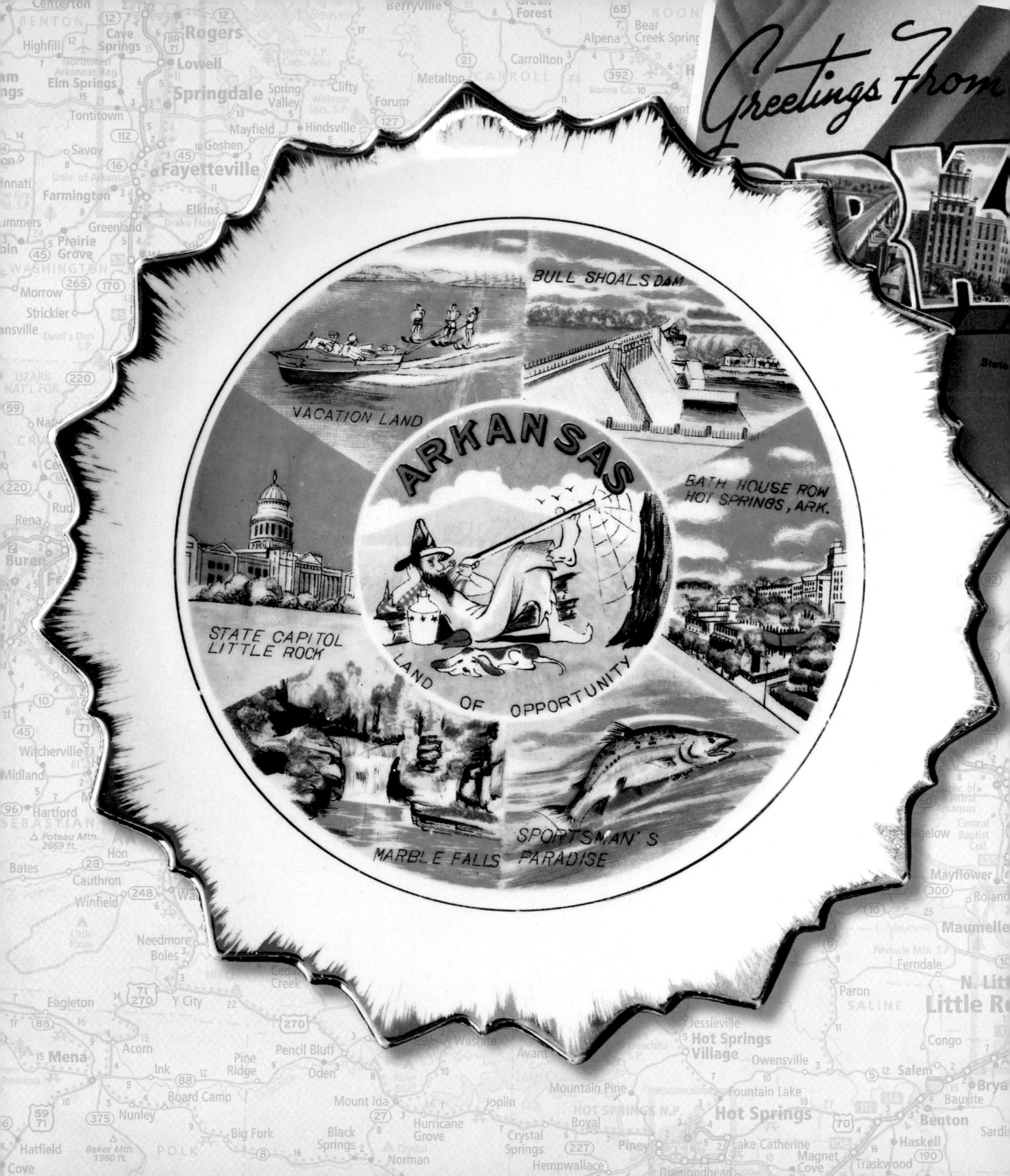

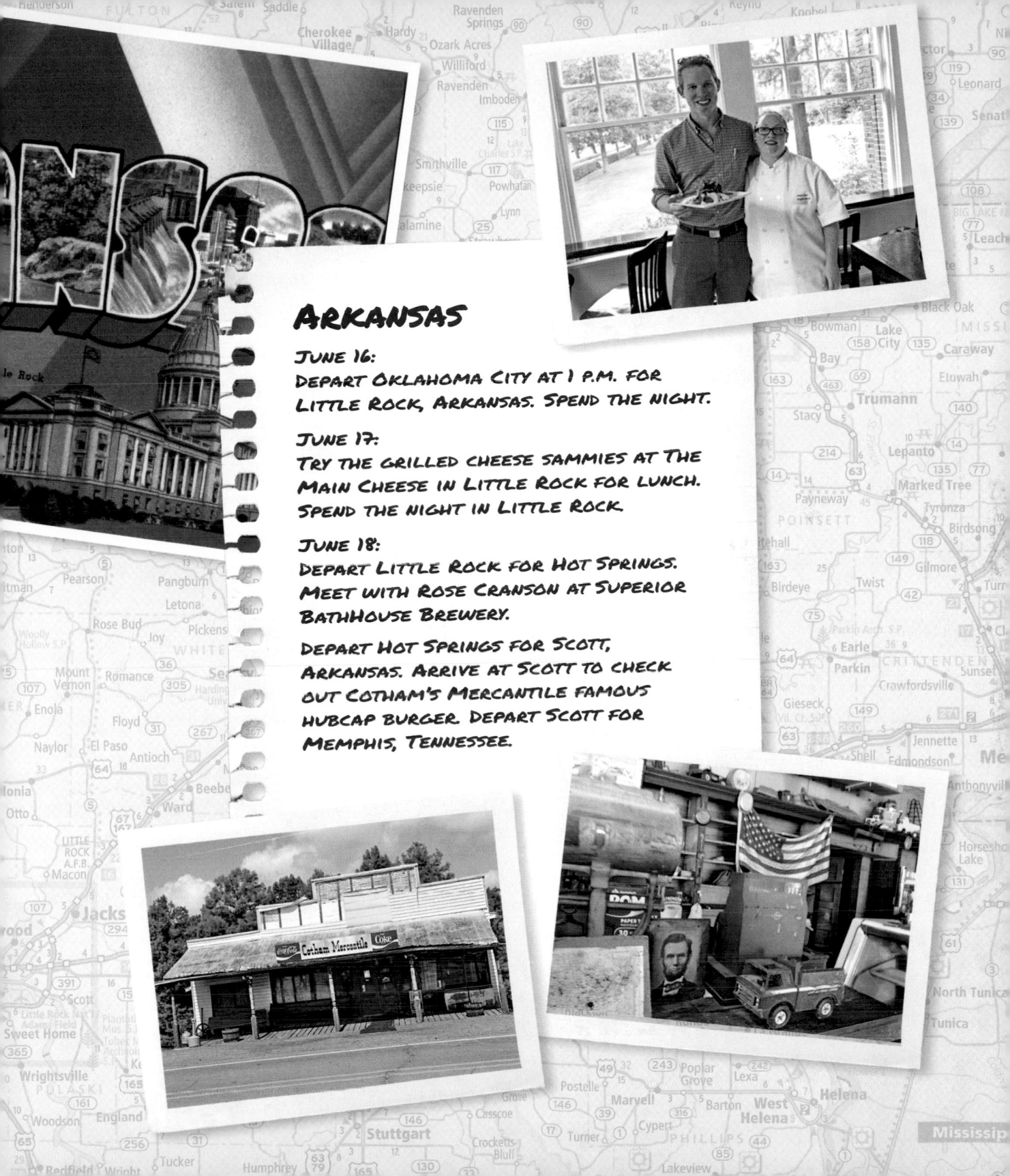

Arkansas

June 16:
Depart Oklahoma City at 1 p.m. for Little Rock, Arkansas. Spend the night.

June 17:
Try the grilled cheese sammies at The Main Cheese in Little Rock for lunch. Spend the night in Little Rock

June 18:
Depart Little Rock for Hot Springs. Meet with Rose Cranson at Superior Bathhouse Brewery.

Depart Hot Springs for Scott, Arkansas. Arrive at Scott to check out Cotham's Mercantile famous hubcap burger. Depart Scott for Memphis, Tennessee.

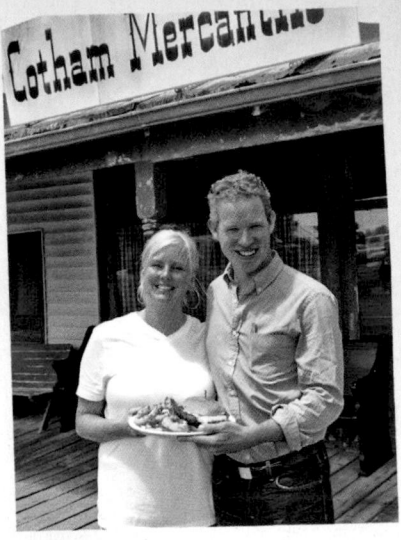

Cotham's Mercantile

5301 Highway 161
Scott, Arkansas 72142
(501) 961-9284
cothamsinthecity.com

I parked under a stately magnolia tree and walked into this tin-roofed shack to order the famous hubcap burger, which weighs in at a whopping 17 ounces. The burger is grand, but it's Cotham's Mercantile's fried green tomatoes and cornbread that you really shouldn't miss. Located in Scott, Arkansas, (population 72), Cotham's sits on the edge of a swamp, and diners drive from miles around to dine here. The old space still boasts remnants of its mercantile days: retro signs, vintage farm equipment, and random Christmas lights. Whatever. It all works, and you won't leave hungry. Just don't lean too heavily on one of the catawampus front porch supports as you wait.

Cornbread

This simple cornbread is a local tradition in Scott and looks like a pancake.

2   cups self-rising cornmeal mix
2   large eggs
1½ cups buttermilk
2   Tbsp. sugar
1   (2-Tbsp.) cube chilled butter

1. Place cornmeal in a medium bowl; make a well in center of mixture. Whisk together eggs, buttermilk, and sugar; add to cornmeal, stirring just until moistened.
2. Heat a griddle or large nonstick skillet over medium heat until a drop of water "dances" on the surface. For each batch of pancakes, use a fork to rub butter cube over hot griddle or skillet to melt a light coating of butter. (Set butter aside between batches.)
3. Quickly pour about ¼ cup batter for each pancake onto lightly buttered griddle or skillet. Cook pancakes over medium heat 3 minutes or until tops are covered with bubbles and edges look dry and cooked; turn and cook other side about 2 minutes. **Makes: 12 servings**

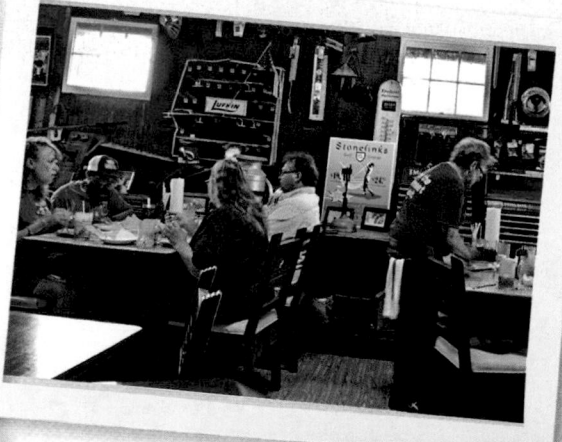

Fried Green Tomatoes

These fried green tomatoes are tart and slightly gritty, but the grand thing about them is the batter holds tight.

1 (12-oz.) green tomato, cut into
   8 (¼-inch) slices
Ice water
1½ cups canola oil
1 cup cornstarch
1 cup seasoned fish fry coating
1 large egg

1. Place tomato slices in a large bowl. Add ice water to cover. Let stand 15 minutes.
2. Heat oil in a 12-inch skillet until hot.
3. Place cornstarch in a shallow bowl; place fish fry coating in another shallow bowl. Whisk egg in a small bowl. Shake water off tomato slices; dredge in cornstarch. Dip in egg; dredge in fish fry coating.
4. Fry, in 2 batches, in hot oil 2 minutes on each side or until browned. Drain on a wire rack over paper towels 2 minutes. Serve immediately. **Makes: 4 servings**

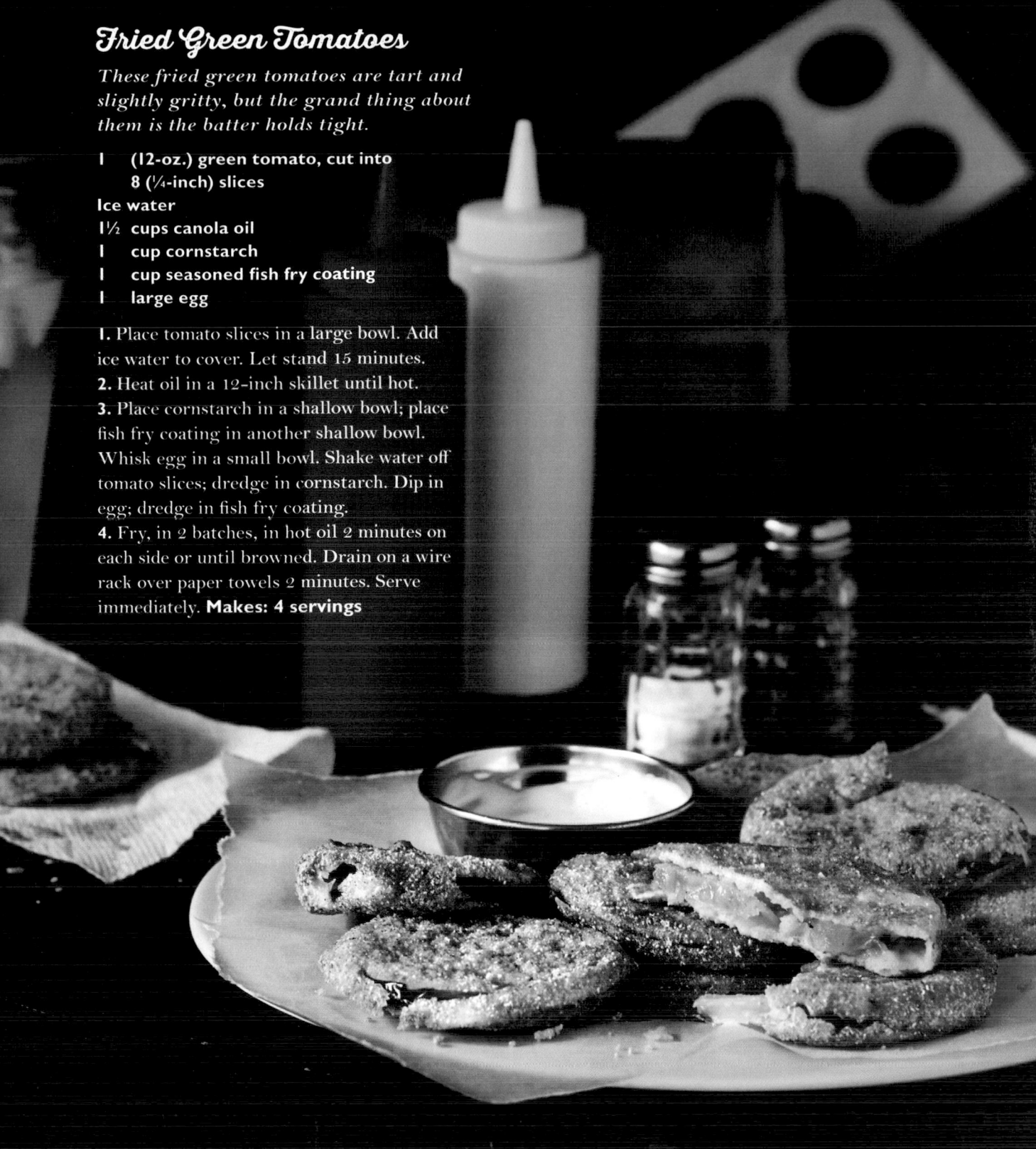

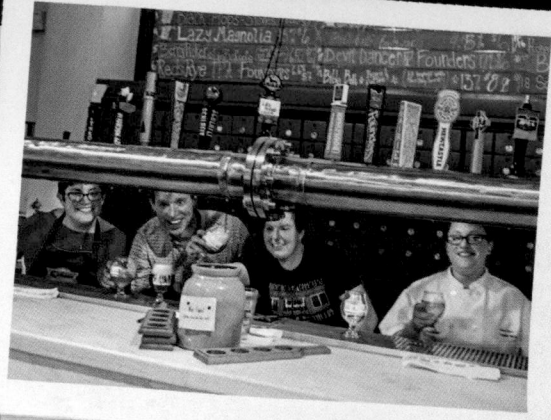

Superior Bathhouse Brewery & Distillery

329 Central Avenue
Hot Springs, Arkansas 71901
(501) 624-2337
superiorbathhouse.com

Professional tuba player Rose Cranson decided to move to Hot Springs, start a restaurant, restore a National Historic Landmark, and build a brewery—all in a national park. Rose is one determined lady. She and her collaborators created a vibrant reason to visit Hot Springs, where many of the original bathhouses remain trapped in a state of decayed grandeur. It's Superior Bathhouse Brewery & Distillery, which features 18-plus beers on tap (the world's only using thermal spring water as its main ingredient), house-made gelato, and a hugely inventive menu with the best fare in town. Don't miss Chef Angela Nardi's mushroom and fig strudel or Rose's homemade root beer. The night I visited, I ended up shutting down the place—it's easy to do when you're having fun.

Black-Eyed Pea Hummus

I'm a big fan of this Southern twist on a Middle Eastern classic.

1½ cups dried black-eyed peas
1 garlic bulb
2 Tbsp. olive oil
½ cup fresh lemon juice (about 3 lemons)
½ cup extra virgin olive oil, divided
¼ cup tahini
1 tsp. table salt
½ tsp. onion powder
½ tsp. freshly ground black pepper
¼ tsp. dried crushed red pepper
Garnishes: arugula, olive oil, freshly ground black pepper
Serve with: pita wedges, pita chips, pretzel chips, or fresh vegetables

1. Soak black-eyed peas in a bowl in water to cover for 20 minutes. Drain.
2. Place black-eyed peas and 3 cups water in a Dutch oven. Bring to a boil; cover, reduce heat, and cook 35 minutes or until very soft. (Black-eyed peas are done when they can easily be mashed with a fork.) Drain and cool completely (about 1 hour).
3. Meanwhile, preheat oven to 400°. Cut off pointed end of garlic; place garlic on a piece of aluminum foil; drizzle with 2 Tbsp. olive oil. Fold foil to seal. Bake at 400° for 40 minutes; cool 20 minutes.
4. Squeeze pulp from garlic cloves into a food processor. Add peas, lemon juice, next 6 ingredients, and ¼ cup water; process 2 minutes or until smooth. Serve with pita wedges, pita chips, pretzel chips, or fresh vegetables. **Makes: 4 cups**

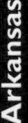

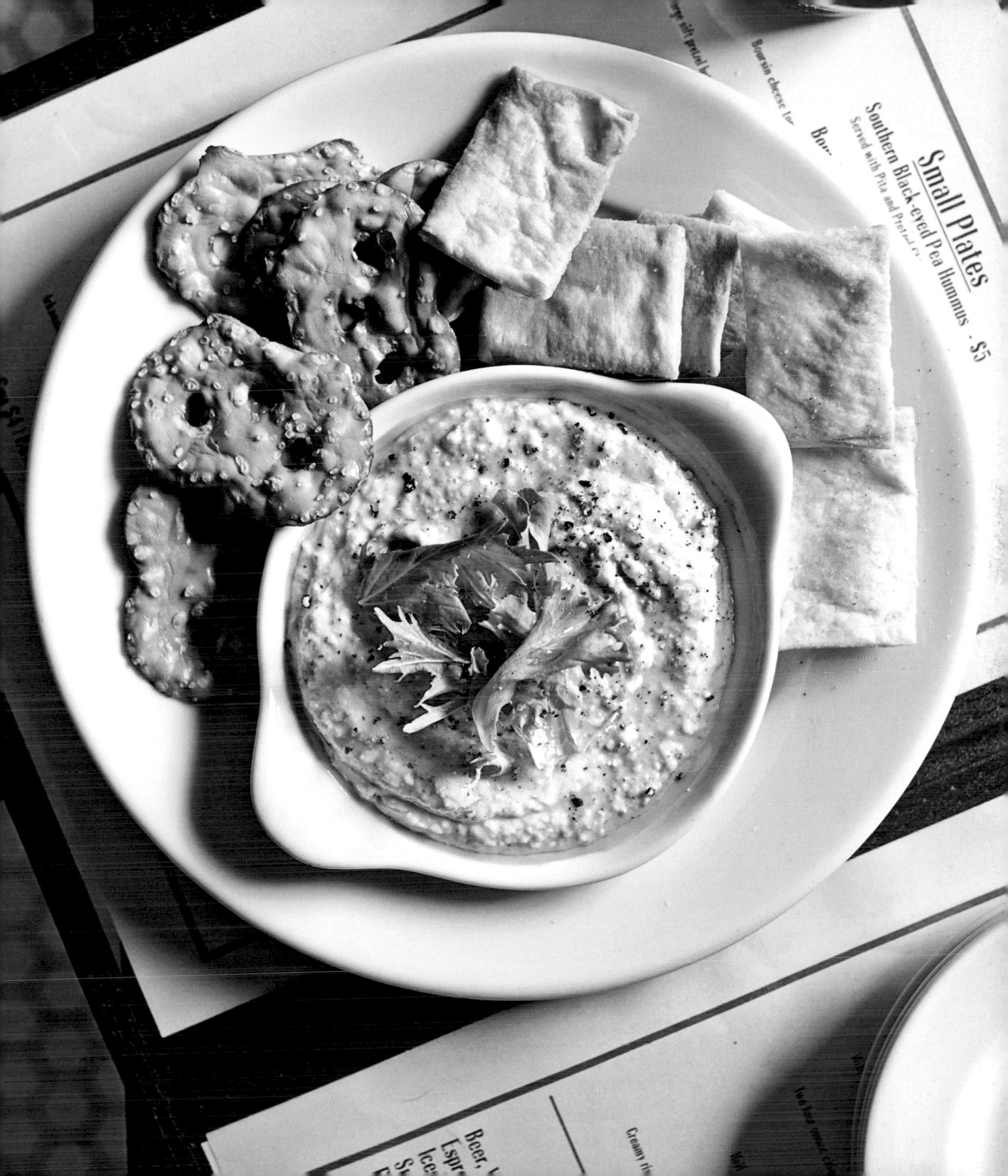

Savory Mushroom Strudel

Earthy mushrooms, sweet figs, and salty Brie come together in this strudel to make a great party appetizer.

½   cup butter
1   (8-oz.) package baby portobello mushrooms, cut into ¼-inch-thick slices
¼   tsp. table salt
¼   tsp. freshly ground black pepper
1   (8-oz.) Brie round, cut into ½-inch cubes with rind
16 small dried figs (figlets), stemmed and chopped
½   (16-oz.) package frozen phyllo pastry, thawed
Parchment paper

1. Melt butter in a small saucepan; set aside.

2. Cook mushrooms in 2 Tbsp. melted butter in a large skillet over medium heat 5 minutes or until tender, stirring occasionally. Sprinkle with salt and pepper. Transfer mushrooms to a large bowl. Stir cheese and figs into warm mushrooms.

3. Preheat oven to 400°. Place 2 phyllo sheets end to end on a work surface, overlapping by 2 inches to make 1 (24-inch-long) sheet. Keep remaining phyllo covered with a damp towel to prevent drying out. Brush long phyllo sheet with melted butter. Repeat procedure, topping with 2 more sheets; brush with butter. Repeat layering and brushing with butter until all sheets are used.

4. Spread mushroom filling on phyllo dough, leaving a 2-inch border. Fold in sides, and roll lengthwise to form a log. Brush log with butter, and place, seam side down, on a parchment paper-lined baking sheet.

5. Bake at 400° for 30 minutes. Place on a cutting board; let stand 10 minutes. Cut into diagonal slices with a serrated knife, using a gentle sawing motion. **Makes: 10 servings**

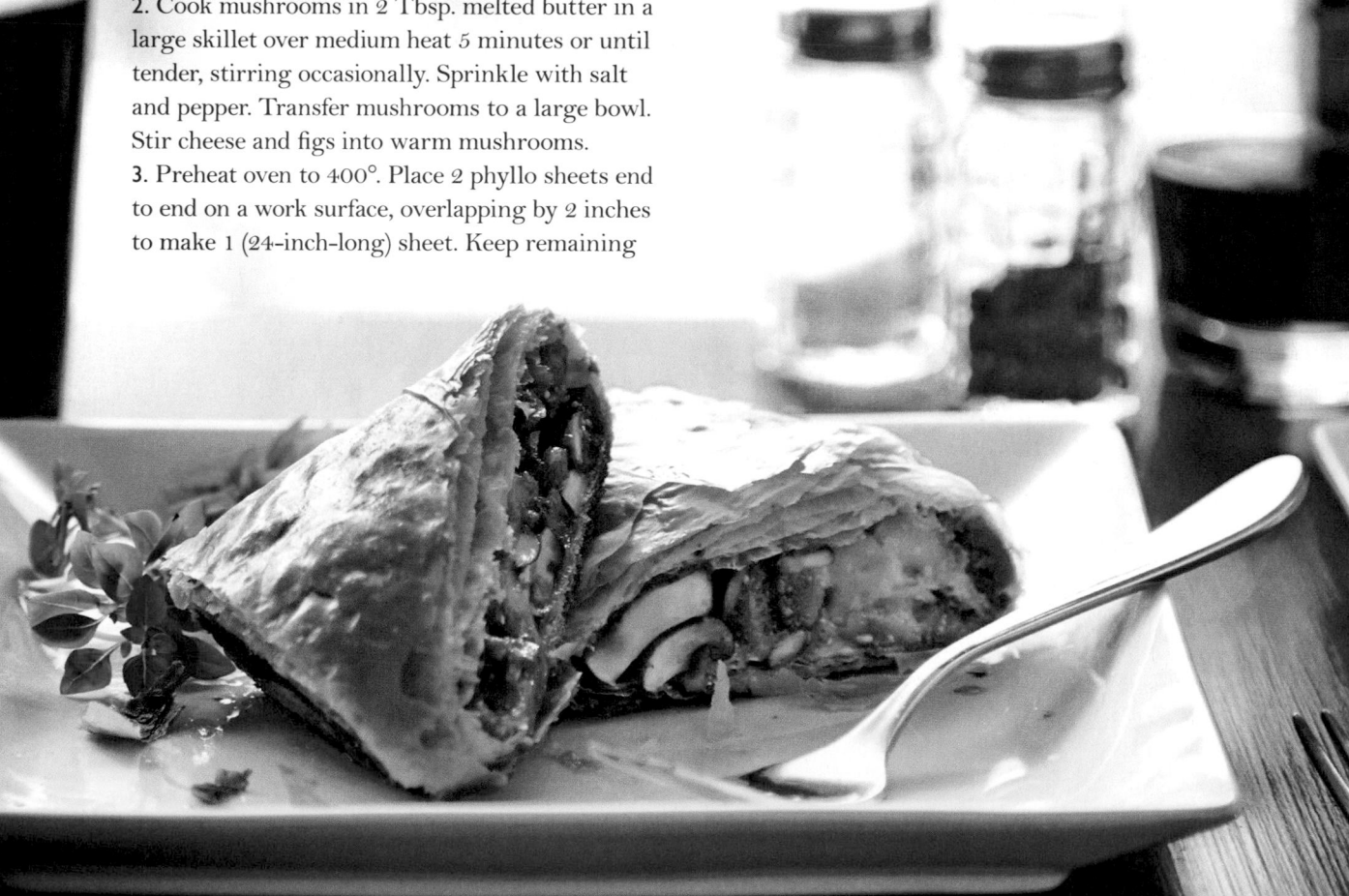

Citrus Quinoa Salad

The super-food ingredients in this salad are not only tasty and healthy, they also combine for a well-balanced side dish.

QUINOA SALAD

I	cup red quinoa
2	oranges, peeled, sectioned, and chopped
I	lemon, peeled, sectioned, and chopped
I	lime, peeled, sectioned, and chopped
2	Tbsp. olive oil
½	tsp. table salt
½	tsp. freshly ground black pepper
I	(5-oz.) package mixed salad greens
12	cherry tomatoes, cut in half
½	cucumber, peeled and cut into half-moon-shaped slices
2	avocados, halved

BASIL-APPLE VINAIGRETTE

6	Tbsp. apple cider vinegar
I	Tbsp. fresh lemon juice
I	Tbsp. bottled minced roasted garlic
¼	tsp. Dijon mustard
2	Tbsp. chopped fresh basil
¾	cup olive oil
⅛	tsp. table salt
⅛	tsp. freshly ground black pepper

1. Prepare Quinoa Salad: Cook quinoa according to package directions. Drain and cool to room temperature (about 30 minutes).

2. Peel and section oranges, lemon, and lime over a bowl to catch juice. Gently combine olive oil, salt, and pepper. Gently stir in quinoa and fruit sections. Cover and refrigerate until thoroughly chilled (about 1 hour).

3. Meanwhile, prepare Basil-Apple Vinaigrette: Combine first 5 ingredients in a blender. Turn blender on high; gradually add oil in a slow, steady stream. Process until thickened. Add salt and pepper.

4. Toss together quinoa mixture and salad greens. Spoon onto salad plates. Arrange tomato halves and cucumber slices around salad. Cut each avocado half into thin slices, and arrange on each salad. Serve with Basil-Apple Vinaigrette.

Makes: 4 servings

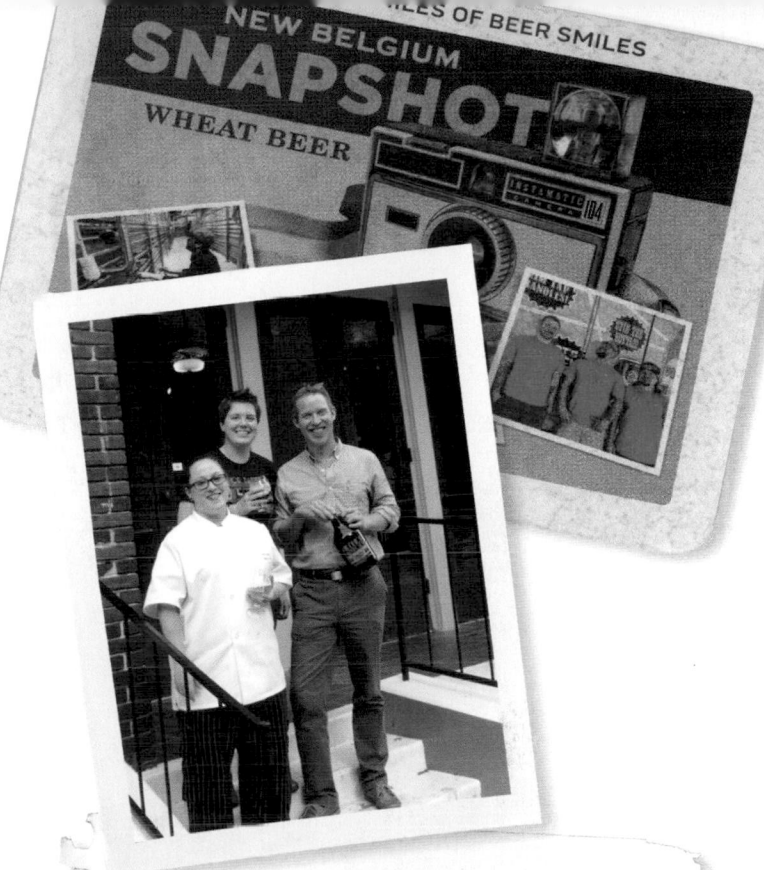

SOUNDTRACK:

"LET THERE BE LOVE"
BY NAT KING COLE

"A SUNDAY KIND OF LOVE"
BY ETTA JAMES

"PAPA WAS A ROLLIN' STONE"
BY THE TEMPTATIONS

"GREEN ONIONS"
BY BOOKER T. & THE M.G.'s

"UPTIGHT (EVERYTHING'S ALRIGHT)"
BY STEVIE WONDER

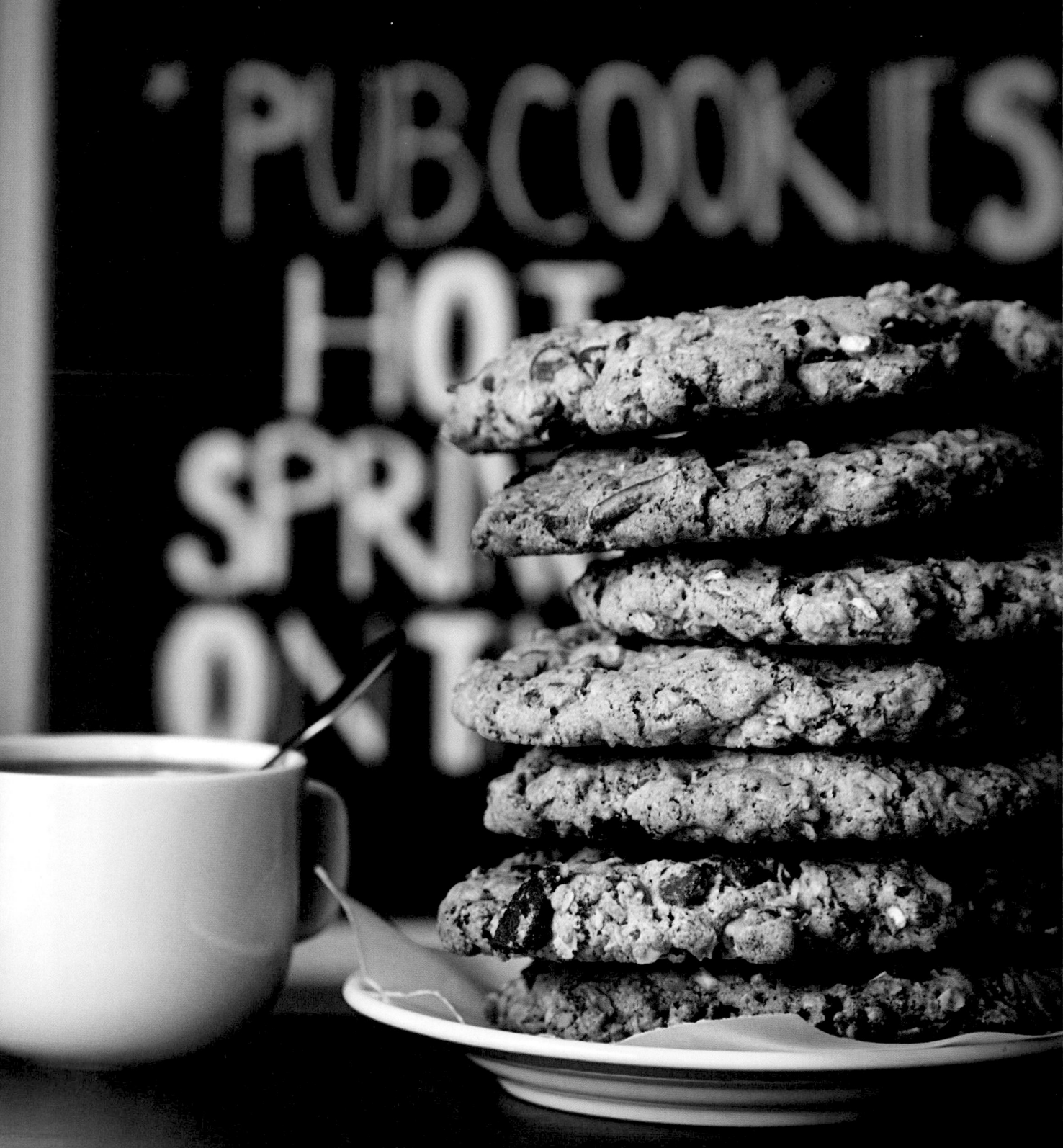

Gelato di Superior Pub Cookie

This crunchy and slightly salty cookie is the signature dessert at Superior Bathhouse. One bite and you'll know why.

1	cup butter, softened
1	cup granulated sugar
1	cup firmly packed brown sugar
2	large eggs
1	tsp. vanilla extract
2	cups all-purpose flour
1	tsp. baking soda
1	tsp. baking powder
1	tsp. kosher salt
2	cups uncooked regular oats
1	cup sweetened flaked coconut
1½	cups semisweet chocolate morsels
1	cup coarsely crushed pretzel sticks
12	chocolate sandwich cookies, chopped

Parchment paper

1. Preheat oven to 350°. Beat first 3 ingredients at medium speed with an electric mixer until creamy. Add eggs and vanilla, beating just until blended.

2. Combine flour and next 3 ingredients in a bowl; gradually add to butter mixture, beating well. Combine oats and next 4 ingredients in a large bowl. Add cookie dough to oat mixture, and blend, using your hands.

3. Roll about ½ cup dough into a ball. Place on a parchment paper-lined baking sheet. Flatten ball to ½-inch thickness with the palm of your hand. Repeat procedure with remaining dough.

4. Bake at 350° for 18 minutes or until golden brown. Cool on pan on a wire rack (about 30 minutes). **Makes: 15 servings**

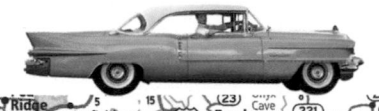

Arkansas bucket list

things to see and do (besides eat) here

1 Take a mineral bath or get a massage at the newly restored **Buckstaff Bath House** in Hot Springs.

2 Marvel in the majesty that is **Thorncrown Chapel** *(pictured)*, architect E. Fay Jones's masterpiece near Eureka Springs.

3 Channel your own version of House of Cards in the **William J. Clinton Presidential Library and Museum** Oval Office in Little Rock.

4 Meet with some of the country's best authors at **Arkansas Literary Festival**, held annually every spring in Little Rock.

5 Immerse yourself in Ozark Mountain culture while listening to the impromptu bluegrass and folk music that takes place (almost) nightly at the **Stone County Courthouse** in Mountain View.

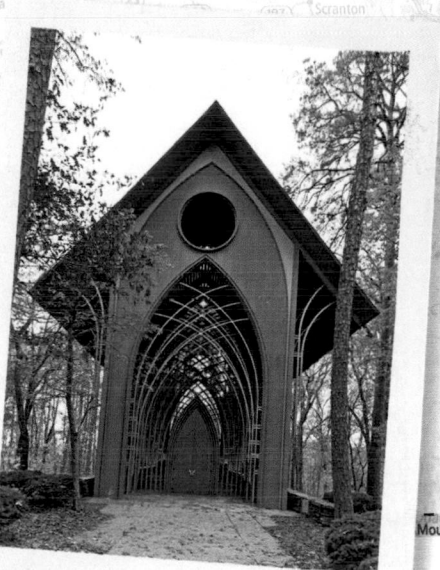

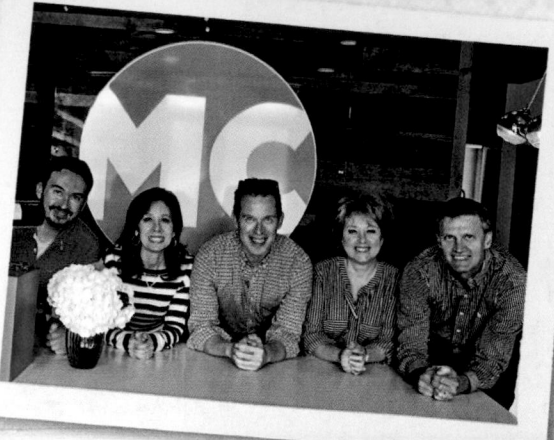

The Main Cheese

14524 Cantrell Road
Little Rock, Arkansas 72223
themaincheese.com
(501) 367-8082

The bright walls and urbane style of this spot make dining here a happy experience. The menu centers around what you might traditionally think of as kiddie fare: the grilled cheese. But these grilled cheeses are no butter-soaked slabs of white bread and processed slices. The Main Cheese takes grilled cheese sammies to a whole new gourmet level. My fave is the Ouachibella, a masterpiece of portobello mushroom, Swiss, provolone, feta, spinach, red onions, sun-dried tomatoes, truffle oil, and red pepper aïoli on toasted rosemary focaccia. Now that's what I call an adult grilled cheese. And if you need to kick it up another notch, order your sandwich with a side of house-made chips and beer or wine.

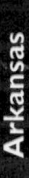
The Main Cheese Farmers Market

AVOCADO MIX

4   Tbsp. mashed avocado (about ½ avocado)
1½ tsp. fresh lemon juice
¼   to ½ tsp. all-purpose seasoning

SPINACH AÏOLI

1   small garlic clove, peeled
1⅓ cups loosely packed fresh baby spinach
3   Tbsp. mayonnaise
Pinch of table salt

SANDWICHES

8   (1.5-oz.) slices multigrain bread
¼   cup butter, softened
3   Tbsp. freshly grated Parmesan cheese
8   (¾-oz.) slices sharp Cheddar cheese
8   (¾-oz.) slices Muenster cheese
8   thin tomato slices
2   cups packed arugula
4   lemon wedges

1. **Prepare Avocado Mix:** Combine all ingredients in a small bowl. Cover and chill until ready to use.

2. **Prepare Spinach Aïoli:** With processor on, drop garlic through food chute; process until minced. Add spinach and next 2 ingredients; process until smooth.

3. **Prepare Sandwiches:** Generously spread 1 side of each slice of bread with butter; sprinkle lightly with Parmesan cheese, spreading with a knife to blend cheese into butter. Heat a large nonstick skillet over medium heat. Place 2 bread slices, buttered side down, in hot skillet. Top 1 bread slice with 2 Cheddar cheese slices; top other bread slice with 2 Muenster cheese slices. Top Cheddar cheese with about 1½ Tbsp. Spinach Aïoli. Cook 2 minutes or until cheeses melt and bread is golden. Transfer to a plate.

4. Top Muenster cheese with 1 Tbsp. Avocado Mix; top with 2 tomato slices and ½ cup arugula.

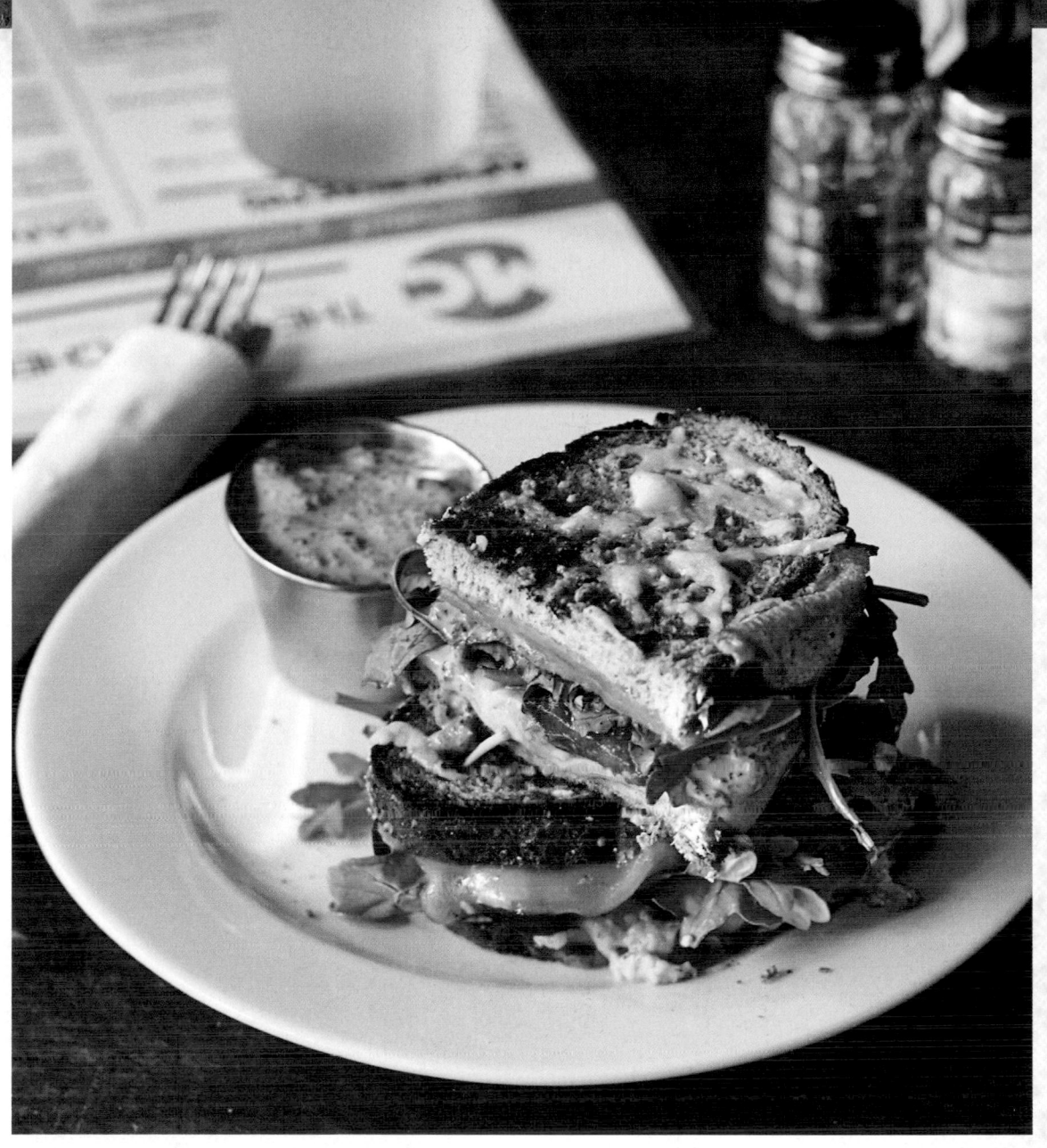

Squeeze 1 lemon wedge over arugula. Top with remaining toasted bread slice, Cheddar cheese-side down.

5. Repeat procedure with remaining bread slices, butter, Cheddar cheese, Muenster cheese, Spinach Aïoli, Avocado Mix, tomato slices, arugula, and lemon wedges. **Makes: 4 servings**

Note: We tested with Spike Original Magic Gourmet Natural Seasoning.

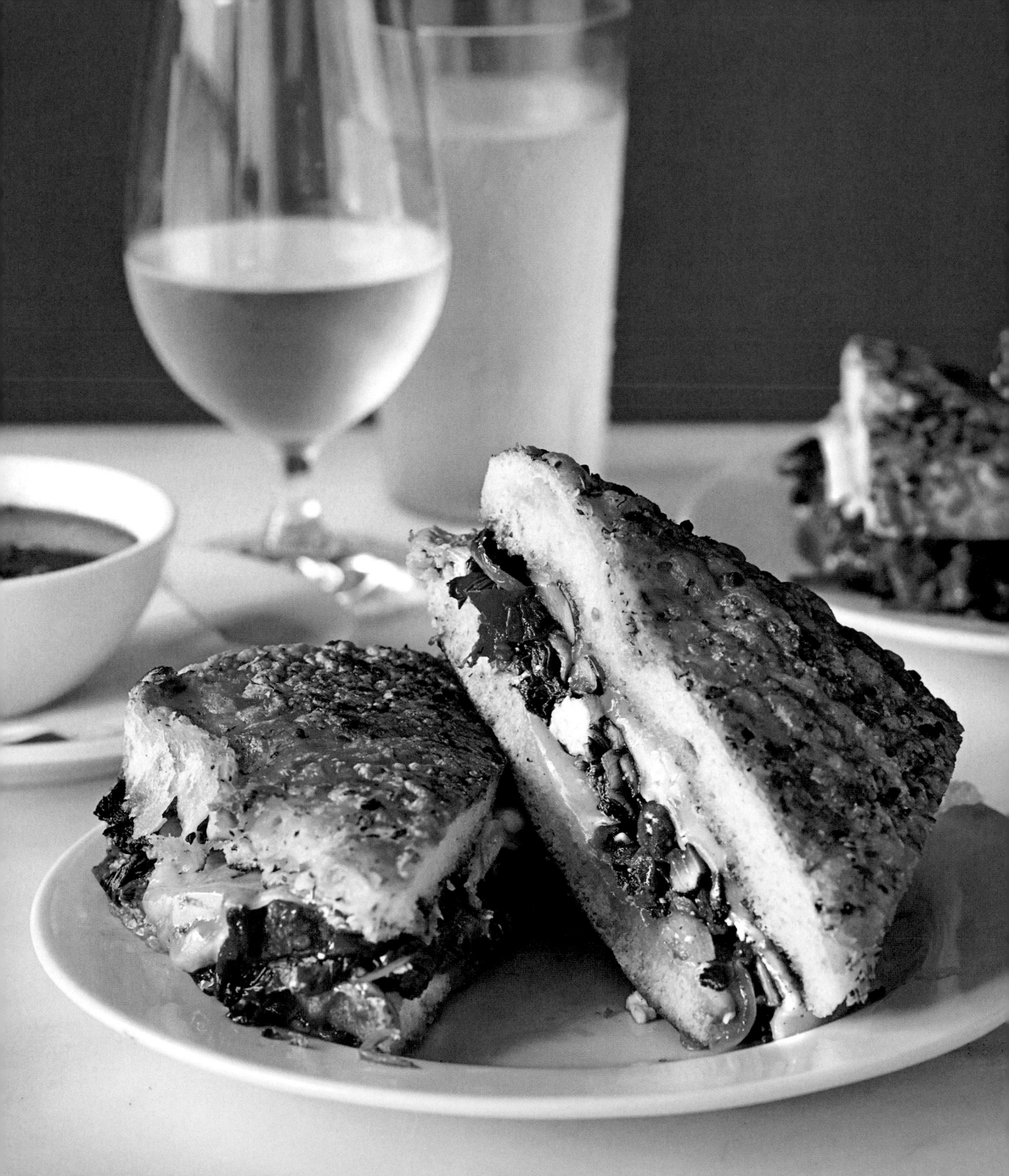

The Ouachibella

If ever I've eaten a sophisticated grilled cheese, this is it. Not many will come close to topping the Ouachibella.

RED PEPPER AÏOLI SAUCE

5	Tbsp. minced drained roasted red bell peppers
¼	cup mayonnaise
1	garlic clove, minced

SANDWICHES

1	large (4½-inch) portobello mushroom cap, stemmed
1	Tbsp. olive oil
¼	tsp. table salt
⅛	tsp. freshly ground black pepper
1	Tbsp. white truffle oil
¼	cup thin vertical slices red onion
7	cups fresh baby spinach
2	Tbsp. coarsely chopped sun-dried tomatoes
1	garlic clove, minced
1	oz. crumbled feta cheese
1	(12- x 5-inch) garlic-herb focaccia bread
2	Tbsp. butter, softened
8	(¾-oz.) slices Swiss cheese

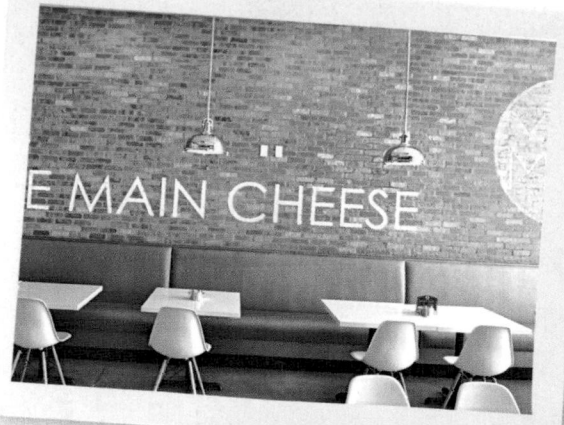

OVERHEARD:

"LA PETITE ROCHE."

FRENCH FOR "LITTLE ROCK," THIS EXPRESSION IS POPULAR AMONG LOCALS TO IDENTIFY THE SMALL OUTCROPPING OF ROCK IN THE ARKANSAS RIVER FIRST OBSERVED BY FRENCH EXPLORERS IN 1722.

1. Prepare Red Pepper Aïoli Sauce: Process all ingredients in a blender until smooth. Reserve 2 Tbsp. aïoli for sandwiches. Cover and store remaining aïoli in refrigerator for another use.

2. Prepare Sandwiches: Brush mushroom with olive oil; sprinkle with salt and pepper. Heat a large nonstick skillet over medium-high heat. Add mushroom; cook 3 minutes on each side or until browned and tender. Transfer to a cutting board; cool slightly. Holding a sharp knife at an angle, cut mushroom into thin slices.

3. Heat truffle oil in a large skillet over medium-high heat. Add onion and next 3 ingredients; sauté 3 minutes or until spinach wilts. Remove from heat. Stir in feta cheese.

4. Cut focaccia in half crosswise. Reserve half of focaccia for another use. Cut remaining half into 2 (5- x 3-inch) rectangles. Cut rectangles horizontally in half.

5. Heat a large nonstick skillet over medium heat. Spread cut sides of rectangles with butter. Place 2 focaccia pieces, buttered side up, in hot skillet.

6. Place 2 cheese slices on each piece of focaccia. Spread 1 Tbsp. aïoli sauce on top of cheese slices. Top aïoli with ½ cup spinach mixture, half of mushroom slices, 2 more cheese slices, and a second focaccia slice, buttered side down. Cook sandwich 1 minute on each side or until cheese melts. Remove sandwich from skillet, and cut diagonally in half. Repeat procedure with remaining ingredients to make a second sandwich. Serve immediately. Makes: 2 servings

Float'n the Buffalo Sandwich

This "buffalo" chicken sandwich is one spicy and hearty grilled cheese.

BUFFALO CHICKEN

1	(8-oz.) boned and skinned chicken breast

Vegetable cooking spray

⅛	tsp. table salt
⅛	tsp. freshly ground black pepper
¼	tsp. dried onion flakes

BUFFALO SAUCE

⅓	cup hot sauce
¼	cup cold salted butter, cut into pieces
2¼	tsp. white vinegar
⅛	tsp. Worcestershire sauce
⅛	tsp. ground red pepper
⅛	tsp. table salt

Pinch of garlic powder

SANDWICHES

2	tsp. canola oil
⅓	cup chopped onion
2	Tbsp. butter, softened
4	(1.5-oz.) sourdough bread slices
2	(¾-oz.) slices fontina cheese (thin sandwich slices)
2	Tbsp. shredded Havarti cheese
2	Tbsp. crumbled blue cheese

1. **Prepare Buffalo Chicken:** Preheat oven to 350°. Coat chicken with cooking spray; sprinkle with salt, pepper, and onion flakes. Place chicken in a small baking pan coated with cooking spray. Cover pan with aluminum foil.

2. Bake at 350° for 30 minutes or until done. Let stand 15 minutes or until cool enough to cut crosswise into ¼-inch-thick medallions.

3. **Meanwhile, prepare Buffalo Sauce:** Combine all ingredients in a small saucepan. Bring just to a simmer over medium heat, whisking constantly; immediately remove from heat.

4. **Prepare Sandwiches:** Heat a large well-seasoned cast-iron skillet over medium heat until hot. Add canola oil. Add onion; sauté 4 minutes or until tender and browned. Remove from skillet. Wipe out skillet with paper towels.

5. Lightly spread butter on 1 side of bread slices. Place 2 slices, buttered side down, in skillet; top each slice with 1 fontina cheese slice. Spread fontina with half of Buffalo Sauce. Sprinkle 1 Tbsp. Havarti cheese, 1 Tbsp. blue cheese and half of onion over Buffalo Sauce. Top with half of chicken slices over onion on bread slice containing the blue cheese.

6. Cook 2 minutes or until cheese melts and bread is golden brown. Invert bread slice topped with fontina cheese and sauce onto chicken to close sandwich. Remove from griddle.

7. Cut sandwich diagonally in half, and serve immediately. **Makes: 2 servings**

The Main Cheese Sandwich

There's nothing simple about the basic house grilled cheese at The Main Cheese.

1	Tbsp. softened butter
2	(1.5-oz.) slices sourdough bread
1	(¾-oz.) slice fontina cheese
2	(¾-oz.) slices sharp Cheddar cheese
2	(¾-oz.) slices Muenster cheese

1. Heat a large nonstick skillet over medium heat. Spread 1½ tsp. butter on 1 side of each bread slice. Place bread, buttered side down, in skillet. Top 1 bread slice with fontina and Cheddar cheeses; top other bread slice with Muenster cheese.

2. Cover skillet. Cook 2 to 3 minutes or until cheese melts and bread is golden. Uncover and place 1 bread slice, cheese side down, on top of the other. Remove from skillet; serve immediately. **Makes: 1 serving**

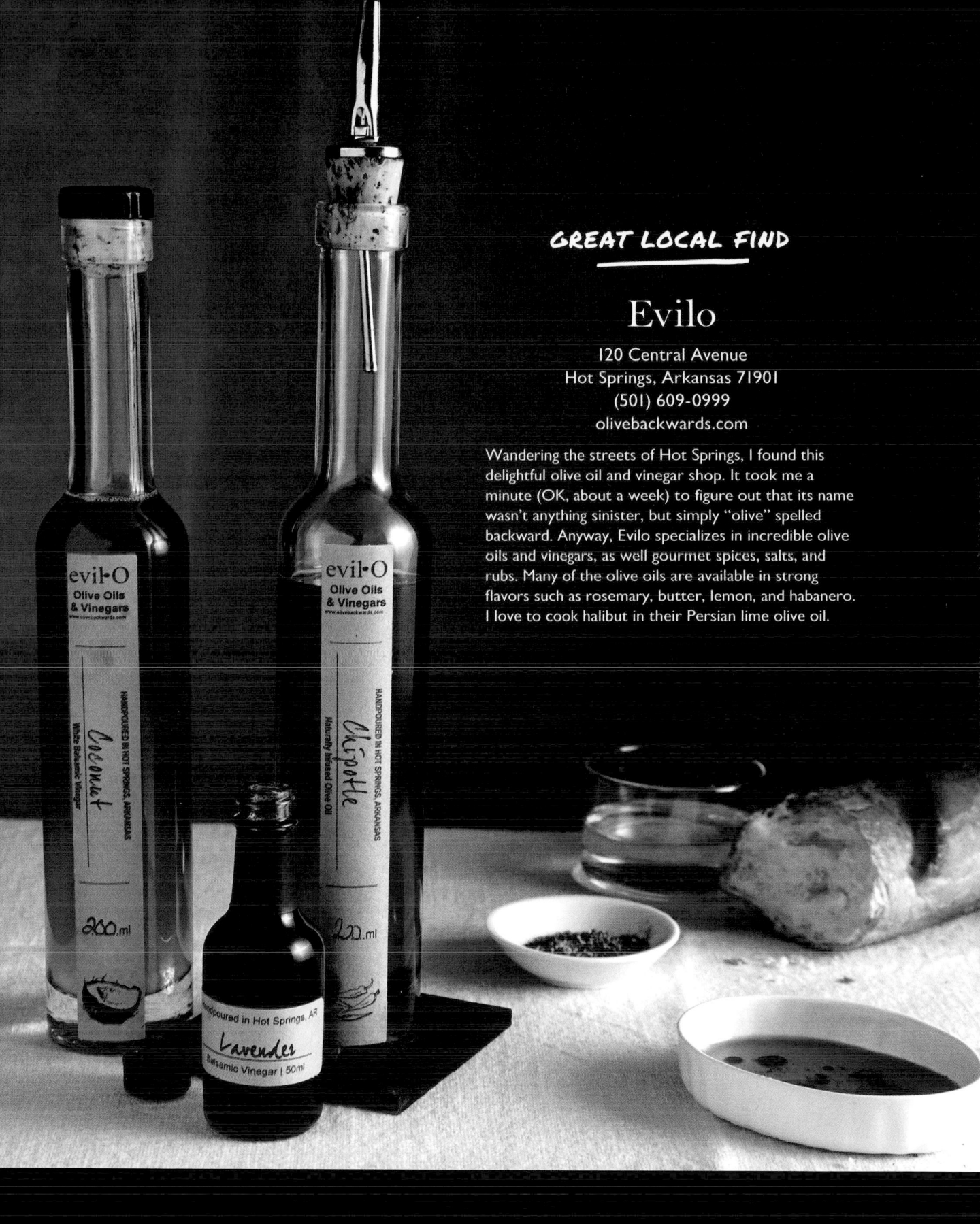

GREAT LOCAL FIND

Evilo

120 Central Avenue
Hot Springs, Arkansas 71901
(501) 609-0999
olivebackwards.com

Wandering the streets of Hot Springs, I found this delightful olive oil and vinegar shop. It took me a minute (OK, about a week) to figure out that its name wasn't anything sinister, but simply "olive" spelled backward. Anyway, Evilo specializes in incredible olive oils and vinegars, as well gourmet spices, salts, and rubs. Many of the olive oils are available in strong flavors such as rosemary, butter, lemon, and habanero. I love to cook halibut in their Persian lime olive oil.

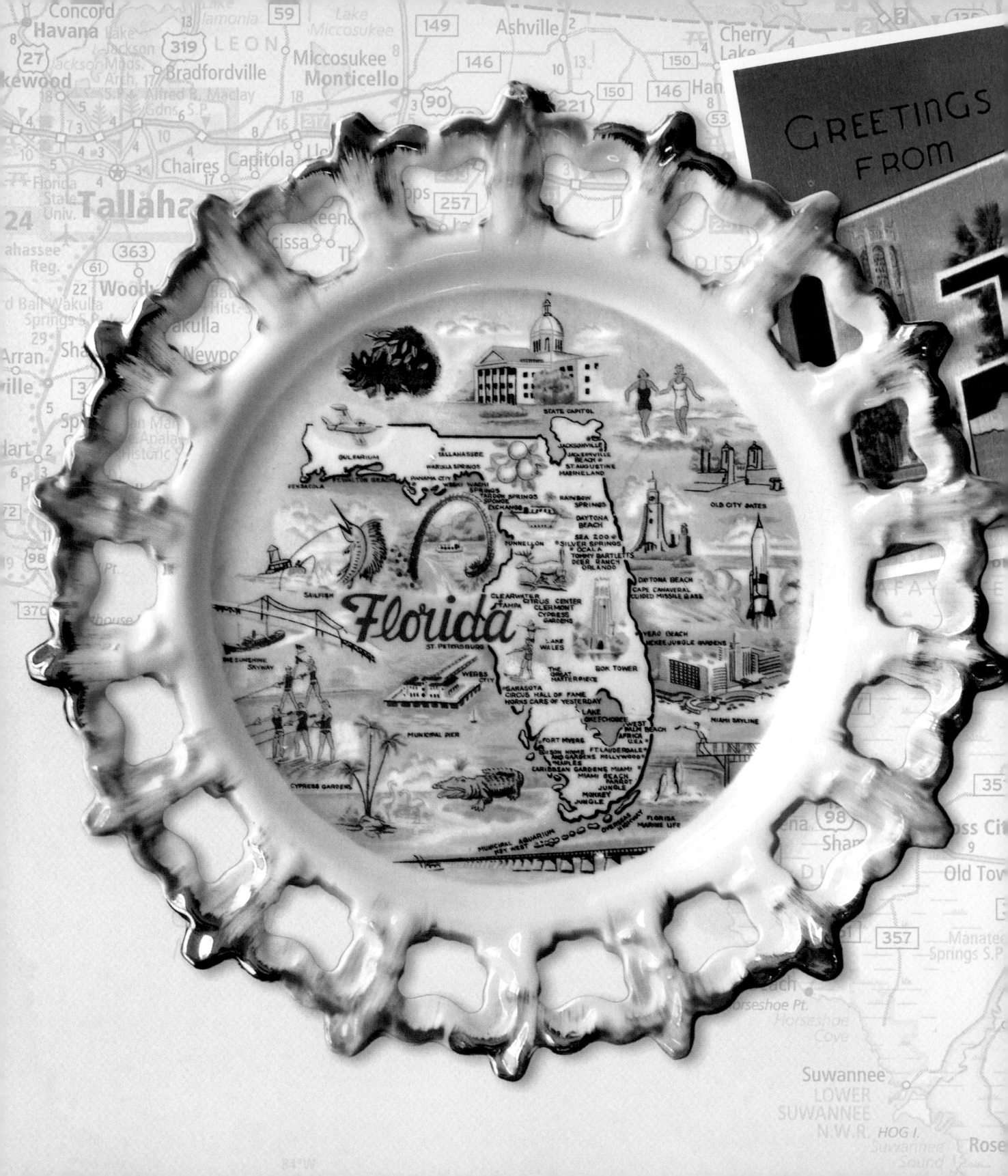

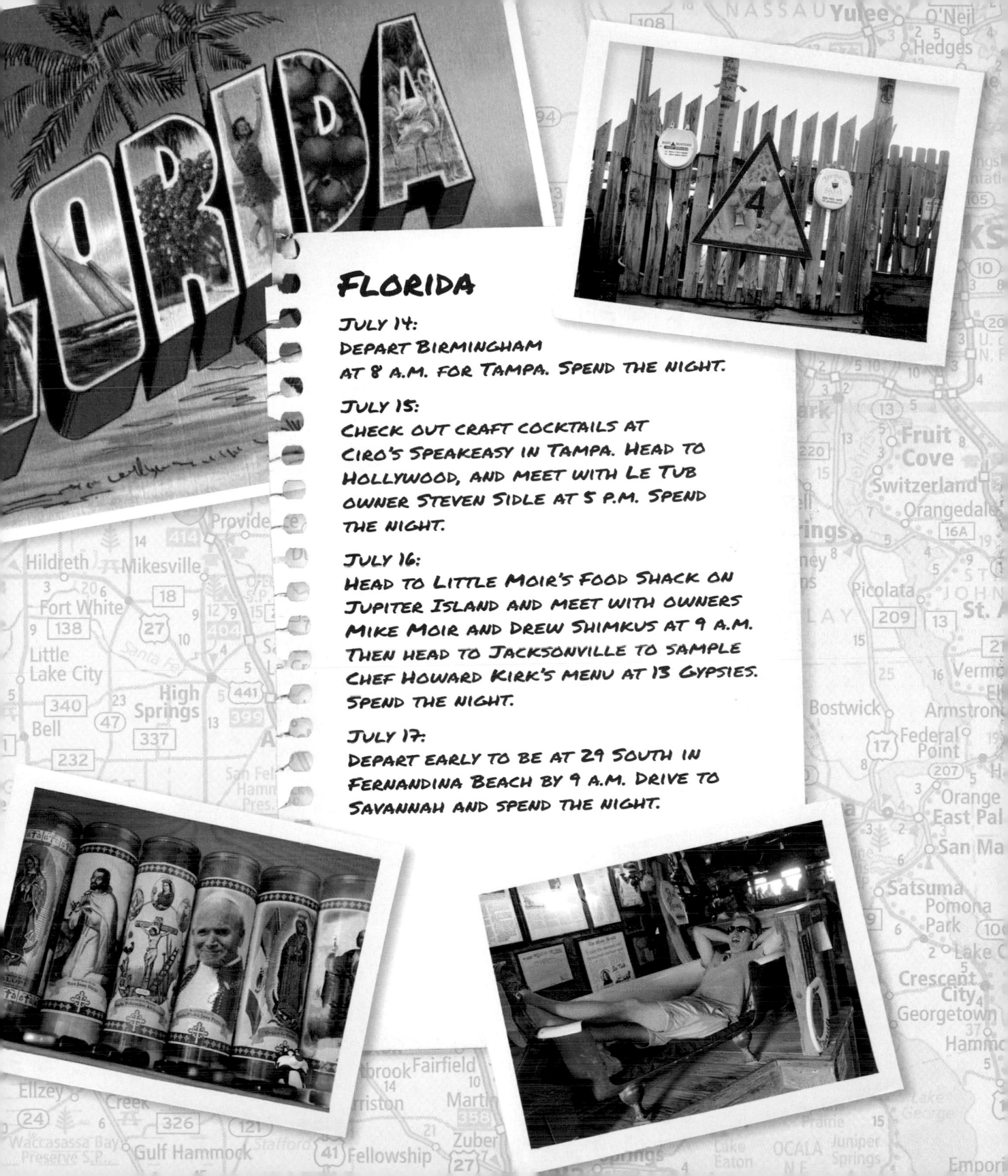

FLORIDA

JULY 14:
DEPART BIRMINGHAM AT 8 A.M. FOR TAMPA. SPEND THE NIGHT.

JULY 15:
CHECK OUT CRAFT COCKTAILS AT CIRO'S SPEAKEASY IN TAMPA. HEAD TO HOLLYWOOD, AND MEET WITH LE TUB OWNER STEVEN SIDLE AT 5 P.M. SPEND THE NIGHT.

JULY 16:
HEAD TO LITTLE MOIR'S FOOD SHACK ON JUPITER ISLAND AND MEET WITH OWNERS MIKE MOIR AND DREW SHIMKUS AT 9 A.M. THEN HEAD TO JACKSONVILLE TO SAMPLE CHEF HOWARD KIRK'S MENU AT 13 GYPSIES. SPEND THE NIGHT.

JULY 17:
DEPART EARLY TO BE AT 29 SOUTH IN FERNANDINA BEACH BY 9 A.M. DRIVE TO SAVANNAH AND SPEND THE NIGHT.

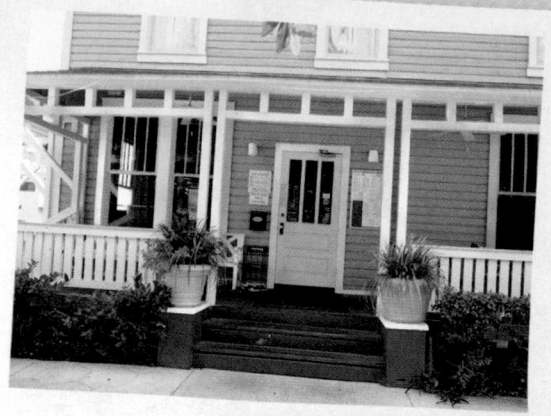

29 South

29 South 3rd Street
Fernandina Beach, Florida 32034
(904) 277-7919
29southrestaurant.com

When you dig into dinner at 29 South, chances are at least one of the ingredients in your meal was plucked from the garden just hours before it landed on your plate. Chef Scotty Schwartz, a culinary mastermind, is fanatical about freshness. So much so, he turned the restaurant's parking lot into a garden, and what he doesn't grow himself he buys exclusively from four local farms. But don't expect to find a menu full of organic shrubs and berries. You will leave full when you eat here. Plates of pork belly, pork chops, and grits flew out of the kitchen the day I visited. But Schwartz did me in with his coffee and doughnuts dessert. The indulgent bread pudding is made of glazed doughnuts and coffee ice cream. It's as memorable as the city of Fernandina itself.

29 South Sweet Tea Brined Pork Chops

A sweet, herby brine tenderizes these massive pork chops.

BRINED PORK CHOPS

2	qt. cold unsweetened tea
1	cup sugar
½	cup kosher salt
2	Tbsp. black peppercorns
6	garlic cloves, smashed
6	(3-inch) thyme sprigs
2	(3-inch) rosemary sprigs
6	bay leaves
6	(12- to 14-oz.) bone-in center-cut pork chops

GINGER-BLACKBERRY PRESERVES

2	cups sugar
2	cups blackberries
¼	cup rice vinegar
1	(1-inch) piece fresh ginger, unpeeled and halved

1. Prepare Brined Pork Chops: Combine first 3 ingredients in a large bowl, stirring until sugar dissolves. Pour half of tea mixture into each of 2 large zip-top plastic freezer bags. Add half each of peppercorns and next 4 ingredients to each bag. Add 3 pork chops to each bag. Seal bags; marinate in refrigerator 12 hours.

2. Prepare Ginger-Blackberry Preserves: Bring all ingredients to a boil in a medium saucepan; reduce heat, and simmer, uncovered, 30 to 45 minutes or until thickened and reduced to about 1½ cups. Remove from heat. Remove and discard ginger.

3. Preheat grill to 350° to 400° (medium-high) heat. Remove pork from marinade, discarding marinade. Grill pork, covered with grill lid, 10 minutes, turning once, or until a meat thermometer inserted in pork chop registers 145°. Remove from grill; cover with aluminum foil, and let stand 10 minutes.

4. Serve with preserves. Makes: 6 servings

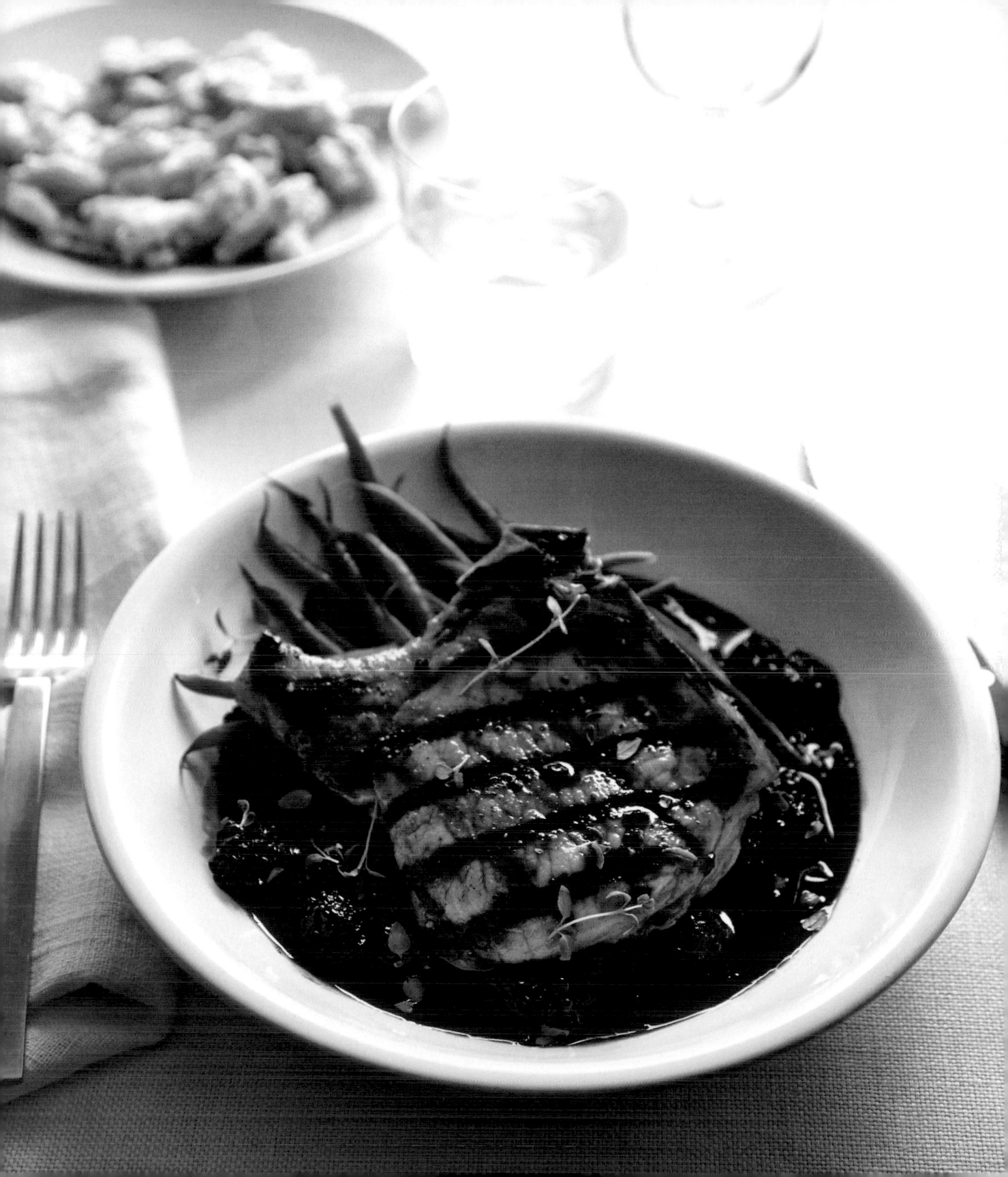

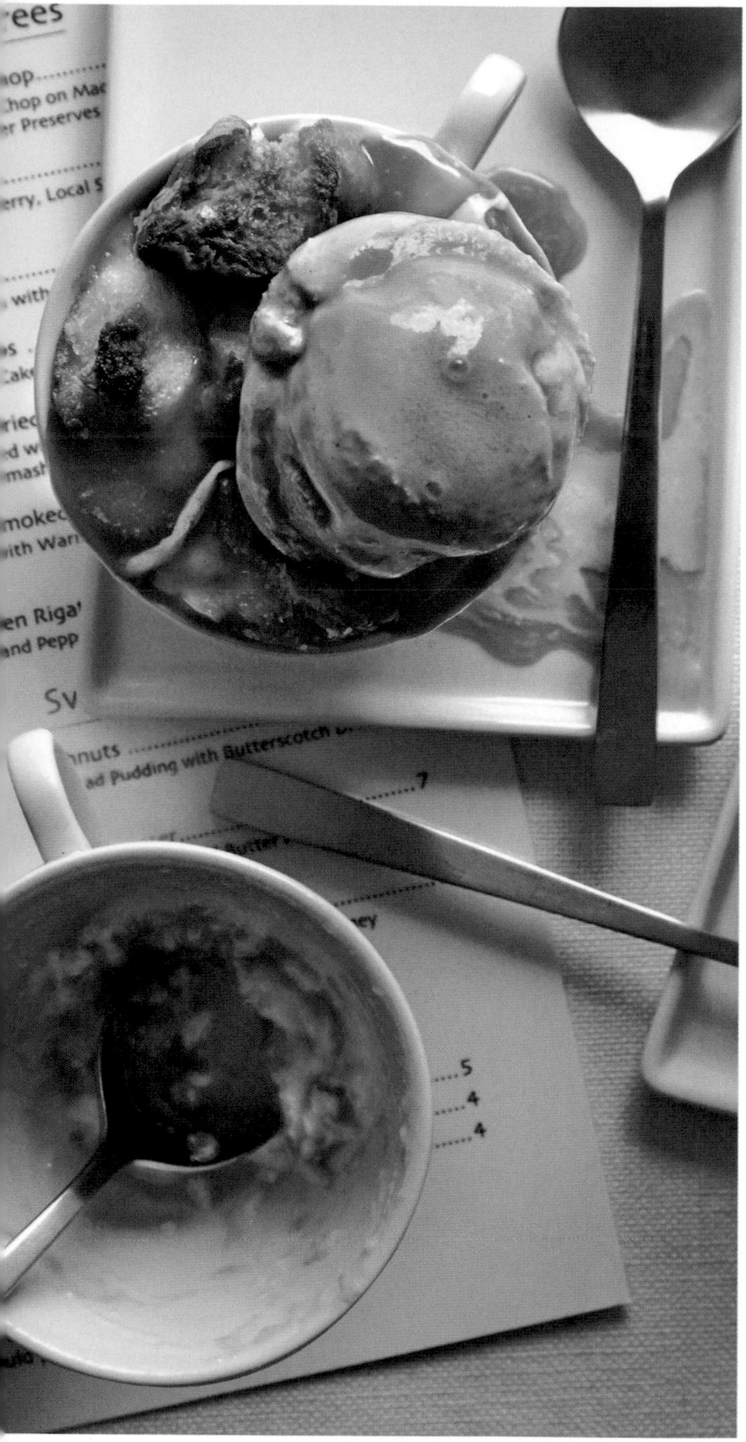

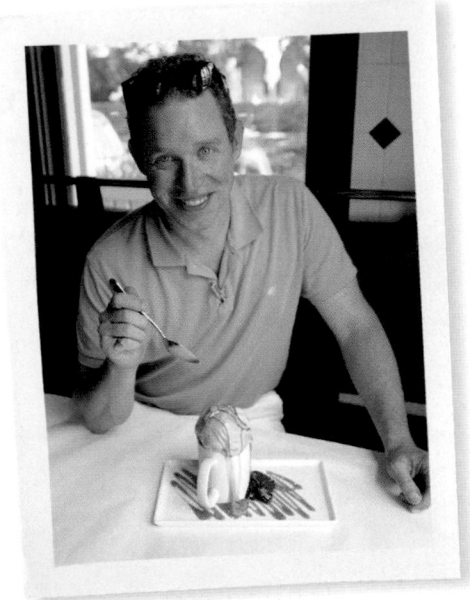

Coffee and Doughnuts

If you're on a diet, don't even read this recipe.

CUSTARD
6   store-bought glazed yeast doughnuts
Vegetable cooking spray
2   cups heavy cream
2   cups half-and-half
1   cup sugar
6   large eggs
1   qt. coffee ice cream

CARAMEL SAUCE
1   cup heavy cream
Pinch of sea salt
2   cups sugar
2   Tbsp. bourbon

1. **Prepare Custard:** Preheat oven to 350°. Tear each doughnut into bite size pieces, and place into each of 6 (10-oz.) coffee cups or ramekins coated with cooking spray. Place cups in a 15- x 10- inch pan.

2. Bring heavy cream, half-and-half, and 1 cup sugar to a simmer in a large saucepan, stirring until sugar dissolves. Remove pan from heat. Whisk eggs in a medium bowl. Gradually whisk about one-fourth of hot cream mixture into eggs; add egg mixture to remaining hot cream mixture, whisking constantly. Pour mixture through a wire-mesh strainer into a bowl. Ladle half of custard evenly over doughnuts in cups. Let stand 10 minutes. Ladle remaining half of custard into cups. (Doughnuts will not be submerged.)

3. Add hot water to pan with cups to depth of 1 inch. Bake, uncovered, at 350° for 48 minutes or until a knife inserted in center comes out clean. (Unsubmerged doughnut pieces will become browned and crisp.)

4. **Meanwhile, prepare Caramel Sauce:** Bring cream and salt to a simmer in a small saucepan; remove from heat, and keep warm.

5. Combine sugar and 1 cup water in a heavy 4-qt. saucepan; cook over medium heat 17 to 19 minutes or until sugar caramelizes, tipping pan to swirl mixture in pan to evenly caramelize sugar. Remove pan from heat. Slowly whisk in half of hot cream mixture (mixture will bubble vigorously). Whisk in remaining half of cream mixture and bourbon. Continue whisking 2 minutes or until thick and smooth. Cool until warm, about 20 minutes.

6. When custards are done, transfer cups to a wire rack. Cool until warm (20 minutes).

7. Top each custard with ⅔ cup ice cream; drizzle with Caramel Sauce, and serve immediately.

Makes: 6 servings

Note: Cool any remaining caramel sauce completely. Cover and store in refrigerator up to 1 month.

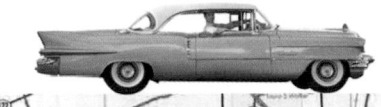

Florida bucket list

things to see and do (besides eat) here

1 Take a dip in the bubbling blue waters at the **Ocala National Forest's** Juniper Springs.

2 Get in 18 holes on the Donald Ross-designed championship course at **The Biltmore in Coral Gables** *(pictured)*.

3 Explore the shops of Apalachicola, where the quaint streets and friendly Floridians make this part of the Panhandle worth the drive.

4 Go horseback riding in the surf, or try Horse-Surfing at **Beach Horses** in Bradenton.

5 Throw down some serious cash shopping on **Ocean Drive** in Miami.

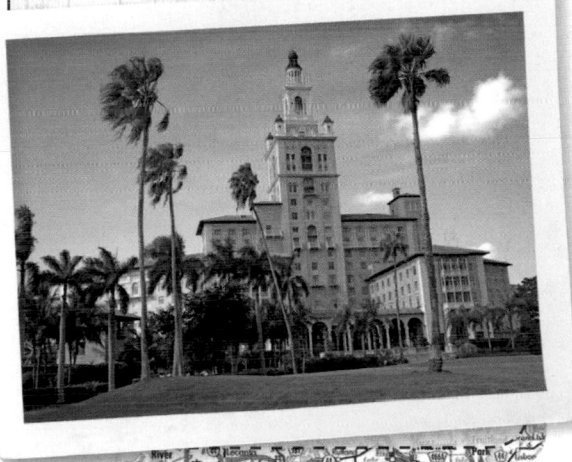

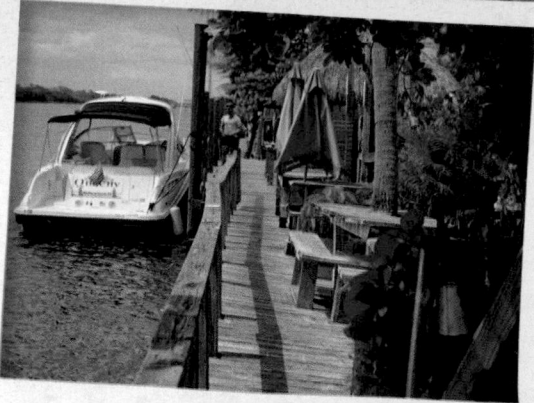

Le Tub Saloon

1100 North Ocean Drive
Hollywood, Florida 33019
(954) 921-9425
theletub.com

Perched on the Intracoastal Waterway, this little restaurant is festooned with vintage bathtubs, various decks, lots of signage, and a kitchen the size of a Kia. But from that tiny kitchen comes one whopper of a burger, weighing in at 13 ounces. The story behind Le Tub Saloon is equally perfect. "The original owner had a bunch of junk in this vacant lot. The city told him to clean it up, so he made a restaurant out of it," says Le Tub's salty owner Steven Sidle. And don't let the lack of A/C deter you: This place is cool. Sit on the deck, have one of the amazing cocktails, and take in a glorious sunset over the water. You'll feel like you're in the islands when you're just a few minutes from downtown Miami.

Bloody Marys

These bloodies are just right to spice up your morning brunch (or to recover from an overindulgent night on the town).

BLOODY MARY MIX
1   (48-oz.) bottle tomato juice, chilled
1½ Tbsp. Greek seasoning
¼   cup dill pickle juice
¼   cup fresh lime juice (about 3 large limes)
2   Tbsp. prepared horseradish
1½ Tbsp. Worcestershire sauce

BLOODY MARY SEASONING
3   Tbsp. Cajun seasoning
1   tsp. celery salt

BLOODY MARYS
2   cups vodka
Garnishes: celery leaf sprigs, dill pickle slices, lime wedges

1. Prepare Bloody Mary Mix: Combine all ingredients in a large container. Cover and chill until ready to serve.
2. Prepare Bloody Mary Seasoning: Stir together all ingredients in a small shallow bowl.
3. Prepare Bloody Marys: For each cocktail, dip rims of 8 (8-oz.) glasses in water. Dip rims in Bloody Mary Seasoning to coat. Fill glasses with ice. Pour ¼ cup vodka into each glass. Add about ¾ cup Bloody Mary Mix to each glass; stir.
Makes: 8 servings
Note: We tested with Cavender's Greek Seasoning and Emeril's Cajun Seasoning.

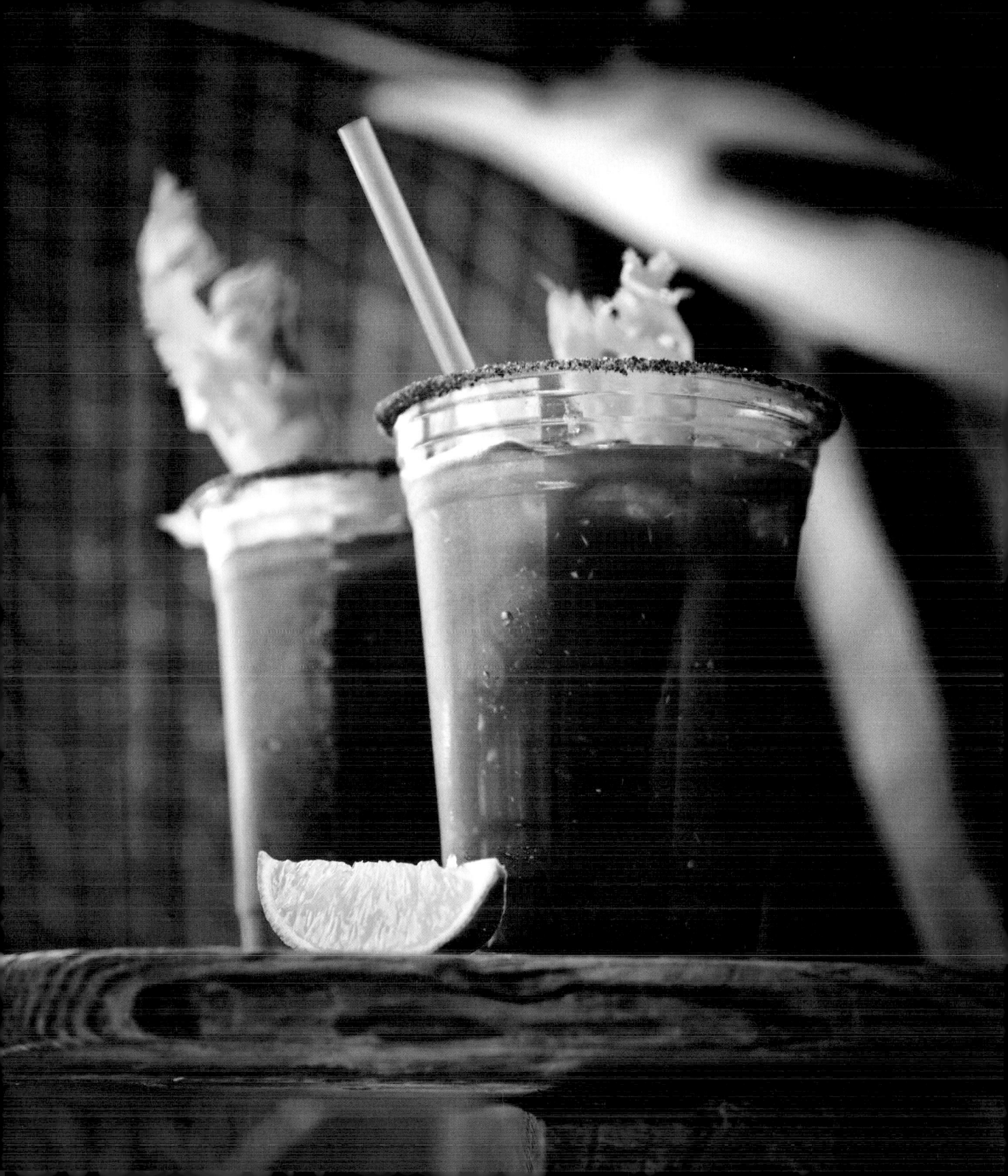

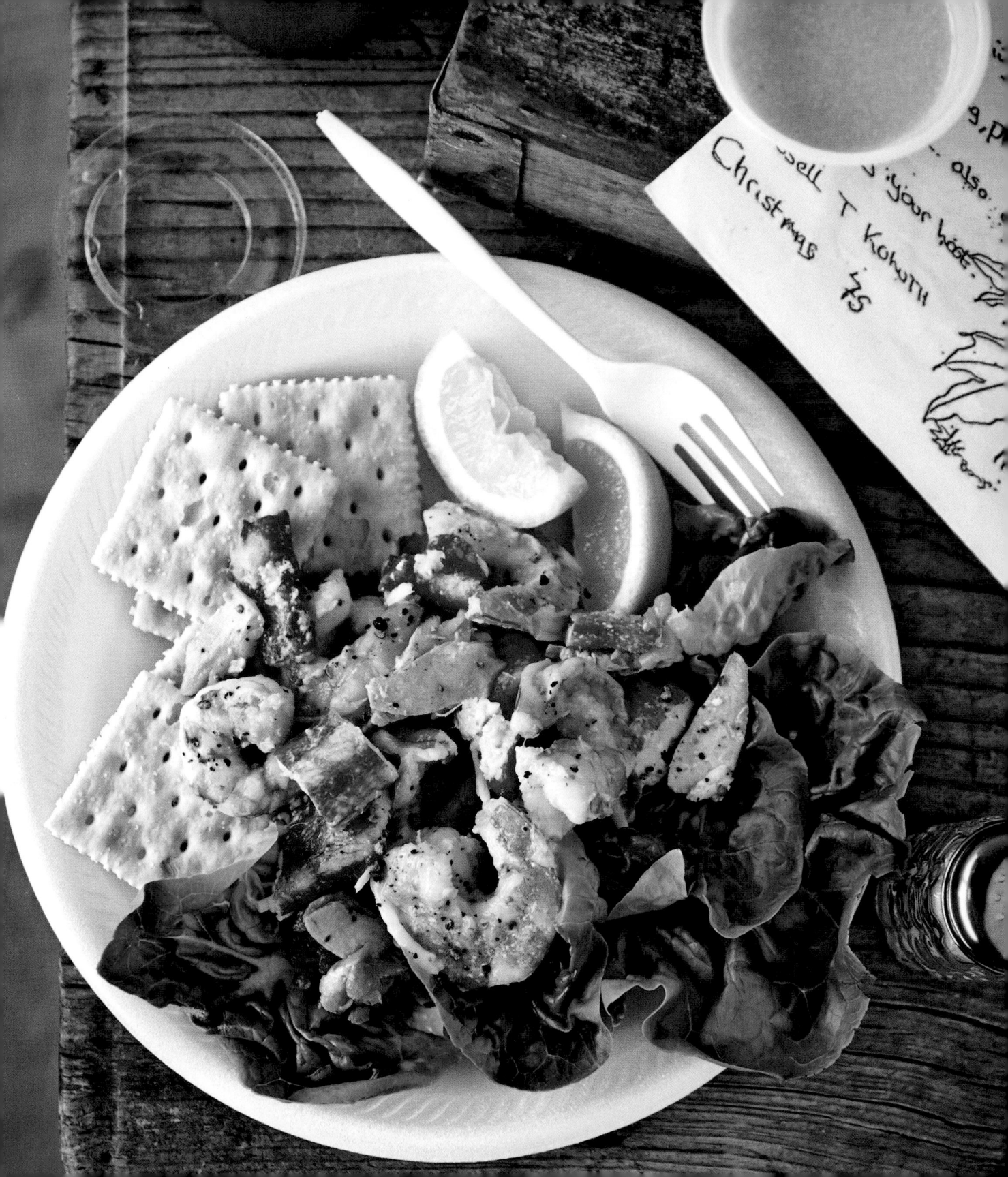

Seafood Salad

This hearty salad is full of shrimp, salmon, and Alaskan king crab legs, and makes a killer beachside appetizer.

SEAFOOD SALAD

1	Tbsp. sea salt
6	fresh parsley sprigs
1	lemon, sliced
8	oz. peeled and deveined medium-size raw shrimp
1	(8-oz.) skinless salmon fillet (1 inch thick)
2	(4-oz.) thawed frozen cooked Alaska king crab legs, cracked
4	iceberg lettuce leaves

Lemon wedges
Saltine crackers

DRESSING

⅔	cup red wine vinegar
½	cup coarsely chopped onion
¼	cup loosely packed fresh dill
3	peeled garlic cloves
2	drained anchovy fillets
1	cup extra virgin olive oil

1. **Prepare Seafood Salad:** Pour water to depth of 2½ inches into a Dutch oven. Add first 3 ingredients; bring to a boil over medium-high heat. Add shrimp. Boil 2 minutes or just until shrimp turn pink. Remove shrimp from poaching liquid with a slotted spoon, reserving liquid in Dutch oven. Plunge shrimp into ice water to stop the cooking process. Let stand 2 minutes; drain. Cool completely. Place shrimp in a bowl; cover and chill.
2. Return liquid in Dutch oven to a boil; add salmon. Return liquid to a boil, reduce heat to low, and simmer, uncovered, 7 to 10 minutes or until fish flakes with a fork. Remove salmon from Dutch oven. Cool completely (30 minutes). Wrap in plastic wrap, and chill.
3. **Meanwhile, prepare Dressing:** Process first 5 ingredients in a blender until pureed. Turn blender on high; gradually add oil in a slow, steady stream. Cover and chill.

4. Break salmon into large chunks; place in a bowl. Remove crabmeat from shell; cut into large pieces. Add crabmeat to salmon; add shrimp. Add ⅓ to ½ cup dressing to taste, reserving remaining dressing for another use. Sprinkle with table salt and black pepper to taste; toss gently.
5. Line each of 4 salad plates with 1 lettuce leaf. Spoon seafood mixture evenly onto lettuce leaves. Serve each salad with lemon wedges and crackers.
Makes: 4 servings

OVERHEARD:

"THE REDNECK RIVIERA"

COINED IN THE LATE 1970S BY FORMER NEW YORK TIMES EDITOR HOWELL RAINES, THE REDNECK RIVIERA REFERS TO FLORIDA'S PANHANDLE AND ALABAMA'S GULF COAST. OF COURSE WITH TODAY'S MONEYED VISITORS TO 30A, THOSE BEACHES MAY ACTUALLY BE CLOSER TO THE RIVIERA'S WEALTH AND STYLE THAN RAINES EVER IMAGINED.

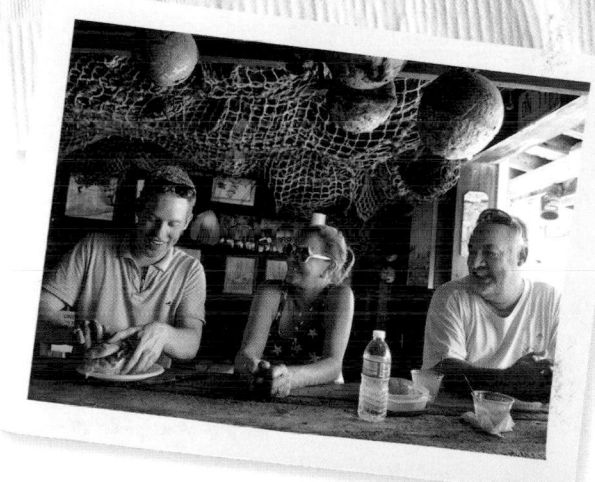

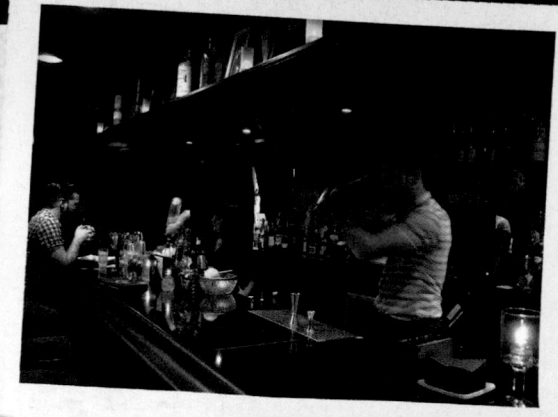

Ciro's Speakeasy and Supper Club

2109 Bayshore Blvd.
Tampa, Florida 33606
(813) 251-0022
cirostampa.com

In the back of a high-rise condo building along Tampa's elegant Bayshore Boulevard you'll find a nondescript wooden door. Beside it a small brass sign says, "Please knock & speak easy." You'll need a password—the night I visited it was el diablo. Once inside this retro bar, a reverence for classic and craft cocktails reigns: The spirits are primarily bourbon, gin, and rum. Bartender Robby Wages only recently added vodka as an option, God bless him. The dining menu is equally as impressive. The chocolate ganache with candied walnut crust will blow whatever is left of your mind, provided you've survived the cocktail list. Ciro's, named to honor the famed bar in Hollywood, can also host a small party in a secret room, accessible only by tugging on a copy of Charles Dickens's Great Expectations.

Chocolate Ganache with Candied Walnut Crust

This sweet treat is über-rich and the ultimate dessert for the chocoholic in all of us. Just take it slow and steady and you'll be able to tackle it like a champ.

CANDIED WALNUT CRUST
1   Tbsp. table salt
½   tsp. ground red pepper
4   cups sugar, divided
2   cups walnuts plus 16 walnut halves, toasted
Vegetable cooking spray
Parchment paper
1   Tbsp. butter

GANACHE
4   cups semisweet chocolate morsels
2   cups heavy cream
1   Tbsp. butter
Sea salt flakes (optional)

1. **Prepare Walnut Crust:** Stir together salt, ground red pepper, and 2 cups sugar in a bowl until blended. Bring remaining 2 cups sugar and 2 cups water to a boil in a medium saucepan. Add walnuts; boil for 2 minutes. Remove saucepan from heat. Remove walnuts with a slotted spoon, in batches, and add to sugar mixture, tossing to coat. Remove walnuts from sugar mixture with a slotted spoon, shaking spoon to remove excess sugar mixture. Place on a wire rack set over a baking sheet. Let stand 30 minutes.

2. Coat a 9-inch springform pan with cooking spray; line pan with parchment paper. Coat parchment paper with cooking spray.

3. Reserve 16 walnut halves. Process remaining sugared walnuts and 1 Tbsp. butter in a food processor until consistency of coarse wet sand. Press walnut mixture into bottom and 1 inch up sides of springform pan.

4. **Prepare Ganache:** Place chocolate morsels in a medium bowl. Heat cream in a medium saucepan

over medium heat 6 minutes or just until it begins to simmer, stirring often. Pour over chocolate morsels; add 1 Tbsp. butter, and let stand 1 minute. Whisk until smooth. Pour ganache into prepared walnut crust. Cover and chill at least 6 hours.

5. Run a sharp knife around sides of pan. Remove sides of pan. Cut Ganache into 16 wedges. Top each wedge with 1 reserved candied walnut, and if desired, sprinkle with sea salt. **Makes: 16 servings**

Sautéed Shrimp with Oyster Mushrooms

This shrimp dish goes light-years beyond the basic "shrimp cocktail" of the 1930s.

1	cup (1-inch) cubed French bread baguette
3	Tbsp. extra virgin olive oil, divided
1½	cups oyster mushrooms
½	tsp. table salt, divided
½	tsp. freshly ground black pepper, divided
1	Tbsp. diced shallots
2	garlic cloves, sliced
10	large raw shrimp, peeled and deveined
¼	cup mezcal
2	Tbsp. fresh lemon juice
½	cup diced seeded plum tomatoes
2	Tbsp. butter

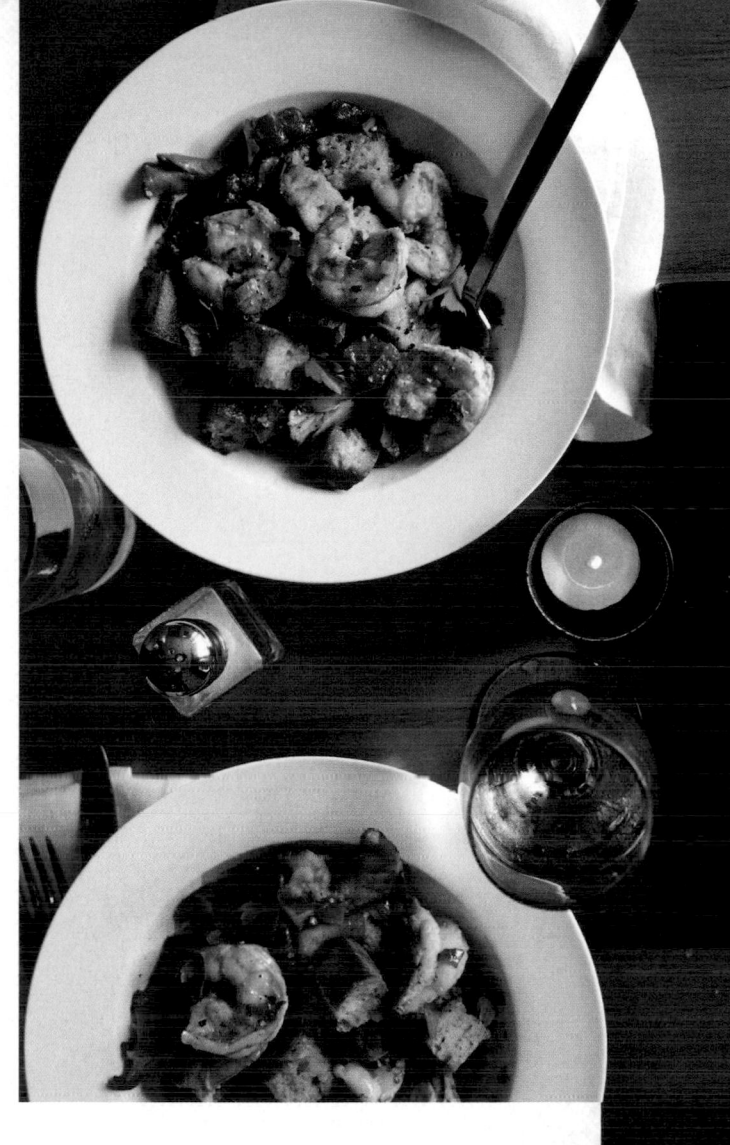

1. Preheat oven to 450°. Place bread in a bowl; drizzle with 1 Tbsp. olive oil, tossing to coat. Spread bread cubes in a single layer on a baking sheet. Bake at 450° for 3 to 4 minutes or until browned and crisp, turning once.

2. Heat 1 Tbsp. oil in a medium skillet over medium-high heat. Add mushrooms, ¼ tsp. salt, and ¼ tsp. pepper; sauté 3 minutes or until tender. Keep warm.

3. Heat remaining 1 Tbsp. oil in a large skillet over medium-high heat. Add shallots, garlic, and shrimp. Sauté 3 minutes or just until shrimp turn pink. Remove from heat. Add mezcal, lemon juice, remaining ¼ tsp. salt, and remaining ¼ tsp. pepper, stirring to loosen browned bits from bottom of skillet.

4. Add tomato and butter; return skillet to medium-high heat, stirring until butter melts. Add bread cubes; toss gently. Divide shrimp mixture between 2 plates. Top shrimp mixture evenly with mushrooms. **Makes: 2 servings**

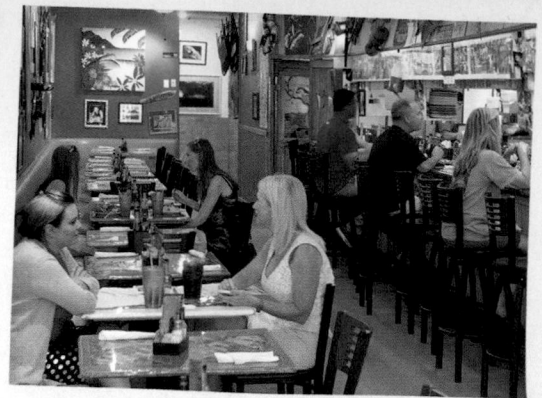

Little Moir's Food Shack

103 South U.S. Highway 1 #D3
Jupiter, Florida 33477
(561) 741-3626
littlemoirs.com

In a strip mall near posh Jupiter Island, right next to a grocery store, diners line up to visit Little Moir's Food Shack. Step inside, and you'll hear the beats of reggae music and be surrounded by the colorful flair of the Caribbean. Owners Mike Moir and Drew Shimkus infuse their food with that vibe, too. Locals love them for the fresh seafood and indulgent desserts. "Our best seller is the sweet potato-encrusted fish that we made up on day four," Moir says. Don't miss the chocolate mash—a sort of primitive mousse that looks like a cross between mashed potatoes and ice cream. Sure there are fancier places on the island, but none is more creative. And after a long day of fishing or surfing, nothing is more relaxing than kicking back with a beer at the Food Shack.

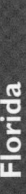

Dark Mash

While this sweet treat may look similar to ice cream, it's far lighter, and actually isn't frozen.

12 oz. semisweet chocolate morsels
¾ cup chopped toasted pecans
¾ tsp. vanilla extract
2 large pasteurized eggs, well beaten
1 cup heavy cream
Garnishes: fresh berries, whipped cream, chocolate shavings

1. Pour water to depth of 1 inch into bottom of a double boiler over medium heat; bring to a boil. Reduce heat, and simmer; place chocolate morsels in top of double boiler over simmering water. Cook, stirring occasionally, 2 to 3 minutes or until melted. Remove from heat.
2. Stir in nuts, vanilla, and eggs; cool 5 minutes.
3. Beat cream until soft peaks form. Fold whipped cream into chocolate mixture. Cover and chill 30 minutes or until set. Scoop mixture into serving bowls. Garnish with fresh berries, whipped cream, and chocolate shavings. **Makes: 6 servings**

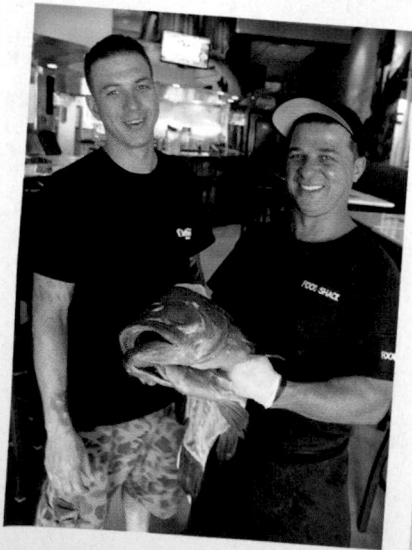

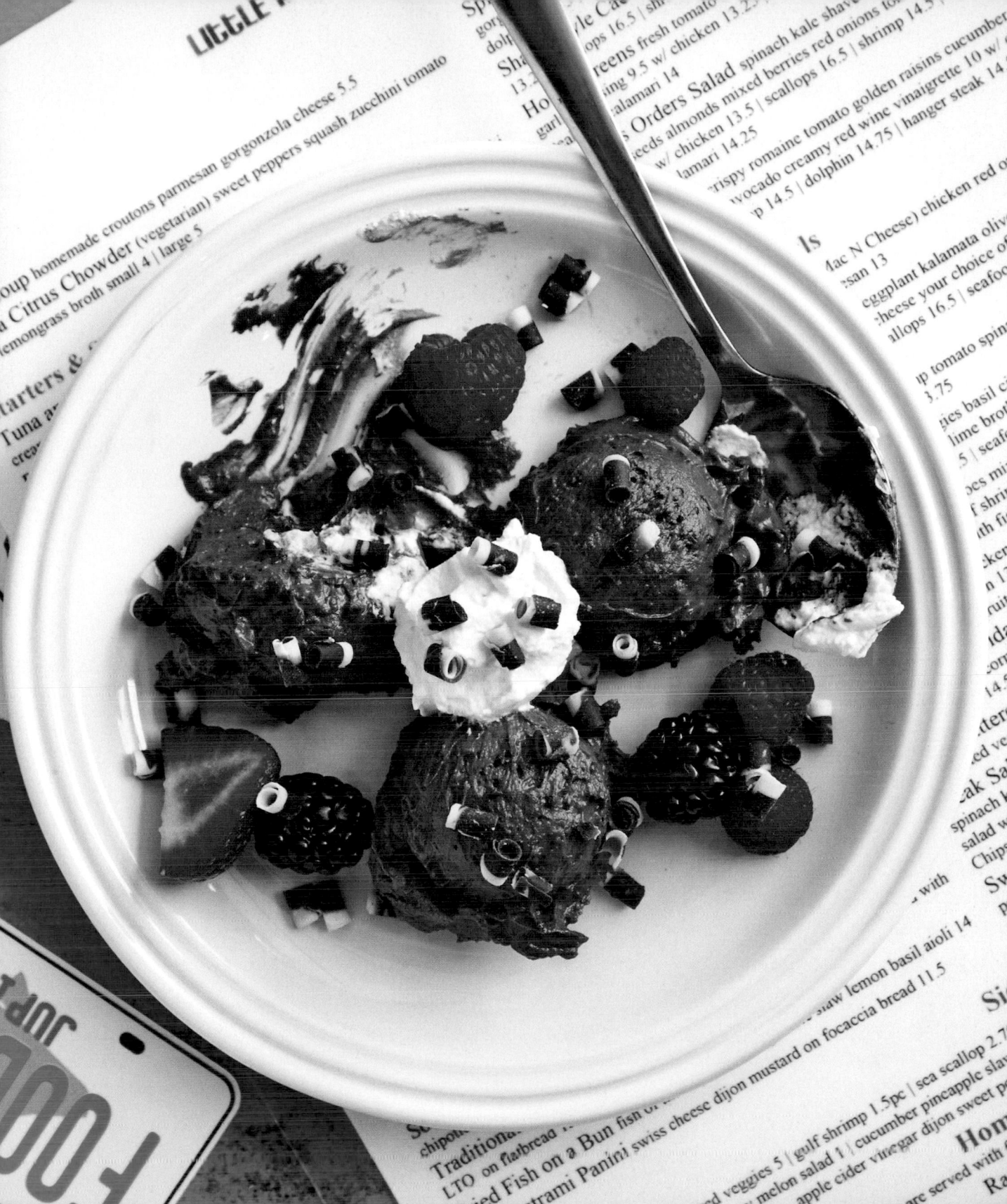

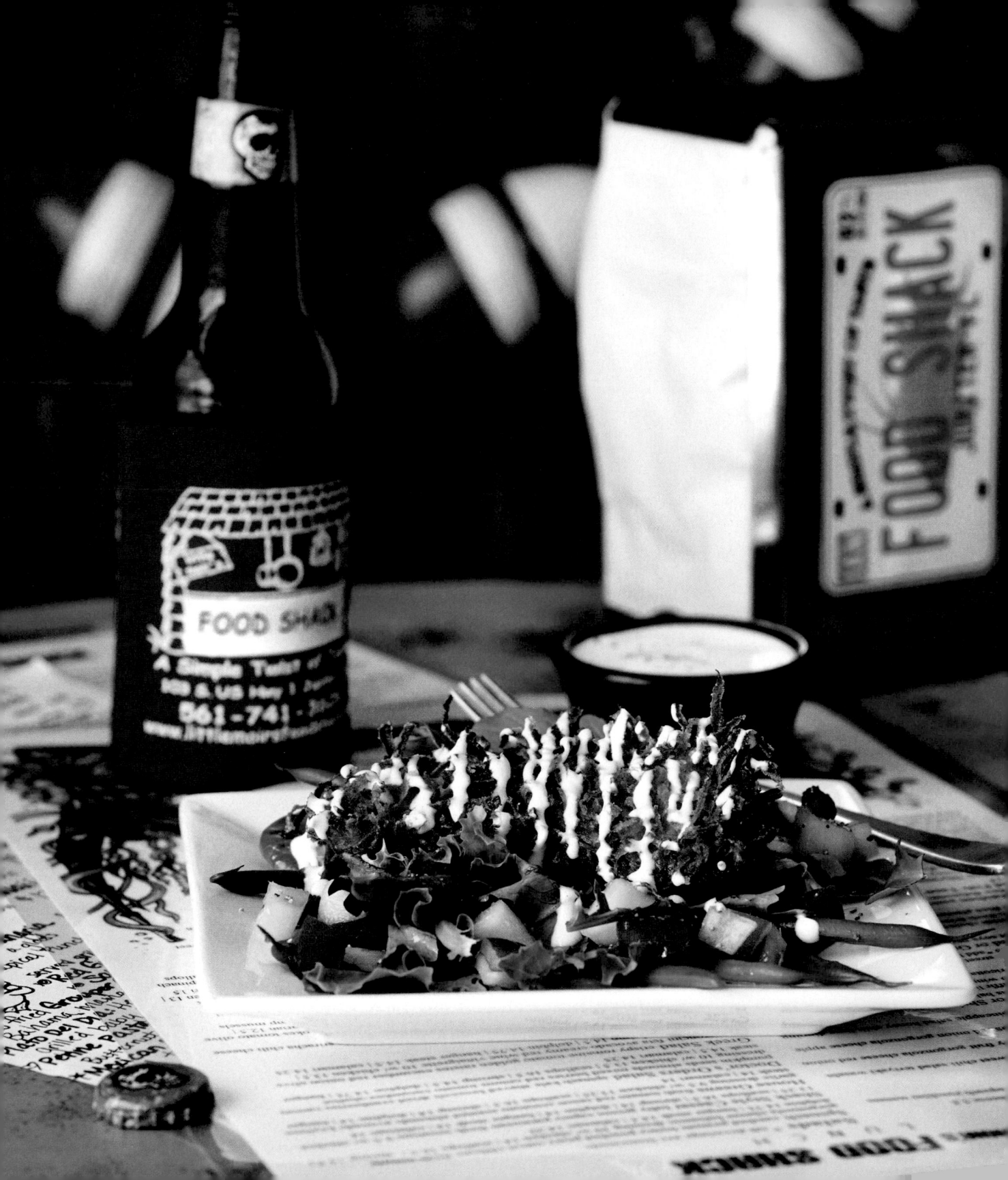

Sweet Potato-Crusted Chicken with Green Bean-Mango Salad

This dish is full of fresh flavors and textures—it's sure to be an instant classic if you make it for friends and family.

KEY LIME-GARLIC DRESSING
¼ cup rice wine vinegar
¼ cup fresh Key lime juice
1 Tbsp. Dijon mustard
Dash of table salt
Dash of freshly ground black pepper
Dash of Worcestershire sauce
2 garlic cloves
1 large pasteurized egg
2 cups canola oil

SWEET POTATO-CRUSTED CHICKEN
1½ cups canola oil
½ cup all-purpose flour
2 large eggs
2½ cups shredded peeled sweet potato (about ½ lb.)
12 chicken breast tenders (about 1½ lb.)*
½ tsp. table salt
¼ tsp. freshly ground black pepper

GREEN BEAN-MANGO SALAD
1 (8-oz.) package microwave-in-bag haricots verts (thin green beans)
1 (1-lb.) mango, peeled and diced
1 (12-oz.) tomato, peeled, seeded, and chopped
¼ cup finely chopped red onion
¼ tsp. table salt
¼ tsp. freshly ground black pepper
2 tsp. olive oil
6 cups mixed salad greens

1. Preheat oven to 350°. **Prepare Key Lime-Garlic Dressing:** Process first 8 ingredients and 2 Tbsp. water in a blender until combined. With blender on, gradually add oil in a slow, steady stream; process until blended. Transfer to a container. Cover and chill.

2. **Prepare Sweet Potato-Crusted Chicken:** Pour 1½ cups oil to depth of ⅛ inch deep in a large nonstick skillet; heat over medium-high heat. Place flour in a shallow dish. Place eggs in a bowl; beat well with a fork. Place sweet potato in another shallow dish.

3. Sprinkle chicken with salt and pepper. Dredge chicken in flour; dip in egg. Coat with shredded sweet potato, pressing to adhere. Fry chicken, in batches, 1 to 2 minutes on each side or until browned, adding oil to maintain ⅛-inch depth as needed. (Heat oil until hot before adding chicken.) Transfer chicken to a baking pan. Bake at 350° for 7 minutes or until chicken is done.

4. **Meanwhile, prepare Green Bean-Mango Salad:** Microwave haricots verts according to package directions. Plunge into ice water until chilled; drain well. Place beans, mango, and next 2 ingredients in a large bowl; sprinkle with salt and pepper, and drizzle with olive oil. Toss well.

5. Divide greens among 4 large plates. Top evenly with green bean mixture and chicken. Serve with Key Lime-Garlic Dressing. **Makes: 4 servings**
*You may substitute 1½ lb. redfish fillets for the chicken.

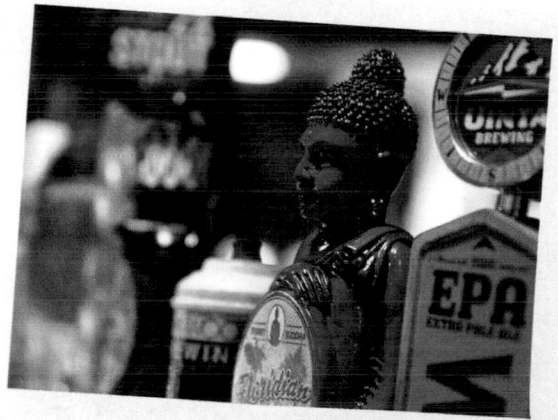

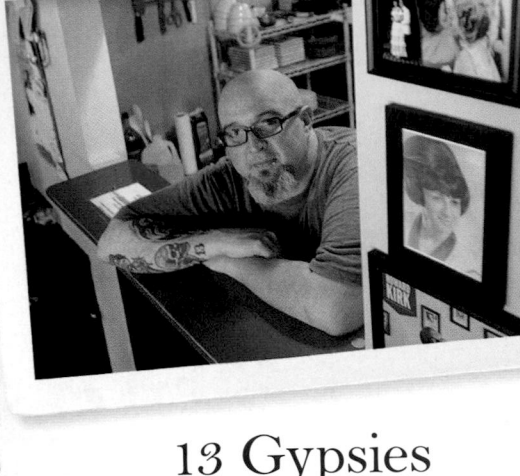

13 Gypsies

887 Stockton Street
Jacksonville, Florida 32204
(904) 389-0330
13gypsies.com

If you look closely at the pictures on the walls at 13 Gypsies, you'll see a snappy sailor and an exotic beauty looking back at you." Those are my parents—my dad was stationed in Rota, Spain, where he met my mother", says Chef Howard Kirk. Mama's gypsy blood inspired the name of the restaurant and much of the menu. Like Spain itself, 13 Gypsies is a collision of flavors from Morocco, the Mediterranean, and Europe (and Kirk chucks in some Asian spice every now and then to keep things interesting). His savory mushroom crêpe is soft and buttery. Or try his pickled tuna, a lighter option that comes with a refreshing apple arugula salad.

Bacon and Swiss Empanadas

DOUGH

3 cups all-purpose flour
¾ cup cold butter, cut up
½ tsp. table salt
1 large egg

DIPPING SAUCE

1 cup mayonnaise
3 Tbsp. sugar
3 Tbsp. apple cider vinegar
1½ Tbsp. ketchup
½ tsp. garlic powder

EMPANADAS

6 oz. Swiss cheese, diced
6 hickory-smoked bacon slices, cooked and crumbled
Vegetable oil
Asian hot chili sauce (such as Sriracha)

1. **Prepare Dough:** Pulse all ingredients and 5 Tbsp. water in a food processor 12 to 15 times or until a rough dough forms. Transfer to a lightly floured work surface; shape into a flat disk, kneading lightly. Cover in plastic wrap, and chill 1 hour.
2. **Prepare Dipping Sauce:** Whisk together all ingredients in a bowl.
3. **Prepare Empanadas:** Roll out dough on a lightly floured surface. Cut dough into 6-inch circles, rerolling scraps once. Place 2 Tbsp. cheese and 1 Tbsp. bacon in center of each circle. Brush edges of circles with water. Fold dough over filling, and crimp edges with a fork to seal.
4. Pour oil to depth of 2 inches in a Dutch oven; heat to 375°. Fry empanadas, in batches, 6 minutes until golden brown. Drain on paper towels. Squirt Sriracha sauce in a zig-zag pattern on top of empanadas; serve with Dipping Sauce.
Makes: 4 to 5 servings

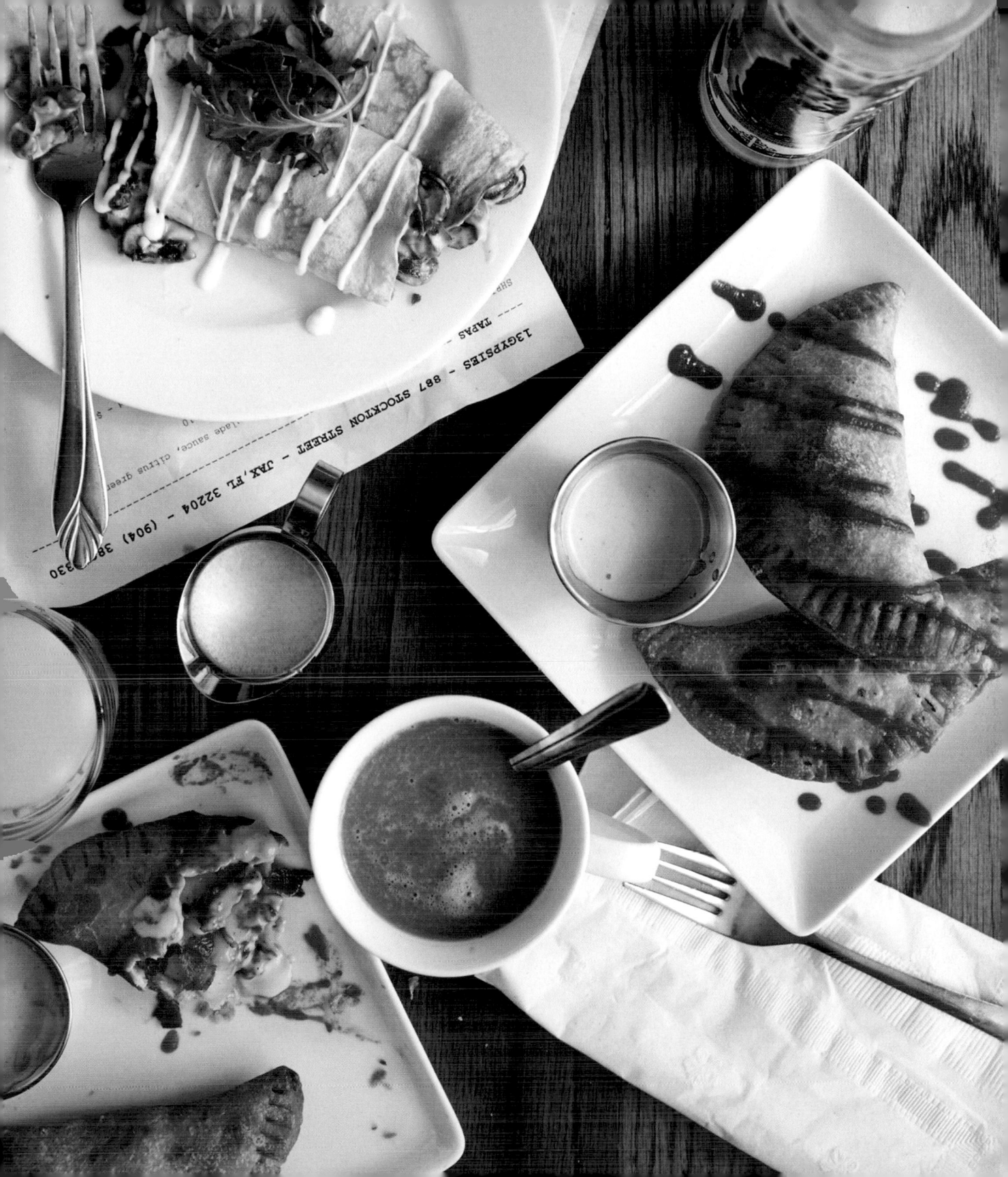

Mushroom Crêpes

I swear I could eat 10 of these savory little crêpes at one sitting.

CRÊPES

1¼ cups all-purpose flour
1 tsp. sugar
¼ tsp. table salt
3 large eggs
¼ cup butter, melted and divided
1½ cups milk
Wax paper

MUSHROOM FILLING

24 cremini mushrooms, sliced
1 large garlic clove, minced
1 Tbsp. olive oil
6 Tbsp. frozen petite peas
⅓ cup butter
⅓ cup all-purpose flour
3 cups milk
¼ tsp. freshly ground black pepper
10 thin slices prosciutto (about 4 oz.), cooked and crumbled

TOPPING

⅓ cup sour cream
1 to 2 Tbsp. heavy cream

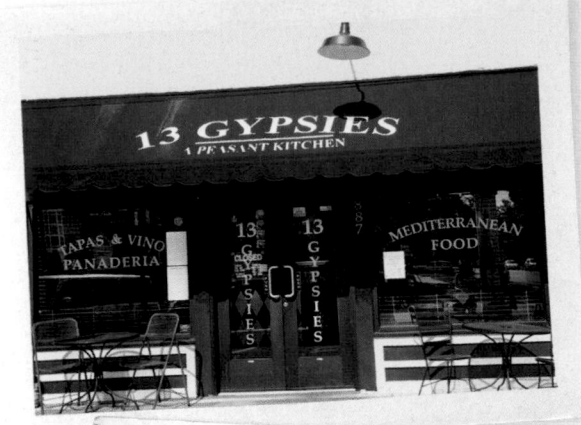

1. **Prepare Crêpes:** Whisk together first 3 ingredients. Beat eggs, 2 Tbsp. melted butter, and 1½ cups milk at medium speed with an electric mixer until blended. Gradually add flour mixture, beating until smooth. Cover and chill 1 hour.

2. Brush bottom of an 8-inch nonstick skillet lightly with some of remaining 2 Tbsp. melted butter; place skillet over medium heat until hot. Pour 3 Tbsp. batter into skillet; quickly tilt in all directions so batter covers bottom of skillet.

3. Cook 1 minute or until crêpe can be shaken loose from skillet. Turn crêpe over, and cook about 30 seconds. Repeat procedure with remaining melted butter and batter. Stack crêpes between sheets of wax paper.

4. **Prepare Mushroom Filling:** Sauté mushrooms and garlic in hot olive oil in a large skillet 9 minutes or until tender and liquid evaporates. Add peas; sauté 1 minute or until thoroughly heated. Remove from heat; set aside, and keep warm.

5. Melt ⅓ cup butter in a 2-qt. heavy saucepan over low heat; whisk in ⅓ cup flour until smooth. Cook 1 minute, whisking constantly. Gradually whisk in 3 cups milk; cook over medium heat, whisking constantly, until mixture is thickened and bubbly. Stir in pepper. Stir in mushroom mixture and prosciutto.

6. **Prepare Topping:** Stir together sour cream and heavy cream in a small bowl until smooth and drizzling consistency.

7. Spoon ⅓ cup filling down center of each crêpe. Roll up. Drizzle with sour cream mixture, and serve immediately. **Makes: 4 to 6 servings**

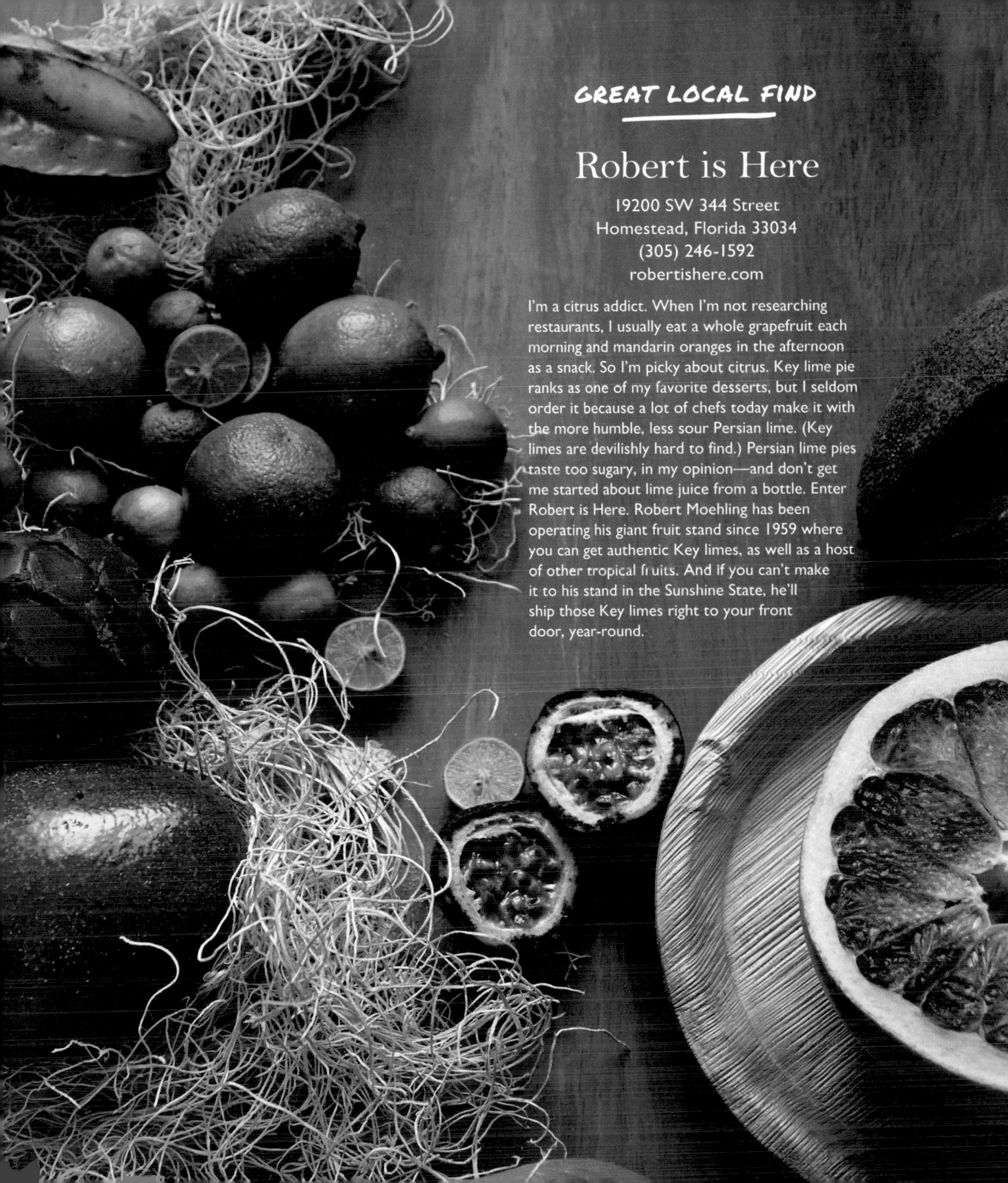

Robert is Here

19200 SW 344 Street
Homestead, Florida 33034
(305) 246-1592
robertishere.com

I'm a citrus addict. When I'm not researching restaurants, I usually eat a whole grapefruit each morning and mandarin oranges in the afternoon as a snack. So I'm picky about citrus. Key lime pie ranks as one of my favorite desserts, but I seldom order it because a lot of chefs today make it with the more humble, less sour Persian lime. (Key limes are devilishly hard to find.) Persian lime pies taste too sugary, in my opinion—and don't get me started about lime juice from a bottle. Enter Robert is Here. Robert Moehling has been operating his giant fruit stand since 1959 where you can get authentic Key limes, as well as a host of other tropical fruits. And if you can't make it to his stand in the Sunshine State, he'll ship those Key limes right to your front door, year-round.

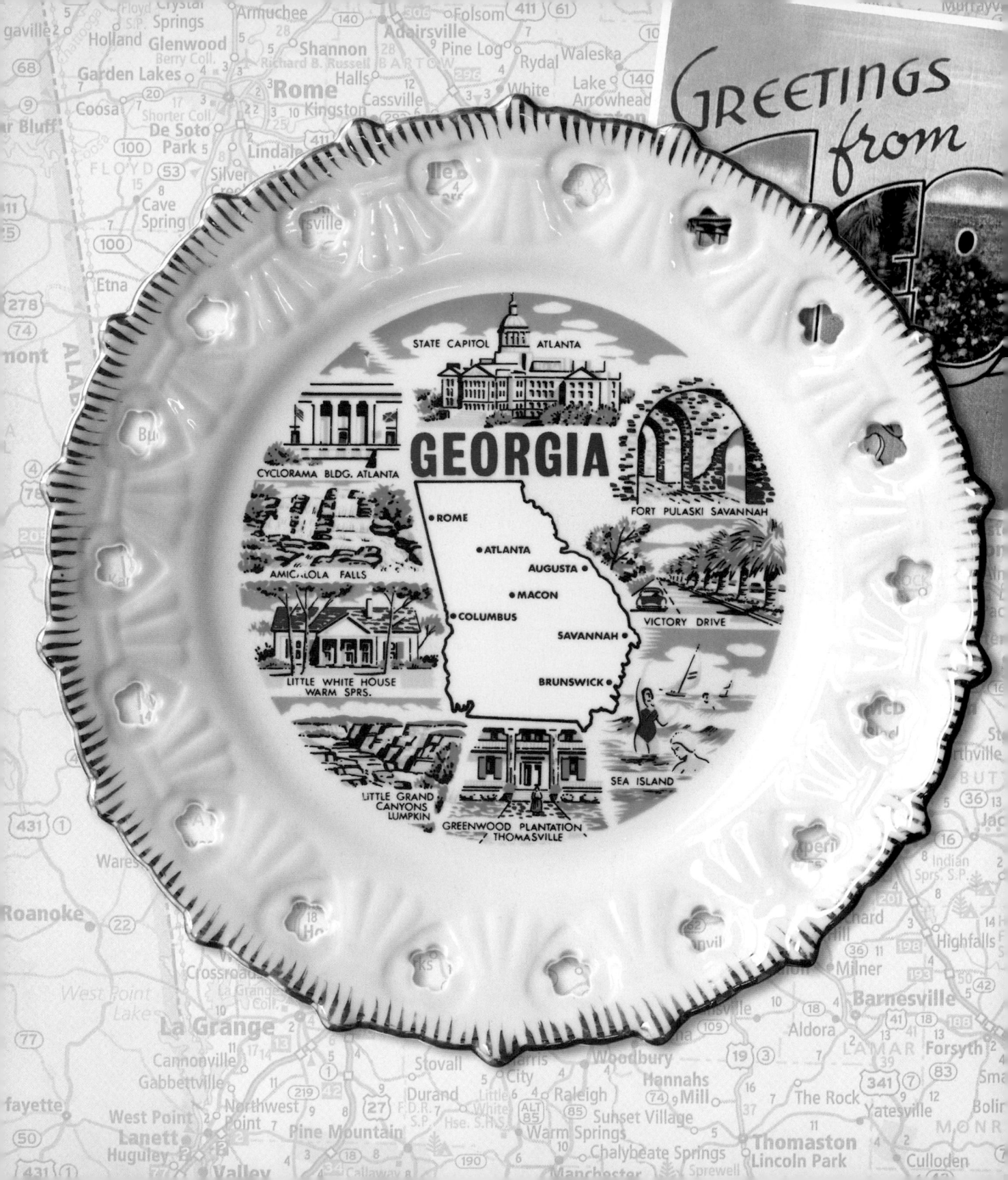

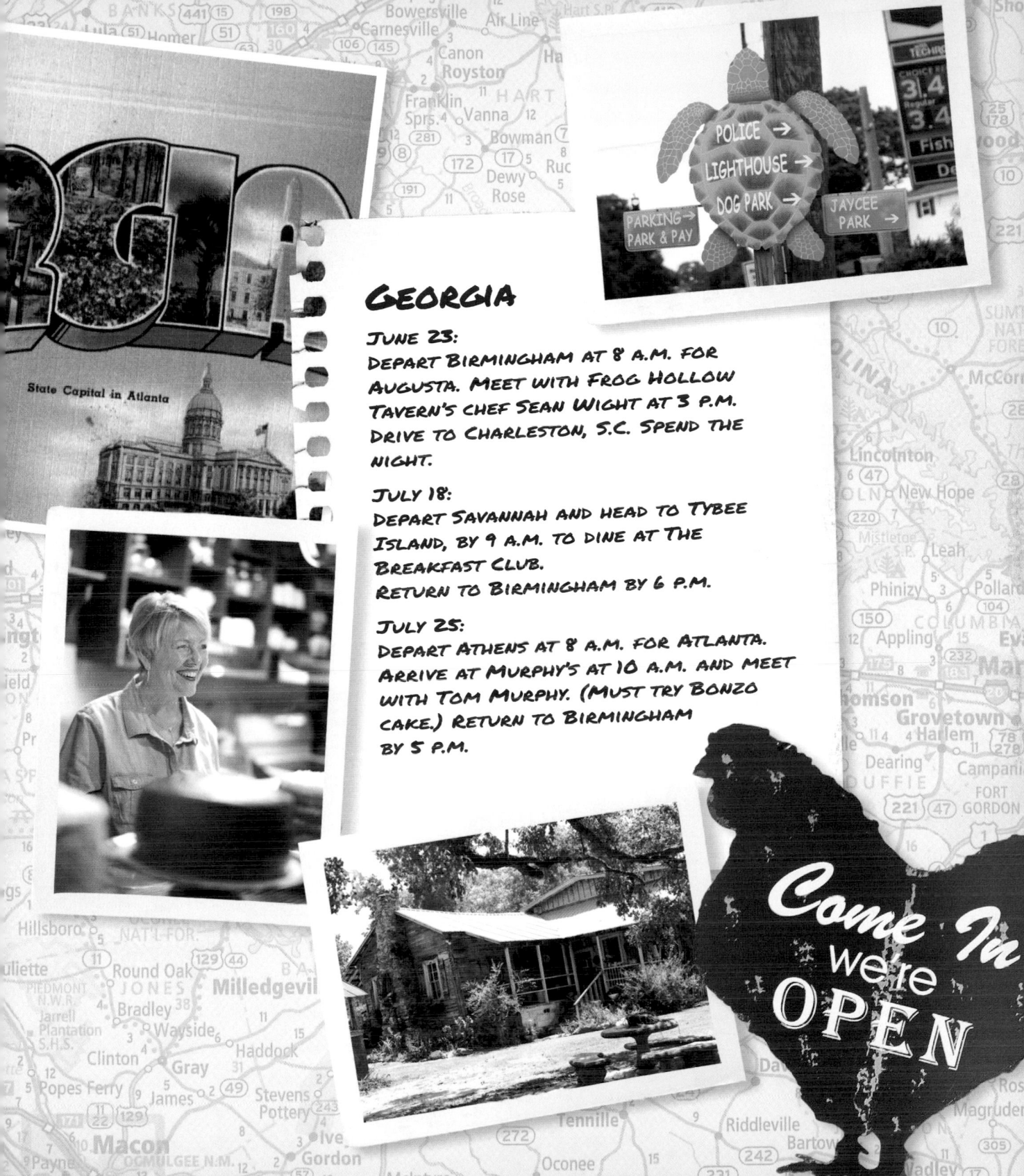

Georgia

June 23:
Depart Birmingham at 8 a.m. for Augusta. Meet with Frog Hollow Tavern's chef Sean Wight at 3 p.m. Drive to Charleston, S.C. Spend the night.

July 18:
Depart Savannah and head to Tybee Island, by 9 a.m. to dine at The Breakfast Club.
Return to Birmingham by 6 p.m.

July 25:
Depart Athens at 8 a.m. for Atlanta. Arrive at Murphy's at 10 a.m. and meet with Tom Murphy. (Must try Bonzo cake.) Return to Birmingham by 5 p.m.

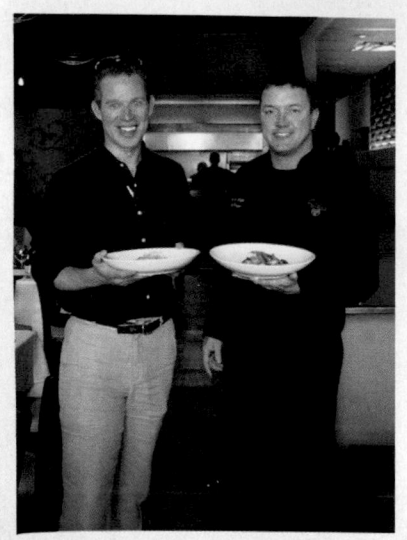

Frog Hollow Tavern

1282 Broad Street
Augusta, Georgia 30901
(706) 364-6906
froghollowtavern.com

When you're dining in a restaurant where the chef calls the local farmers by name, you know you're in for a good meal. Chef Sean Wight speaks about his suppliers as if they're rare coins or stamps—he's a collector of farmers. It's a difference you can taste in his posh Southern dishes. From the sweet corn risotto to the peach carpaccio, everything on the restaurant's menu is made from scratch and with beautiful attention to detail. Frog Hollow Tavern is housed in what was once a shoe repair store and is named for an old Augusta neighborhood; charming photos of both line the walls. Tip: If you want a reservation during The Masters, you need to call weeks (if not months) in advance.

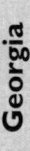
Frog Hollow Tavern Sweet Corn Risotto

CORN STOCK

2   ears fresh corn
¼   tsp. black peppercorns
1   small parsley sprig
1   small thyme sprig
¼   bay leaf

SWEET CORN RISOTTO

1   Tbsp. butter
1   cup Arborio rice
3   Tbsp. dry white wine
¼   cup heavy cream
2   Tbsp. grated Asiago cheese
½   tsp. table salt
¼   tsp. freshly ground black pepper
Shaved Asiago cheese
Fresh flat-leaf parsley leaves

1. **Prepare Corn Stock:** Cut tips of corn kernels into a large bowl; scrape milk and remaining pulp from cobs, reserving cobs, corn, and milk. Break scraped cobs in half, and place in a 4-qt. saucepan. Add peppercorns, next 3 ingredients, and 4 cups water. Bring to a boil; reduce heat, and simmer, covered, 45 minutes. Pour stock through a wire-mesh strainer into a bowl, discarding solids. If necessary, add water to yield 3½ cups stock.

2. **Prepare Sweet Corn Risotto:** Melt butter in a large saucepan over medium heat. Add rice; cook, stirring constantly, 1 minute. Add wine, and cook, stirring often, 30 seconds or until almost absorbed. Add 1 cup corn stock, and cook, stirring constantly, until liquid is absorbed. Repeat with remaining stock, ½ cup at a time, until all liquid is absorbed (about 22 minutes).

3. Stir in reserved corn and corn milk, cream, 2 Tbsp. grated cheese, salt, and pepper. Cook 1 minute or until thoroughly heated. Sprinkle with shaved Asiago and parsley leaves. Serve immediately. **Makes: 4 servings**

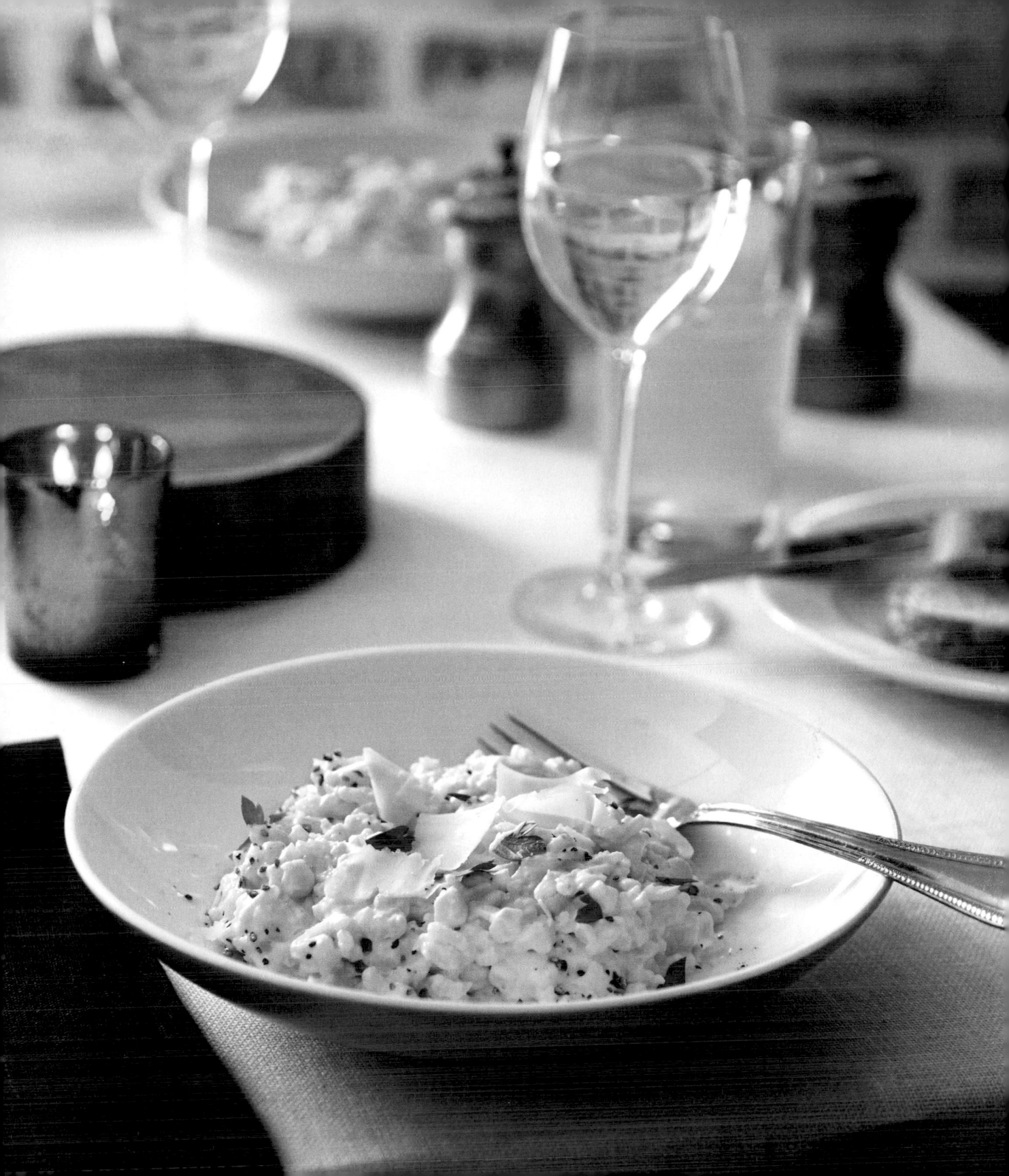

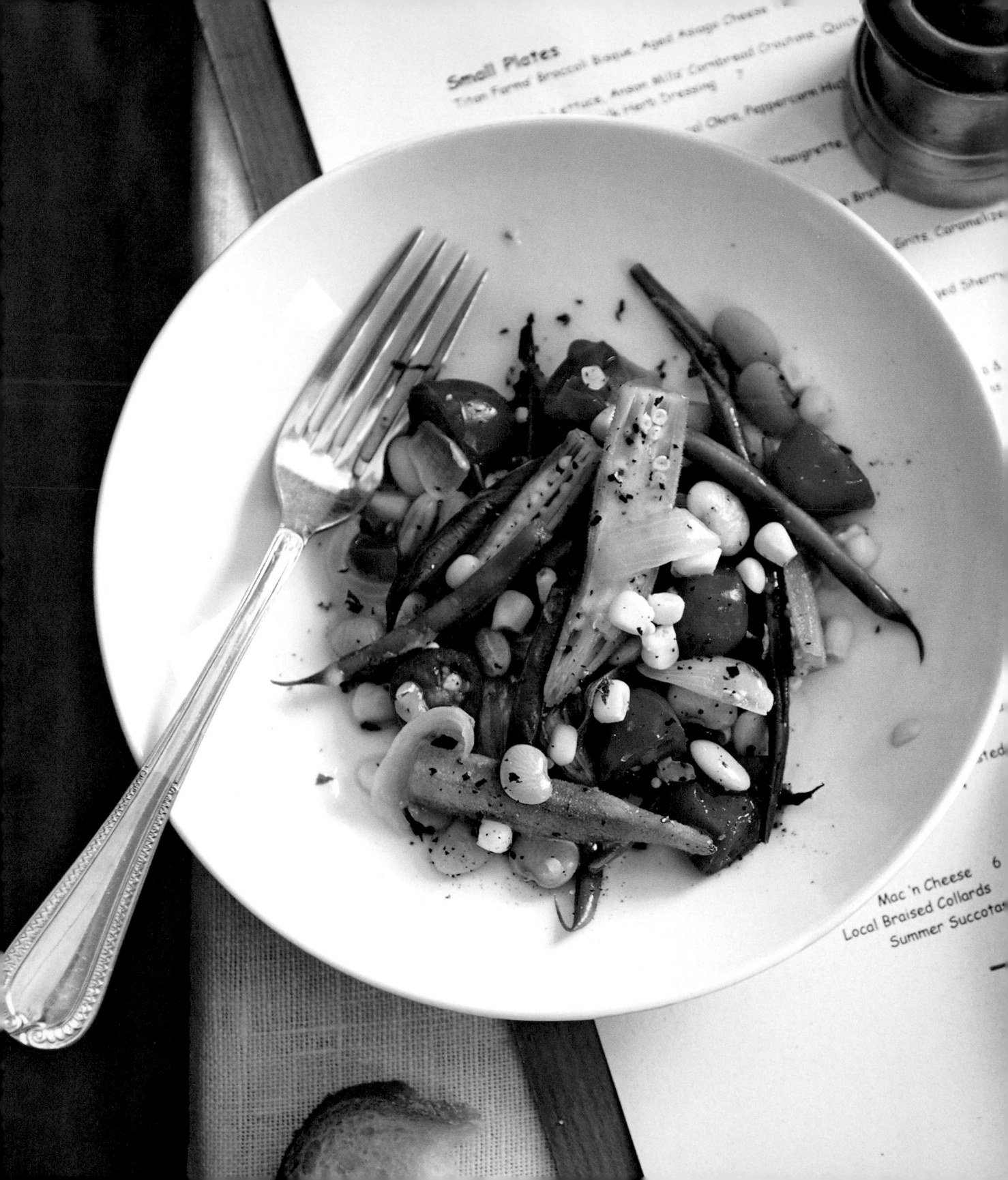

Summer Succotash

VEGETABLE STOCK

2	leeks
4	medium celery ribs, coarsely chopped
4	medium carrots, coarsely chopped
1	large Vidalia onion, coarsely chopped
6	fresh flat-leaf parsley sprigs
5	fresh thyme sprigs
2	bay leaves

SUCCOTASH

1	cup fresh lima beans
2	Tbsp. kosher salt
¼	lb. fresh green beans, trimmed and cut into 2-inch pieces (1 cup)
2	ears fresh corn
1	Tbsp. butter
⅔	cup vertically sliced Vidalia onion
⅓	lb. small okra pods, trimmed and cut in half lengthwise (2 cups)
1	cup Vegetable Stock
1	cup grape tomatoes, halved
2	Tbsp. Chardonnay or other dry white wine
¾	tsp. table salt
⅛	tsp. freshly ground black pepper
2	Tbsp. fresh parsley leaves

HONEY-THYME BUTTER

¼	cup unsalted butter, softened
½	tsp. finely chopped fresh thyme
1½	tsp. honey

1. Prepare Vegetable Stock: Cut off 1½ inches of green tops of leeks; cut leeks in half lengthwise. Rinse leeks under cold running water to remove grit and sand; cut into large pieces. Combine leek, celery, remaining ingredients, and 3 qt. water in a large Dutch oven or stockpot. Bring to a boil; reduce heat, and simmer, partially covered, 1 hour. Pour stock through a wire-mesh strainer into a large bowl; discard solids. Cool completely (1 hour). Cover and refrigerate, or freeze until ready to use.

2. Prepare Succotash: Cook lima beans and kosher salt in 6 cups boiling water in a large saucepan 10 minutes; add green beans, and cook 2 more minutes. Drain. Plunge vegetables into ice water to stop the cooking process; drain.

3. Cut tips of corn kernels into a large bowl; scrape milk and remaining pulp from cobs.

4. Melt 1 Tbsp. butter in a Dutch oven over medium heat. Add onion, and sauté 4 minutes or until tender, but not browned. Add beans, corn (and corn milk), okra, and next 5 ingredients. Bring to a boil; reduce heat, cover, and simmer 10 minutes or until okra is tender, stirring occasionally.

5. Meanwhile, prepare Honey-Thyme Butter: Stir together all ingredients until blended.

6. Add Honey-Thyme Butter to hot vegetable mixture, stirring until butter melts. Sprinkle with parsley. **Makes: 6 to 8 servings**

Georgia

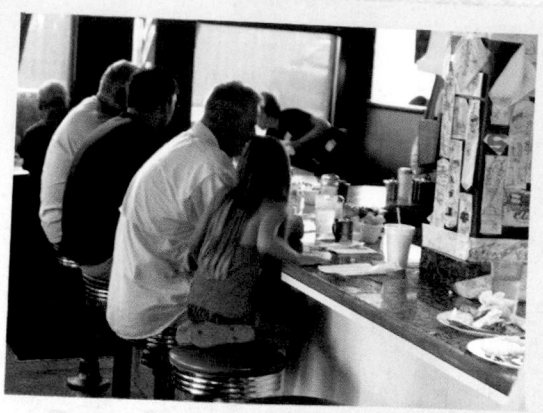

The Breakfast Club

1500 Butler Avenue
Tybee Island, Georgia 31328
(912) 786-5984
thebreakfastclubtybee.com

The day I visited The Breakfast Club on Tybee Island, the town's civil defense sirens blared and a giant thunderstorm threatened. Yet nobody left the line that wrapped around this breakfast institution. Try just about anything on the menu and you'll understand why. Owner Jodee Sadowsky trained at the Culinary Institute of America and brings a gourmand's sensibility to breakfast. For instance, his omelets are stuffed with Parmesan and Asiago cheeses. "Each bite takes seven years off your life, but it's worth it," says Jodee's son, Ryan, who also works here. The tiny restaurant grinds its own Polish sausage and bakes its own buns. Food like this has gained The Breakfast Club loyal local followers that have been breakfasting here for nearly 40 years.

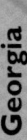

Helen's Solidarity aka Grille Cleaner's Special

1   cup thinly sliced andouille sausage or spicy kielbasa
2   tsp. bacon drippings or canola oil
1½ cups finely diced cooked potatoes
⅔   cup diced onion
2   large eggs
1   Tbsp. finely chopped onion
1   Tbsp. finely chopped red bell pepper
1   Tbsp. finely chopped green pepper
½   tsp. table salt
⅛   tsp. freshly ground black pepper
2   (¾-oz.) slices pepper Jack cheese
2   (¾-oz.) slices Cheddar cheese
Serve with: hot sauce, grits, sliced tomatoes, toasted English muffin halves

1. Preheat oven to 400°. Fry sausage in an 8-inch nonstick skillet over medium-low heat 4 minutes or until partially cooked. Remove from skillet.
2. Add bacon drippings. Spread potatoes evenly over bottom of skillet; sprinkle potatoes with ⅔ cup diced onion. Cook 8 minutes or until bottom is golden brown, pressing down occasionally with a spatula. Turn potato over; cook 8 minutes or until golden brown. Transfer to a plate. Arrange sausage pieces in bottom of skillet. Spoon potatoes over sausages.
3. Whisk eggs in a bowl; add 1 Tbsp. finely chopped onion and bell peppers. Pour egg mixture over potato mixture. Sprinkle with salt and pepper. Place pepper Jack slices diagonally on lower left and upper right of mixture; place Cheddar cheese slices diagonally across upper left and lower right of egg mixture.
4. Place skillet in oven, and bake at 400° for 5 minutes or until cheese is bubbly. Serve with hot sauce, grits, sliced tomatoes, and toasted English muffin halves. **Makes: 1 serving**

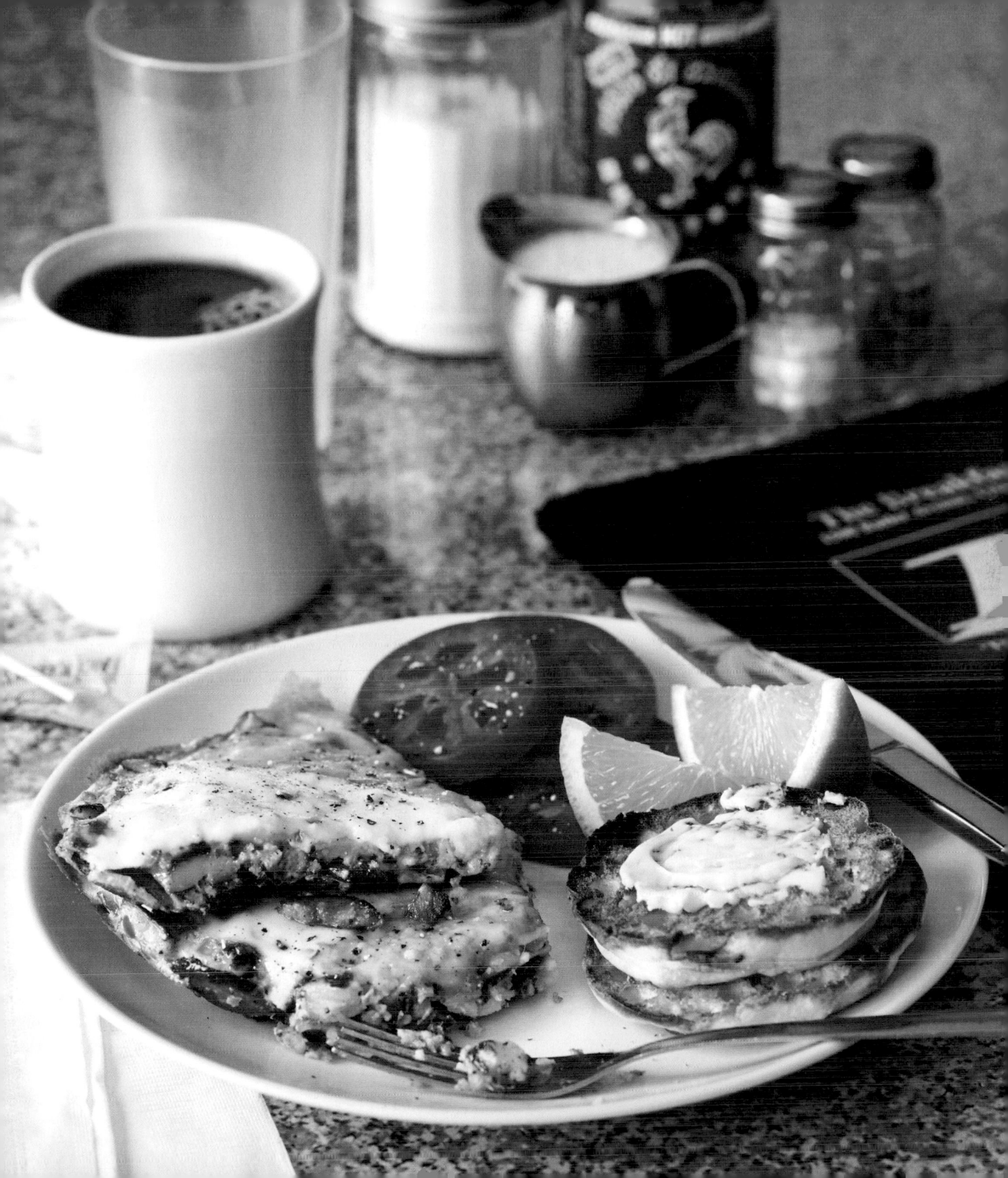

Egg Florentine aka House Special

Chef Jodee Sadowsky says this house special dish is a twist on a traditional Escoffier egg recipe—he changes it up with fresh salmon patties, béarnaise sauce, hollandaise sauce, and even sushi-grade tuna.

2   Tbsp. minced shallots
3   Tbsp. finely chopped mushrooms
3   Tbsp. bacon drippings, divided
2   cups firmly packed fresh baby spinach
1   extra-large egg
¼   tsp. seasoned salt
2   ice cubes
2   (¾-oz.) slices Swiss cheese
Serve with: buttered whole wheat toast points, tomato slices

1. Sauté shallots, mushrooms, and table salt and black pepper to taste in 1 Tbsp. hot drippings in a 9-inch nonstick skillet over medium-high heat 2 minutes or until tender. Transfer to a small bowl.
2. Heat 1 Tbsp. drippings in same skillet. Add spinach; sauté 1 minute or until spinach begins to wilt. Make a hole in center of spinach mixture. Add remaining 1 Tbsp. bacon drippings to center of spinach mixture. Crack egg into drippings; sprinkle with seasoned salt and pepper to taste. Place 2 ice cubes on opposite sides of skillet. Cook, covered, 30 seconds to 1 minute or until eggs are lightly poached. Spoon mushroom mixture on top of egg; top with cheese. Remove skillet from heat, and let stand 1 minute or until cheese melts.
3. Carefully lift egg-spinach mixture out of skillet, using 2 wide spatulas and letting excess liquid drain into skillet. Transfer to a plate. Serve with toast points and tomato slices. **Makes: 1 serving**

SOUNDTRACK:

"GEORGIA" BY EMILY KING
"WHY GEORGIA" BY JOHN MAYER
"RAINY NIGHT IN GEORGIA" BY RAY CHARLES
"NIGHTTIMING" BY COCONUT RECORDS
"RIGHT MOVES" BY JOSH RITTER

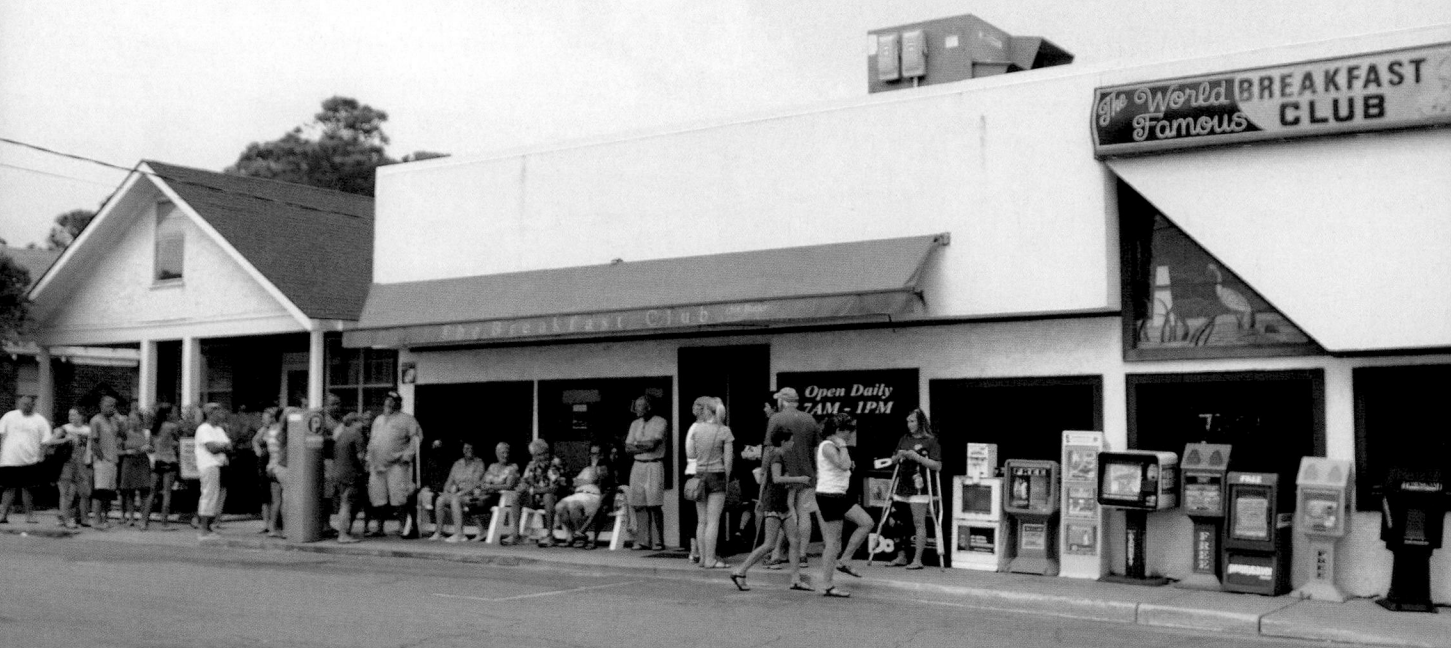

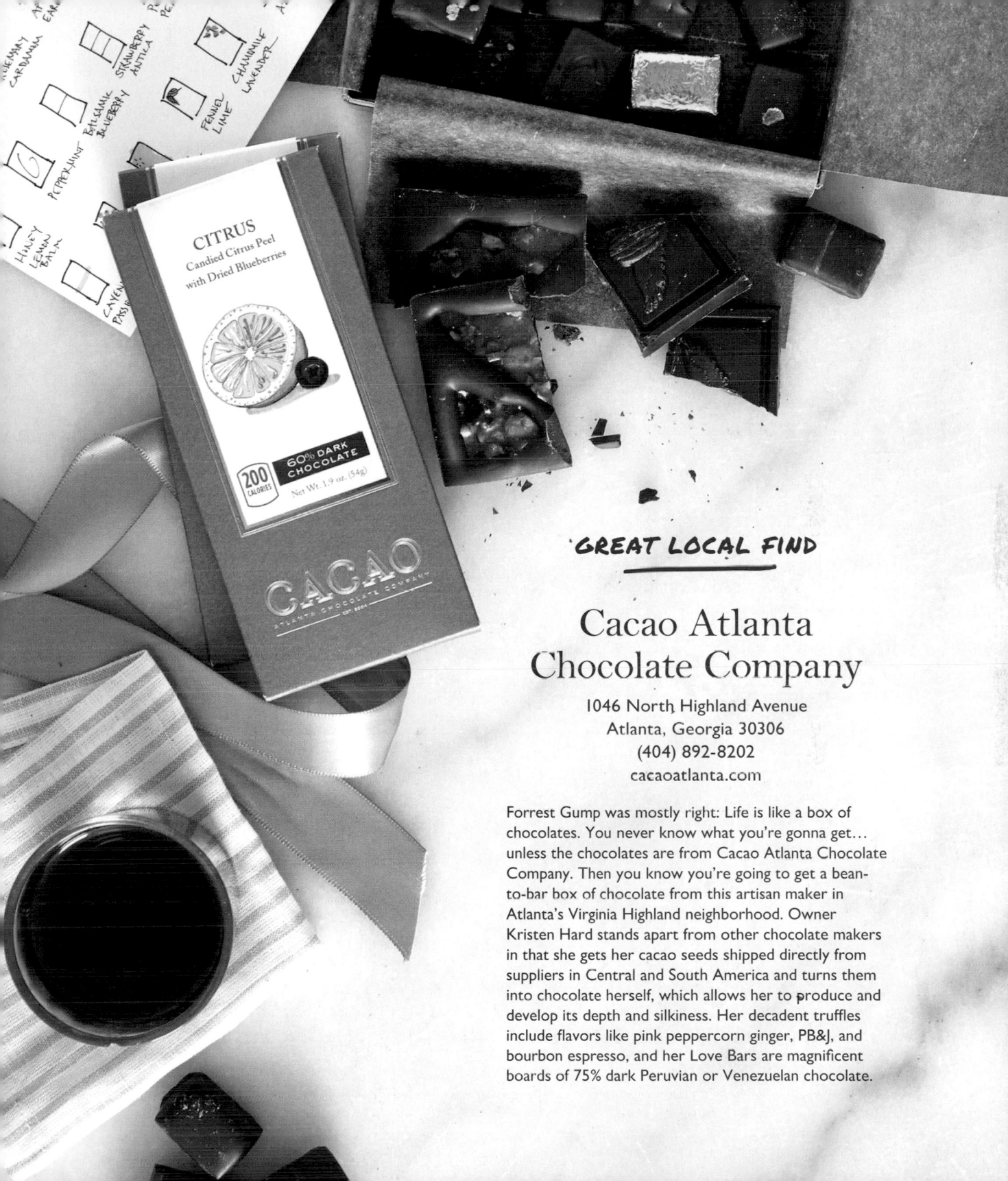

CITRUS

Candied Citrus Peel
with Dried Blueberries

200 CALORIES

60% DARK CHOCOLATE

Net Wt. 1.9 oz. (54g)

CACAO
ATLANTA CHOCOLATE COMPANY · EST 2004

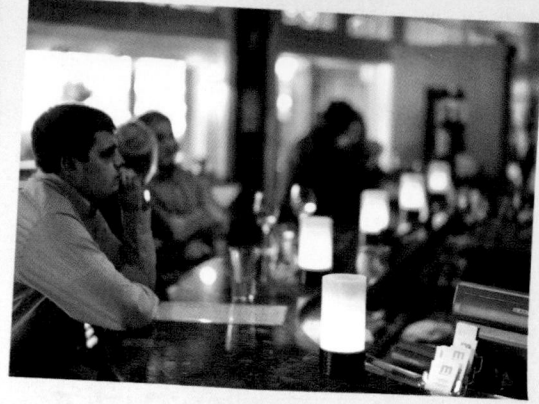

Murphy's

997 Virginia Avenue NE
Atlanta, Georgia 30306
(404) 872-0904
murphys-atlanta-restaurant.com

For years I've ventured to this Virginia Highland institution for brunch. A Murphy omelet, bloody Mary, and a good paper makes for an outstanding way to begin any day. Tom Murphy, who began selling hot dogs at the age of 13, has an Irishman's charm and sense of theater. Murphy's lighting, its service, menu, and enormous wine list all work together in harmony. The food here is unpretentious and hearty—you won't leave hungry. Take Tom's Guinness Braised Beef Brisket, for example. It's so tender you could eat the entire dish with a spoon (OK, you need a fork for the green beans). My server admitted, sheepishly, he eats it every night. And end your meal with Murphy's Bonzo Cake—think chocolate mousse, brownie, and cheesecake all in one, topped by a bit of whipped cream to keep it real. This dessert's got my name all over it.

Guinness Braised Beef Brisket

This brisket is so tender and delicious, it proves not all should be barbecued.

1	(7-lb.) beef brisket, trimmed and cut into 2 equal pieces
1	tsp. table salt
2½	tsp. freshly ground black pepper
1	Tbsp. canola oil
2	qt. chicken stock
1	cup tomato paste
½	cup soy sauce
¼	cup Dijon mustard
¼	cup molasses
3	Tbsp. chopped fresh thyme
2	(12-oz.) bottles stout beer
1	(14½-oz.) can diced tomatoes
1	bay leaf

Hot mashed potatoes

1. Preheat oven to 350°. Sprinkle brisket with salt and pepper. Heat oil in a large ovenproof Dutch oven. Brown brisket, in 2 batches, in hot oil on both sides. Remove from Dutch oven.
2. Add chicken stock to Dutch oven, stirring to loosen browned bits from bottom of Dutch oven. Stir in tomato paste and next 7 ingredients. Bake, covered, at 350° for 5 to 6 hours or until fork-tender. Cool completely in pan (1 hour).
3. Remove brisket from Dutch oven. Skim fat from brisket liquid. Bring to a boil; reduce heat, and simmer 20 minutes or until sauce is reduced to 3½ cups and coats the back of a spoon. Discard bay leaf. Serve brisket with sauce and mashed potatoes. **Makes: 8 to 10 servings**
Note: We tested with Guinness Extra Stout Beer.

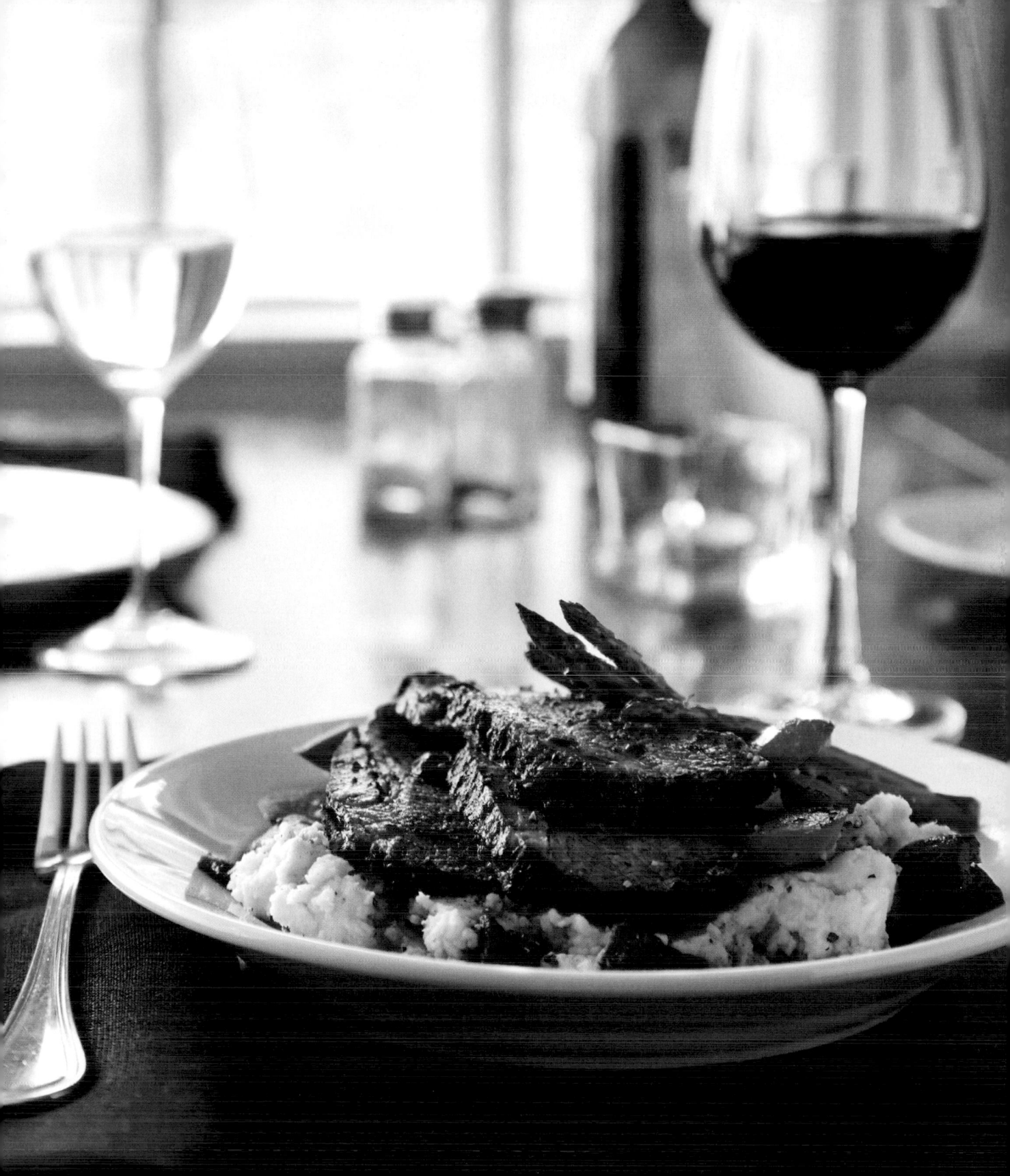

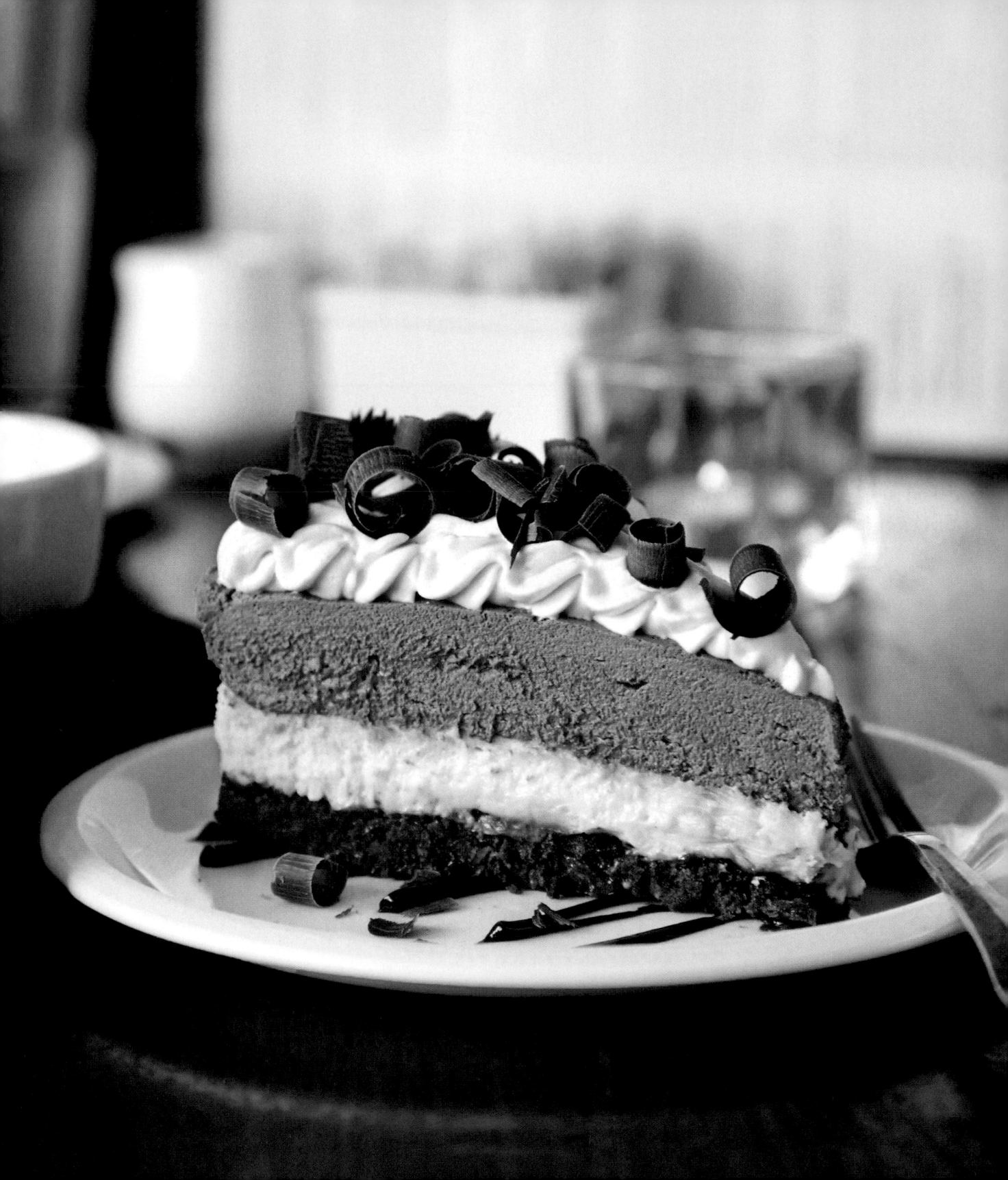

Murphy's Bonzo Cake

Tom recommends preparing the brownie and cheesecake day one, the mousse day two, and unmolding the Bonzo at least three hours after the mousse is prepared and the cake is assembled.

BROWNIE

Vegetable cooking spray
Parchment paper
1 cup unsalted butter, cut up
½ cup semisweet chocolate morsels
1⅓ cups sugar
3 large eggs
1 cup cake flour
3 Tbsp. unsweetened cocoa
¼ tsp. table salt

CHEESECAKE

2½ (8-oz.) packages cream cheese
¾ cup sugar
2 large eggs
1 tsp. vanilla extract

CHOCOLATE MOUSSE

⅓ cup sugar
9 large egg yolks
14 oz. semisweet chocolate, chopped
2 cups heavy cream

Sweetened whipped cream
Shaved chocolate

1. Prepare Brownie: Preheat oven to 325°. Lightly grease a 10-inch springform pan with cooking spray. Line bottom of pan with parchment paper. Set pan aside.

2. Place butter and chocolate morsels in a large microwave-safe bowl. Microwave at HIGH 1 to 1½ minutes or until melted and smooth, stirring at 30-second intervals. Whisk in sugar. Add 3 eggs, 1 at a time, whisking well after each addition.

3. Whisk together flour, cocoa, and salt. Add flour mixture to egg mixture; whisk until blended. Pour batter into prepared pan. Bake at 325° for 40 minutes or until a wooden pick inserted in center comes out clean. Cool brownie completely in pan on a wire rack (1 hour).

4. Meanwhile, prepare Cheesecake: Beat cream cheese at medium speed with a heavy-duty electric stand mixer until smooth. Gradually add ¾ cup sugar, beating until smooth, scraping bowl as needed. Add eggs, 1 at a time, beating until blended after each addition. Beat in vanilla. Pour cream cheese mixture over brownie layer.

5. Bake at 325° for 40 minutes or until set. Transfer pan to a wire rack. Cool cake completely in pan (2 hours). Cover and chill overnight.

6. Prepare Chocolate Mousse: Beat ⅓ cup sugar and egg yolks at medium speed with a heavy-duty electric stand mixer until thick and pale.

7. Pour water to depth of 1 inch into bottom of a double boiler over medium heat; bring to a boil. Reduce heat, and simmer; place chocolate in top of double boiler over simmering water. Cook, stirring often, 3 to 4 minutes or until melted. Gradually add hot melted chocolate to egg mixture alternately with cream, beating until stiff peaks form. Scrape down sides of bowl as needed. Pour chocolate mousse over cheesecake, spreading in an even layer with an offset spatula. Cover and chill thoroughly.

8. Gently run a knife around outer edge of cheesecake to loosen from sides of pan. Remove sides of pan. Carefully transfer cake to a serving plate using 2 wide spatulas. Decorate with sweetened whipped cream and chocolate shavings. Cut into wedges. **Makes: 12 servings**

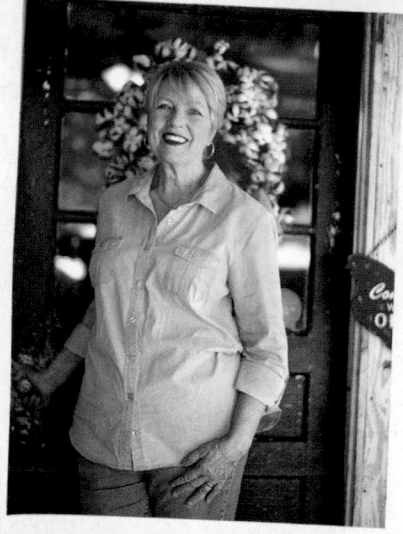

The Farm House

469 Farmhouse Road
Ellerslie, Georgia 31807
(706) 561-3435
ilovethefarmhouse.com

Drive down Farmhouse Road in Ellerslie and you'll come upon a 200-year-old former sharecropper's house. It is now The Farm House, run by Beckie and Mike McKenzie. They welcome diners on Fridays and Saturdays for lunch and dinner. The helpings of Southern favorites—meatloaf, squash casserole, Country Captain Chicken, and fresh cornbread—have stuffed customers since 1981. But it's Beckie's cakes that really wowed me. Her caramel cake is a four-layer masterpiece. "My mother was the 'cake lady', and I've just followed her recipes," Beckie says. Modesty aside, she serves one of the best meals in South Georgia.

Country Captain Chicken

President Franklin D. Roosevelt purportedly ate this dish in Warm Springs, Georgia, where he shared it with General George Patton. It became a favorite dish of both men.

¼	cup olive oil, divided
¾	cup all-purpose flour
2	tsp. table salt, divided
1	tsp. freshly ground black pepper, divided
2¾	lb. chicken breast tenders (about 21 tenders)
3	cups finely chopped onion
2	cups chopped green bell pepper
1	small garlic clove, minced
¼	cup currants
1	Tbsp. curry powder
½	tsp. ground thyme
3	(14½- oz.) cans diced tomatoes, undrained

Hot cooked rice
4   oz. blanched almonds, toasted and chopped
Chopped fresh parsley

1. Heat 3 Tbsp. oil in a large nonstick skillet over medium-high heat. Combine flour, ½ tsp. salt, and ½ tsp. pepper in a shallow dish.
2. Dredge chicken in flour mixture; shake off excess. Cook chicken, in 3 batches, in hot oil 2 to 3 minutes on each side or until browned. Drain on paper towels; keep warm. Wipe skillet clean.
3. Heat remaining olive oil in skillet over medium-high heat. Add onion, bell pepper, and garlic; sauté 6 minutes or until tender. Stir in currants, next 3 ingredients, and remaining salt and pepper.
4. Place chicken in a Dutch oven; add tomato mixture. Bring to a boil over medium-high heat; reduce heat, cover, and simmer 40 minutes, stirring occasionally. Uncover and simmer 10 more minutes or until chicken is tender and sauce is thickened.
5. Serve chicken and sauce over rice. Sprinkle with almonds and parsley. **Makes: 6 servings**

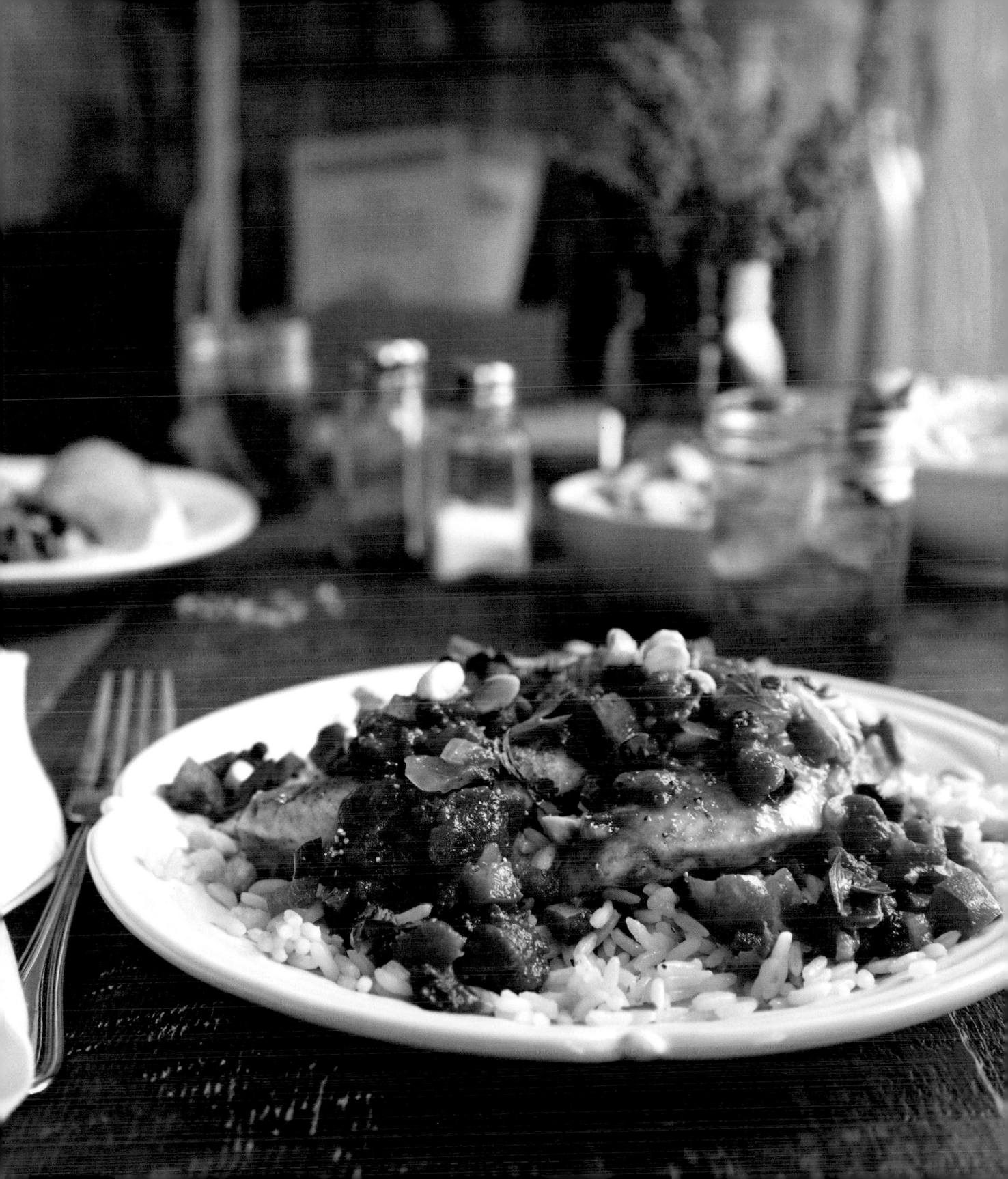

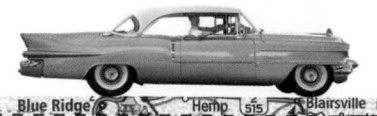

Georgia bucket list

things to see and do (besides eat) here

❶ Furnish your entire house at **Scott Antique Market**, which takes place the second weekend of every month in Atlanta.

❷ Take a selfie at one of Savannah's most famous landmarks, the **Forsyth Park Fountain** *(pictured)*, which was built in 1858.

❸ Climb the 178 steps of the **Tybee Island Light Station** and marvel at the views of the Atlantic from the 18th-century lighthouse.

❹ Snag a refurbished retro stove, fridge, or range at **Antique Appliances** in Clayton.

❺ See **Rock City**. Seriously. The commanding views (and iconic birdhouses) are worth the trip alone to Lookout Mountain, Georgia.

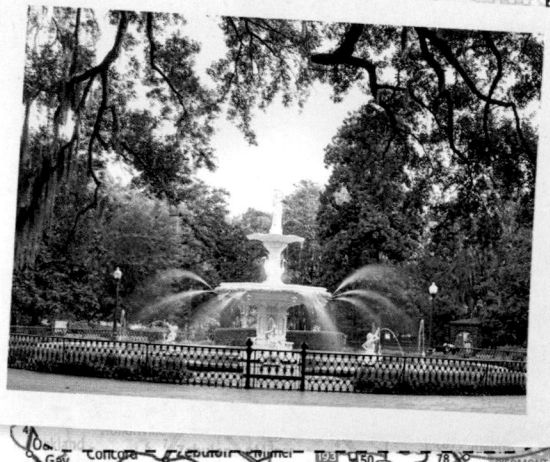

Mamaw's Farm House Meatloaf

A lot of meatloaf can be dry or greasy; not this one. The sauce makes it moist.

MEATLOAF

Vegetable cooking spray

2	lb. ground sirloin
1½	cups crushed round buttery crackers crumbs (about 25 crackers)
1	cup finely chopped green bell pepper
1	cup finely chopped onion
½	cup tomato juice
1	Tbsp. table salt
1	tsp. dried oregano
1	tsp. freshly ground black pepper
1	tsp. garlic powder
2	large eggs, beaten

SAUCE

½	cup canned condensed tomato soup, undiluted
1	Tbsp. brown sugar
1	Tbsp. yellow mustard
1½	tsp. white vinegar
1½	tsp. soy sauce

1. Prepare Meatloaf: Preheat oven to 350°. Lightly grease a 9- x 5-inch loaf pan with cooking spray. Combine beef and next 9 ingredients in a large bowl, using hands. Pack mixture into prepared pan.

2. Bake at 350° for 45 minutes. Remove meatloaf from oven; pour off drippings.

3. Prepare Sauce: Stir together all ingredients and ¼ cup water in a bowl.

4. Pour sauce over meatloaf, and bake 20 more minutes. Let stand 15 minutes before serving.

Makes: 8 servings

Caramel Cake

This cake is so moist and delicious, but the real treat is the frosting.

CAKE

Parchment paper

I	cup unsalted butter, softened
3	cups sugar
4	large eggs
3	cups all-purpose flour
I	tsp. baking soda
½	tsp. table salt
I ½	cups buttermilk
I	Tbsp. vanilla extract

FROSTING

4	cups sugar, divided
I	cup milk
I	cup butter
2	tsp. white vinegar
I	tsp. baking soda
I	cup finely chopped toasted pecans

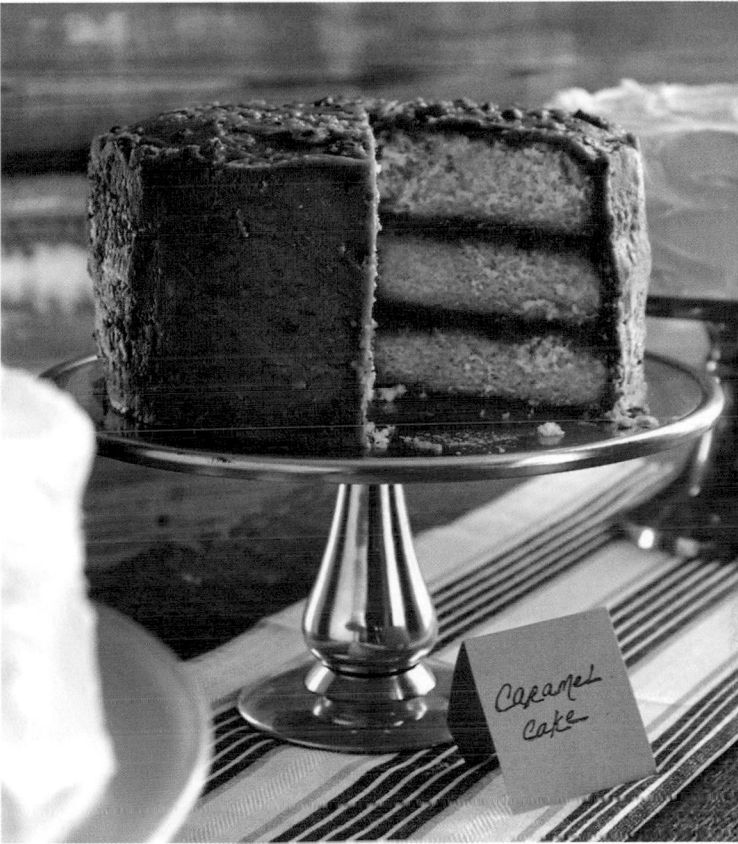

1. **Prepare Cake:** Butter 3 (9-inch) round cake pans. Line pans with parchment paper. Butter parchment paper; dust pans with flour.

2. Preheat oven to 350°. Beat butter at medium speed with an electric mixer until creamy; gradually add sugar, beating well. Add eggs, 1 at a time, beating just until blended after each addition.

3. Combine flour, baking soda, and salt; add to butter mixture alternately with buttermilk, beginning and ending with flour mixture. Beat at low speed just until blended after each addition, stopping to scrape bowl as needed. Stir in vanilla. Pour batter into prepared pans.

4. Bake at 350° for 23 minutes or until a wooden pick inserted in center comes out clean. Cool in pans on wire racks 10 minutes; remove from pans to wire racks, and cool completely (about 1 hour).

5. **Meanwhile, prepare Frosting:** Combine 3½ cups sugar, milk, and butter in a 4-qt. saucepan. Bring to a boil over medium heat. Keep hot over low heat, stirring occasionally.

6. Sprinkle remaining ½ cup sugar in a 10-inch stainless steel skillet; place over medium heat, and cook, shaking skillet constantly, 6 minutes or until sugar melts and turns a light golden brown. Remove from heat. Pour caramelized sugar into hot milk mixture. Bring to a boil; cook until a candy thermometer registers 234° to 240° (syrup forms a soft ball when a small amount is dropped in cold water, but flattens on removal from water). Remove from heat; stir in vinegar and soda. Beat until foam settles down. Stir in pecans. Let frosting stand, stirring occasionally, about 15 minutes or until frosting cools slightly and begins to thicken.

7. Quickly spread frosting between layers and on top and sides of cooled cake. Let cake stand 2 hours before slicing. **Makes: 12 servings**

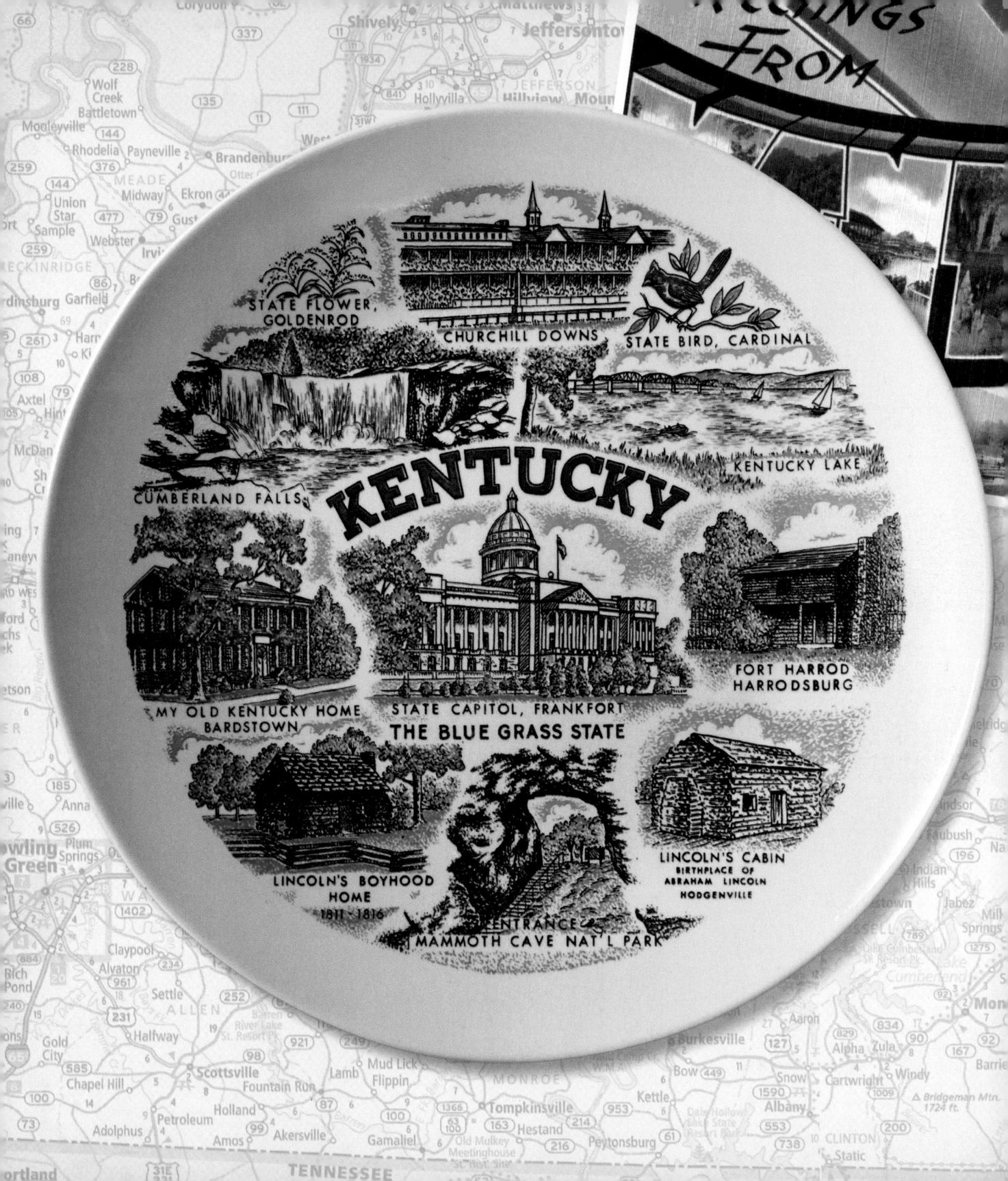

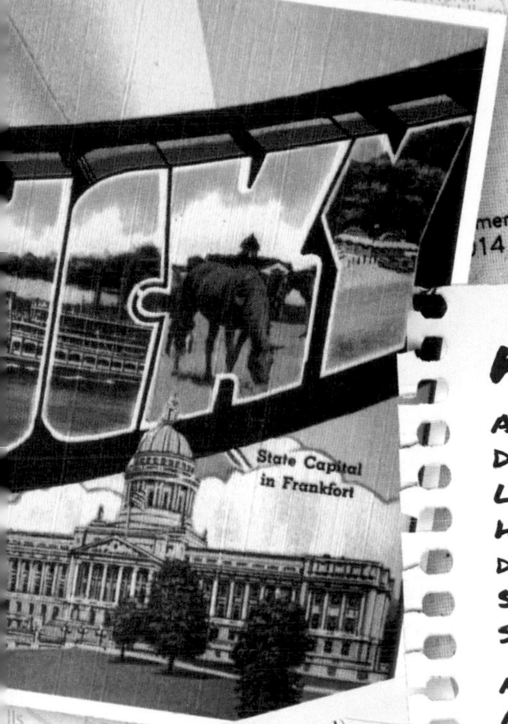

Kentucky

August 5:
Depart Bloomdale, Missouri for Louisville, Kentucky by 4 p.m. Head to Harvest Louisville for dinner with Chef Coby Ming at 5 p.m. (Order the fried chicken.) Spend the night.

August 6:
Meet with Hillbilly Tea owners, Karter Louis and Arpad Lengyel at 8 a.m. Drive to Lexington. Spend the night.

August 7:
Check out Ashley Minton's tiny Minton's @760 in Lexington (just four tables).

Head to Chattanooga, Tennessee. Spend the night.

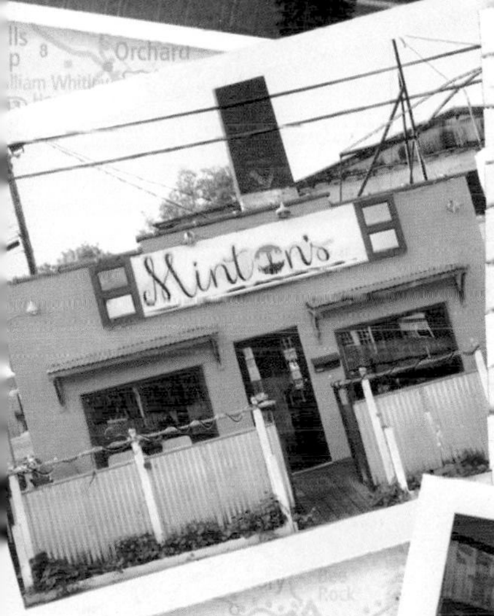

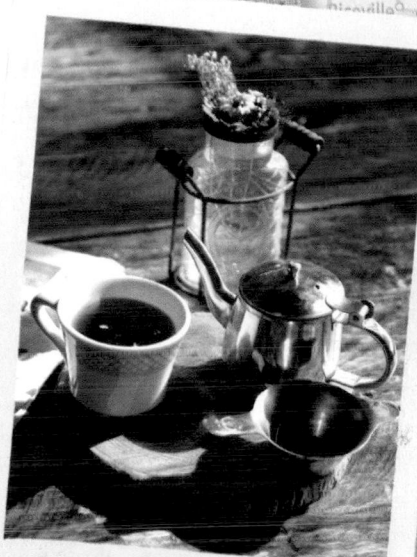

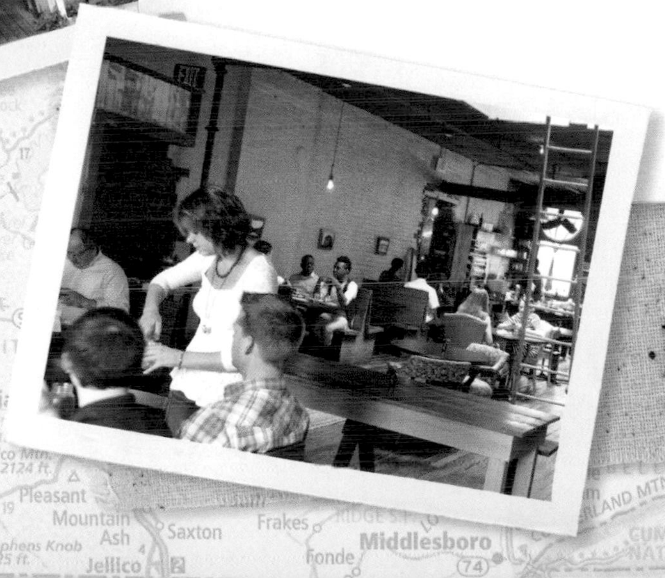

State Capital in Frankfort

dinner served 5-10

·hillbilly tea·

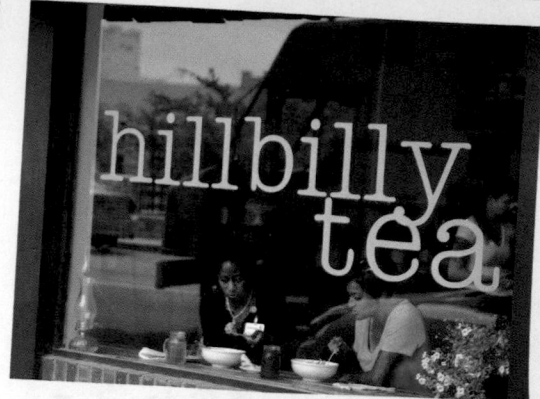

Hillbilly Tea

120 South 1st Street
Louisville, Kentucky 40202
(502) 587-7350
hillbillytea.com

Southerners' love of tea remains unsur-
passed by anyone except perhaps the
British. Hillbilly Tea's owners, Karter
Louis and Arpad Lengyel, deepen that
passion with an enormous and varied
selection of teas. You'll find no grocery store varieties here. Instead Karter
combs China for the very best green
and black teas to bring home. I normally
don't order anything more adventur-
ous than Earl Grey, but after scanning
Hillbilly's menu, I opted for a tea called
"Morning Dew." Its rich flavor and floral
notes needed no milk or sugar. Chef
Arpad uses tea on his menu as well.
Don't know oolong from osthmanthus?
No problem." The idea behind Hillbilly Tea
is to make tea approachable and unpretentious," Karter says. They've done more
than that: They've made tea cool.

Big Earl's Chocolate Torte

Parchment paper
Vegetable cooking spray
1½ cups semisweet chocolate morsels
1 cup plus 2 Tbsp. butter
2 regular-size Earl Grey tea bags
6 large eggs, separated
¾ cup granulated sugar
6 Tbsp. firmly packed light brown sugar
½ tsp. table salt
1 cup almond meal
½ tsp. cream of tartar
Garnishes: whipped cream, fresh blueberries,
fresh mint sprigs

1. Preheat oven to 350°. Line bottom of a 10-inch
springform pan with parchment paper; coat pan
and parchment paper with cooking spray.
2. Pour water to depth of 1 inch into bottom of
a double boiler over medium heat; bring to a
boil. Reduce heat, and simmer; place chocolate
morsels and butter in top of double boiler. Cook,
stirring often, 2 to 3 minutes or until melted.
Remove from heat, and cool 10 minutes.
3. Remove tea from tea bags. Beat egg yolks and
granulated sugar at medium-high speed with an
electric mixer 3 minutes or until thick and pale.
Gradually add chocolate mixture, brown sugar,
and salt, beating at low speed until blended. Fold
in almond meal and tea.
4. Beat egg whites and cream of tartar at high
speed with an electric mixer until soft peaks
form. Fold egg whites into chocolate mixture.
Pour batter into prepared pan.
5. Bake at 350° for 45 to 50 minutes or until a
wooden pick inserted in center comes out clean.
Cool completely in pan on a wire rack (1½ hours).
Run a sharp knife around sides of pan. Remove
sides of pan. Cut torte into wedges. **Makes:**
12 servings

Kentucky

* veggie
** vegan

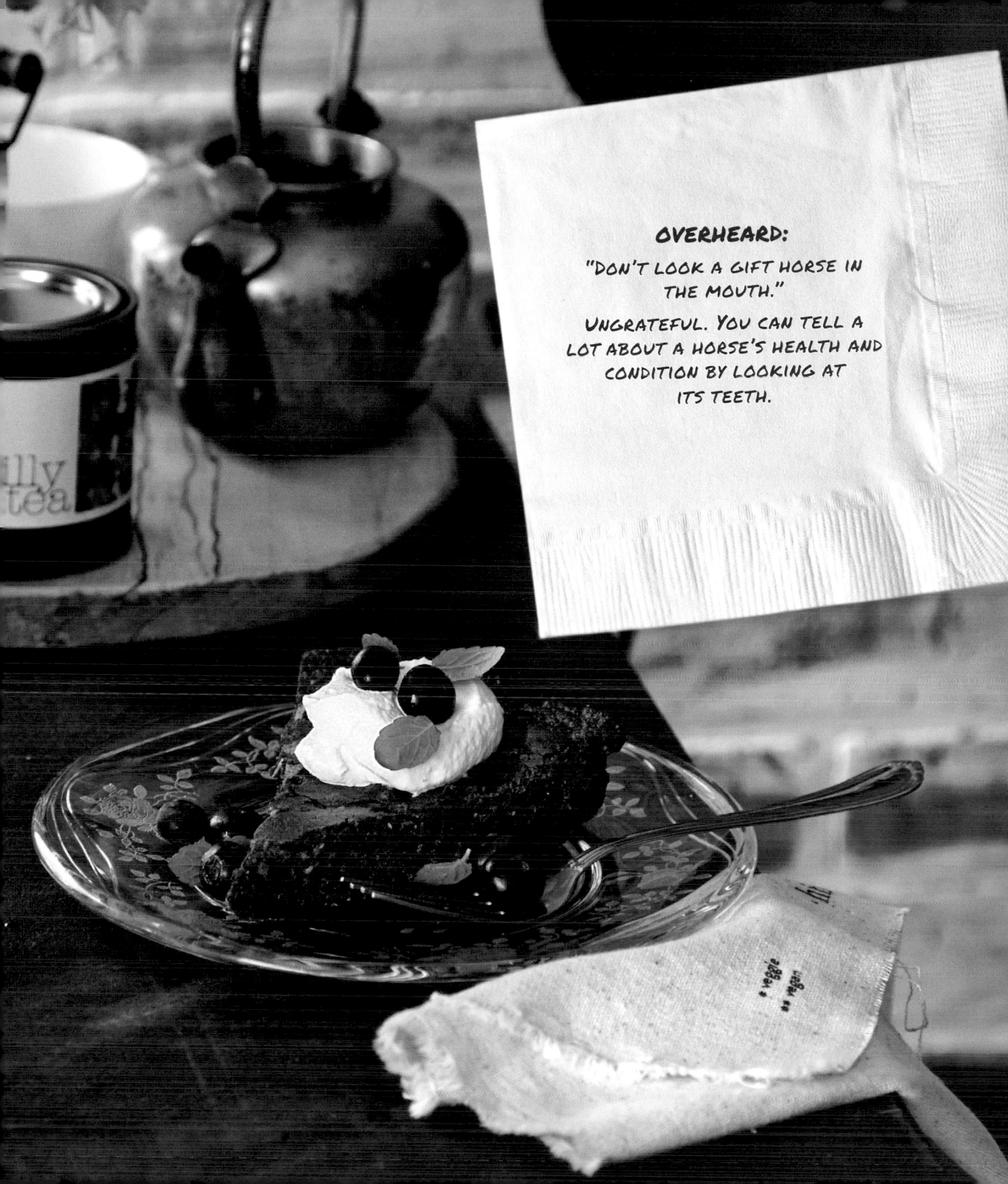

Corn Pone

These tasty treats have a hint of extra flavor from being kissed by the grill right before service.

Shortening
1¼ cups cake flour
1 cup plain yellow cornmeal
¼ cup sugar
2½ tsp. baking powder
1 tsp. table salt
3 large eggs
1½ cups sour cream
¾ cup canola oil
1 (14¾-oz.) can cream-style corn

1. Preheat oven to 350°. Grease (with shortening) a 13- x 9-inch pan. Combine flour and next 4 ingredients in a medium bowl; make a well in center of mixture.

2. Whisk together eggs and next 3 ingredients; add to flour mixture, whisking until smooth. Spread batter in prepared pan. Bake at 350° for 30 minutes or until a wooden pick inserted in center comes out clean. Cool in pan 10 minutes. Remove from pan; cool completely on a wire rack (about 1 hour). Cut into 24 squares.

3. If desired, cut squares in half horizontally. Place halves, cut side down, on a hot, lightly greased grill pan. Cook 1 to 2 minutes on each side or until grill marks appear. Serve immediately. **Makes: 12 servings**

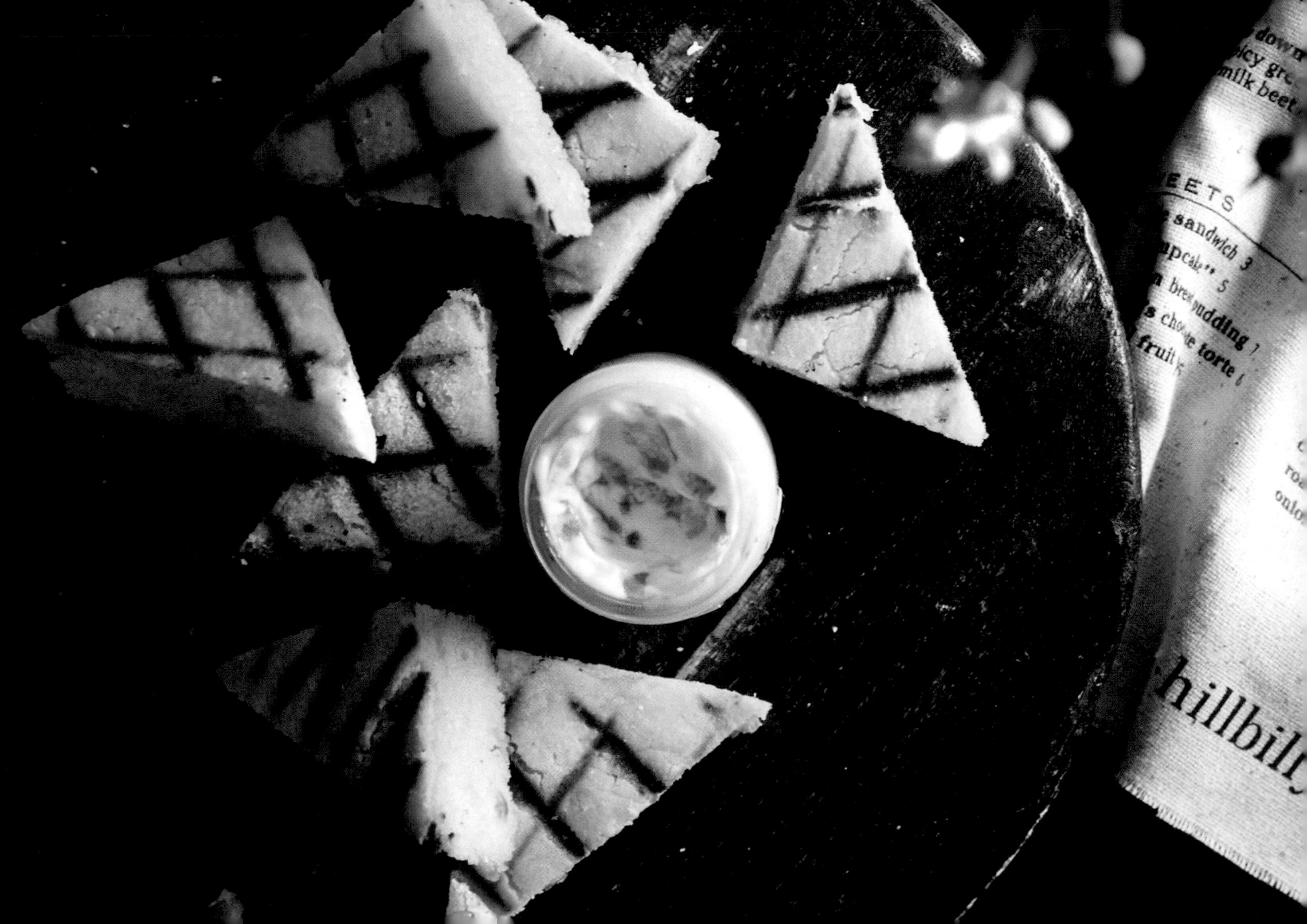

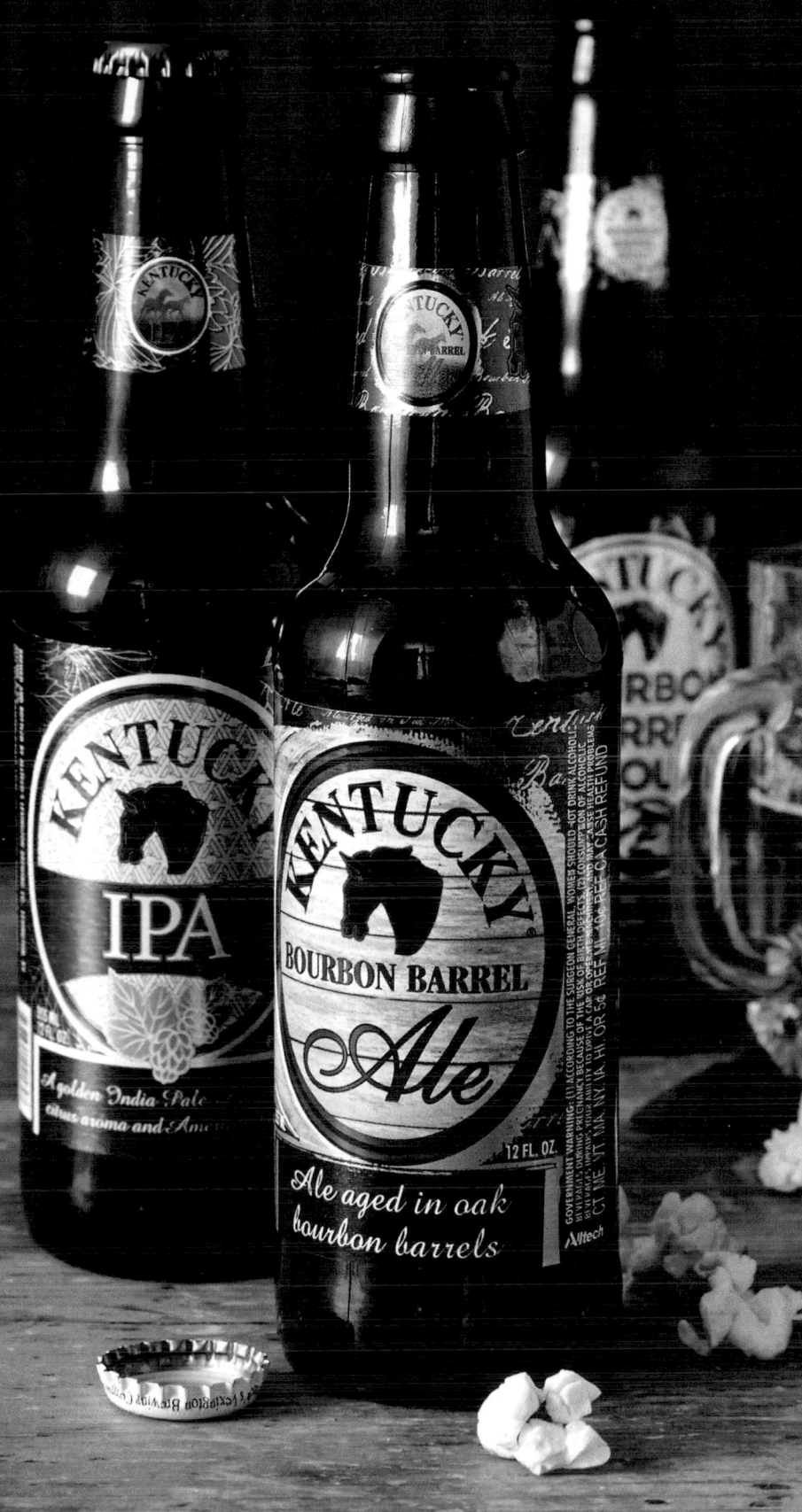

GREAT LOCAL FIND

Lexington Brewing and Distilling Company

401 Cross Street
Lexington, Kentucky 40508
(859) 255-2337
kentuckyale.com

You know Kentucky's famed horses and bourbon, but the state hosts another delightful concoction: beer aged six weeks in a used bourbon barrel. If you've not had Lexington Brewing and Distilling Co.'s Kentucky Ale, you're missing out. I met the company's founder, Pearse Lyons, who is a supremely enthusiastic Irishman, and fell hoops over bungs for his hearty, rich beer. The company brews several other beers, as well, including Kentucky Kölsch, Kentucky Bourbon Barrel Ale, Kentucky Bourbon Barrel Stout, and Kentucky IPA, and I pick some up whenever I'm in Kentucky. Lyons began his career working for Guinness and Harp, so it feels right that he should bring fine craft beer to the South.

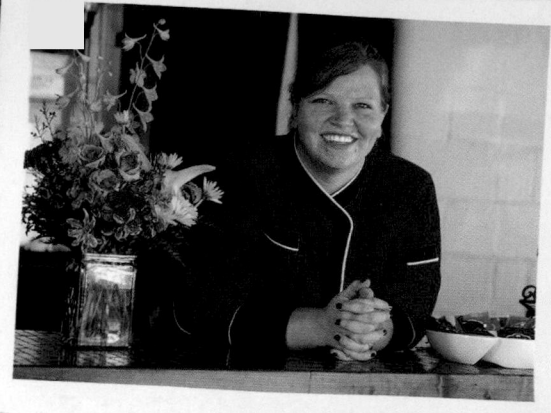

Minton's @ 760

760 N. Limestone Street
Lexington, Kentucky 40508
(859) 948-1874
mintonsat760.com

In a tiny cinderblock building next to a tattoo parlor, Minton's @ 760 brings a heaping helping of creativity and fun to the neighborhood. Chef and owner, Ashley Minton, attended culinary school in Lexington. After graduating, she began teaching cooking classes, and then opened a food truck. Soon fans of her food grew, and loyal devotees followed her to this permanent four-table location. And it's a family affair at Minton's. Dad built the counters, mom meets and greets, and her brother now runs the food truck, aptly named Little Brother. When it comes to the food, the French toast is a must try; while most French toast is soggier than an English afternoon, Ashley's flaxseed bread gives hers a crispy, crunchy texture. The spareribs on mac and cheese are spicy and creamy, and each rib alone is big enough for a meal.

Apple-Cinnamon French Toast

6	Tbsp. butter, divided
2	(8-oz.) Gala apples, unpeeled, cored, and sliced
¼	cup firmly packed light brown sugar
⅔	cup maple syrup
½	tsp. ground cinnamon
4	large eggs
1½	cups milk
8	(1.5-oz.) slices multigrain bread with flaxseed
1	(3.62-oz.) bottle cinnamon-sugar

1. Melt 2 Tbsp. butter in a large skillet over medium-high heat. Add apple slices; sauté 7 minutes or until tender and lightly browned. Add brown sugar; cook 1 minute or until sugar melts and slices are coated. Stir in maple syrup and cinnamon. Remove from heat, and keep warm.

2. Whisk together eggs and milk in a shallow dish.

3. Melt 1 Tbsp. butter in a large nonstick skillet over medium heat. Lightly press 2 bread slices, 1 at a time, into egg mixture, coating both sides of bread. Cook bread slices in melted butter 1 minute on each side; sprinkle tops generously with cinnamon-sugar. Turn slices over; cook 30 seconds or until sugar caramelizes. Sprinkle tops with desired amount of cinnamon-sugar; turn slices back over, and cook 30 seconds or until sugar caramelizes. Remove from skillet; keep warm. Wipe skillet clean with paper towels. Repeat procedure with remaining butter, bread slices, egg mixture, and cinnamon-sugar. Serve with apple mixture. **Makes: 4 servings**

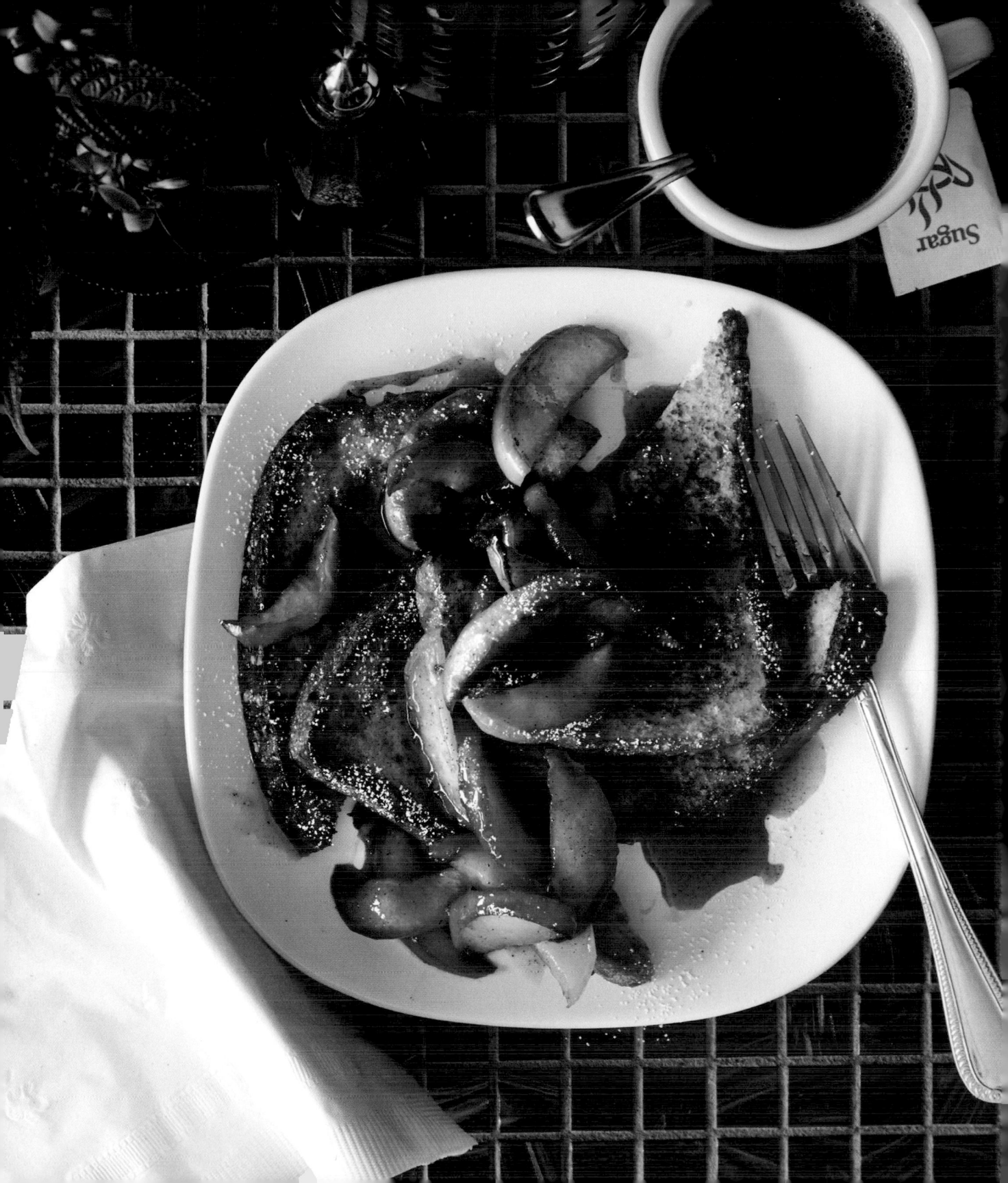

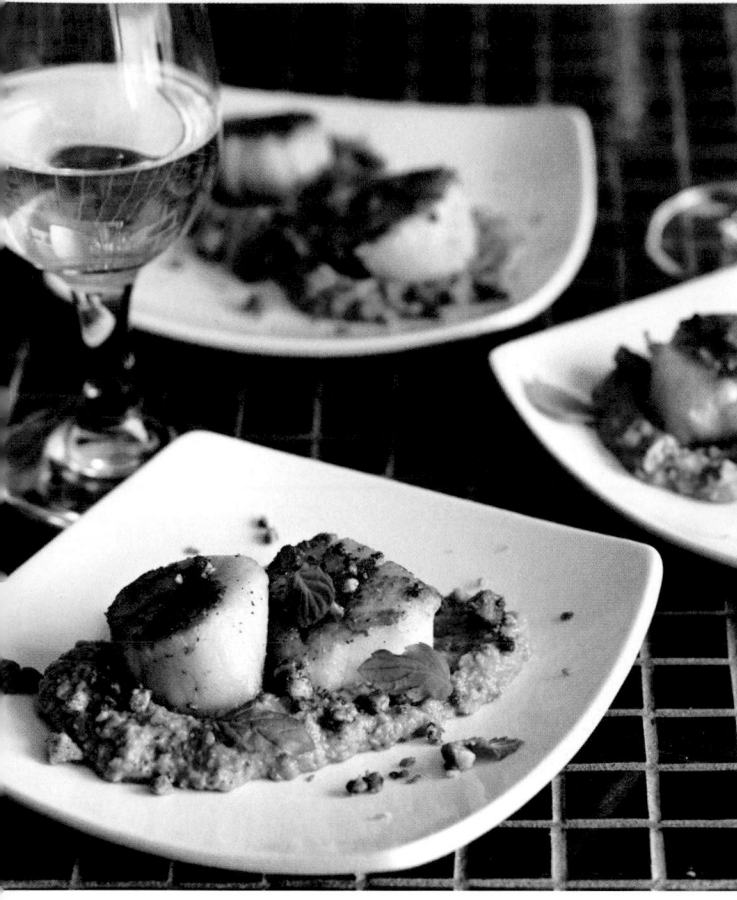

1. Heat nuts in a small nonstick skillet over medium-low heat, stirring often, 2 to 3 minutes or until lightly toasted and fragrant. Add ¼ tsp. olive oil, stirring to coat. Stir in curry powder and ½ tsp. salt. Remove nuts from skillet; let stand 10 minutes.

2. Rinse scallops, and pat dry with paper towels. Sprinkle scallops with pepper and remaining ¼ tsp. salt.

3. Heat 1½ tsp. olive oil in a large nonstick skillet over medium-high heat. Cook 6 scallops in hot skillet 2 to 3 minutes on each side or until golden brown. Remove from skillet. Repeat procedure with remaining 1½ tsp. olive oil and 6 scallops. Sprinkle scallops with macadamia nuts, and serve with Pea Pesto. **Makes: 6 appetizer servings**

Pea Pesto

2	garlic cloves
¼	cup loosely packed fresh basil leaves
¼	cup loosely packed fresh mint leaves
1	(12-oz.) package frozen petite peas, thawed
½	cup (2 oz.) freshly grated Parmesan cheese
⅓	cup olive oil
1	tsp. kosher salt
½	tsp. lemon zest
5	tsp. fresh lemon juice
¼	tsp. freshly ground black pepper

With processor running, drop garlic cloves through food chute; process until minced. Add basil and mint; process until minced. Add peas and remaining ingredients; process until smooth. Cover and chill up to 1 week. **Makes: 2 cups**
Note: Pesto can be frozen.

Seared Sea Scallops with Pea Pesto

The fresh pea pesto and macadamia nuts pair perfectly with the sweet sea scallops—the flavor combinations really make this little dish addictive.

¼	cup chopped salted macadamia nuts
¼	tsp. olive oil
1	tsp. madras curry powder
¾	tsp. table salt, divided
12	large sea scallops (about 1½ lb.)
¼	tsp. freshly ground pepper
1	Tbsp. olive oil
Pea Pesto	

Garnish: fresh mint sprigs

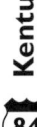

Chocolate Chip Donut Bread Pudding with Warm Bourbon Sauce

Loaded with bourbon, donuts, and chocolate, this bread pudding may have your guests gnawing on their plates to get every last morsel.

BREAD PUDDING
Butter

1	dozen commercial glazed yeast donuts
½	cup semisweet chocolate morsels
½	cup coarsely chopped pecans
3	large eggs
½	cup sugar
1½	cups heavy cream
½	cup milk
2	tsp. vanilla extract
½	tsp. ground cardamom

BOURBON SAUCE

¾	cup bourbon
¾	cup firmly packed light brown sugar
1	cup heavy cream
3	Tbsp. light corn syrup
2	tsp. vanilla extract

1. Prepare Bread Pudding: Butter a 13- x 9-inch baking dish. Tear each donut into 6 to 8 pieces; place in prepared pan. Sprinkle with chocolate morsels and pecans.

2. Whisk together eggs and sugar in a large bowl until slightly thick and pale. Whisk in cream and next 3 ingredients. Pour egg mixture over donut pieces. Let stand 45 minutes.

3. Preheat oven to 350°. Bake bread pudding at 350° for 35 minutes or until set, slightly puffed, and browned. Cool in pan on a wire rack until warm (20 minutes).

4. Meanwhile, prepare Bourbon Sauce: Bring bourbon to a boil in a heavy saucepan. Reduce heat, and simmer 4 minutes or until reduced by half. Add sugar; cook until mixture begins to bubble. Add cream, corn syrup, and vanilla. Simmer 10 minutes or until sauce coats the back of a metal spoon. Pour over warm bread pudding.

Makes: 8 servings

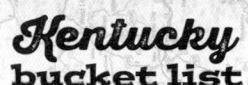

Kentucky bucket list
things to see and do (besides eat) here

1. Deck yourself in prep and watch a race from Keeneland's posh clubhouse in Lexington.

2. Go whiskey tasting in the distilleries on the **Kentucky Bourbon Trail** or **Urban Bourbon Trail**.

3. Land an original piece of art from **Berea**, which is full of local artists, and hosts several crafts festivals annually.

4. Buy a custom-made baseball bat from the **Louisville Slugger Museum & Factory** in Louisville.

5. Don your best hat and sip too many mint juleps at the **Kentucky Derby** *(pictured)*.

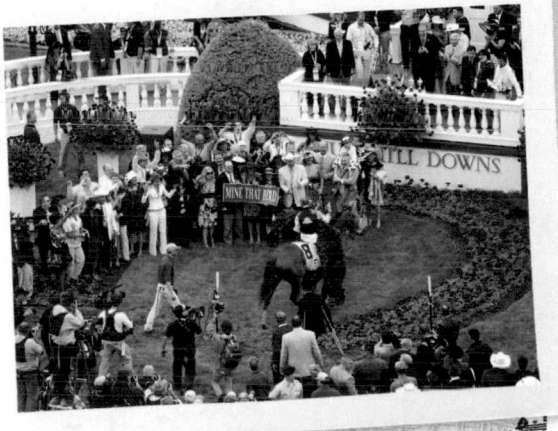

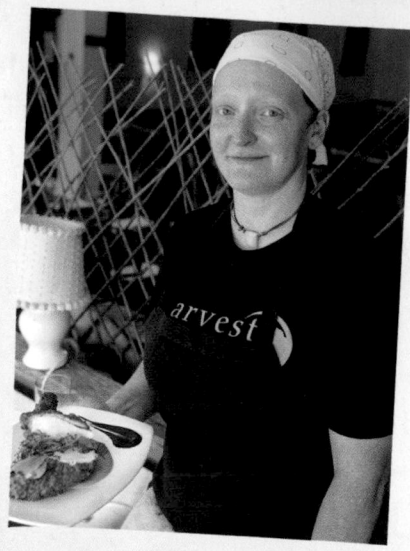

Harvest

624 East Market Street
Louisville, Kentucky 40202
(502) 384-9090
harvestlouisville.com

I found this magical little spot while researching my book *Bourbon & Bacon*. Open for breakfast, lunch, and dinner, Harvest has yet to serve me a meal I didn't love. The produce Chef Coby Ming uses is so fresh, it's as if she hand-picked every vegetable just for you. And her fried chicken—it's moist, tender, and served atop vegetable bread pudding. If the menu doesn't win you over, the bar will. Co-owner Patrick Kuhl also owns a liquor store, so he knows his booze. Best of all, Harvest celebrates local farmers. Every wall of the restaurant is adorned with black-and-white pictures of the people who grow and cultivate the food on your plate.

Fried Chicken

Fried chicken is a huge deal in Kentucky and you don't have to be a colonel to boast your own secret recipe. Harvest's spice blend varies by season, but usually is made with local ground peppers, onions, and garlic. Use your favorite barbecue spice blend as a substitute.

1½   cups buttermilk
1½   tsp. garlic oil
4¾   tsp. barbecue seasoning, divided
2   tsp. table salt, divided
2   tsp. freshly ground black pepper, divided
4   lb. chicken pieces
2   cups all-purpose flour
Canola oil

1. Combine first 2 ingredients, ¾ tsp. barbecue seasoning, ½ tsp. salt, and ½ tsp. pepper in a large bowl. Add chicken pieces, turning to coat. Cover and chill 12 to 24 hours.

2. Remove chicken from buttermilk mixture, discarding buttermilk mixture. Drain chicken well.

3. Whisk together flour, remaining 4 tsp. barbecue seasoning, remaining 1½ tsp. salt, and remaining 1½ tsp. pepper in a large bowl. Spoon flour mixture into a brown paper bag or large zip-top plastic freezer bag. Place half of chicken in bag; seal bag, and shake to coat. Remove chicken from flour mixture, shaking off excess; transfer to a wire rack. Repeat procedure with remaining chicken. Let chicken stand 30 minutes to form a crust.

4. Pour oil to depth of 1½ inches into a cast-iron Dutch oven; heat to 325°. Fry chicken, in batches, 10 to 15 minutes or until browned and done, turning occasionally. Drain on a wire rack over paper towels. **Makes: 4 servings**

Note: If using a 12-inch-wide (2¼-inch-deep) cast-iron skillet, pour oil to depth of 1 inch. We tested with Paul Prudhomme's Magic Seasoning Blends Barbecue Magic.

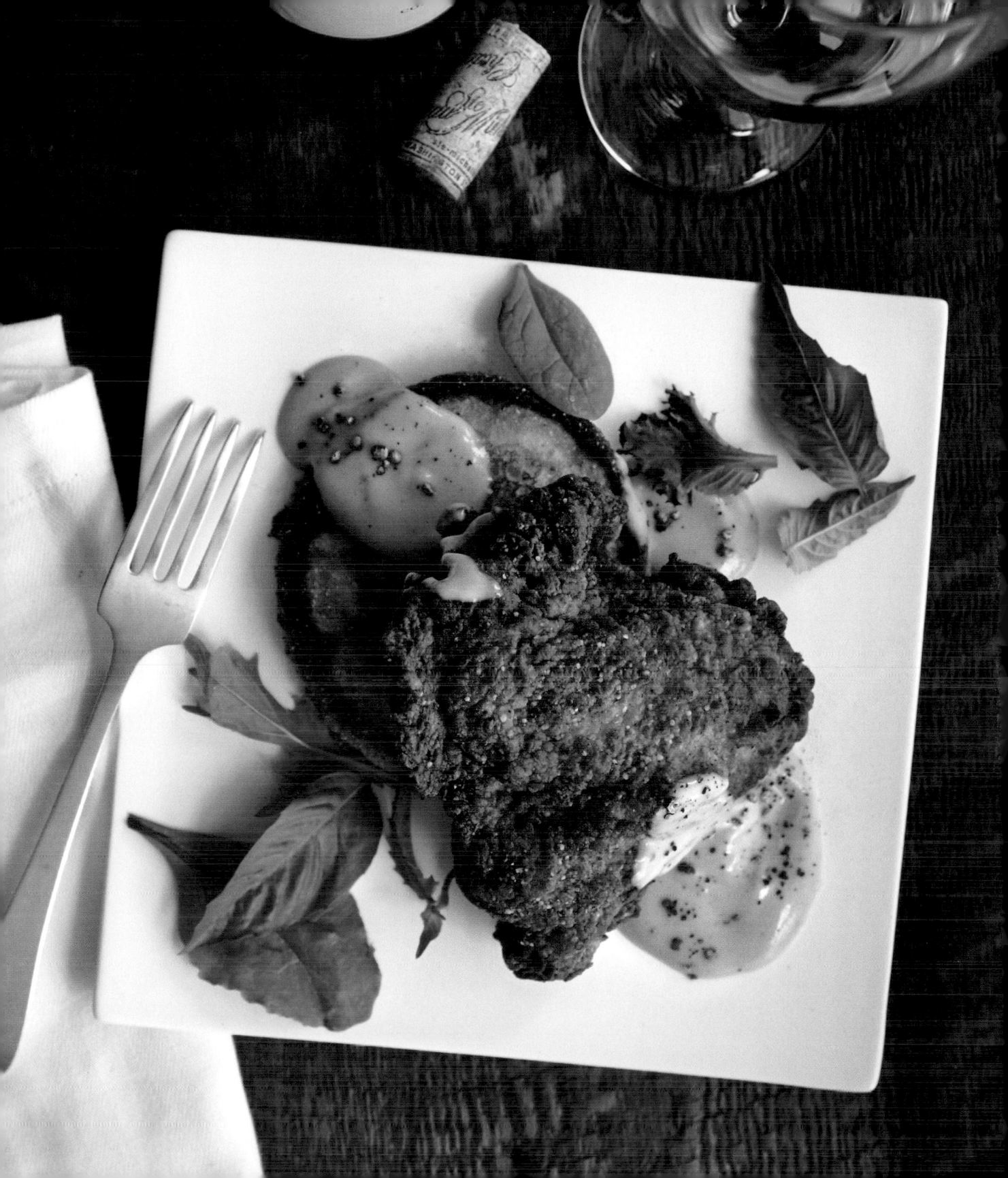

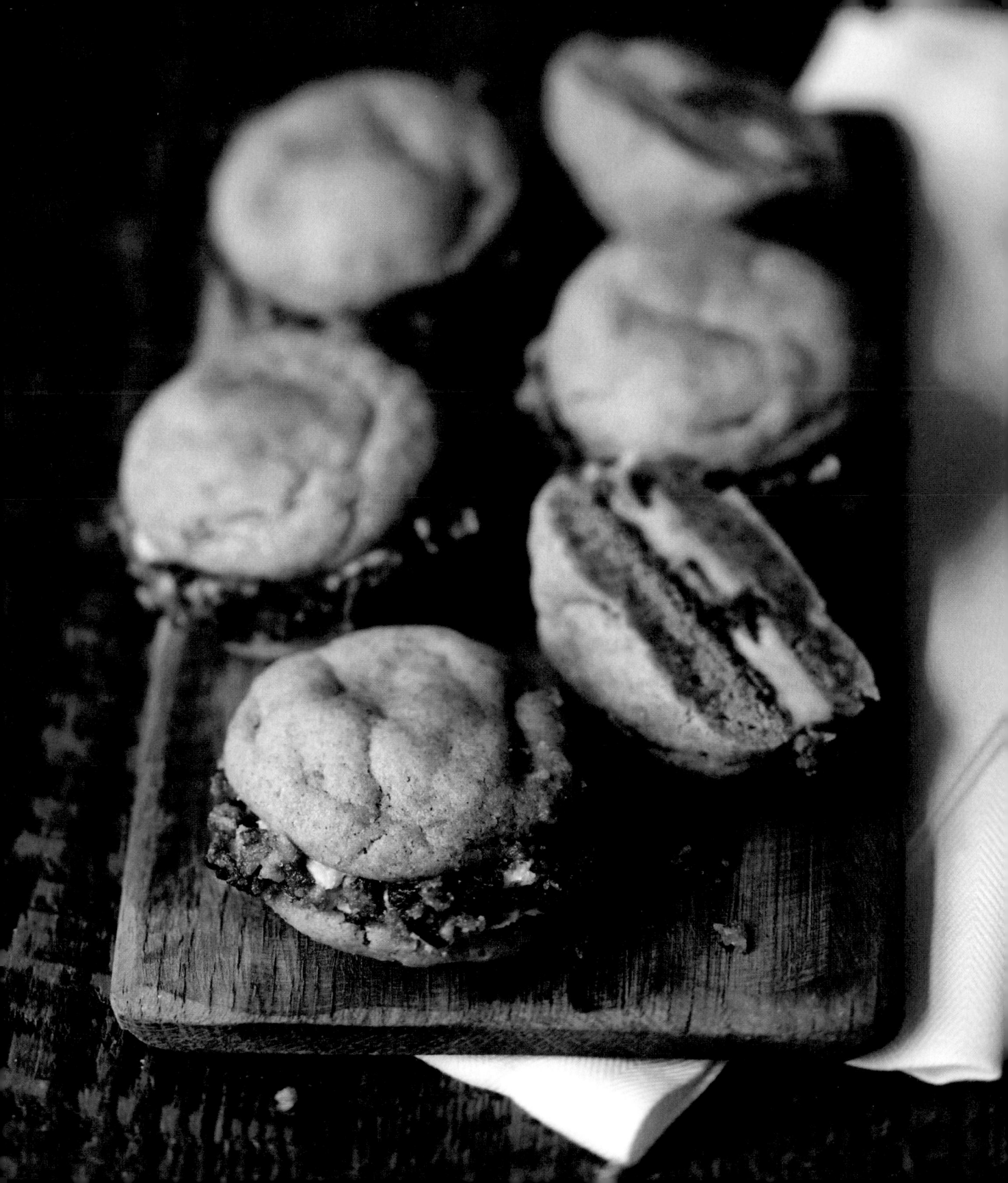

Sorghum Bacon Cookie

These deliciously decadent cookies contain my favorite ingredient—bacon.

CANDIED BACON

12 slices (1 lb.) thick-cut hickory-smoked
   bacon slices
½ cup firmly packed light brown sugar
¼ cup maple syrup

BACON FILLING

1 cup butter
1 Tbsp. bacon drippings
1½ cups powdered sugar
¼ tsp. ground white pepper

COOKIE DOUGH

½ cup butter, softened
¼ cup granulated sugar
¼ cup firmly packed brown sugar
1 large egg yolk
⅓ cup sorghum syrup
2 Tbsp. milk
½ tsp. vanilla extract
1¾ cups all-purpose flour
¾ tsp. baking soda
¾ tsp. ground cinnamon
¾ tsp. ground ginger
⅛ tsp. ground white pepper
⅛ tsp. ground allspice
⅛ tsp. table salt
Parchment paper

1. Prepare Candied Bacon: Preheat oven to 375°. Arrange bacon in a single layer on a wire rack in an aluminum foil-lined 17- x 12-inch rimmed baking sheet. Bake at 375° for 10 minutes or just until bacon begins to curl at ends.

2. Meanwhile, combine brown sugar and maple syrup in a small bowl. Remove bacon from oven. Brush both sides of bacon with brown sugar mixture. Bake at 375° for 30 to 35 more minutes or until bacon is crisp around edges and browned, brushing both sides of bacon with brown sugar mixture after 15 minutes. Cool completely on

rack (about 30 minutes). Finely chop bacon.

3. Prepare Bacon Filling: Beat 1 cup butter and 1 Tbsp. bacon drippings at medium speed with an electric mixer until fluffy. Gradually add powdered sugar and white pepper, beating until smooth. Stir in ¾ cup Candied Bacon.

4. Prepare Cookie Dough: Preheat oven to 350°. Beat ½ cup butter and sugars at medium speed with an electric mixer until creamy. Add egg yolk and next 3 ingredients, beating until blended.

5. Combine flour and next 6 ingredients in a small bowl; gradually add to butter mixture, beating well. Drop dough in 24 portions (about 2 Tbsp. each) 2 inches apart onto baking sheets lined with parchment paper. Bake at 350° for 10 minutes or until cookies looked cracked on top and edges are light golden brown. (The insides of the cracks will appear slightly underdone.) Cool on pans 2 minutes. Transfer cookies to wire racks; cool completely (15 minutes).

6. Spread 2 Tbsp. of filling on bottoms of 12 cookies. Top with remaining cookies, pressing until filling is even with edges. Roll edges of cookies in remaining Candied Bacon, pressing to adhere. Chill until firm. **Makes: 12 servings**

SOUNDTRACK:

"KENTUCKY RAIN" BY ELVIS PRESLEY

"BOURBON IN KENTUCKY" BY DIERKS BENTLEY

"WHISKEY IN MY WHISKEY" BY THE FELICE BROTHERS

"HAVE LOVE WILL TRAVEL" BY THE BLACK KEYS

"THAT'LL BE THE PLAN" BY DANIEL MARTIN MOORE

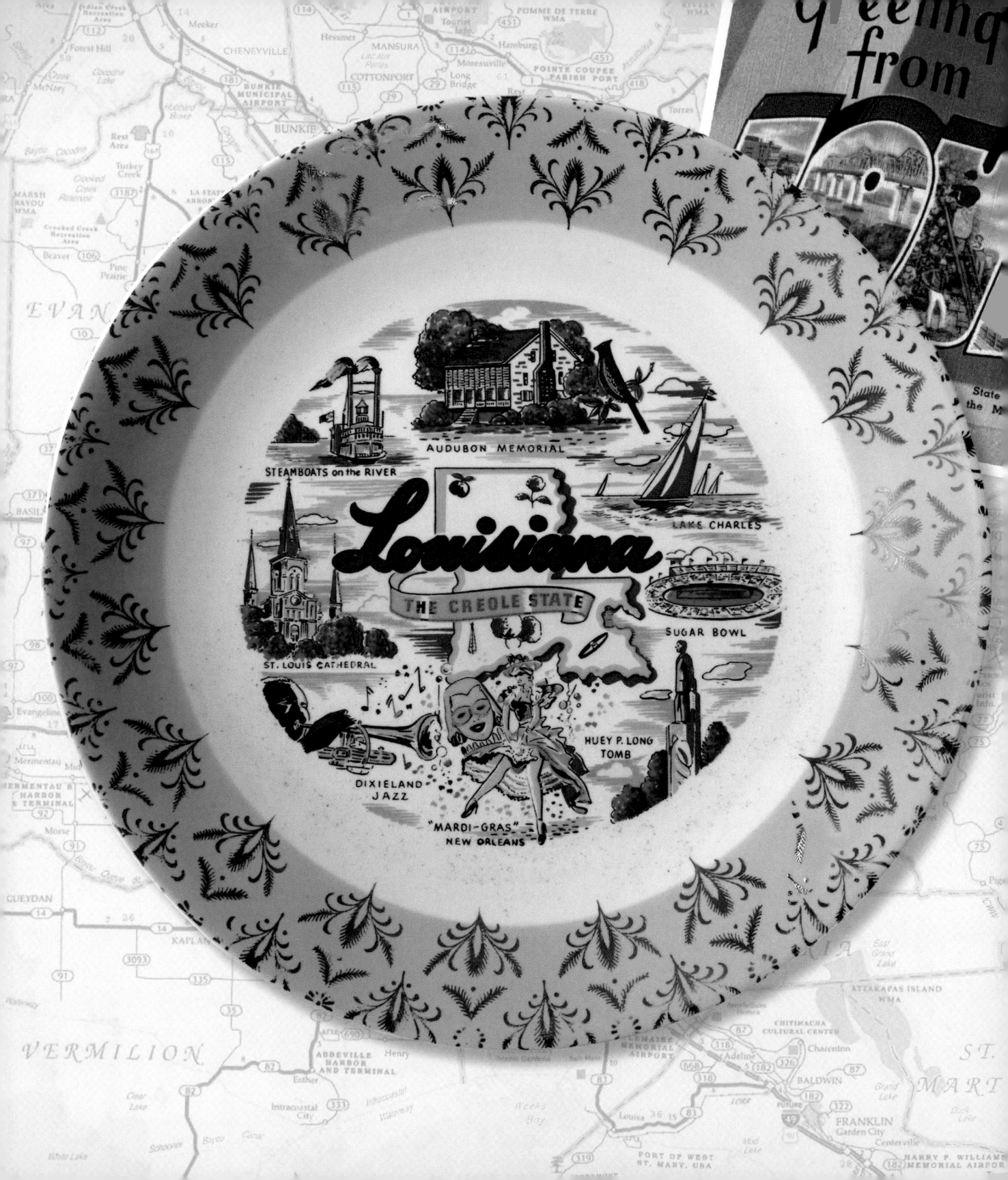

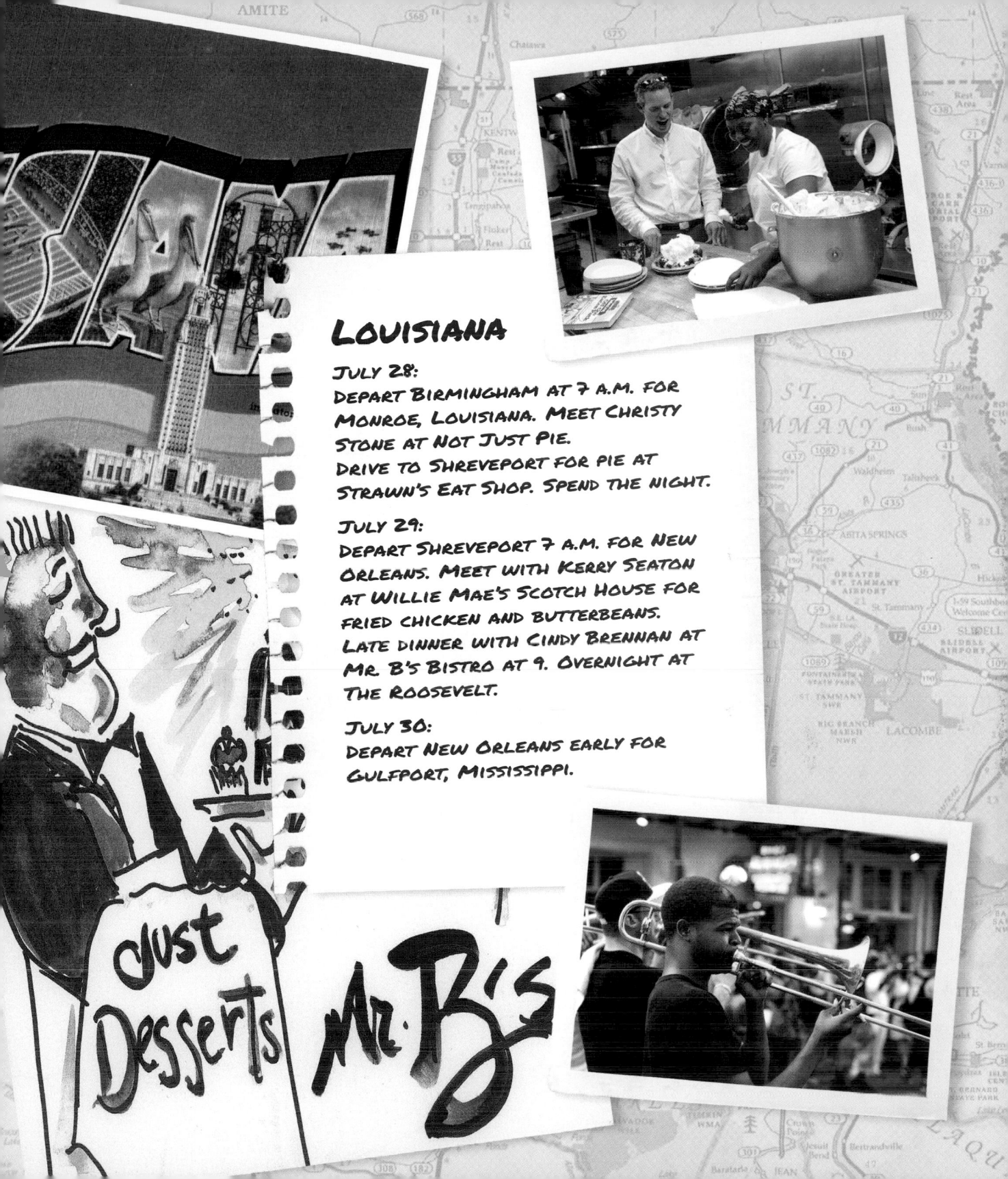

LOUISIANA

JULY 28:
Depart Birmingham at 7 a.m. for Monroe, Louisiana. Meet Christy Stone at Not Just Pie.
Drive to Shreveport for pie at Strawn's Eat Shop. Spend the night.

JULY 29:
Depart Shreveport 7 a.m. for New Orleans. Meet with Kerry Seaton at Willie Mae's Scotch House for fried chicken and butterbeans.
Late dinner with Cindy Brennan at Mr. B's Bistro at 9. Overnight at The Roosevelt.

JULY 30:
Depart New Orleans early for Gulfport, Mississippi.

Just Desserts

Mr. B's

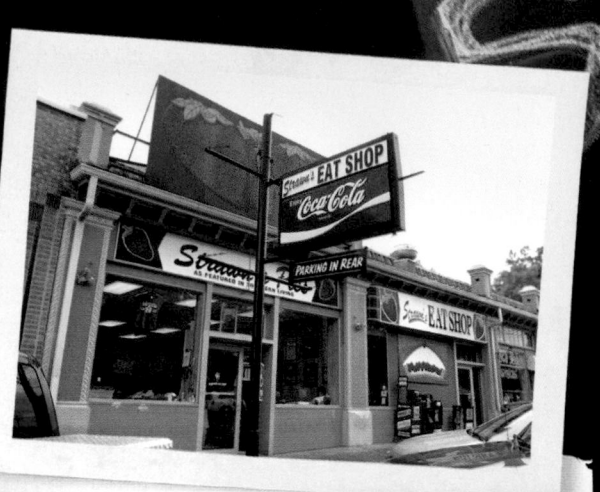

Strawn's Eat Shop

125 Kings Highway
Shreveport, Louisiana 71104
(318) 868-0634
strawnseatshop.com

Once you taste anything from Strawn's Eat Shop, you'll never drive through Shreveport again without stopping here. Its classic counter and red bar stools create just the right ambiance for eating massive amounts of pie. Strawn's makes its own piecrusts, fillings, and whipped cream. The strawberry pie is simple to make, but don't let that fool you. It's a masterpiece of fresh flavors. "If I could ship these pies, I'd be shipping them from a beach somewhere," says Wes Gauthier, who along with his dad, Buddy, are co-owners. And I thought I'd had good pancakes, but these buttery, golden flapjacks put others to shame—they don't even need syrup. Strawn's is the ultimate mom and pop shop, but the commitment to cooking puts it in the big leagues.

Pancakes

3   large eggs
2   cups half-and-half
½   cup buttermilk
1   Tbsp. vanilla extract
3   cups all-purpose flour
½   cup sugar
1   Tbsp. baking powder
½   tsp. baking soda
½   tsp. table salt
Butter, softened
Maple syrup

1. Beat eggs at medium speed with an electric mixer until foamy. Add half-and-half and next 2 ingredients, beating at low speed until blended. Combine flour and next 4 ingredients; add to egg mixture, beating at low speed 5 minutes or until light and airy. Let batter stand 10 minutes.
2. Pour about ¼ cup batter for each pancake onto a hot, lightly greased griddle or large nonstick skillet. Cook pancakes over medium-high heat 2 minutes or until tops are covered with bubbles and edges look dry and cooked; turn and cook other side. Serve with softened butter and maple syrup. **Makes: 8 servings**

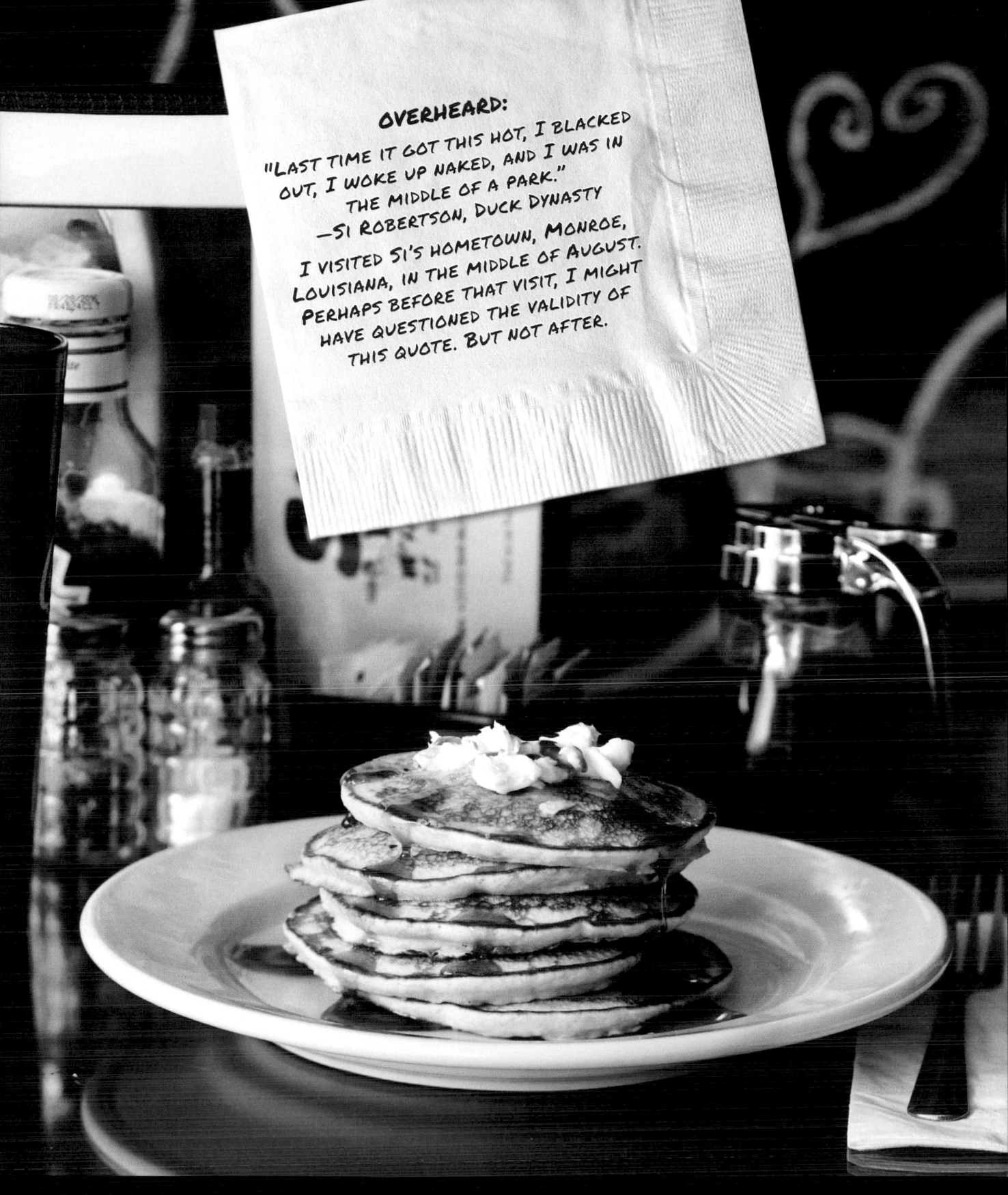

OVERHEARD:

"LAST TIME IT GOT THIS HOT, I BLACKED OUT, I WOKE UP NAKED, AND I WAS IN THE MIDDLE OF A PARK."
—SI ROBERTSON, DUCK DYNASTY

I VISITED SI'S HOMETOWN, MONROE, LOUISIANA, IN THE MIDDLE OF AUGUST. PERHAPS BEFORE THAT VISIT, I MIGHT HAVE QUESTIONED THE VALIDITY OF THIS QUOTE. BUT NOT AFTER.

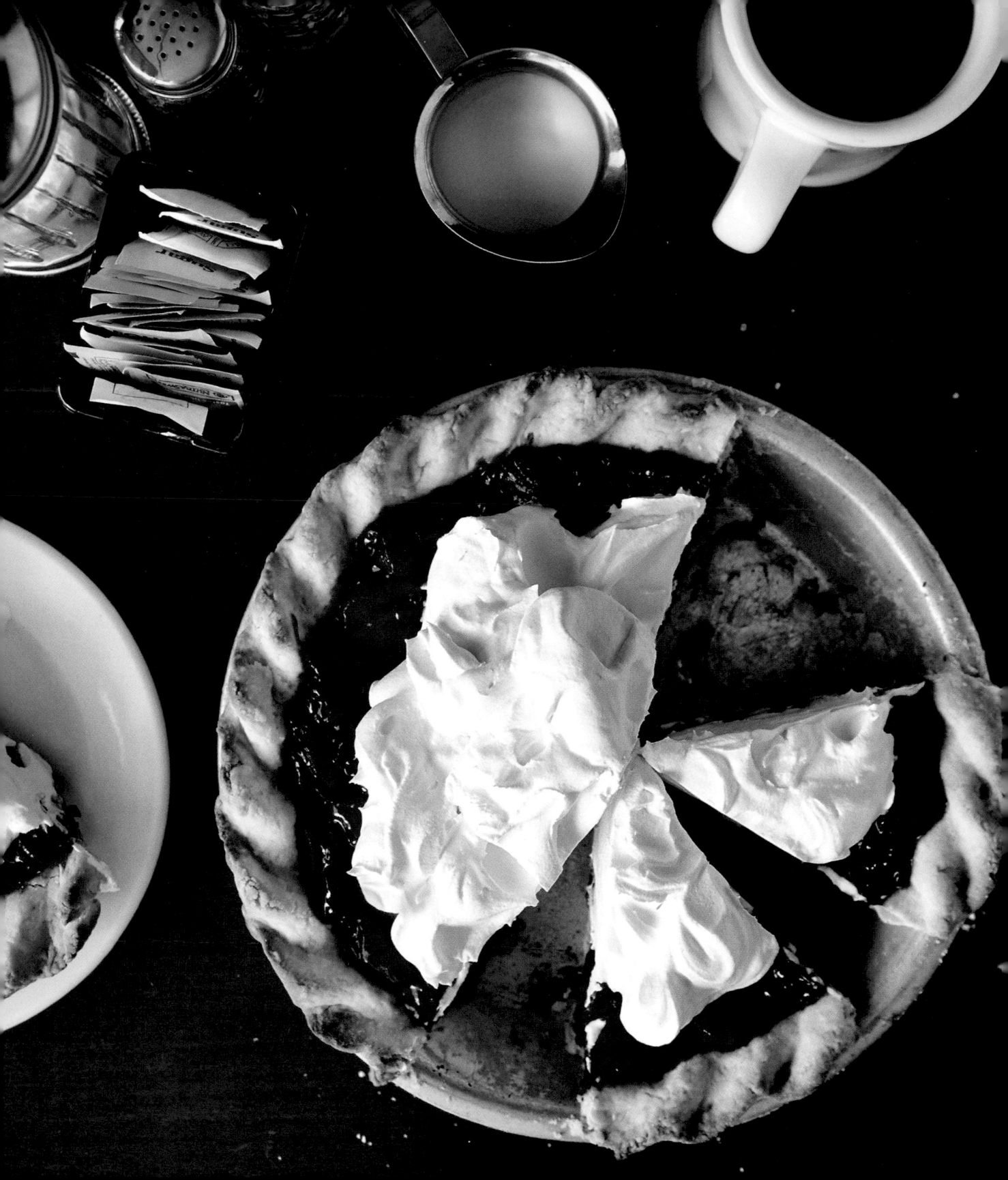

Strawberry Pie

This is a simple recipe but it's the freshness of the ingredients that make this pie world famous.

PASTRY

1½ cups all-purpose flour
¼ cup cold butter, cut into pieces
¼ cup cold shortening, cut into pieces
2 Tbsp. sugar
½ tsp. table salt
3 Tbsp. ice water

STRAWBERRY FILLING

¾ cup sugar
3 Tbsp. cornstarch
Pinch of table salt
1 Tbsp. lemon juice
½ tsp. red liquid food coloring
3 cups fresh strawberries, sliced
1 cup heavy whipping cream
1 Tbsp. sugar

1. Prepare Pastry: Combine first 5 ingredients in a bowl with a pastry blender until mixture resembles small peas. Sprinkle ice water, 1 Tbsp. at a time, over surface of mixture in bowl; stir with a fork until dry ingredients are moistened. Gather dough into a flat disk; cover and chill 1 hour.

2. Preheat oven to 425°. Roll dough into a 13-inch circle on a lightly floured surface. Fit into a 9-inch pie plate; fold edges under, and crimp.

3. Line pastry with aluminum foil, and fill with pie weights or dried beans. Bake at 425° for 15 minutes. Remove weights and foil; bake 15 to 20 more minutes or until golden brown, shielding edges if necessary. Cool completely on a wire rack.

4. Prepare Strawberry Filling: Combine first 3 ingredients in a saucepan; stir in 3 Tbsp. water until a paste forms. Slowly stir in 1 cup water. Bring to a boil over medium heat; boil 1 minute or until thickened. Stir in lemon juice and food coloring. Remove from heat. Fill a large bowl with ice; place pan in ice, and let stand, stirring occasionally, 15 minutes or until cool. Stir in strawberries.

5. Beat whipping cream until foamy; gradually add sugar, beating until soft peaks form.

6. Spread filling in piecrust. Top with whipped cream. Chill at least 2 hours. **Makes: 8 servings**

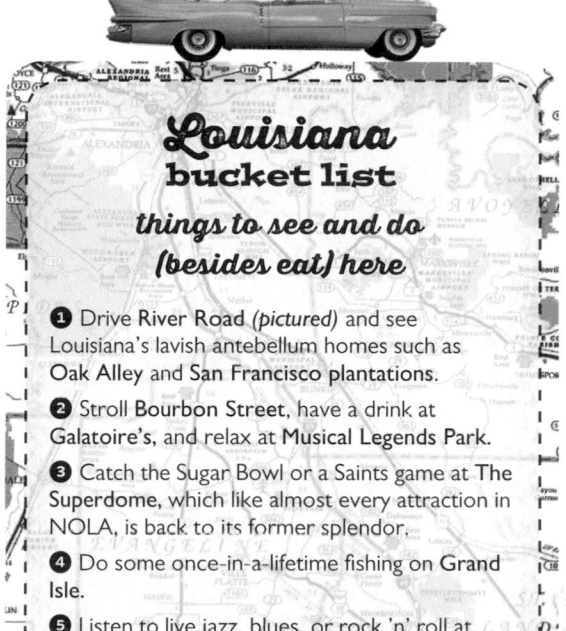

Louisiana bucket list
things to see and do (besides eat) here

❶ Drive River Road *(pictured)* and see Louisiana's lavish antebellum homes such as Oak Alley and San Francisco plantations.

❷ Stroll Bourbon Street, have a drink at Galatoire's, and relax at Musical Legends Park.

❸ Catch the Sugar Bowl or a Saints game at The Superdome, which like almost every attraction in NOLA, is back to its former splendor.

❹ Do some once-in-a-lifetime fishing on Grand Isle.

❺ Listen to live jazz, blues, or rock 'n' roll at Preservation Hall in the Big Easy.

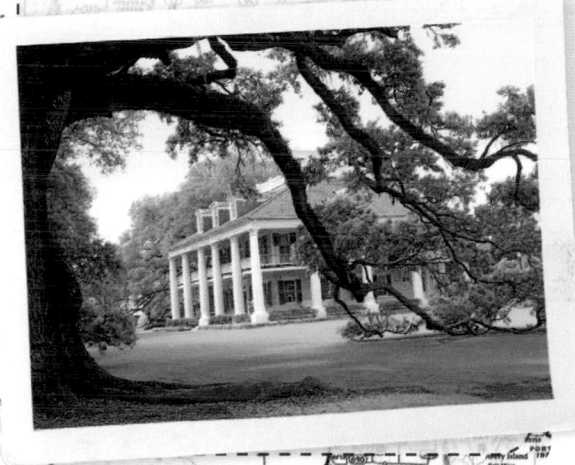

Mr. B's Bistro

201 Royal Street
New Orleans, Louisiana 70130
(504) 523-2078
mrbsbistro.com

The Big Easy's dining culture, cast by centuries of travelers, tradition, and taste, boasts a top tier of grand classic restaurants—spots so revered that many families have boasted the same tables and waiters for generations. Mr. B's Bistro, though open only since 1979, belongs in that exclusive club. Now, no resident of New Orleans would call "Mr. B's" an undiscovered spot. Cindy Brennan's restaurant (and those of her family) remains firmly on the eaten path. Yet sometimes foodies skip a dearly loved spot in their quest for what's hot and new. That's a shame. You'll miss out if you visit New Orleans and don't dine here. From the barbecue shrimp to the fried oysters, Mr. B's cuisine is NOLA all the way. It's one of my favorite spots to have a Sazerac, tie on a bib, and go to work on a plate of shrimp.

Gumbo Ya-Ya

This super-rich, dark brown roux gumbo is one of my favorite dishes in the Big Easy.

- ½ cup unsalted butter
- ¾ cup all-purpose flour
- ½ cup diced onion
- ½ cup diced red bell pepper
- ½ cup diced green bell pepper
- ½ cup diced celery
- 5 cups Chicken Stock or canned chicken stock
- ¼ lb. andouille sausage, cut into ¼-inch slices
- 1½ tsp. Creole seasoning
- 1½ tsp. kosher salt
- ¼ tsp. freshly ground black pepper
- ¼ tsp. dried crushed red pepper
- ¼ tsp. chili powder
- ¼ tsp. dried thyme
- 1 garlic clove, minced
- ½ bay leaf
- 3½ cups coarsely chopped cooked chicken
- 2 tsp. hot sauce (optional)
- Hot cooked rice
- Garnish: chopped fresh parsley

1. Melt butter in a 3-qt. saucepan over medium-low heat. Gradually add flour in 3 additions; cook, stirring constantly, 30 seconds after each addition. Cook, stirring constantly, 55 minutes or until roux is the color of milk chocolate.
2. Add onion and next 3 ingredients, stirring constantly, 30 seconds. Gradually stir in 5 cups Chicken Stock, reserving remaining stock for another use. Add sausage and next 8 ingredients. Bring to a boil; reduce heat, and simmer, uncovered, 40 minutes, stirring and skimming fat occasionally, until slightly thickened and coats the back of a spoon.
3. Stir in chicken; simmer 15 minutes. Stir in hot sauce, if desired. Discard bay leaf. Spoon rice into bowls; ladle gumbo over rice. **Makes: 7½ cups**

Chicken Stock

- 3 lb. chicken leg quarters
- 4 celery ribs, coarsely chopped
- 3 carrots, coarsely chopped
- 2 onions, coarsely chopped
- 1 bay leaf
- 1 tsp. black peppercorns
- 2 garlic cloves, peeled
- 1 fresh thyme sprig

1. Bring all ingredients and 3 qt. water to a boil in a large Dutch oven; reduce heat, and simmer, partially covered, 3 hours, adding water as needed to cover.

2. Pour broth through a wire-mesh strainer into a large bowl; discard solids. Cool completely (2 hours). Pour stock into freezer containers. Cover and chill up to 3 days, or freeze up to 3 months. **Makes: 9½ cups**

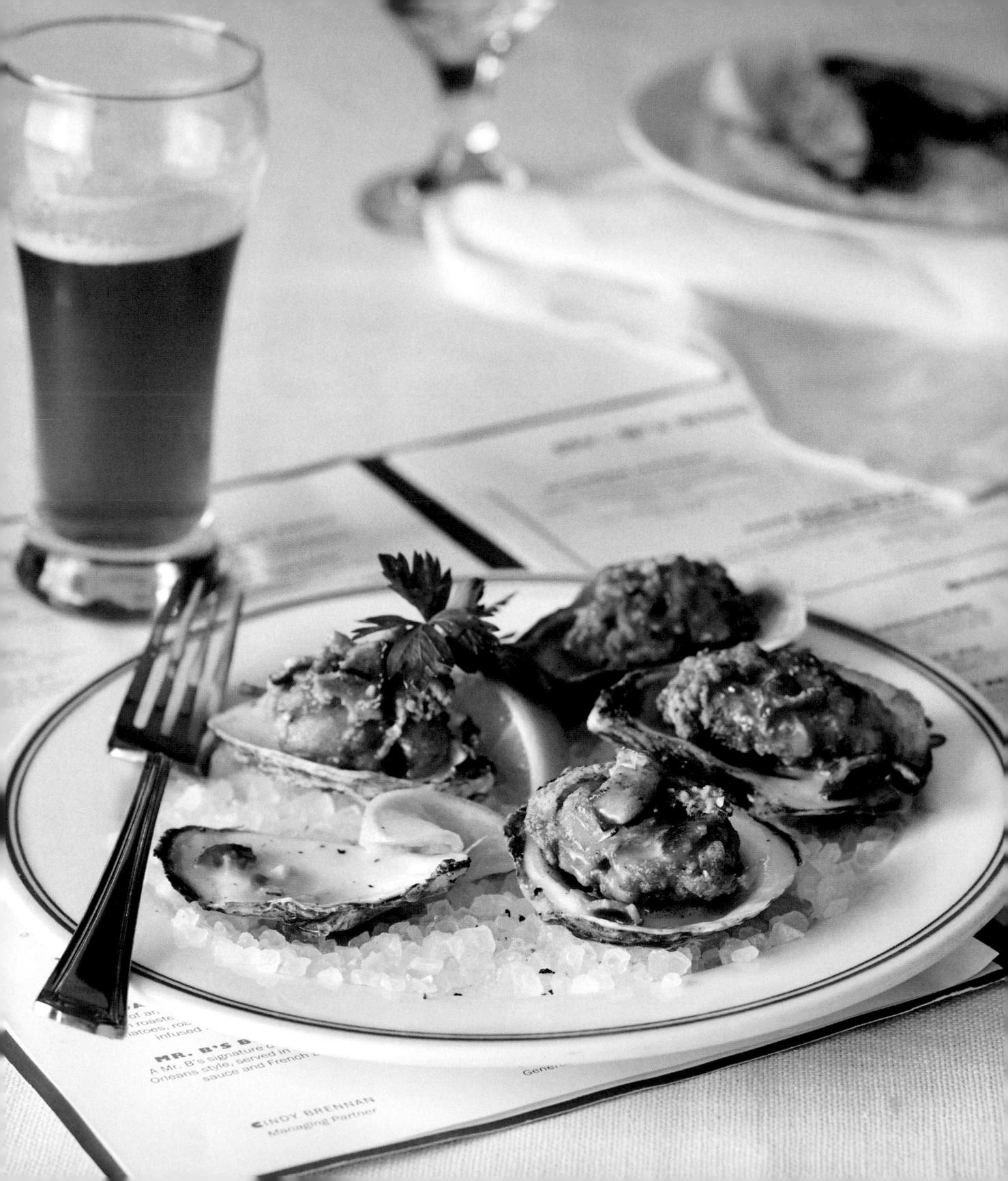

Fried Oysters on the Half Shell with Bacon Horseradish Hollandaise Sauce

The breading on these oysters gives just enough crunch to make them a meal, but it doesn't overpower the delicious taste of the sea.

FRIED OYSTERS

2	dozen fresh select oysters (about 1 pt.), drained
⅔	cup hot sauce
1	large egg, lightly beaten
	Canola oil
¼	tsp. table salt

BREADING

¾	cup all-purpose flour
½	cup instant masa harina (corn flour)
½	cup cornstarch
¼	cup plain yellow cornmeal
1	tsp. kosher salt
¾	tsp. granulated onion
¾	tsp. granulated garlic
¾	tsp. paprika
½	tsp. ground white pepper
½	tsp. chili powder

BACON HORSERADISH HOLLANDAISE SAUCE

1	large egg yolk
1	tsp. white wine
¼	cup cold unsalted butter, cut up
¼	tsp. table salt
1	hickory-smoked bacon slice, cooked and crumbled
¼	tsp. prepared horseradish
¼	tsp. hot sauce (optional)
6	cups rock salt
2	dozen oyster shells

Garnishes: lemon wedges, fresh parsley sprigs

1. Prepare Fried Oysters: Combine oysters, hot sauce, and egg in a large bowl. Cover and marinate in refrigerator 2 hours or up to overnight.

2. Pour oil to depth of 2 inches in a large heavy saucepan; heat to 350°.

3. Prepare Breading: Combine all ingredients in a shallow bowl. Drain oysters, discarding marinade. Dredge oysters in Breading, shaking off excess. Fry oysters in hot oil, in batches, 1½ minutes or until golden brown. Drain on paper towels; sprinkle with ¼ tsp. table salt.

4. Prepare Bacon Horseradish Hollandaise Sauce: Whisk together egg yolk, wine, and 2 tsp. water in a small bowl. Place over hot water (do not boil). Add butter, 1 Tbsp. at a time, whisking until smooth; whisk in salt. Cook, whisking constantly, 4 to 5 minutes or until thickened and a thermometer registers 160°. Remove bowl from over simmering water. Whisk in bacon and horseradish and, if desired, ¼ tsp. hot sauce.

5. Place 1½ cups rock salt on each of 4 plates. Place 1 fried oyster in each oyster shell. Top each oyster with about ½ tsp. Bacon Horseradish Hollandaise Sauce. Serve immediately. **Makes:** 4 servings

SOUNDTRACK:

"DOWN BY THE WATER" BY THE DECEMBERISTS

"BLUE TURNING GREY OVER YOU" BY LOUIS ARMSTRONG

"DE TEMPS EN TEMPS" BY JOSEPHINE BAKER

"IKO IKO" BY DR. JOHN

"KILLING ME SOFTLY" BY YOUNGBLOOD BRASS BAND

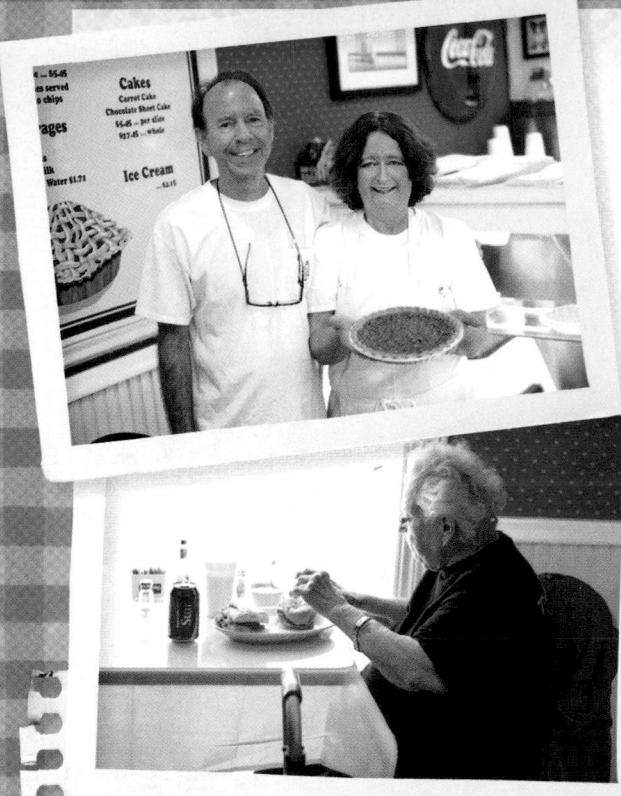

Not Just Pie

2117 Forsythe Avenue
Monroe, Louisiana 71201
(318) 322-9928

As the name of Christy, Jimmy, and their son J. Walter Stone's restaurant implies, Not Just Pie also serves other food. But let's be serious: It's mostly pie. And it's really unbelievably tasty pie. Like the big, fluffy slices of peach cream pie, or luscious pecan pie, banana chocolate cream pie, and fresh apple pie. Choosing just one slice is impossible. I suggest adopting what I call the "Give a Moose Diabetes Plan" and eating a slice of each at one sitting. And order a glass of milk for good measure.

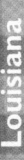

Quiche

Real men do eat quiche—at least the quiche at Not Just Pie. This flavorful version is hearty enough for any Y chromosome.

PIECRUST

1⅓ cups all-purpose flour
¼ cup cold butter, cut into pieces
¼ cup cold shortening, cut into pieces
¼ tsp. table salt
¼ cup ice water

FILLING

3 hickory-smoked bacon slices
1 (8-oz.) package fresh mushrooms, sliced
½ cup sliced green onions
6 oz. Swiss cheese, shredded
1 cup (¼-inch) cubed smoked fully cooked ham
3 large eggs
⅓ cup half-and-half
¼ tsp. table salt
¼ tsp. freshly ground black pepper
¼ tsp. dry mustard

1. **Prepare Piecrust:** Combine first 4 ingredients in the bowl of a food processor. Pulse until mixture resembles coarse meal but some larger, pea-sized pieces remain.
2. Sprinkle ice water, 1 Tbsp. at a time, over flour mixture, pulsing until dry ingredients are moistened. Shape dough into a flat disk; wrap in plastic wrap, and chill 1 hour.
3. Preheat oven to 350°. Roll dough into a 13-inch circle on a lightly floured surface. Fit piecrust into a 9-inch pie plate; fold edges under, and crimp. Line pastry with aluminum foil, and fill with pie weights or dried beans.
4. Bake at 350° for 15 minutes. Remove weights and foil, and bake 10 minutes or until bottom is golden brown. Cool completely on a wire rack (25 minutes).
5. **Prepare Filling:** Cook bacon in a large nonstick skillet over medium heat 7 minutes or until

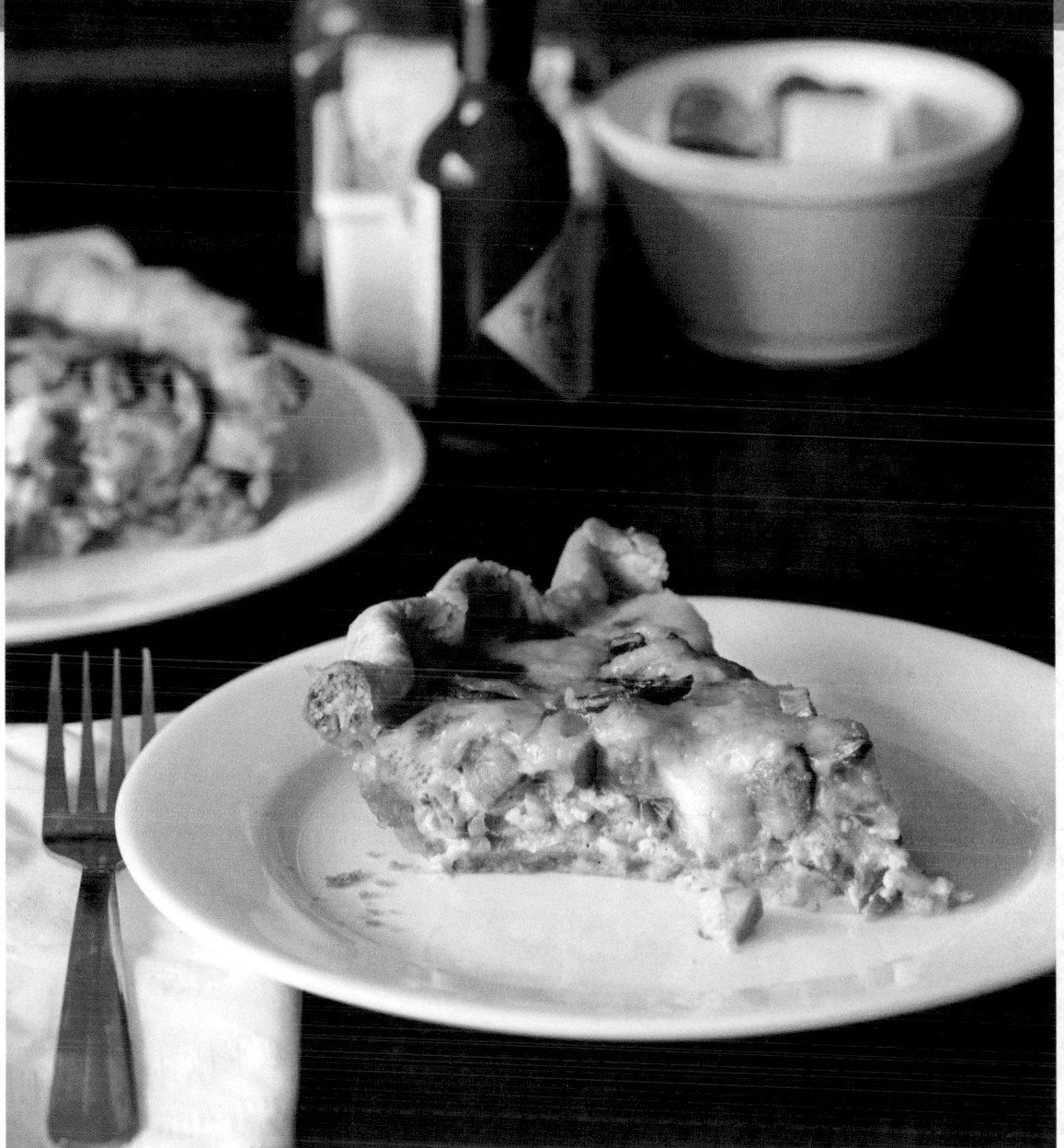

crisp; remove bacon, and drain on paper towels, reserving 1 Tbsp. drippings in skillet. Sauté mushrooms in hot drippings 6 minutes or until lightly browned. Stir in green onions.

6. Sprinkle half of cheese in bottom of crust; top with mushrooms, ham and remaining cheese.

7. Whisk together eggs and next 4 ingredients. Pour egg mixture over cheese mixture. Bake at 350° for 40 minutes or until set and top is browned. **Makes: 6 servings**

Pecan Pie

This simple pecan pie can be whipped up in a flash. Christy's trick of placing the pecans in the piecrust first keeps them evenly distributed.

PIECRUST
- 1⅓ cups all-purpose flour
- ¼ cup cold butter, cut into pieces
- ¼ cup cold shortening, cut into pieces
- ¼ tsp. table salt
- ¼ cup ice water

FILLING
- 1 cup sugar
- 1 Tbsp. all-purpose flour
- ½ cup butter, melted
- 2 large eggs
- ½ cup light corn syrup
- 1 tsp. vanilla extract
- 1½ cups chopped pecans

1. Prepare Piecrust: Combine first 4 ingredients in the bowl of a food processor. Pulse until mixture resembles coarse meal but some larger, pea-sized pieces remain.

2. Sprinkle ice water, 1 Tbsp. at a time, over flour mixture, pulsing just until dry ingredients are moistened. Shape dough into a flat disc; wrap in plastic wrap, and chill 1 hour.

3. Preheat oven to 350°. Roll dough into a 13-inch circle on a lightly floured surface. Fit into a 9-inch pie plate; fold edges under, and crimp.

4. Prepare Filling: Whisk together sugar and flour in a large bowl. Whisk in melted butter. Add eggs, 1 at a time, whisking until blended after each addition. Whisk in corn syrup and vanilla.

5. Sprinkle pecans in bottom of pie crust. Pour egg mixture over pecans. Bake at 350° for 48 minutes or until set and browned. Cool completely on a wire rack (2 hours). **Makes: 8 servings**

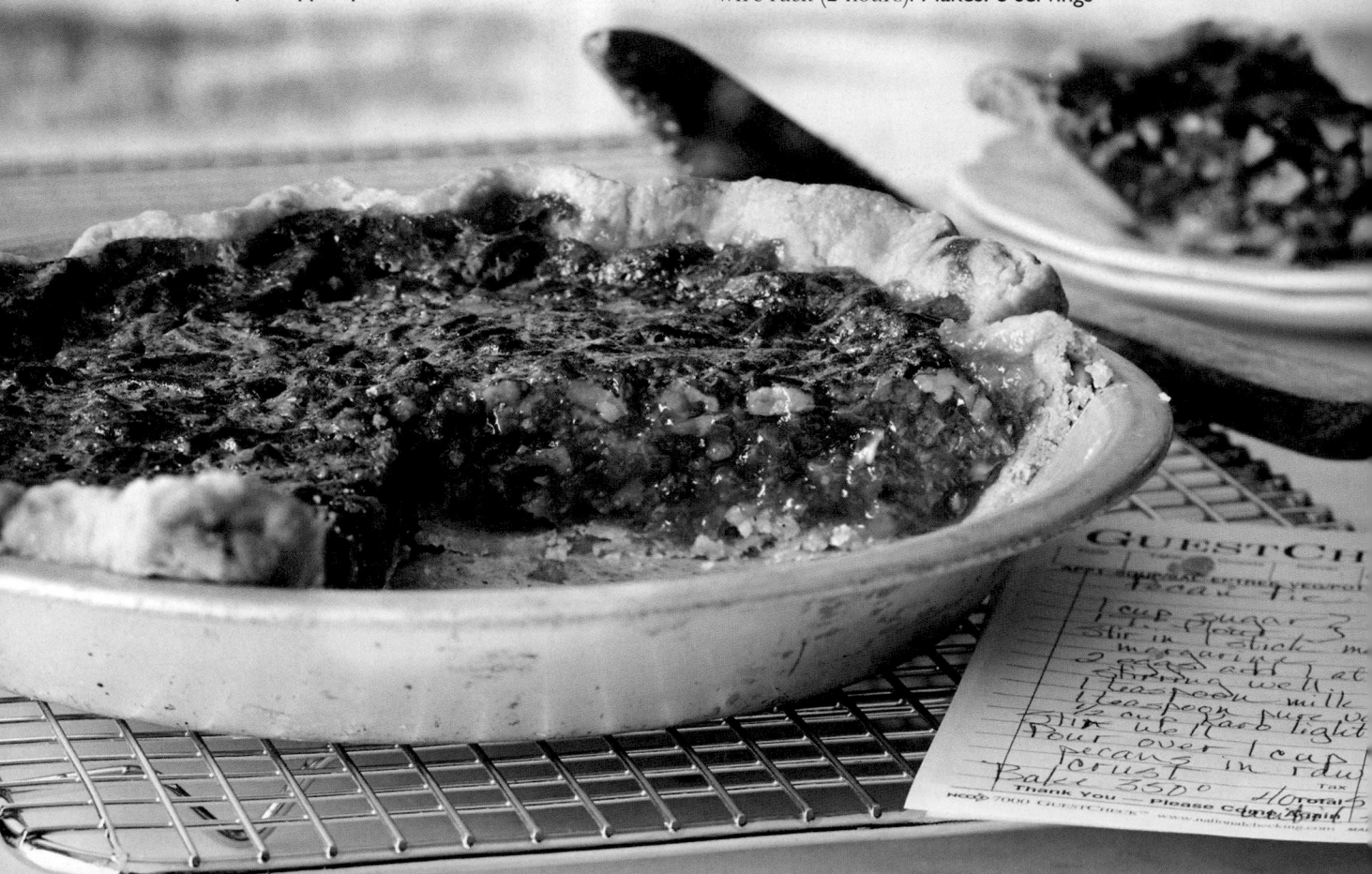

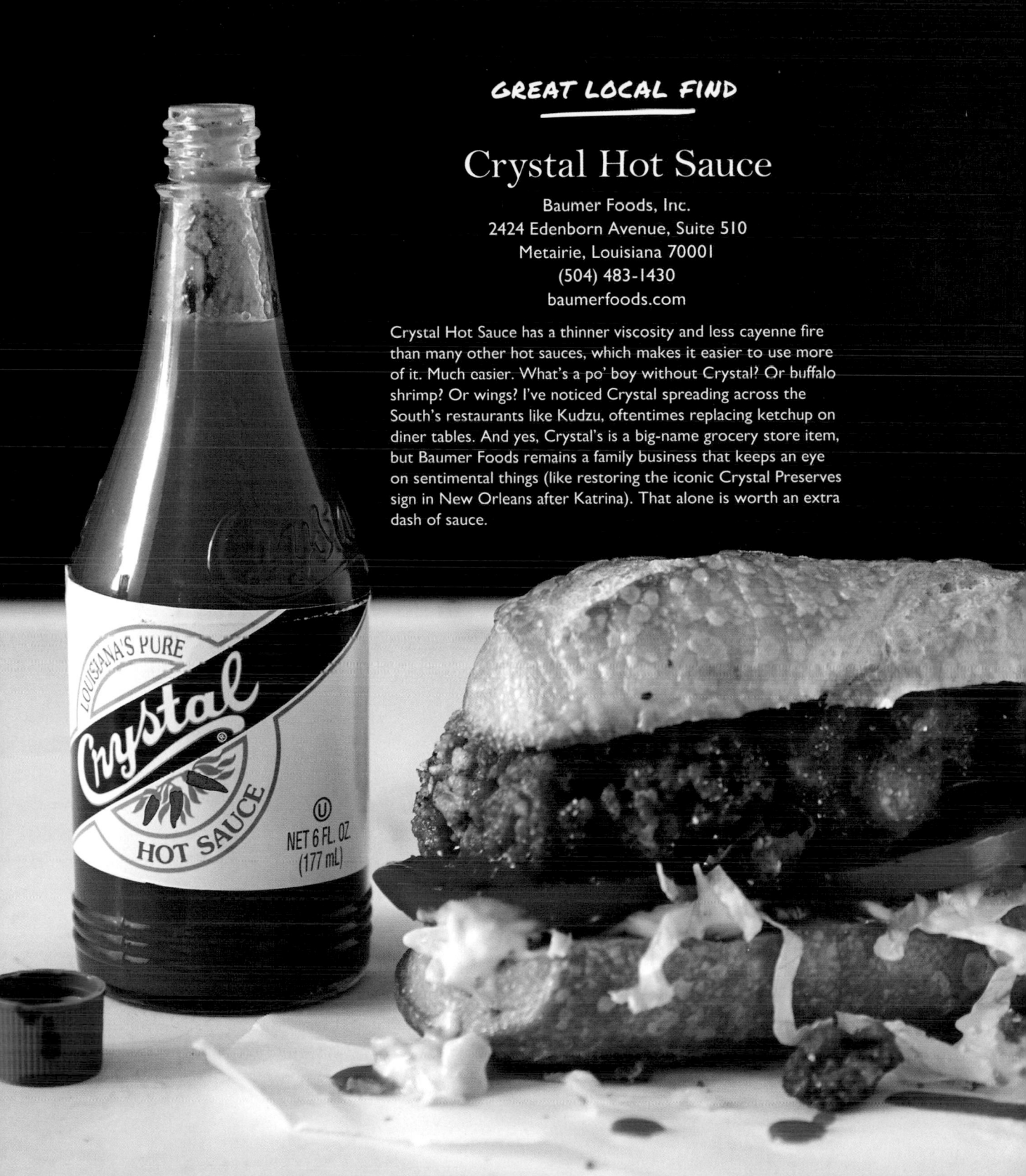

Crystal Hot Sauce

Baumer Foods, Inc.
2424 Edenborn Avenue, Suite 510
Metairie, Louisiana 70001
(504) 483-1430
baumerfoods.com

Crystal Hot Sauce has a thinner viscosity and less cayenne fire than many other hot sauces, which makes it easier to use more of it. Much easier. What's a po' boy without Crystal? Or buffalo shrimp? Or wings? I've noticed Crystal spreading across the South's restaurants like Kudzu, oftentimes replacing ketchup on diner tables. And yes, Crystal's is a big-name grocery store item, but Baumer Foods remains a family business that keeps an eye on sentimental things (like restoring the iconic Crystal Preserves sign in New Orleans after Katrina). That alone is worth an extra dash of sauce.

Willie Mae's Scotch House

2401 St. Ann Street
New Orleans, Louisiana 70119
(504) 822-9503

My friend Kerry Seaton comes from a long line of cooks—her great-grandmother, Willie Mae Seaton, opened her doors in New Orleans in 1957. Although Willie Mae, who is approaching a century of living, doesn't come into the restaurant any longer, Kerry continues her tradition of wowing diners in the culinary capital of the South. The fried chicken, which is made with her great-grandmother's secret wet batter, defies the hot sauce and sticky sweet trends. It is simple, but incredibly moist, tender, and flaky with a little touch of Creole heat. "You can wait or you can go, baby," Willie Mae says. And there will be a wait at the Scotch House—word is out among foodies, but the wait is worth it. For the fried chicken, or for Kerry's own bread pudding recipe, which cajoles with white chocolate, rum, and New Orleans's fabulous French bread. And it's worth waiting for Willie Mae's butter beans. The Scotch House elevates this humble Southern staple to a plane all its own. They taste meaty, despite being cooked vegetarian. They'll be a new staple in my house for sure.

Willie Mae's Butter Beans

Serve these big beans with a little rice and cornbread, like they do at Willie Mae's, and you've got yourself a simple, Southern meal.

1	lb. large dried lima beans
3	Tbsp. olive oil, divided
1¼	tsp. table salt, divided
3	bay leaves
1½	cups chopped onion
1	cup chopped green bell pepper
½	cup chopped celery
½	tsp. ground white pepper
½	tsp. Cajun seasoning
2	Tbsp. chopped fresh parsley

1. Rinse and sort beans according to package directions. Place beans in a Dutch oven; cover with water 2 inches above beans. Let soak 8 hours. Drain.
2. Return beans to Dutch oven; add 2 Tbsp. oil, 1 tsp. salt, bay leaves, and 6 cups water. Bring to a boil; reduce heat, partially cover, and cook 1 hour or until beans are creamy.
3. Heat remaining 1 Tbsp. oil in a large skillet. Add onion and next 4 ingredients; sauté 6 minutes or until vegetables are tender. Stir vegetable mixture and remaining ¼ tsp. salt into beans. Bring to a boil; cover, reduce heat, and cook 15 minutes, stirring often. Gradually add about ½ cup water, stirring until mixture is thinned slightly and creamy. Stir in parsley. **Makes: 8 servings**

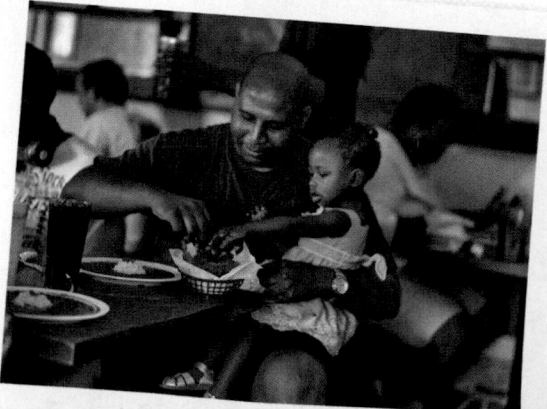

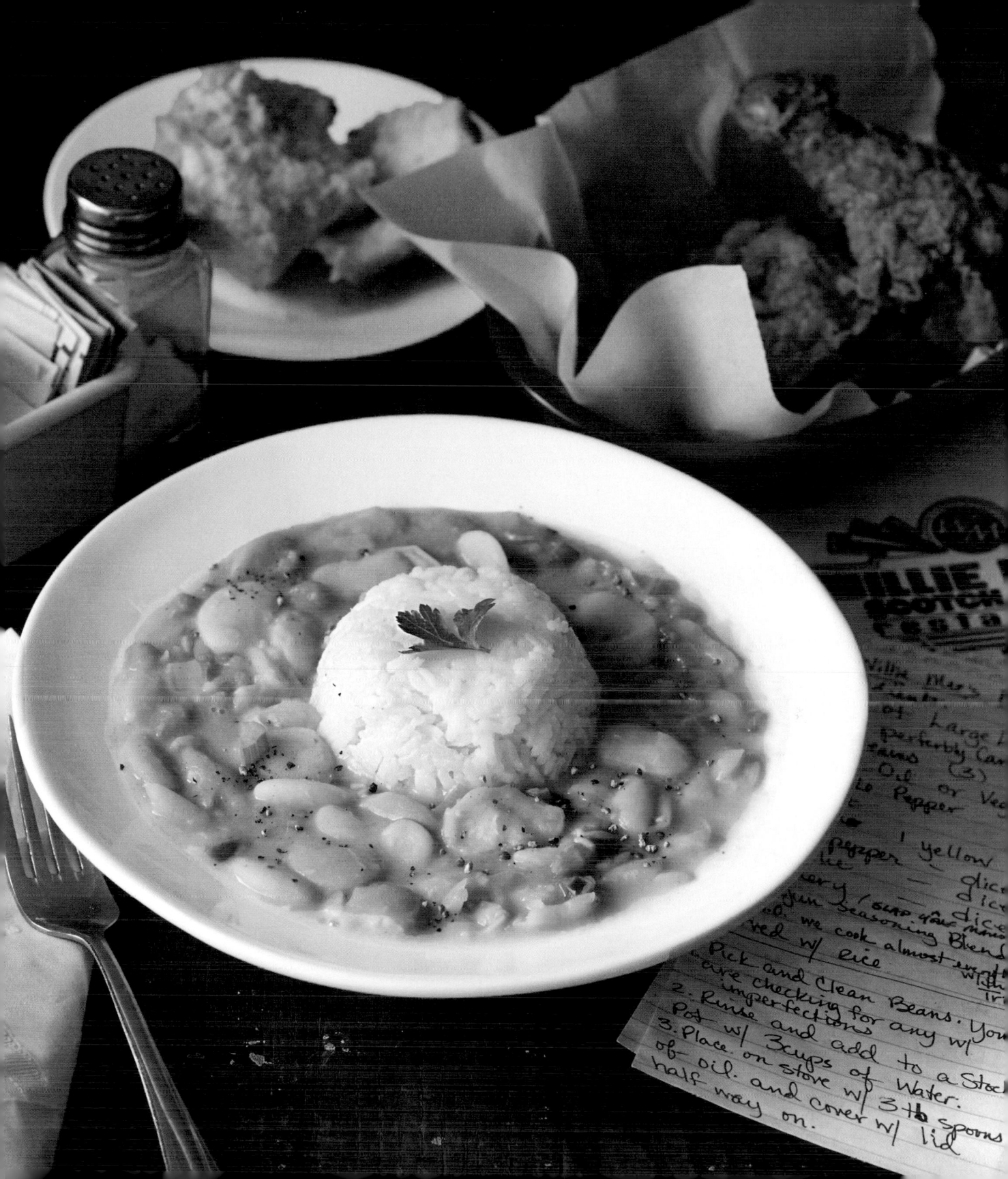

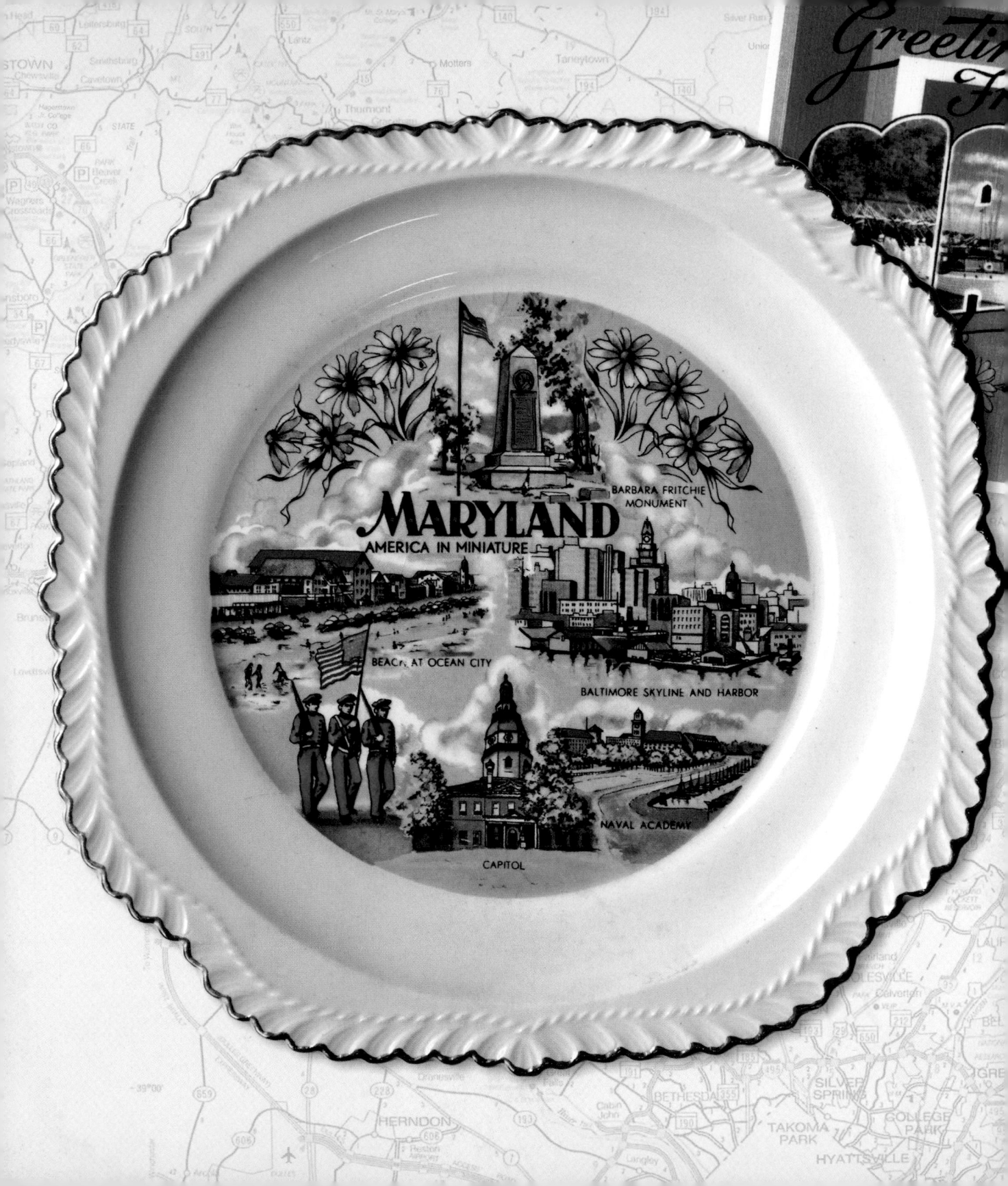

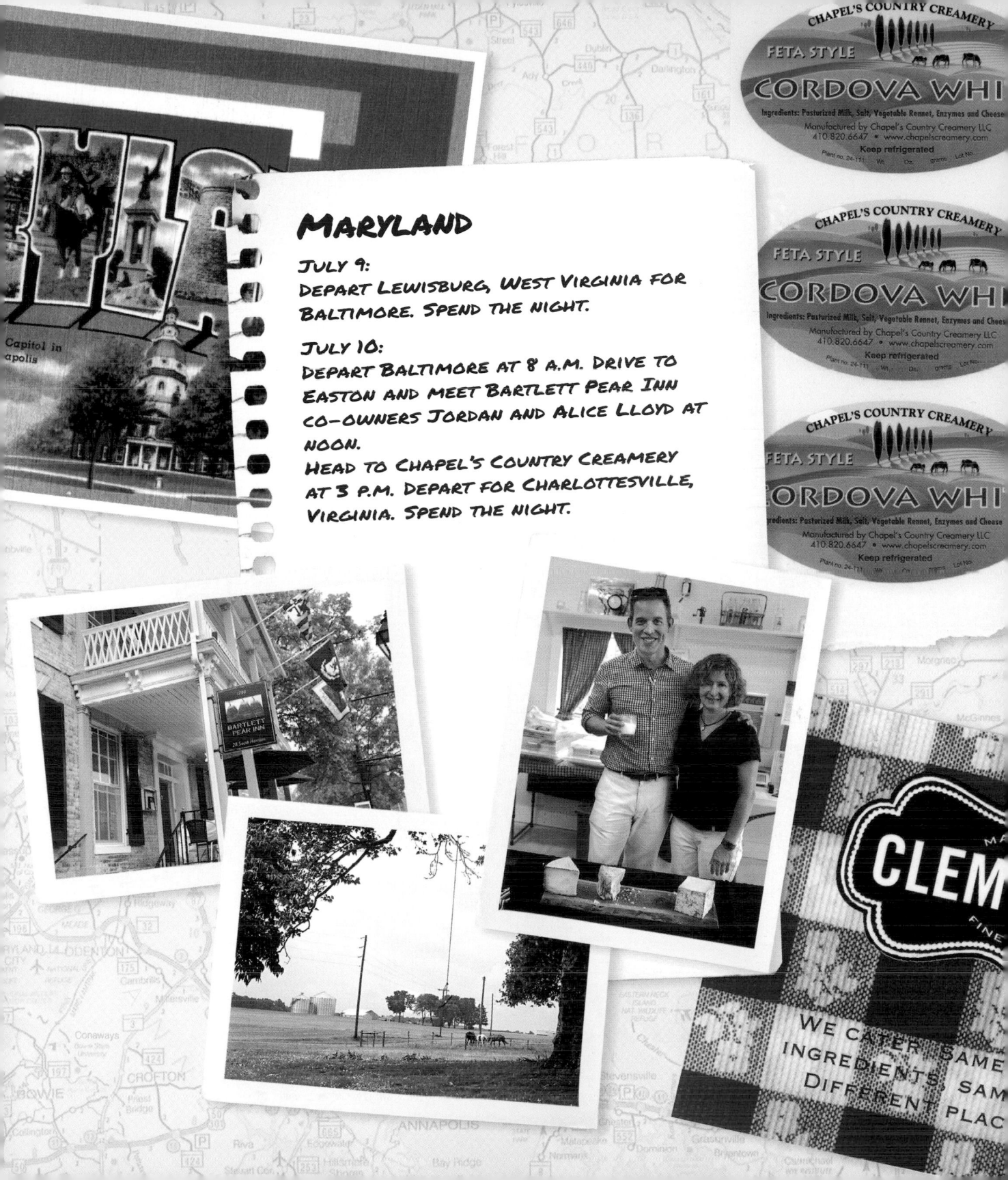

MARYLAND

JULY 9:
DEPART LEWISBURG, WEST VIRGINIA FOR BALTIMORE. SPEND THE NIGHT.

JULY 10:
DEPART BALTIMORE AT 8 A.M. DRIVE TO EASTON AND MEET BARTLETT PEAR INN CO-OWNERS JORDAN AND ALICE LLOYD AT NOON.
HEAD TO CHAPEL'S COUNTRY CREAMERY AT 3 P.M. DEPART FOR CHARLOTTESVILLE, VIRGINIA. SPEND THE NIGHT.

CHAPEL'S COUNTRY CREAMERY
FETA STYLE
CORDOVA WHI
Ingredients: Pasturized Milk, Salt, Vegetable Rennet, Enzymes and Cheese
Manufactured by Chapel's Country Creamery LLC
410.820.6647 • www.chapelscreamery.com
Keep refrigerated
Plant no. 24-111

CLEM

WE CATER SAME
INGREDIENTS, SAM
DIFFERENT PLAC

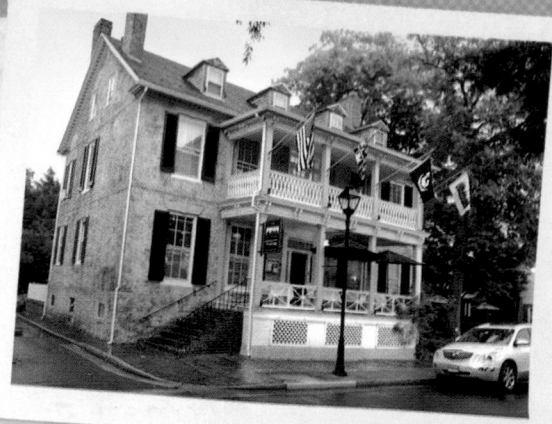

Bartlett Pear Inn

28 South Harrison Street
Easton, Maryland 21601
(410) 770-3300
bartlettpearinn.com

If you want to create a romantic restaurant, it helps to be a romantic at heart. Bartlett Pear Inn co-owners Jordan and Alice Lloyd met in the fourth grade, became childhood sweethearts, and reunited in the restaurant business years later. Jordan brings inventive passion to the plate. He's a dynamo with his own garden, bakery, and ice cream operation. Alice designed the Bartlett Pear in a home built during George Washington's presidency to be sophisticated and inviting. Though the menu changes daily, most everything is fresh and local. Jordan concentrates on the food, not the latest trends. "There are some guys who know how to float a piece of meat in a bag for 36 hours but can't braise," he says. An emphasis on classic cuisine and local farmers makes the Bartlett Pear Inn a must-stop on the Eastern Shore.

Wild Striped Bass Meunière

Striped bass is one of my favorite fishes, and this recipe ranks up there with some of the best I've tried.

2	(10-oz.) skin-on striped bass fillet (½ inch thick)
½	Tbsp. kosher salt
2	Tbsp. canola oil
¾	cup unsalted butter
2	Tbsp. lemon juice
3	Tbsp. chopped fresh flat-leaf parsley

Potato Gnocchi (facing page)

1. Let fish stand at room temperature 20 minutes to ensure even cooking and to prevent fish from sticking to pan when searing.
2. Pat fish dry with paper towels, and sprinkle with salt. Heat oil in a heavy skillet over medium-high heat. Add fish to pan, skin side down. Cook 3 minutes or until browned. Reduce heat to medium. Turn fish over; cook 2 minutes or until fish flakes easily with a fork. Transfer fish to a serving platter; cover with aluminum foil to keep warm. Discard oil in pan.
3. Return pan to medium heat; add butter. Cook 4 minutes or just until butter browns and develops a nutty aroma. Remove from heat; stir in lemon juice and parsley. Drizzle fish with browned butter mixture. Serve fish with Potato Gnocchi. **Makes: 4 servings**

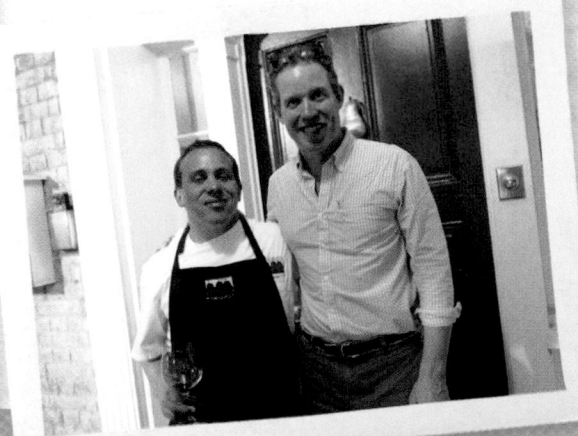

Potato Gnocchi

Heat is your friend when it comes to making gnocchi. If the potato mixture gets cold or even lukewarm before the finished dough is made, the resulting product will be gummy and disappointing.

1   (13-oz.) russet potato
Table salt
½   cup (2 oz.) freshly grated Parmigiano-Reggiano cheese
1   large egg, room temperature
1   large egg yolk, room temperature
½   cup plus 2 Tbsp. all-purpose flour
½   tsp. table salt

1. Preheat oven to 450°. Scrub potato under cold running water. Pat damp dry with paper towels. Generously rub surface of potato with desired amount of salt, and place in a small baking pan lined with aluminum foil. Bake at 450° for 1 hour or until tender.

2. Scoop out hot potato pulp and press through a potato ricer into a warm bowl. Whisk together cheese, egg, and egg yolk. Add to potato. Add flour and ½ tsp. salt; stir, adding additional flour if needed, until dough is pliable and not too dry, but not sticky. Divide dough into 4 equal portions. Roll each portion into a 12-inch-long rope, approximately ½ inch in diameter. Cut ropes at 1-inch intervals.

3. Cook gnocchi, in 2 batches, in boiling salted water in a large Dutch oven 3 minutes or until gnocchi float to surface. Remove gnocchi from boiling water with a long-handled strainer or large slotted spoon, and place on a well-oiled baking pan. Reheat with desired sauce.

Makes: 4 servings

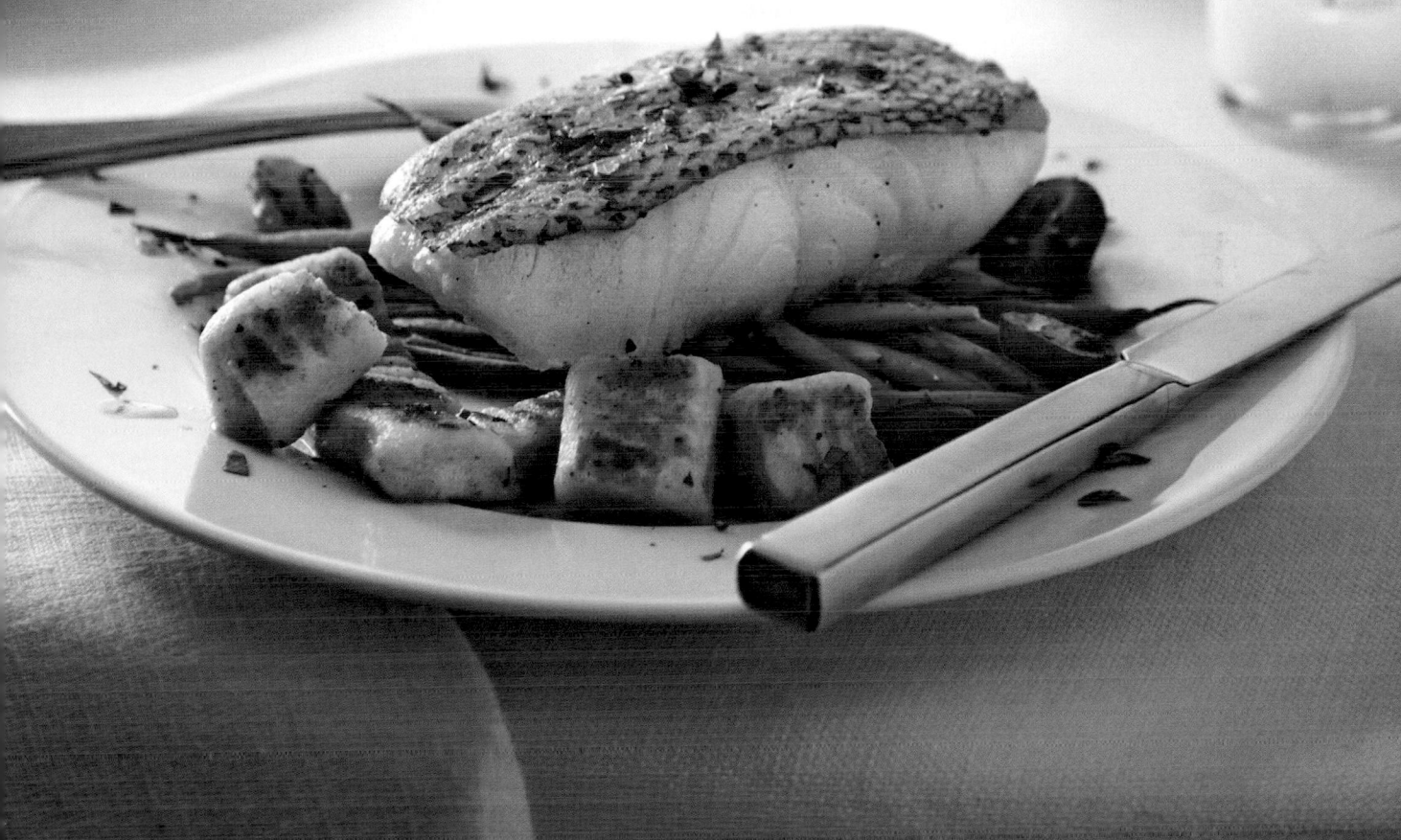

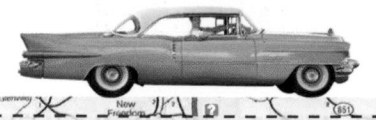

Maryland
bucket list
things to see and do (besides eat) here

1 Tour the gorgeous grounds at the **United States Naval Academy** at Annapolis, or simply wander the quaint streets of the capital.

2 Charter a **sailboat** *(pictured)* in St. Michaels to see the beauty of Maryland's Eastern Shore from the water.

3 Hike up **South Mountain** in Middletown to see the first Washington Monument, erected 58 years before the National Mall's version.

4 Stroll **Fell's Point**, a Colonial-era and waterfront neighborhood in Baltimore with great shopping, cool bars, and magnificent architecture.

5 Catch an Orioles game at **Camden Yards**, the stunning brick Major League Baseball stadium. It sits just a few blocks from Baltimore's **Inner Harbor**, a post-industrial waterfront redevelopment where you can shop, eat, and explore.

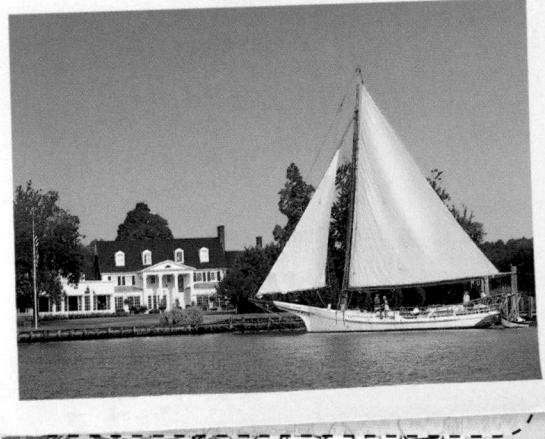

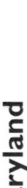 **Maryland**

Hummingbird Farms Tomato Gazpacho

RED GAZPACHO

4	cups chopped red tomato (1½ lb.)
1¼	cups chopped red bell pepper
¾	cup chopped peeled cucumber
½	cup sliced celery
⅓	cup chopped red onion
¼	cup extra virgin olive oil
3	Tbsp. red wine vinegar
1	Tbsp. tomato paste
1	tsp. Espelette spice
2	tsp. Dijon mustard
¾	tsp. table salt
15	fresh cilantro leaves
2	garlic cloves

YELLOW GAZPACHO

4	cups chopped yellow tomato (1½ lb.)
1¼	cups chopped yellow bell pepper
¾	cup chopped peeled cucumber
½	cup sliced celery
⅓	cup chopped red onion
2	garlic cloves
¼	cup extra virgin olive oil
2	Tbsp. white wine vinegar
1	tsp. Dijon mustard
15	fresh cilantro leaves
½	tsp. Espelette spice
1	tsp. table salt

Accompaniments: tomato-and-garlic-rubbed baguettes

1. **Prepare Red Gazpacho:** Combine all ingredients in a blender. Blend on high speed until smooth. Cover and chill at least 2 hours.

2. **Prepare Yellow Gazpacho:** Repeat procedure as for Red Gazpacho.

3. About 30 minutes before serving, place soups in freezer until super cold. Carefully pour both soups into 8 bowls to create yin and yang design. Serve with baguettes. **Makes: 8 servings**

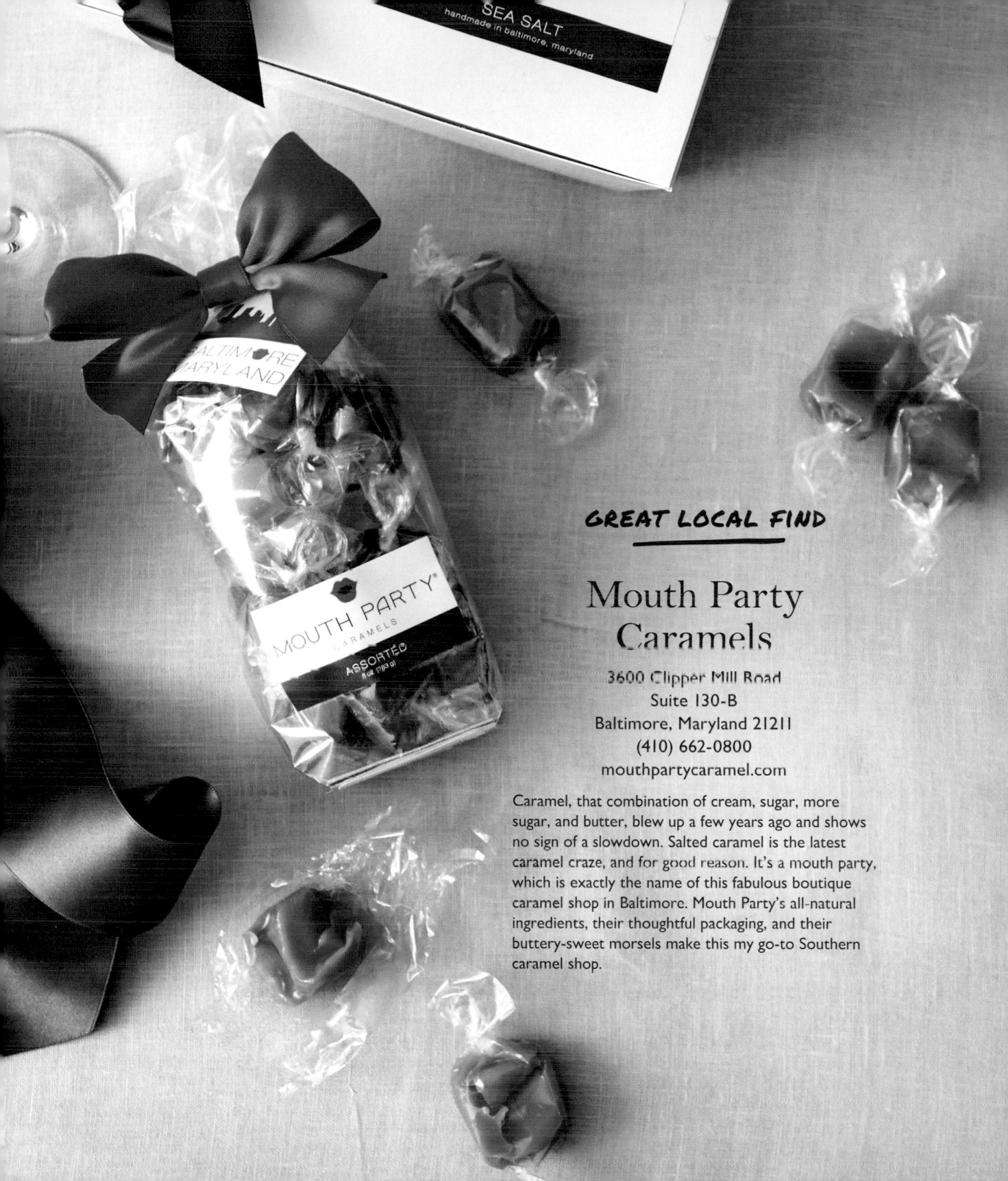

GREAT LOCAL FIND

Mouth Party
Caramels

3600 Clipper Mill Road
Suite 130-B
Baltimore, Maryland 21211
(410) 662-0800
mouthpartycaramel.com

Caramel, that combination of cream, sugar, more sugar, and butter, blew up a few years ago and shows no sign of a slowdown. Salted caramel is the latest caramel craze, and for good reason. It's a mouth party, which is exactly the name of this fabulous boutique caramel shop in Baltimore. Mouth Party's all-natural ingredients, their thoughtful packaging, and their buttery-sweet morsels make this my go-to Southern caramel shop.

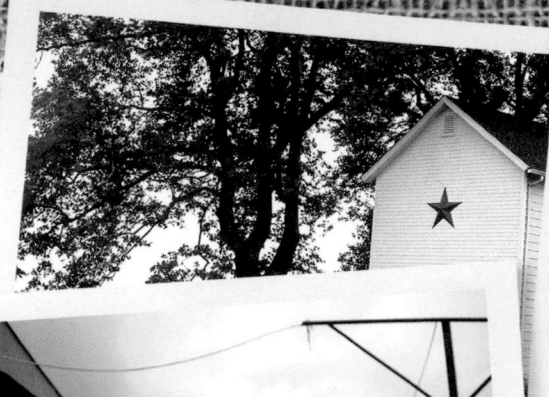

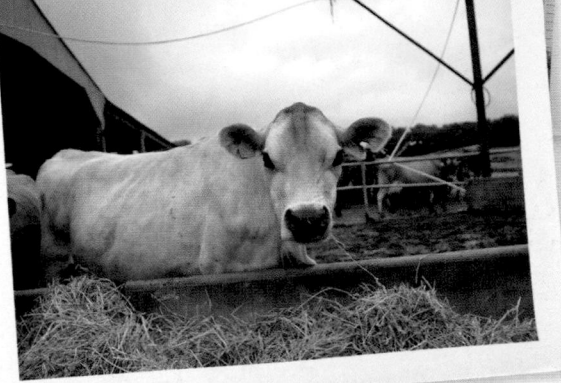

Chapel's Country Creamery

10380 Chapel Road
Easton, Maryland 21601
(410) 820-6647
chapelscreamery.com

Walk around this dairy farm with owner and mother of four, Holly Foster and you'll wonder how she does so much. Her 60 happy cows provide the milk for some of the best cheeses I've ever tasted. The cave-aged Cheddar pleases with a creamy earthiness; the classic blue thumps the back of your throat with a crisp tang; but the Chapelle is my favorite. Holy cow. It's salty and creamy, and made me put Holly on speed dial. These results come from a healthy farm—go see for yourself.

Cheddar Ale Soup

¼	cup butter
1¼	cups finely diced onion
½	cup finely diced celery
¾	cup finely diced carrot
⅓	cup all-purpose flour
1¾	cups milk
1¾	cups chicken stock
1	(12-oz.) bottle ale
2	tsp. Worcestershire sauce
1½	tsp. dry mustard
8	oz. Chapel Cave Aged Cheddar cheese, grated
8	oz. Chapel Cheddar or Chapel Colby, grated
4	oz. Chapel Crab Spice Cheddar cheese, grated
½	tsp. Old Bay seasoning
½	tsp. table salt
¼	tsp. ground red pepper

Crushed pretzel sticks

1. Melt butter in a large Dutch oven over medium-low heat. Add onion, celery, and carrot; cook, stirring constantly, 10 minutes or until very tender. Stir in flour; cook, stirring constantly, 3 minutes.

2. Increase heat to medium high; whisk in milk and chicken stock. Bring to a simmer, stirring constantly. Cook, stirring often, 5 minutes or until mixture coats the back of a spoon.

3. Process soup in a blender (with center cap removed to allow steam to escape) until smooth; strain and return to pan. Stir in ale, Worcestershire sauce, and dry mustard. Simmer 5 minutes. Remove from heat.

4. Add cheeses, ½ cup at a time, whisking constantly until cheese melts, after each addition. Whisk in Old Bay seasoning, salt, and ground red pepper. Ladle into bowls; top with desired amount of crushed pretzels. **Makes: 6 cups**

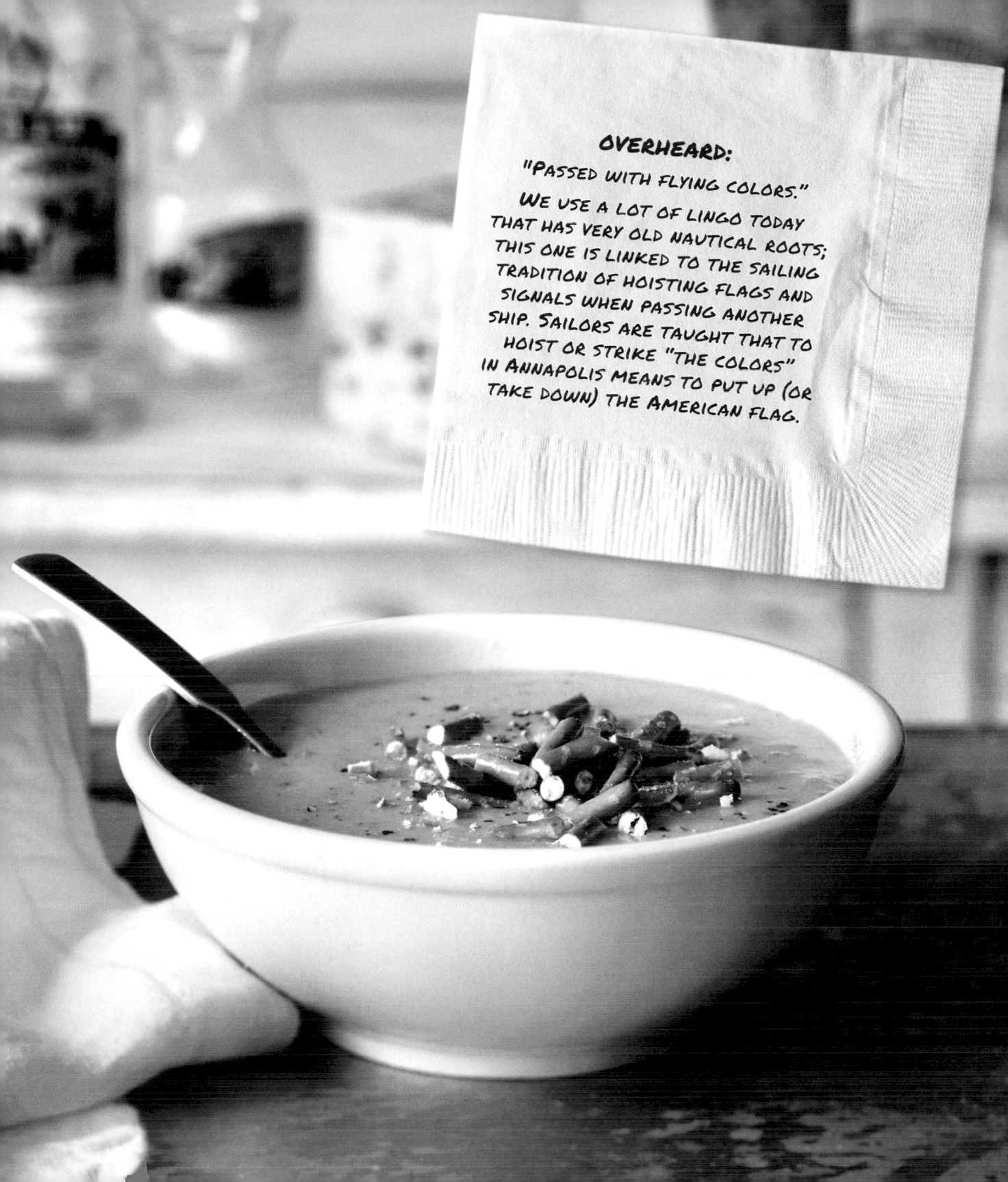

OVERHEARD:
"PASSED WITH FLYING COLORS."
WE USE A LOT OF LINGO TODAY THAT HAS VERY OLD NAUTICAL ROOTS; THIS ONE IS LINKED TO THE SAILING TRADITION OF HOISTING FLAGS AND SIGNALS WHEN PASSING ANOTHER SHIP. SAILORS ARE TAUGHT THAT TO HOIST OR STRIKE "THE COLORS" IN ANNAPOLIS MEANS TO PUT UP (OR TAKE DOWN) THE AMERICAN FLAG.

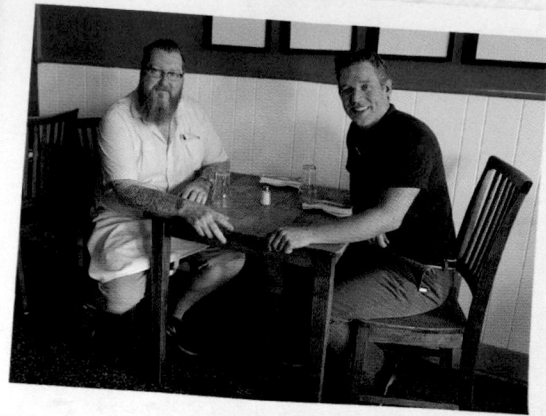

Clementine

5402 Harford Road
Baltimore, Maryland 21214
clementinebaltimore.com
(410) 444-1497

"This is poor people food, and I like that," says Clementine's co-owner Winston Blick. He and wife, Cristin Dadant (one of the state's finest bartenders), co-founded this urban hotspot in 2008. Clementine, with its heart-pine floors, warm-colored walls, and easy-chair feel, is my favorite spot to eat in Baltimore. And the foods Winston is passionate about are classics like sausage, pâté, and even sloppy Joes. Sure, there's crab on the menu, but there are also hearty dishes of pheasant, duck, pork, and the most amazing homemade ice cream. Large portions attract loyal customers (players on the Baltimore Orioles are regulars). Winston scours Maryland for the finest vegetables, meats, and cheeses, and you will definitely taste the results of his culinary scavenger hunts.

Mashed Potatoes

¾ cup (¼-inch) diced onion
4 Yukon gold potatoes (2 lb.), peeled and cut into 1½-inch chunks
1 (10-oz.) russet potato, peeled and cut into 1½-inch chunks
2 garlic cloves, peeled
½ cup heavy cream, warmed
3 Tbsp. butter
1 tsp. kosher salt
2 oz. smoked Gouda cheese, shredded
Garnish: chopped fresh chives

1. Cook first 4 ingredients in a large saucepan in boiling salted water to cover 15 minutes or until potato is tender. Drain and return to pan.
2. Add cream, butter, and salt. Mash with a potato masher to desired consistency. Add cheese, stirring until cheese melts. Serve immediately.
Makes: 6 servings

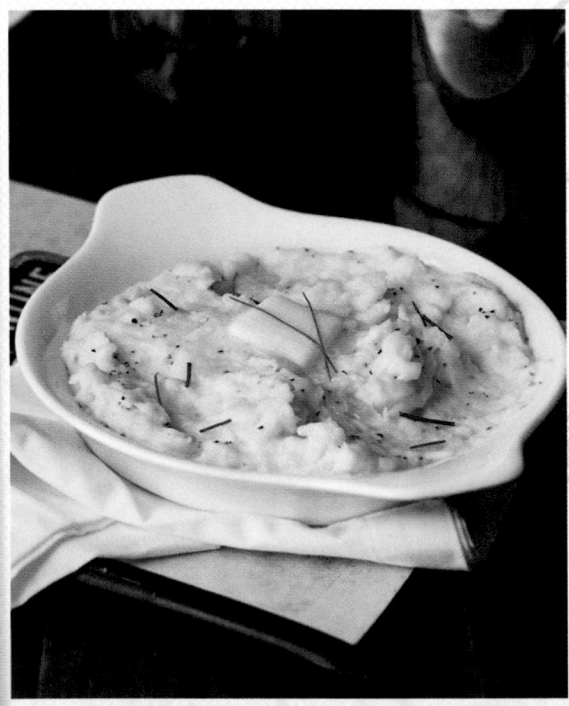

Rabbit Pappardelle

You may think rabbit tastes like chicken, but this is a tad sweeter and more tender.

1.   (3-lb.) whole rabbit, quartered
½   tsp. table salt
¼   tsp. freshly ground black pepper
1   carrot, cut into 1-inch pieces
½   turnip, cut into 1-inch pieces
1   (8.82-oz.) package dried pappardelle pasta
1   Tbsp. olive oil
1   (6-oz.) package assorted colors baby carrots, halved horizontally
½   cup frozen baby sweet peas, unthawed
1   Tbsp. canola oil
¼   cup cold butter, cut up
Chopped fresh chives

1. Sprinkle rabbit quarters with ½ tsp. salt and ¼ tsp. pepper; place on a plate. Chill, uncovered, 1 hour. Bring rabbit legs, carrot pieces, turnip, and water to cover to a boil in a large saucepan; reduce heat to medium, and cook 40 minutes or until rabbit is tender. Remove from heat, and skim off foam. Drain, reserving ¼ cup broth Cool rabbit slightly.

2. Remove meat from rabbit legs; shred meat using 2 forks, and place in a bowl; discard bones.

3. Cook pasta according to package directions in a Dutch oven; drain, reserving pasta water in Dutch oven. Spread drained pasta on a 15- x 10-inch jelly-roll pan. Toss with olive oil. Return pasta water to a boil. Cook baby carrots in boiling pasta water 5 minutes or until tender. Remove vegetables with a slotted spoon. Add baby peas to boiling pasta water; cook 30 seconds. Drain.

4. Heat a medium cast-iron skillet over medium-high heat until hot. Add canola oil to hot skillet, swirling skillet to coat bottom. Add rabbit loins; sear 2 minutes on each side for medium-rare.

Remove skillet from heat. Cover and let rabbit stand 2 minutes.

5. Heat reserved broth in a small skillet over medium heat. Gradually whisk in butter until a sauce forms.

6. Combine pasta, carrots, peas, shredded rabbit, and butter sauce in a bowl. Season with salt and pepper to taste. Top with rabbit loins and chives.

Makes: 4 servings

Maryland

115

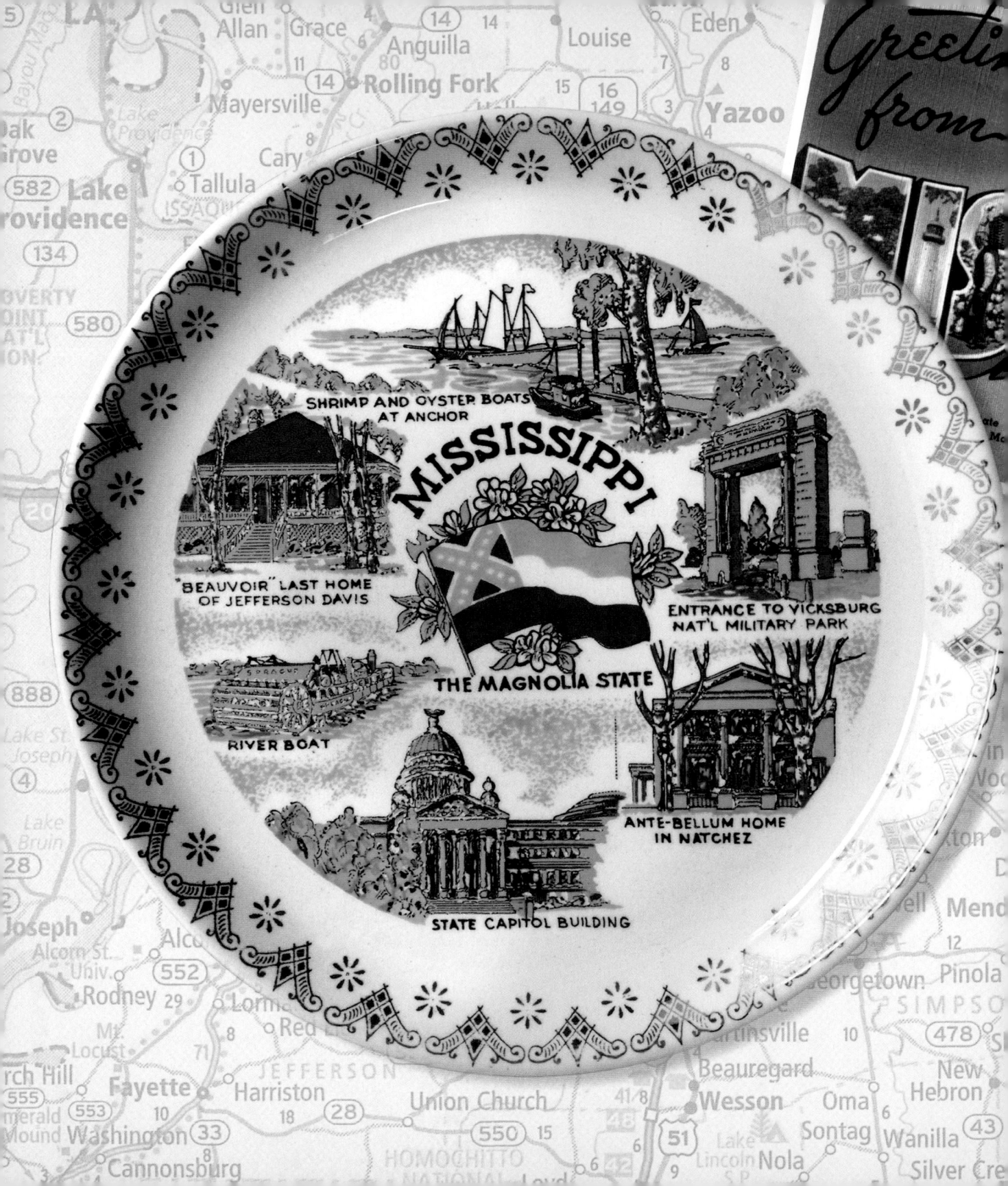

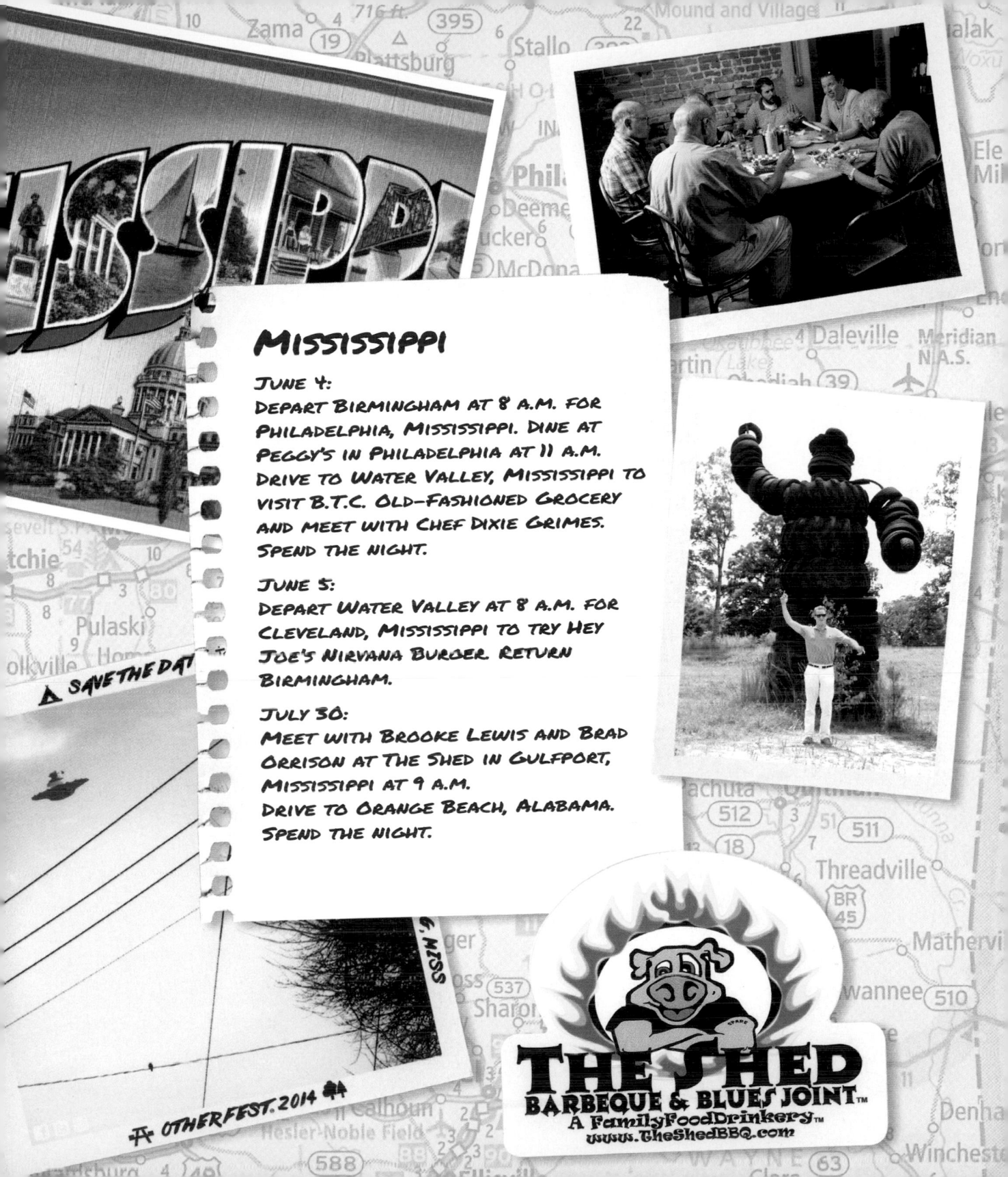

Mississippi

June 4:
Depart Birmingham at 8 a.m. for Philadelphia, Mississippi. Dine at Peggy's in Philadelphia at 11 a.m. Drive to Water Valley, Mississippi to visit B.T.C. Old-Fashioned Grocery and meet with Chef Dixie Grimes. Spend the night.

June 5:
Depart Water Valley at 8 a.m. for Cleveland, Mississippi to try Hey Joe's Nirvana Burger. Return Birmingham.

July 30:
Meet with Brooke Lewis and Brad Orrison at The Shed in Gulfport, Mississippi at 9 a.m. Drive to Orange Beach, Alabama. Spend the night.

THE SHED
BARBEQUE & BLUES JOINT™
A FamilyFoodDrinkery™
www.TheShedBBQ.com

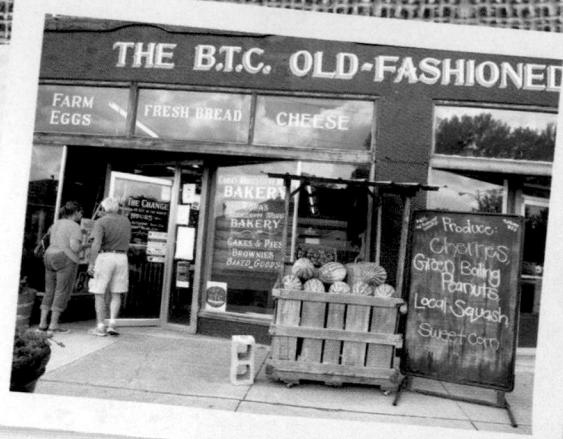

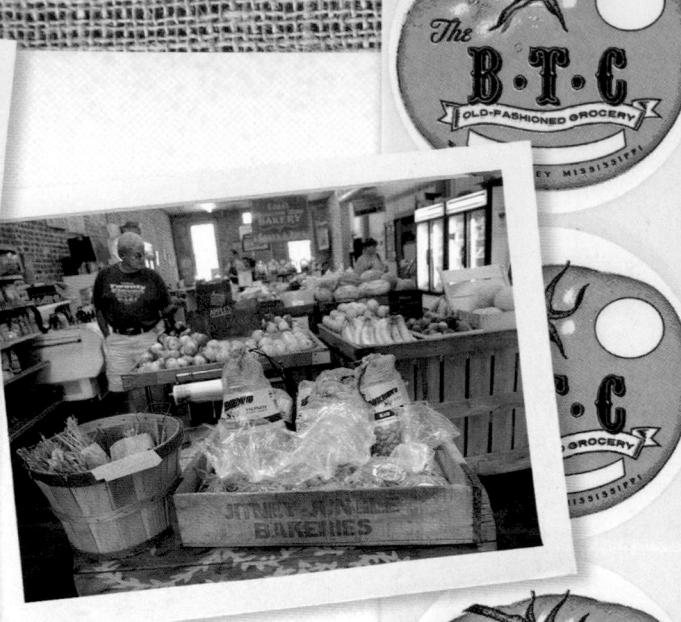

B.T.C.
Old-Fashioned
Grocery

301 North Main Street
Water Valley, Mississippi 38965
(662) 473-4323
btcgrocery.com

Any restaurant with a chef named Dixie, a commitment to making everything from scratch, and a table reserved for "The Old Men's Club" ranks high in my book. B.T.C.'s founder and co-owner, Alexe van Beuren named the neighborhood restaurant/market after Gandhi's quote, "Be the change," and B.T.C. has been a positive change in tiny Water Valley. Linger long enough and you'll probably see most of the town residents—most come for Chef Dixie Grimes's food, like her Delta Grind grits. There's enough butter in these to make Paula Deen blush. The fresh peanuts by the cash register and Coca-Cola in glass bottles complete this authentic grocery.

Tex-Mex Pimiento Cheese

Think of this as your basic pimiento cheese with a kick.

½	cup mayonnaise
¼	cup sour cream
¼	cup chopped drained pimientos
¼	cup chopped seeded jalapeño peppers
1	Tbsp. fresh lime juice
1	tsp. onion powder
¼	tsp. ground cumin
¼	tsp. chili powder
¼	tsp. table salt
¼	tsp. freshly ground black pepper
Pinch of sugar	
1	lb. pepper Jack cheese, shredded

Stir together all ingredients in a medium bowl. Cover and chill 4 hours before serving. Store, covered, in refrigerator up to 1 week.

Makes: 4 cups

Note: We tested with Hellmann's Mayonnaise.

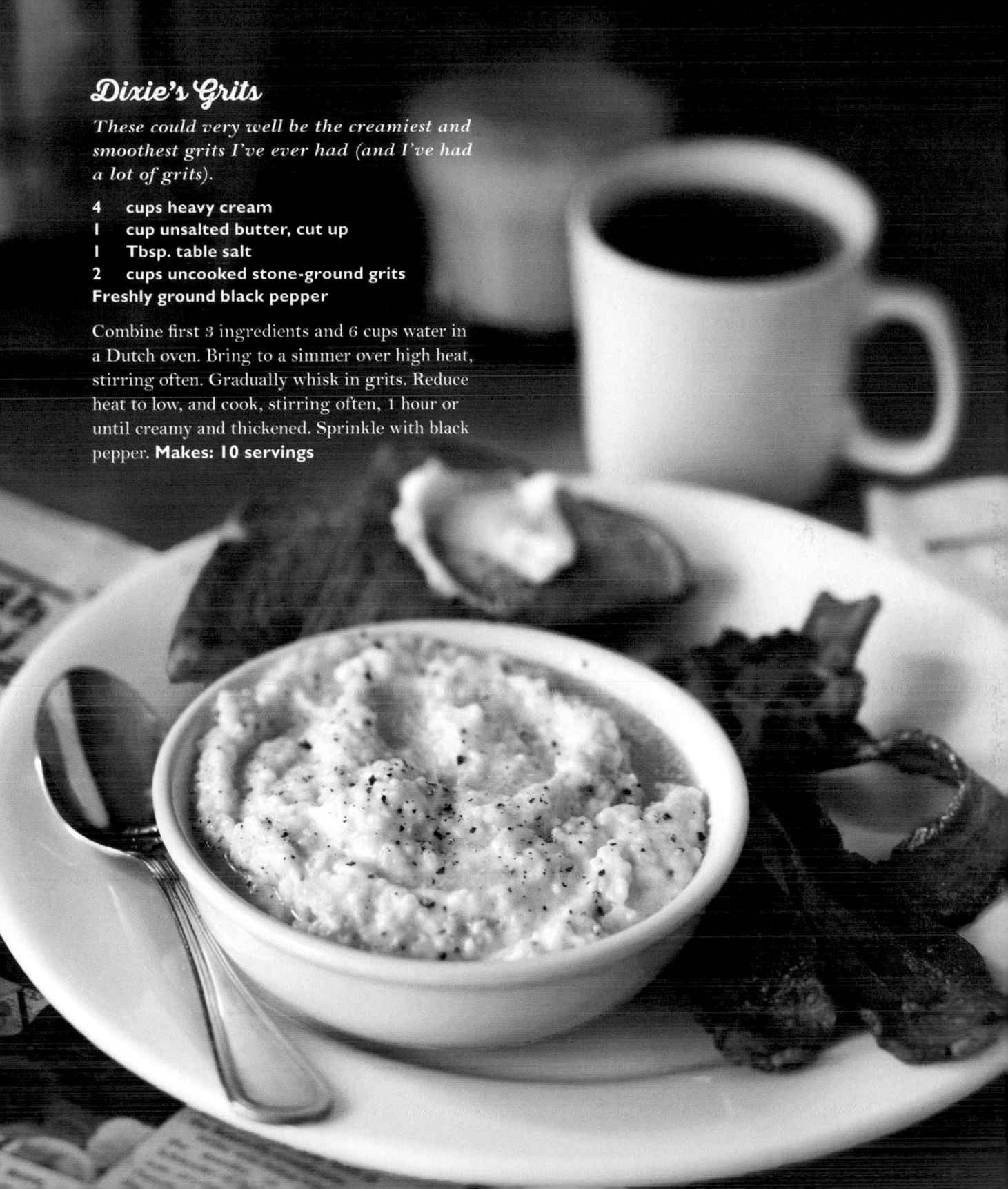

Dixie's Grits

These could very well be the creamiest and smoothest grits I've ever had (and I've had a lot of grits).

4　cups heavy cream
1　cup unsalted butter, cut up
1　Tbsp. table salt
2　cups uncooked stone-ground grits
Freshly ground black pepper

Combine first 3 ingredients and 6 cups water in a Dutch oven. Bring to a simmer over high heat, stirring often. Gradually whisk in grits. Reduce heat to low, and cook, stirring often, 1 hour or until creamy and thickened. Sprinkle with black pepper. **Makes: 10 servings**

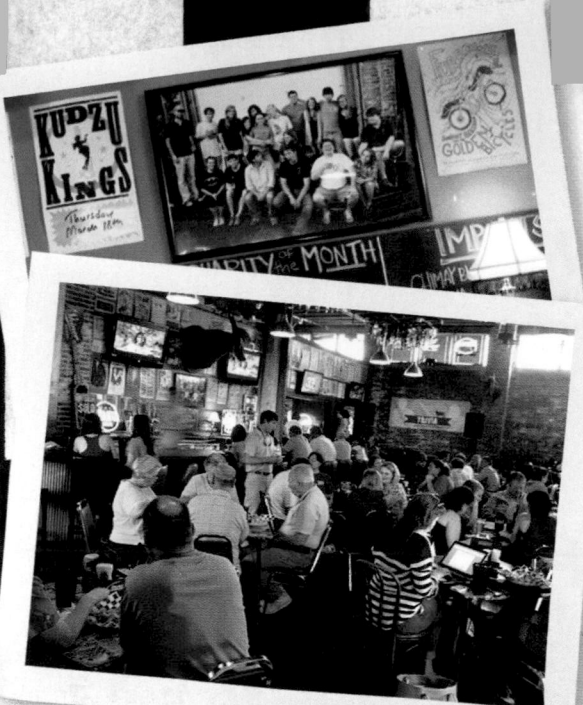

Hey Joe's

118 East Sunflower Road
Cleveland, Mississippi 38732
(662) 843-5425
eatheyjoes.com

Housed in a former tractor warehouse, Hey Joe's was originally meant to be a coffee house until owner Justin Huerta decided burgers and beers would be a better bet. And man, did he and pal Weejy Rogers make a good wager. "We played in a band together in college. We were terrible," Weejy says. The pair has made up for their bad tunes with unforgettable flavor pairings, such as the Nirvana Burger, which features Swiss cheese, onions, and Hey Joe's Burger Juice. Just try it. Trust me. With local beers on tap and a constant stream of events, Hey Joe's is a great spot to chill and devour a week's worth of calories at once.

Nirvana Burger

This is a burger done right. The Nirvana has a crunch, tang, and a sweet finish. Wow.

MARINATED MUSHROOMS AND ONIONS
6	Tbsp. bottled Italian dressing
2	Tbsp. Worcestershire sauce
1	(6-oz.) package portobello mushroom slices
1	cup sliced onion
1	tsp. butter

BURGER JUICE
½	cup Worcestershire sauce
¾	tsp. garlic powder
¾	tsp. freshly ground black pepper
¼	tsp. onion powder

BURGERS
1	lb. ground chuck

Pinch of table salt
Pinch of freshly ground black pepper
Pinch of garlic powder

2	tsp. butter
4	(¾-oz.) slices Swiss cheese
2	(1¼-oz.) potato buns
2	cooked thick-cut applewood-smoked bacon slices, cut in half crosswise
6	dill pickle slices
2	green leaf lettuce leaves

Hey Joe's Sauce (page 122)

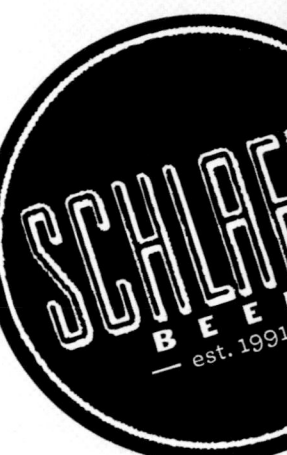

1. **Prepare Marinated Mushrooms and Onions:** Combine Italian dressing and Worcestershire sauce in a bowl. Add mushroom slices and onion, tossing to coat. Cover and marinate in refrigerator 1 hour.
2. **Meanwhile prepare Burger Juice:** Combine all ingredients and ½ cup water in a bowl. Reserve ¼ cup. Pour remaining Burger Juice into a small jar; cover and store in refrigerator.
3. Drain mushroom mixture, discarding marinade. Melt 1 tsp. butter in a large nonstick skillet over medium-high heat. Add mushroom mixture; sauté 12 to 14 minutes or until liquid evaporates and vegetables are tender and beginning to brown.

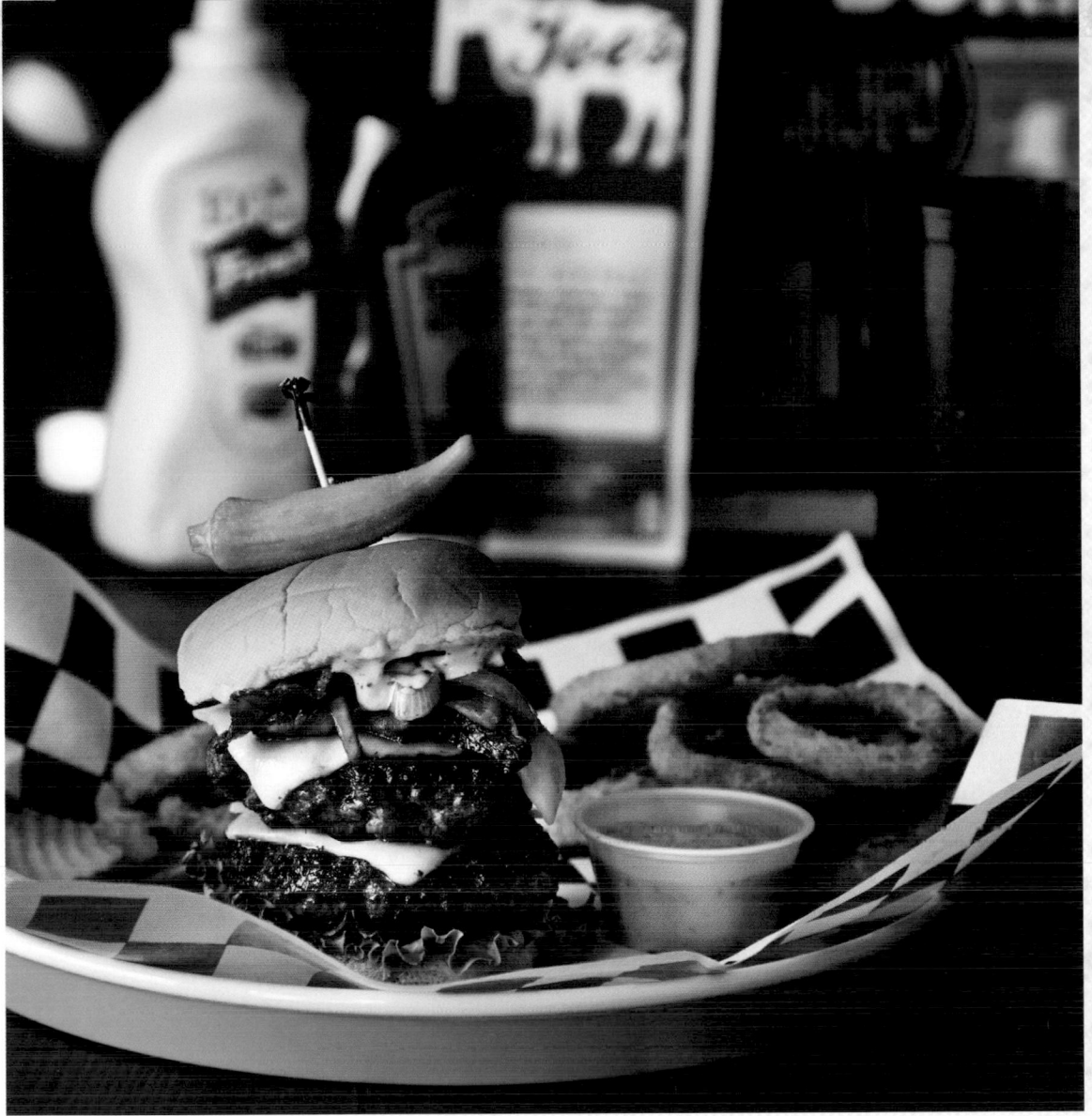

Remove from heat, and keep warm.

4. Prepare Burgers: Combine first 4 ingredients in a medium bowl. Shape into 4 (3½-inch-round, ¾-inch-thick) patties.

5. Melt 2 tsp. butter in a large skillet over medium-high heat. Place patties in skillet; drizzle each with 1 Tbsp. reserved Burger Juice. Cook 6 minutes on each side or to desired degree of doneness.

6. Top each burger patty with 1 slice cheese; place bun bottoms on serving plates. Stack 2 burger patties on each bun bottom. Top each serving with 2 bacon pieces, ½ cup mushroom mixture, 3 pickle slices, 1 lettuce leaf, and top of bun. Serve with Hey Joe's Sauce. **Makes: 2 servings**

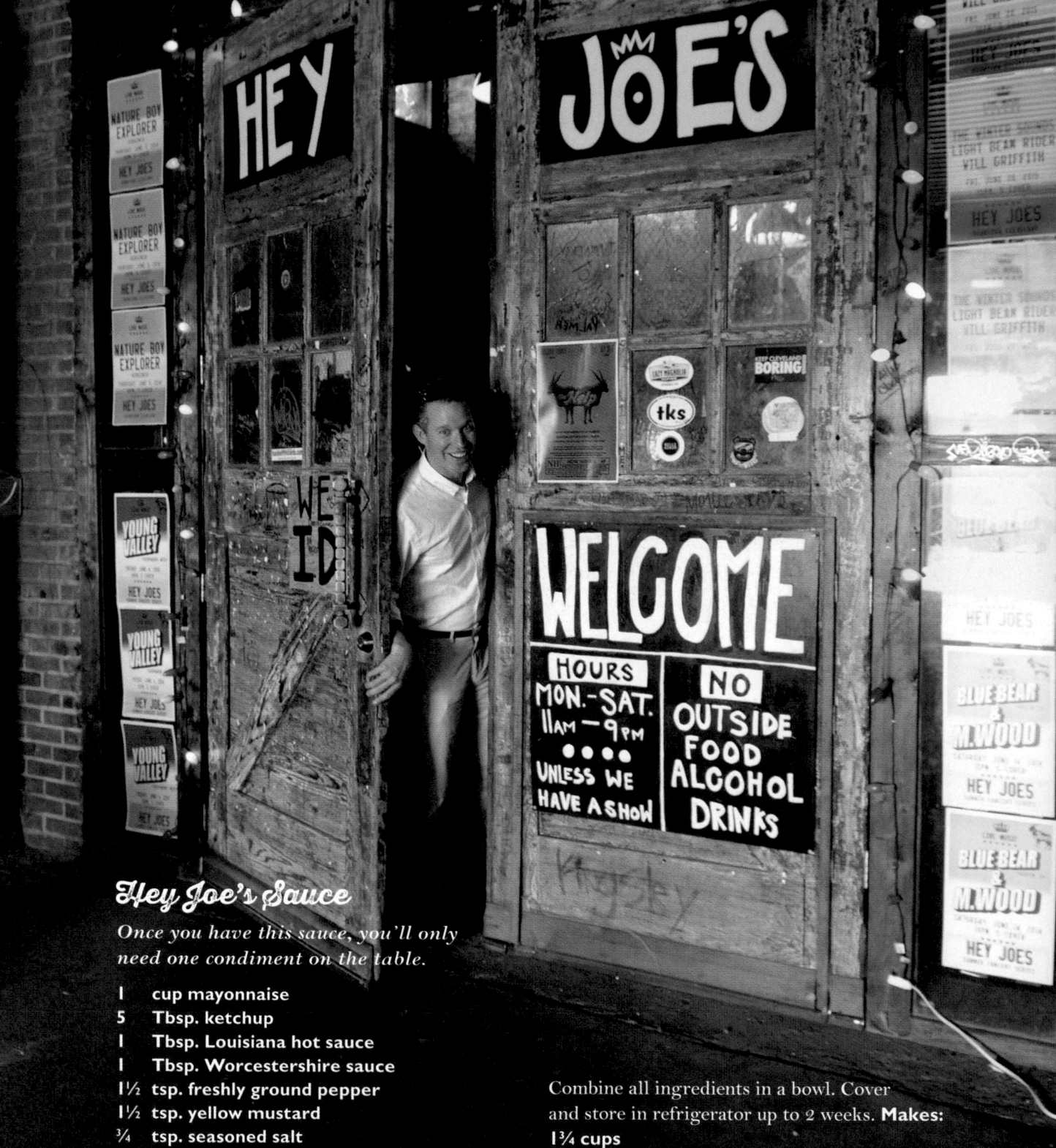

Hey Joe's Sauce

Once you have this sauce, you'll only need one condiment on the table.

1	cup mayonnaise
5	Tbsp. ketchup
1	Tbsp. Louisiana hot sauce
1	Tbsp. Worcestershire sauce
1½	tsp. freshly ground pepper
1½	tsp. yellow mustard
¾	tsp. seasoned salt

Combine all ingredients in a bowl. Cover and store in refrigerator up to 2 weeks. **Makes: 1¾ cups**

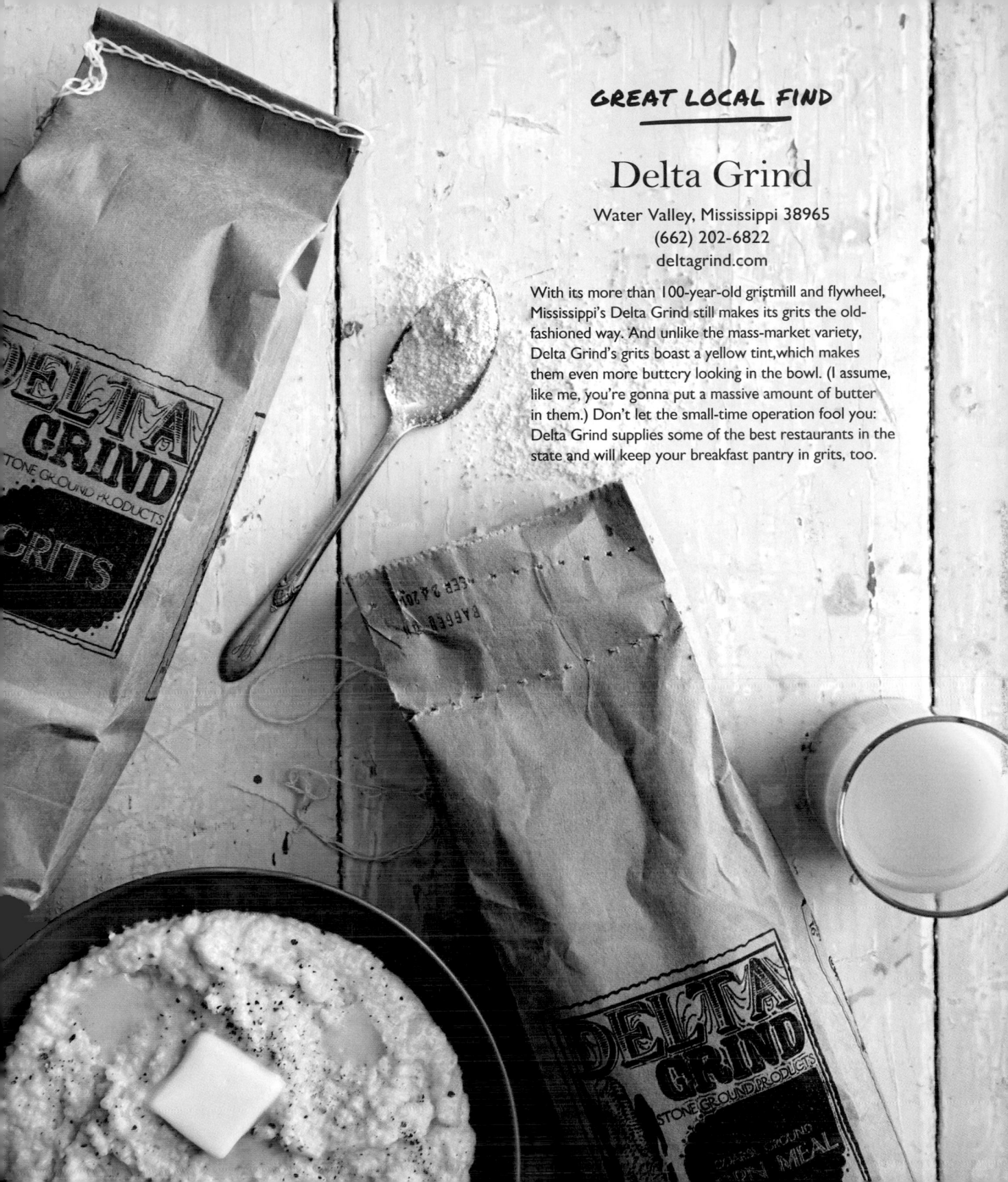

Delta Grind

Water Valley, Mississippi 38965
(662) 202-6822
deltagrind.com

With its more than 100-year-old gristmill and flywheel,
Mississippi's Delta Grind still makes its grits the old-
fashioned way. And unlike the mass-market variety,
Delta Grind's grits boast a yellow tint,which makes
them even more buttery looking in the bowl. (I assume,
like me, you're gonna put a massive amount of butter
in them.) Don't let the small-time operation fool you:
Delta Grind supplies some of the best restaurants in the
state and will keep your breakfast pantry in grits, too.

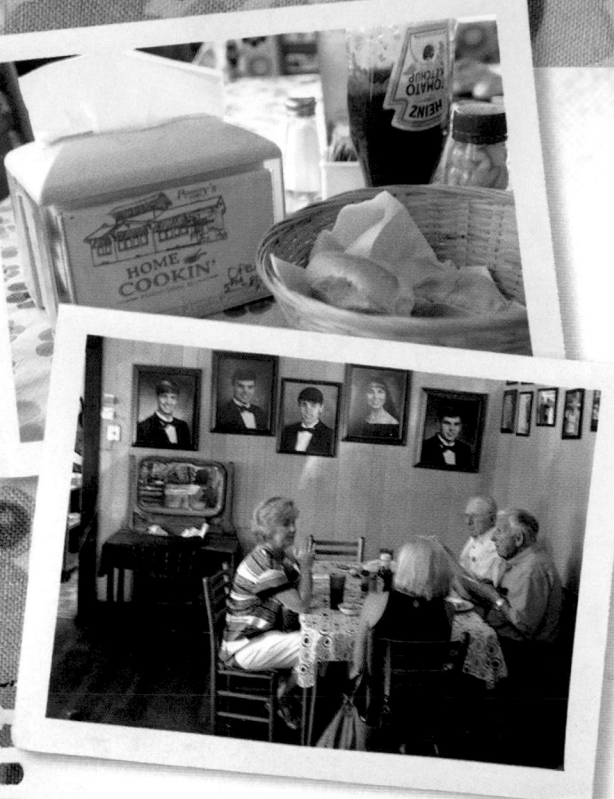

Peggy's

512 Bay Street
Philadelphia, Mississippi 39350
(601) 656-3478

This Philadelphia institution has been serving up Southern staples such as cornbread sticks, fried chicken, and banana pudding in a white, clapboard house on Bay Street since 1961. Regulars dine on Peggy's delicious fare in what used to be the home's living room. Payment is on the honor system—there's not even a cash register. When I visited, I ate with Peggy's youngest son, Stan, who comes in every day for fried chicken drumsticks. "I've put more chickens in wheelchairs than anyone else," says Stan. After one bite of Peggy's crispy fried chicken, you'll understand why.

Peggy's Banana Pudding

It's the homemade custard that makes this sweet treat so special.

- 1⅔ cups granulated sugar
- ⅓ cup all-purpose flour
- 1 (12-oz.) can evaporated milk
- 2 large eggs, lightly beaten
- 3 Tbsp. butter
- 1 tsp. vanilla extract
- 1 (11-oz.) package vanilla wafers
- 4 large bananas
- 2 cups heavy cream
- ½ tsp. vanilla extract
- ¼ cup powdered sugar

1. Whisk together granulated sugar and flour in a 3-qt. saucepan. Whisk in evaporated milk and 1½ cups water until smooth. Bring to a simmer over medium-high heat, whisking constantly; cook 6 minutes or until thickened. Remove from heat.

2. Whisk eggs in a medium bowl. Gradually whisk about one-fourth of hot milk mixture into eggs; add egg mixture to remaining hot milk mixture, whisking constantly. Return to a simmer over medium heat; cook, whisking constantly, 3 minutes. Remove from heat; add butter and vanilla, whisking until butter melts. Cool 20 minutes.

3. Layer half of vanilla wafers in bottom of a 13- x 9-inch baking dish. Slice bananas, and layer half of banana slices over vanilla wafers in dish. Spread half of pudding over banana layer. Repeat layers with remaining vanilla wafers, banana slices, and pudding. Place heavy-duty plastic wrap directly on warm pudding (to prevent a film from forming). Chill 30 minutes.

4. Beat cream and vanilla until foamy; gradually add powdered sugar, beating until soft peaks form. Spread over pudding. Chill 2 hours.
Makes: 12 servings

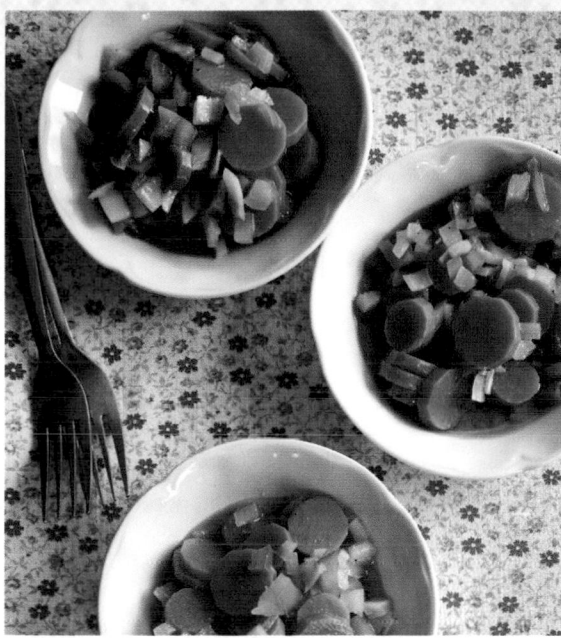

Marinated Carrots

Even if you don't like carrots, you'll love them after they chill overnight in this tangy marinade.

3 cups (¼-inch) sliced carrots
1½ tsp. table salt
1¼ cups chopped onion
1¼ cups chopped green bell pepper
2¼ cups sugar
1 cup apple cider vinegar
1 cup vegetable oil
1½ tsp. freshly ground black pepper
1½ tsp. Worcestershire sauce
1 (10¾-oz.) can condensed tomato soup

1. Bring carrots, salt, and 4 cups water to a boil in a 3-qt. saucepan; cover, reduce heat, and simmer 4 minutes or until tender. Drain. Return carrots to pan. Add onion and bell pepper to carrots; cover pan, and let stand 5 minutes. Transfer carrot mixture to a large bowl.
2. Bring sugar, remaining ingredients, and 1 cup water to a boil in a saucepan; remove from heat.

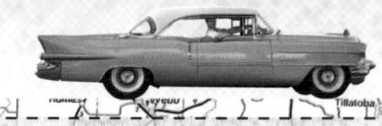

Mississippi bucket list

things to see and do (besides eat) here

❶ Poke around the queen of Southern letters' home at the **Eudora Welty House** in Jackson.

❷ Overnight in a splendid 19th-century antebellum mansion like the **Monmouth Historic Inn** in Natchez.

❸ Listen to some authentic Mississippi Delta Blues at **Ground Zero Blues Club** in Clarksdale.

❹ Take a cooking class at the **Viking Cooking School** in Greenwood.

❺ Drive the **Natchez Trace Parkway** *(pictured)* between Jackson and Tupelo. Make a stop at mile marker 122 near Canton and check out Cypress Swamp where an easy trail crosses a wooden footbridge into a forest of *Baldcypress* and *Water Tupelo*.

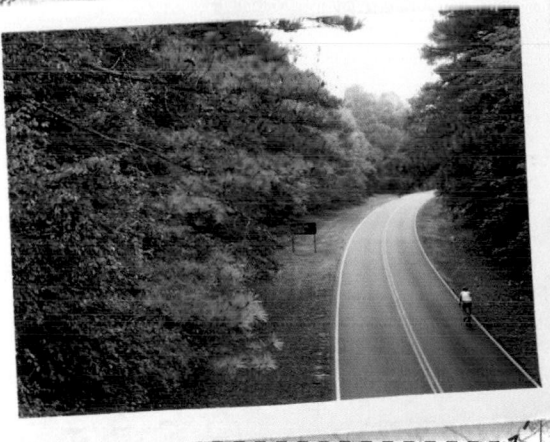

Pour vinegar mixture over carrot mixture. Cool completely (2 hours). Cover and chill 8 hours or overnight. Drain, discarding marinade, before serving. **Makes: 6 servings**

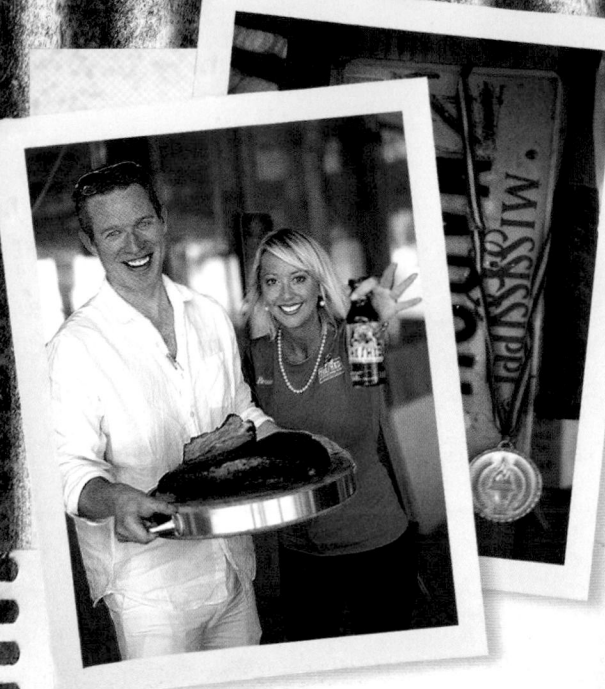

The Shed

7501 Highway 57
Ocean Springs, Mississippi 39565
(228) 875-9590
theshedbbq.com

It doesn't get more Mississippi than barbecue and blues, which is exactly what Brooke Lewis and her brother Brad Orrison serve up at this Ocean Springs joint. The Shed begins with corrugated tin and ends in a smoker. (If your town is missing a road sign, chances are it's here.) The restaurant's walls could have been assembled with pieces from a dumpster, but there's no junk in the food. I'm a huge fan of their barbecue, because as Brooke says, "If you can't pronounce it, it's not in what we serve." There's no gluten, no preservatives, and no MSG. And it tastes awesome.

Mama Mia's Mac Salad

This tart side salad makes an ideal dish for a family reunion, backyard 'cue, or dinner on the grounds.

7	oz. uncooked large pasta shells (2½ cups)
1	Tbsp. canola oil
½	cup mayonnaise
6	Tbsp. sour cream
1½	Tbsp. apple cider vinegar
⅜	tsp. onion powder
⅜	tsp. freshly ground black pepper
¼	tsp. kosher salt
¼	tsp. garlic salt
¾	tsp. Dijon mustard
½	cup chopped red onion
1	cup chopped green bell pepper
1	cup (4 oz.) shredded sharp Cheddar cheese

1. Cook pasta in boiling salted water according to package directions. Drain. Rinse pasta under cold running water; drain. Stir in oil until coated. Cover and chill 30 minutes.
2. Meanwhile, combine mayonnaise and next 7 ingredients in a large bowl, stirring until blended and smooth. Add pasta, stirring until pasta is creamy and coated. Stir in onion and remaining 2 ingredients. Serve immediately, or cover and chill 1 hour. **Makes: 6 servings**

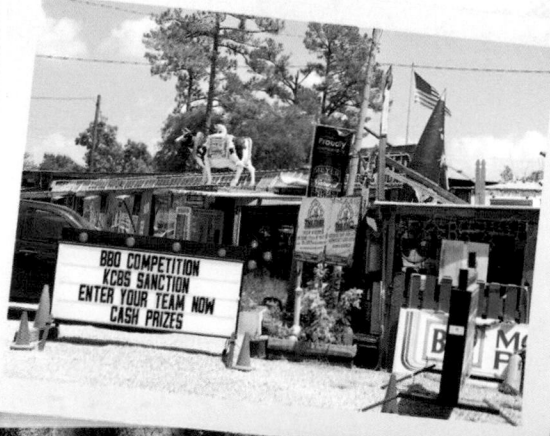

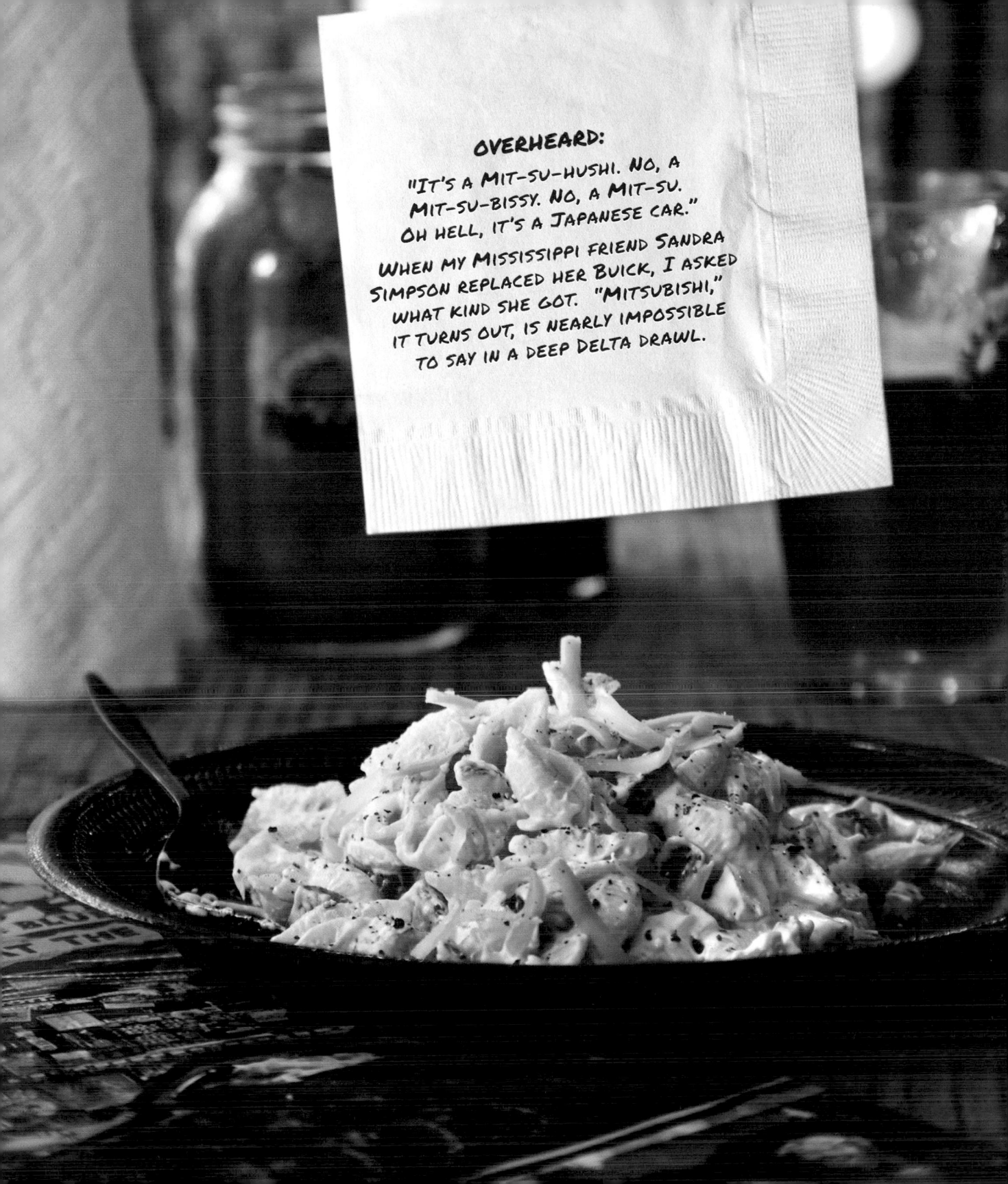

OVERHEARD:

"IT'S A MIT-SU-HUSHI. NO, A MIT-SU-BISSY. NO, A MIT-SU. OH HELL, IT'S A JAPANESE CAR." WHEN MY MISSISSIPPI FRIEND SANDRA SIMPSON REPLACED HER BUICK, I ASKED WHAT KIND SHE GOT. "MITSUBISHI," IT TURNS OUT, IS NEARLY IMPOSSIBLE TO SAY IN A DEEP DELTA DRAWL.

Low and Slow Smoked Brisket

Brad suggests serving his brisket sliced on buttered biscuits with a cup of coffee or bloody Marys while you "enjoy life."

Oak chunks or pecan wood chunks
The Shed's Southern Dry Rub
1   (7-lb.) beef brisket, trimmed

1. Soak wood chunks in water 1 hour. Rub 2 cups The Shed's Southern Dry Rub over all sides of brisket. Cover and let stand at room temperature 30 minutes or up to 1 hour.

2. Prepare smoker according to manufacturer's directions, bringing internal temperature to 225° to 250°; maintain temperature for 15 to 20 minutes.

3. Drain wood chunks, and place on coals. Place brisket on upper cooking grate; cover with smoker lid.

4. Smoke brisket, maintaining temperature inside smoker between 225° and 250°, for 5 to 6 hours or until a meat thermometer inserted into thickest portion registers 170°. Remove brisket from smoker; wrap in aluminum foil, and let stand 1 hour.

5. Cut brisket diagonally across the grain into ¼-inch slices. **Makes: 8 to 10 servings**

The Shed's Southern Dry Rub

This rub is excellent on pork and beef, but if you put it on a roll of paper towels, I'd probably eat those, too.

¼   cup garlic salt
¼   cup paprika
2   Tbsp. ground cumin
1   Tbsp. coarsely ground black pepper
1   Tbsp. chili powder
1½   tsp. dried oregano
1½   tsp. ground white pepper
1   cup firmly packed dark brown sugar

Whisk together first 7 ingredients in a medium bowl. Stir in brown sugar. Store at room temperature in an airtight container.
Makes: 2⅓ cups

SOUNDTRACK:

"AIN'T NO SUNSHINE" BY BUDDY GUY FEATURING TRACY CHAPMAN

"TIGER IN YOUR TANK" BY MUDDY WATERS

"AM I WRONG" BY KEB' MO'

"GRANNY, DOES YOUR DOG BITE" BY NORTH MISSISSIPPI ALLSTARS

"EVER START TO WONDER" BY THE DIRTY GUV'NAHS

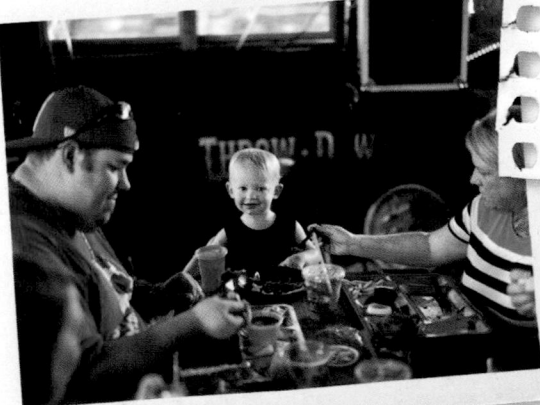

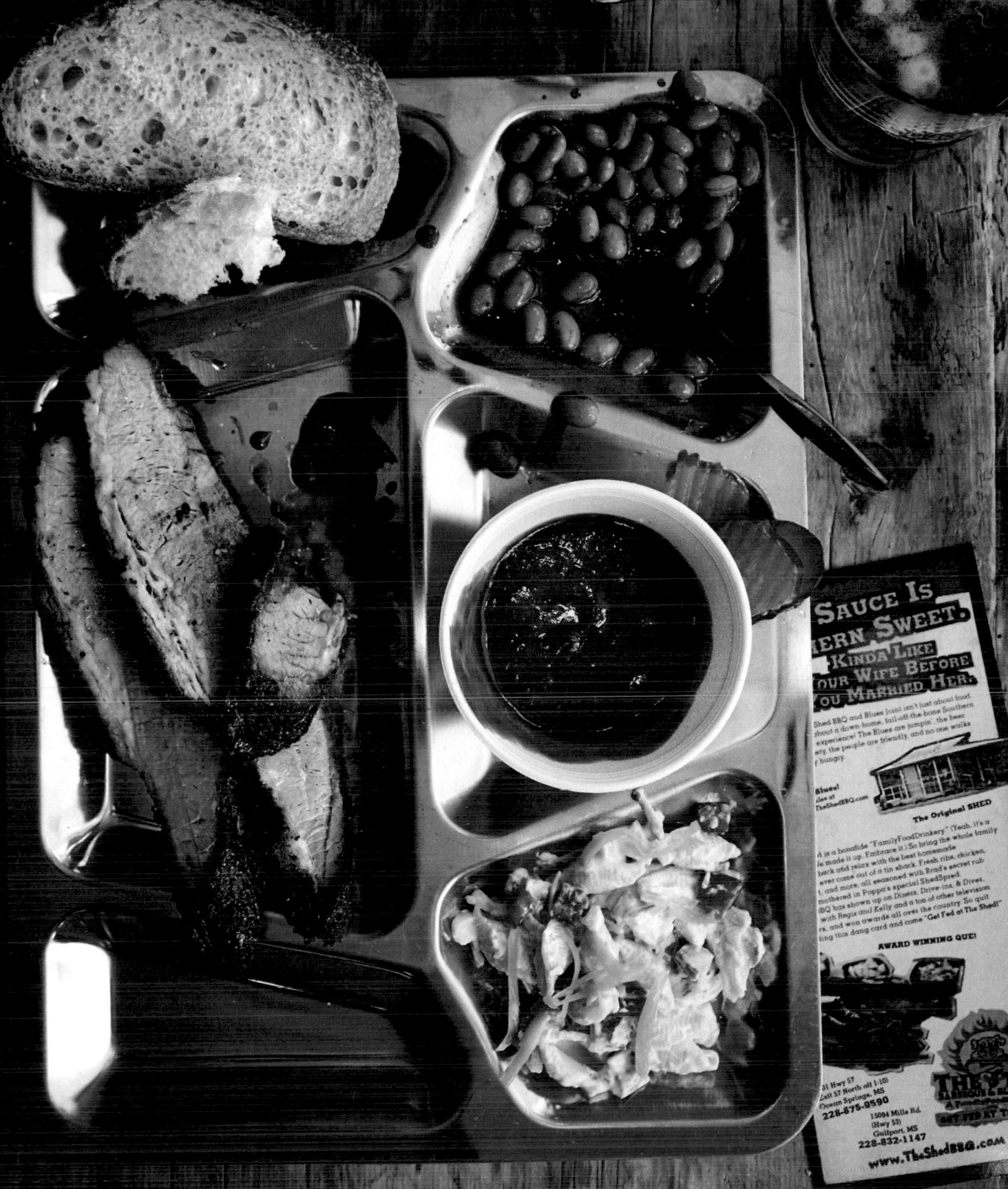

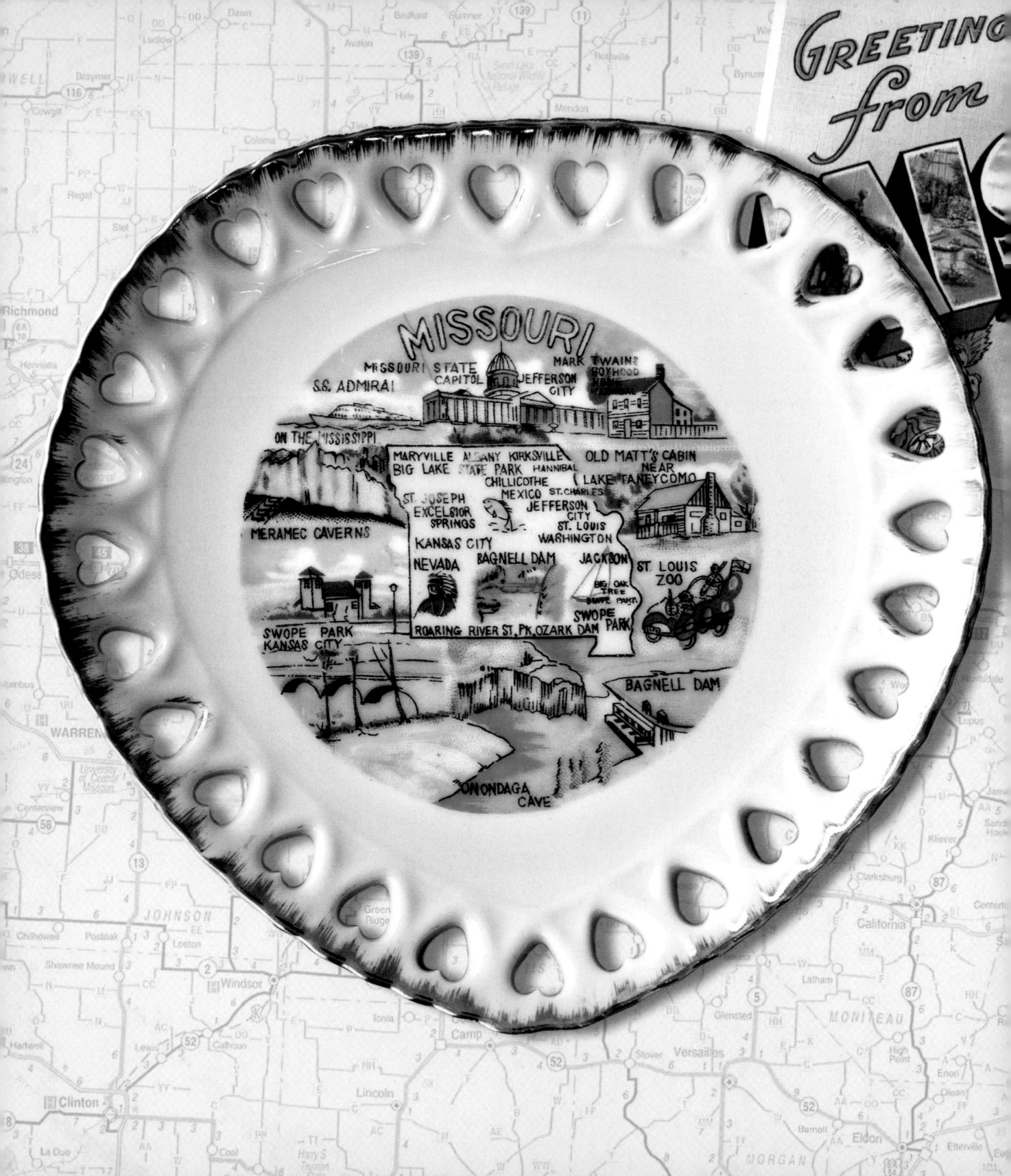

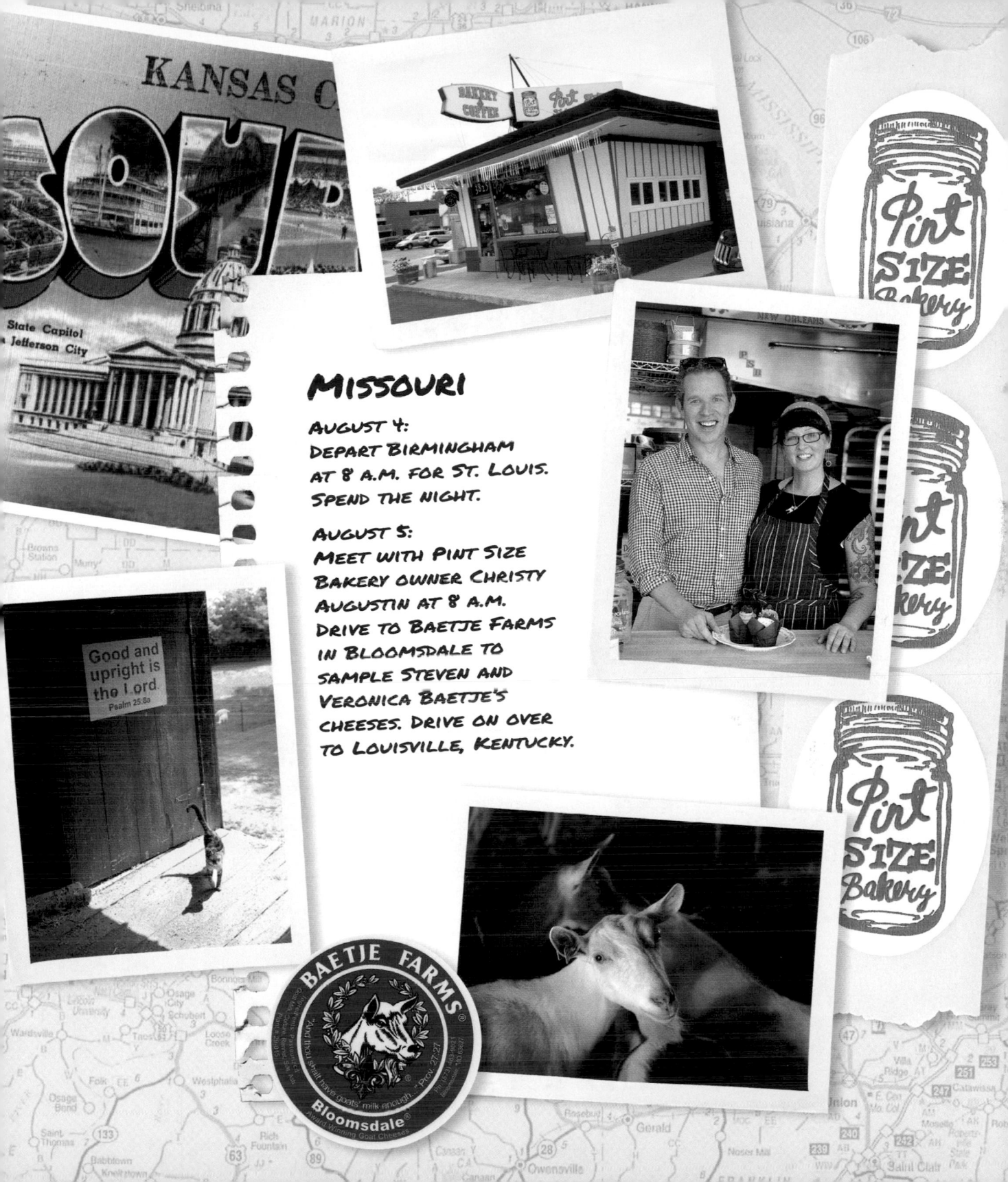

MISSOURI

AUGUST 4:
DEPART BIRMINGHAM
AT 8 A.M. FOR ST. LOUIS.
SPEND THE NIGHT.

AUGUST 5:
MEET WITH PINT SIZE
BAKERY OWNER CHRISTY
AUGUSTIN AT 8 A.M.
DRIVE TO BAETJE FARMS
IN BLOOMSDALE TO
SAMPLE STEVEN AND
VERONICA BAETJE'S
CHEESES. DRIVE ON OVER
TO LOUISVILLE, KENTUCKY.

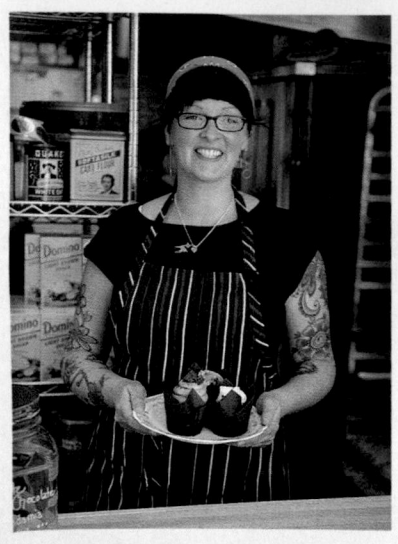

Pint Size Bakery

3825 Watson Road
St. Louis, Missouri 63109
(314) 645-7142
pintsizebakery.com

I am in lurve. Cupcakes and muffins, cookies and pastries, lattes and teas—all this goodness flows out of the tiniest bakery in St. Louis. Owner Christy Augustin welcomes her fans like old friends and talks about her tea cakes like some grandparents gush over grandbabies. "I just love this tea cake. It stays moist and the coconut is just so Southern," she says about her macaroons. There's no place to sit, but you'll love being served across the counters made of an old bowling lane. I'd say to eat your treats in the car, but I ate mine long before I made it back to the Cadillac.

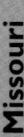

Chewy Oatmeal Cookies

These cookies are one of the bakery's top sellers, and after one bite, it's clear why.

COOKIES
1	cup unsalted butter, softened
1	cup firmly packed light brown sugar
½	cup granulated sugar
1	Tbsp. light molasses
1	tsp. vanilla extract
½	tsp. kosher salt
2	large eggs
2	cups unbleached all-purpose flour
1	tsp. baking soda
¼	tsp. ground cinnamon
2¼	cups uncooked regular oats

Parchment paper

MARSHMALLOW FLUFF BUTTERCREAM
1	cup unsalted butter, softened
½	cup powdered sugar
⅛	tsp. kosher salt
¼	tsp. vanilla extract
1	(7½-oz.) jar marshmallow fluff

1. Prepare Cookies: Preheat oven to 350°. Beat first 6 ingredients at medium speed with an electric mixer until light and fluffy. Add eggs, beating until blended. Combine flour, soda, and cinnamon; add to butter mixture, beating at low speed just until blended. Stir in oats.

2. Using a 1-oz. scoop (about 2 Tbsp.), scoop dough, 3 inches apart, onto parchment paper-lined baking sheets. Chill 20 minutes or until firm.

3. Bake at 350° for 10 to 12 minutes or until a medium golden brown with soft centers. Cool on pans 5 minutes. Transfer cookies to wire racks; cool completely.

4. Prepare Marshmallow Fluff Buttercream: When cookies are cool, beat first 4 ingredients until creamy and smooth. Gradually add marshmallow fluff, beating just until blended. Spoon about 2 Tbsp. buttercream onto bottoms of 20 cookies. Top with remaining 20 cookies, flat sides down.

Place cookie sandwiches in an airtight container; cover and chill 30 minutes or until firm. Serve cold. **Makes: 20 servings**

Coconut Macaroon Tea Cakes

Desiccated coconut is dried coconut, and makes these bite-size tea cakes extra chewy.

2¼   cups powdered sugar
¾   cup unbleached all-purpose flour
¾   cup plus 2 Tbsp. unsalted butter, softened
⅓   cup heavy cream
2   Tbsp. Malibu rum
3   large eggs
¾   cup unsweetened desiccated coconut*
18   brown floret baking cups
18   blackberries
¼   cup sweetened flaked coconut

1. Beat first 3 ingredients at low speed with an electric mixer until a smooth, thick paste forms. Add cream, rum, and eggs, beating at medium speed. Add desiccated coconut; beat until blended.
2. Preheat oven to 375°. Place baking cups on a rimmed baking sheet. Spoon batter evenly into baking cups, filling three-fourths full. Press 1 blackberry into center of each cup. Sprinkle tops with sweetened flaked coconut.
3. Bake at 375° for 20 to 22 minutes or until golden brown and center springs back when lightly pressed (blackberry will sink). Remove from pan. Cool completely on wire racks (about 45 minutes). **Makes: 18 servings**

*You may substitute an equal amount of sweetened flaked coconut, finely chopped, for the desiccated coconut. Reduce powdered sugar to 2 cups.

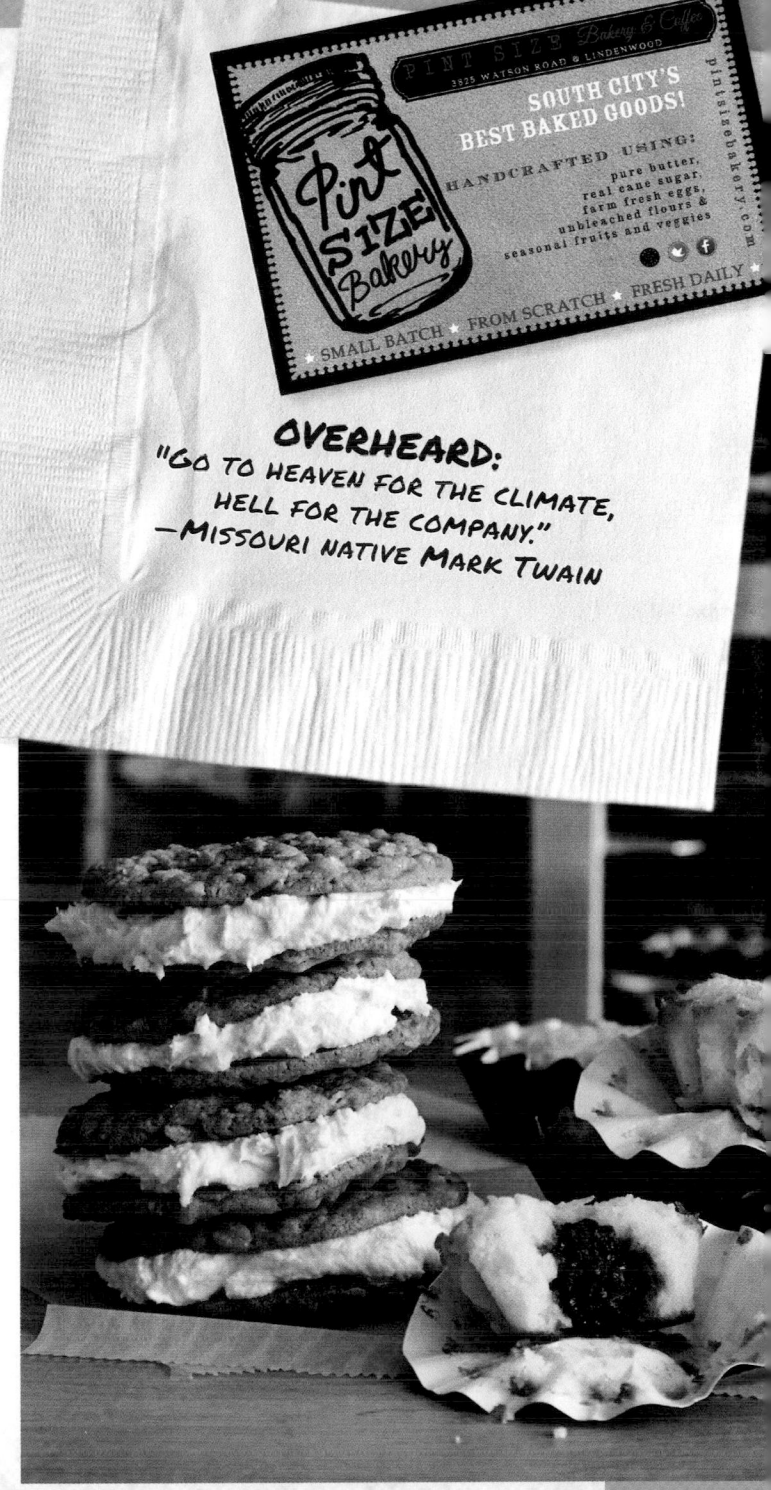

PINT SIZE *Bakery & Coffee*
3325 WATSON ROAD • LINDENWOOD
pintsizebakery.com

SOUTH CITY'S BEST BAKED GOODS!

HANDCRAFTED USING:
pure butter,
real cane sugar,
farm fresh eggs,
unbleached flours &
seasonal fruits and veggies

SMALL BATCH • FROM SCRATCH • FRESH DAILY

OVERHEARD:
"GO TO HEAVEN FOR THE CLIMATE, HELL FOR THE COMPANY."
—MISSOURI NATIVE MARK TWAIN

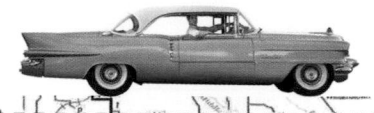

Missouri bucket list

things to see and do (besides eat) here

❶ Take a ride up to the top of the **Gateway Arch** in St. Louis. The 630-foot stainless steel engineering marvel is the tallest man-made monument in the Western Hemisphere.

❷ Bike the beautiful **Katy Trail**, which is mercifully flat, as it runs 240 miles along what was once the Missouri-Kansas-Texas Railroad. Sections also follow the Lewis and Clark National Historic Trail.

❸ Sip your way through **Missouri Wine Country** *(pictured)* and make sure to try a few of the state's famed full-bodied Norton red wines.

❹ Get in some shopping at the upscale stores of **Country Club Plaza**, which opened in 1923. Or take a walking tour of the city's outdoor fountains—Kansas City is home to more fountains than any city outside of Rome, Italy.

❺ Experience a performance in the **Peabody Opera House** in St. Louis. After a $78.7 million restoration—including state-of-the-art upgrades—this Depression-era venue is as grand as ever.

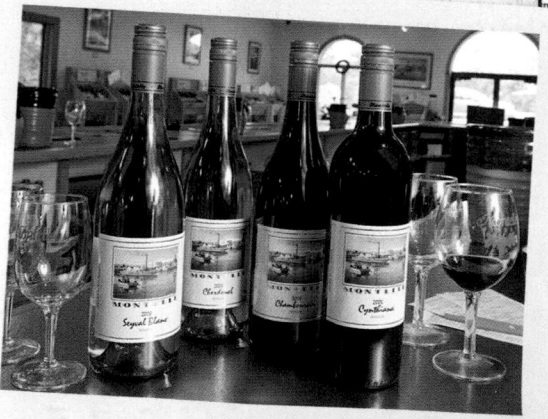

Orange-Ricotta Bundt Cake

This beautiful cake is so moist and orangey from three generous hits of orange—zest, liqueur, and a marmalade glaze.

Shortening
All-purpose flour
1½ cups ricotta cheese
¾ cup unsalted butter, softened
1 Tbsp. orange zest
1¼ cups granulated sugar
2 large eggs
2 Tbsp. orange liqueur
1 tsp. vanilla extract
1½ cups cake flour
2½ tsp. baking powder
1 tsp. kosher salt
Orange Marmalade Glaze or powdered sugar

1. Preheat oven to 350°. Generously grease (with shortening) a 10-cup Bundt pan; dust with flour.
2. Process ricotta cheese in a food processor 20 seconds or until smooth.
3. Beat butter and orange zest at medium speed with an electric mixer until creamy. Gradually add granulated sugar, beating 5 minutes or until light and fluffy. Add eggs, 1 at a time, beating just until yellow disappears. Add liqueur and vanilla, beating until blended.
4. Combine cake flour, baking powder, and salt; add to butter mixture alternately with ricotta cheese, beating at low speed just until blended after each addition. Pour batter into prepared pan.
5. Bake at 350° for 45 minutes or until a long wooden pick inserted in center comes out clean. (Cake will have a golden crust around the edges and begin to pull away from sides of pan.) Cool cake in pan 10 minutes. Invert cake onto a wire rack, and cool completely (about 1½ hours). Spoon Orange Marmalade Glaze over cake.
Makes: 8 to 10 servings
Note: We tested with Grand Marnier.

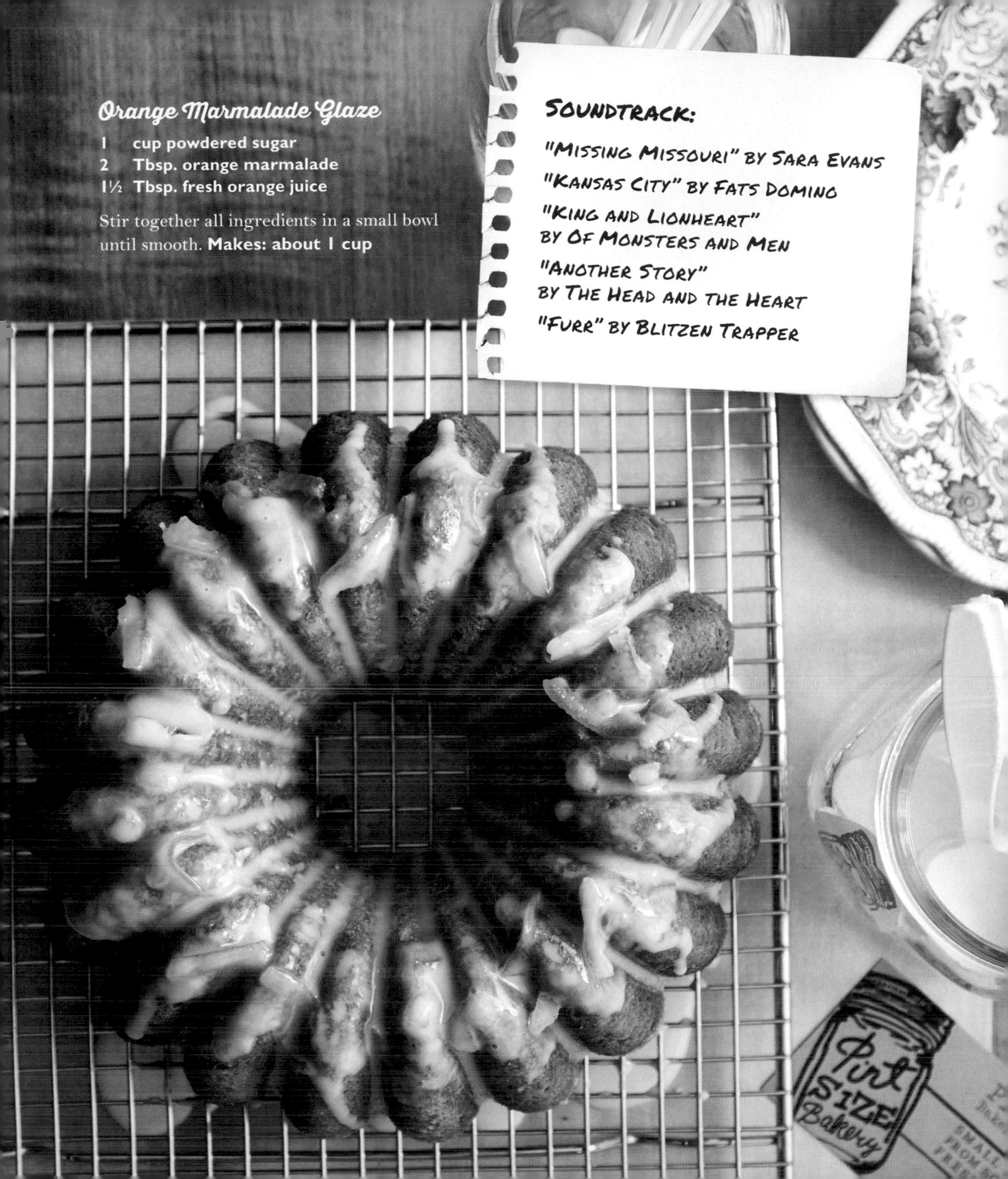

Orange Marmalade Glaze

- 1 cup powdered sugar
- 2 Tbsp. orange marmalade
- 1½ Tbsp. fresh orange juice

Stir together all ingredients in a small bowl until smooth. **Makes: about 1 cup**

SOUNDTRACK:

"MISSING MISSOURI" BY SARA EVANS

"KANSAS CITY" BY FATS DOMINO

"KING AND LIONHEART"
BY OF MONSTERS AND MEN

"ANOTHER STORY"
BY THE HEAD AND THE HEART

"FURR" BY BLITZEN TRAPPER

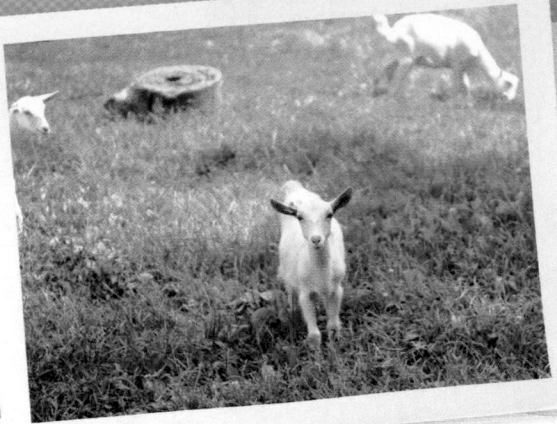

Baetje Farms

8932 Jackson School Road
Bloomdale, Missouri 63627
(573) 483-9021
baetjefarms.com

Steven and Veronica Baetje make cheese that connoisseurs flip for: They hold more than 65 international awards for their artisan fromage. "The awards are starting to just stack up," Stephen told me when I asked about all the blue ribbons adorning the walls of their 1912 red barn. The flagship cheese, the Bloomsdale, holds several prestigious awards, including the 2011, 2012, and 2013 super gold World Cheese Awards. It's a mold-ripened cheese with a hard rind and runny center. You can order it directly from the farm's website (the farm itself is not open for tours). If you're a fan of goat cheese, the Coeur de la Crème line includes nine different varieties. Note the French spelling—the Baetjes have mastered the art of French cheese making's time-honored traditions and labor-intensive practices.

Shells Stuffed with Goat Cheese

Vegetable cooking spray
- ½ (12-oz.) package jumbo pasta shells
- 1 lb. lean ground beef
- ⅔ cup chopped onion
- 2 cups beef broth
- ¼ cup chopped fresh parsley
- 1½ tsp. dried Italian seasoning
- 1 (14½-oz.) can stewed tomatoes, undrained
- 1 (6-oz.) can tomato paste
- 12 oz. Baetje Farms Garlic and Chives Coeur de la Crème Goat Cheese
- 2 cups (8 oz.) shredded mozzarella cheese
- 2 large eggs, lightly beaten

1. Preheat oven to 350°. Lightly grease an 11- x 7-inch baking dish with cooking spray. Prepare pasta according to package directions; drain.
2. Brown ground beef in a large skillet over medium-high heat, stirring often, 5 to 6 minutes or until meat crumbles and is no longer pink; drain and return to skillet. Add onion; cook, stirring often, 5 minutes or until onion is tender. Stir in beef broth and next 4 ingredients. Bring to a boil; reduce heat to low, and simmer, uncovered, 18 minutes or until sauce is thickened, stirring occasionally.
3. Combine goat cheese, ½ cup mozzarella cheese, and eggs in a bowl. Stuff cheese mixture into pasta shells; place in prepared dish. Ladle sauce over shells, and sprinkle with remaining 1½ cups mozzarella cheese.
4. Bake, uncovered, at 350° for 40 minutes or until bubbly and cheese is browned. **Makes:** 6 servings

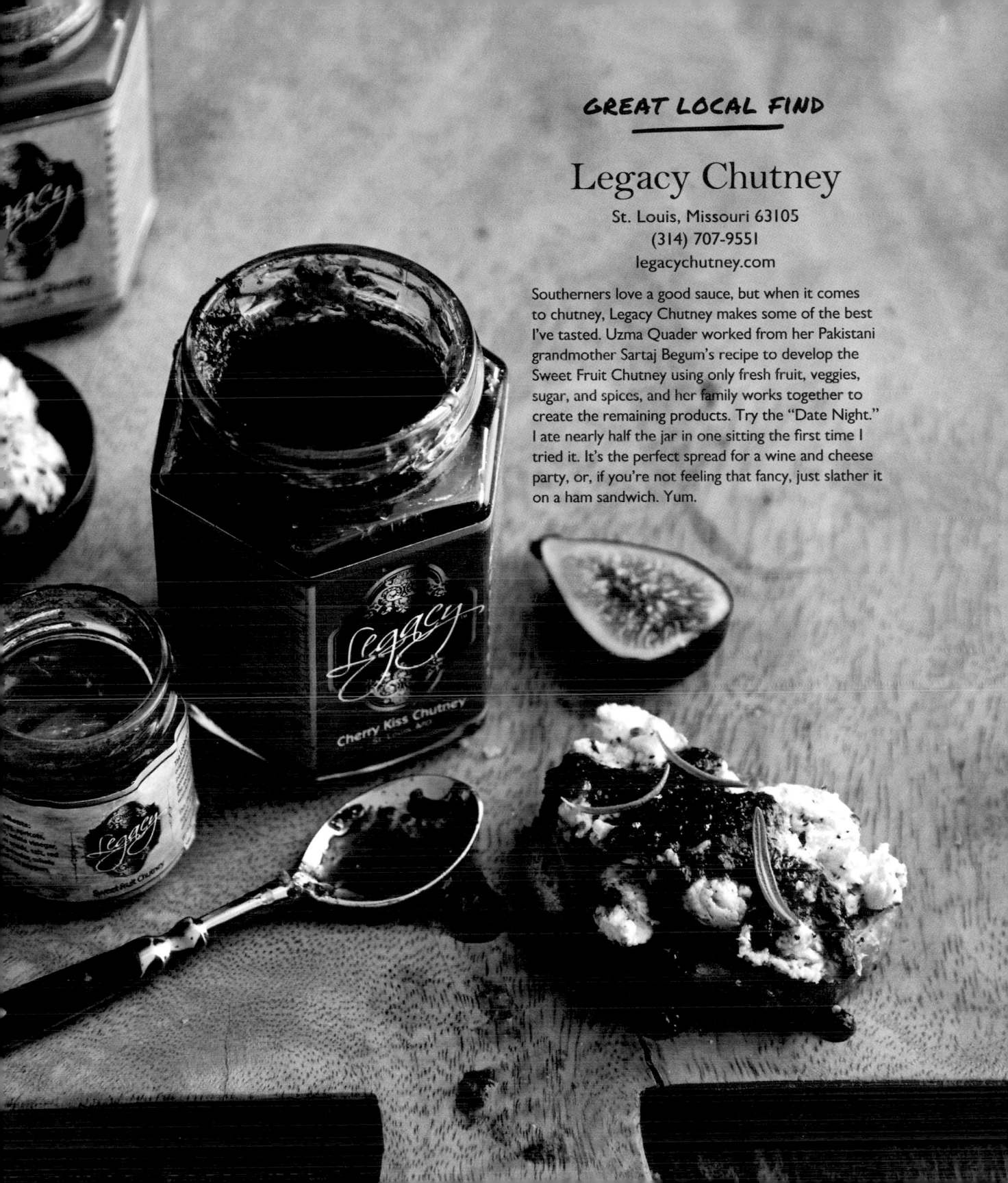

Legacy Chutney

St. Louis, Missouri 63105
(314) 707-9551
legacychutney.com

Southerners love a good sauce, but when it comes to chutney, Legacy Chutney makes some of the best I've tasted. Uzma Quader worked from her Pakistani grandmother Sartaj Begum's recipe to develop the Sweet Fruit Chutney using only fresh fruit, veggies, sugar, and spices, and her family works together to create the remaining products. Try the "Date Night." I ate nearly half the jar in one sitting the first time I tried it. It's the perfect spread for a wine and cheese party, or, if you're not feeling that fancy, just slather it on a ham sandwich. Yum.

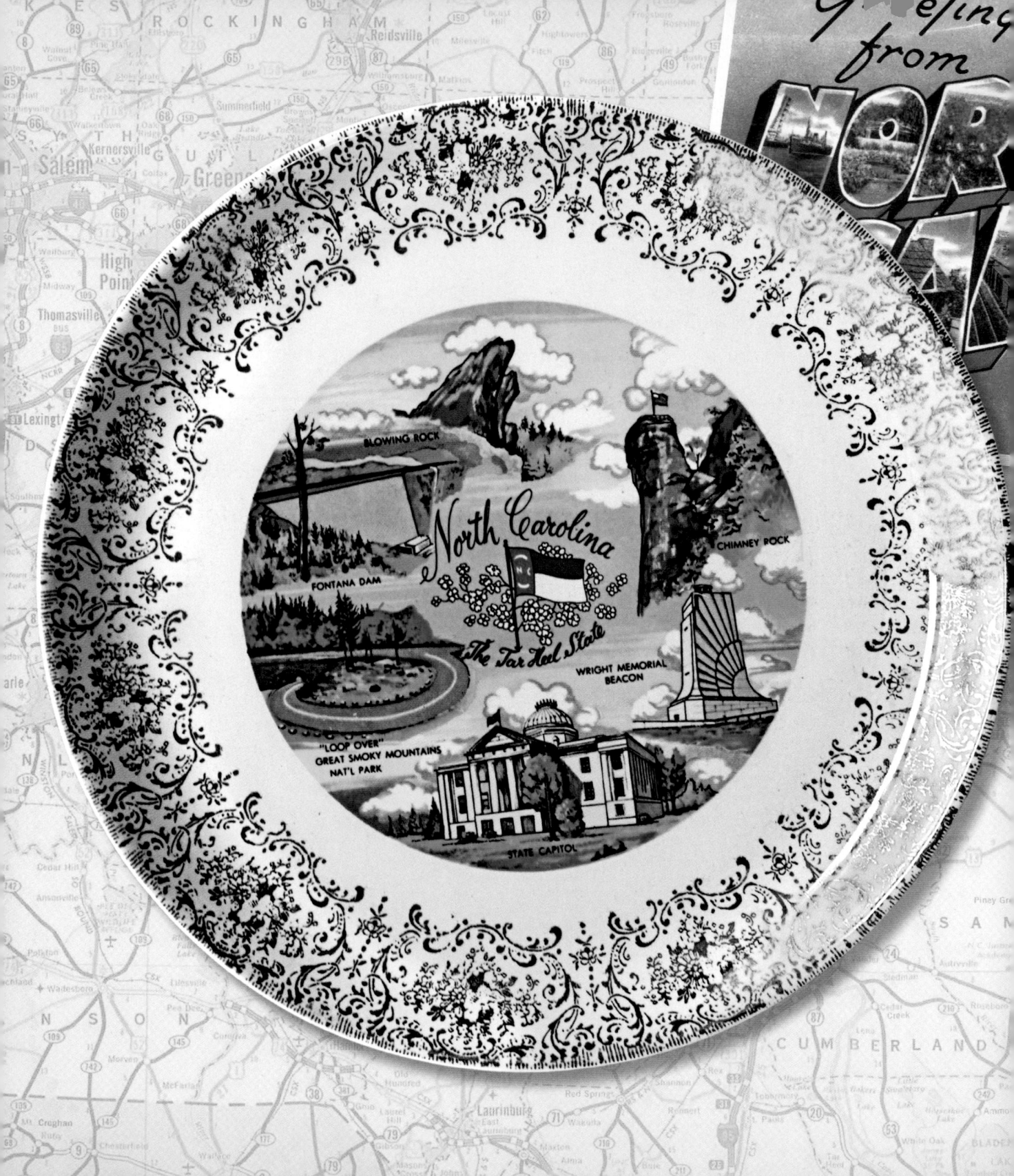

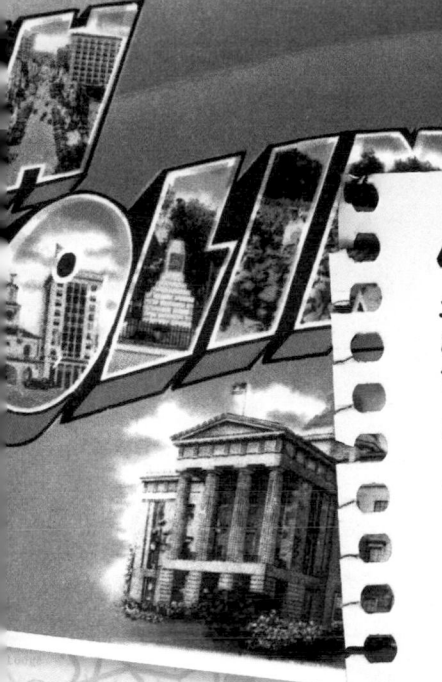

North Carolina

July 21:
Depart Birmingham at 8 a.m. for
Brevard and Rocky's Grill & Soda Shop

Drive to Asheville. Spend the night.

July 22:
Breakfast at Early Girl Eatery in
Asheville at 8 a.m.
Drive to Raleigh. Meet Niall Hanley
at the Station at 3 p.m. Spend the
night.

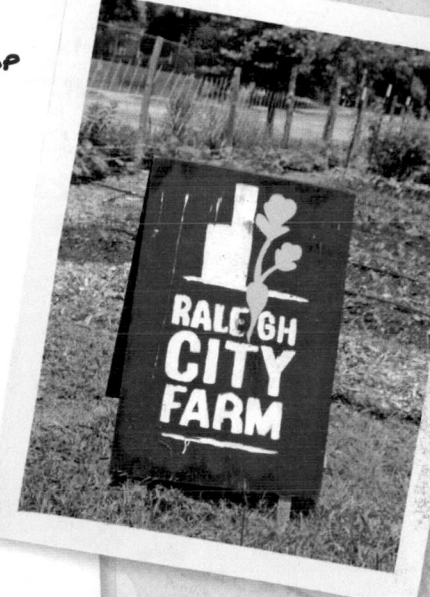

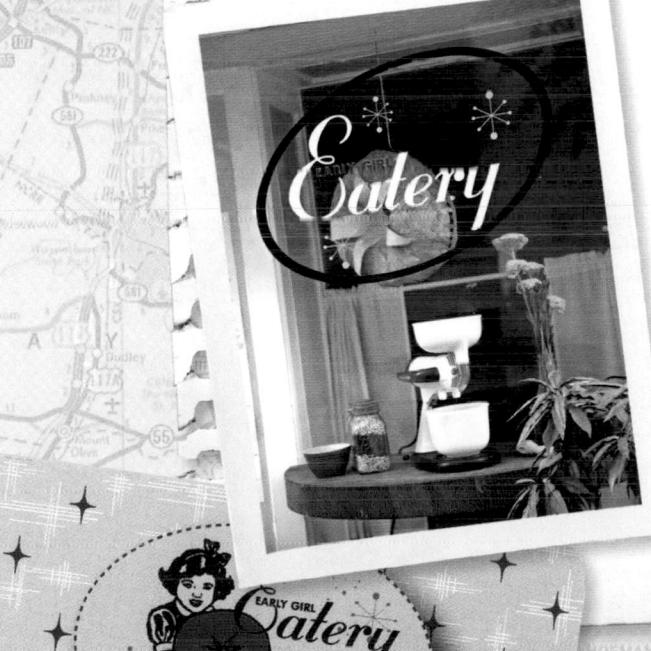

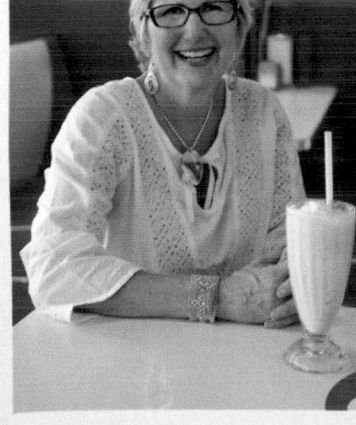

A Farm to Table Southern Comfort Food Experience

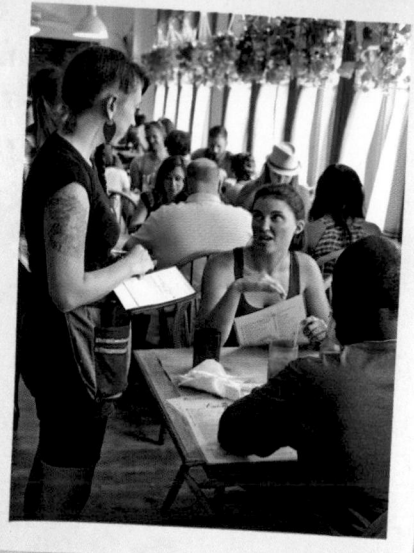

Early Girl Eatery

8 Wall Street
Asheville, North Carolina 28801
(828) 259-9292
earlygirleatery.com

Biscuits, herbed-cream gravy, fried chicken, and yam scrambles will brighten up any morning. This sunny, cheerful restaurant in downtown Asheville welcomes those seeking creative fare at a reasonable price. "We don't do anything fancy, we just do it right," says owner John Stehling. He runs the kitchen with his wife, Julie, who handles the front of the house. The two met while working at Charleston, South Carolina, landmark Hominy Grill, which John's brother owns. Today, though John and Lisa work 70 to 90 hours a week together, their playful relationship pervades the restaurant. They serve lunch and dinner, too, but if you want breakfast, get here, well, early.

Sweet Potato–Black Bean Cakes

These sweet and rich potato cakes are an Early Girl classic.

- 1 medium sweet potato (1 lb.), peeled and cut into 1½-inch pieces
- 1 Tbsp. light brown sugar
- 1½ tsp. ground cumin
- ⅜ tsp. garlic powder
- Dash of hot sauce
- 1 cup fine, dry breadcrumbs
- 1 cup black beans, drained and rinsed
- ¼ cup chopped green onions
- ¼ cup (1 oz.) shredded Cheddar cheese
- 1 large egg, beaten
- Canola oil

1. Cook sweet potato in boiling water to cover 18 minutes or until very tender; drain. Return potato to pan; add brown sugar and next 3 ingredients. Mash well with a potato masher. Cool completely (30 minutes).
2. Stir in breadcrumbs and next 4 ingredients. Shape into 10 (3-inch) patties. Chill 30 minutes.
3. Pour oil to depth of ½ inch into a large skillet; heat to 350°. Fry cakes, 5 at a time, 2 minutes on each side or until golden. Drain on paper towels.
Makes: 5 servings

Avocado Relish

- 2 avocados, diced
- 2 jalapeño peppers, seeded and minced
- 1 Tbsp. finely chopped fresh cilantro
- 1 Tbsp. fresh lime juice
- 1 Tbsp. olive oil
- ½ tsp. table salt

Combine all ingredients in a bowl, stirring gently. (Mixture should be chunky.) **Makes: 1½ cups**

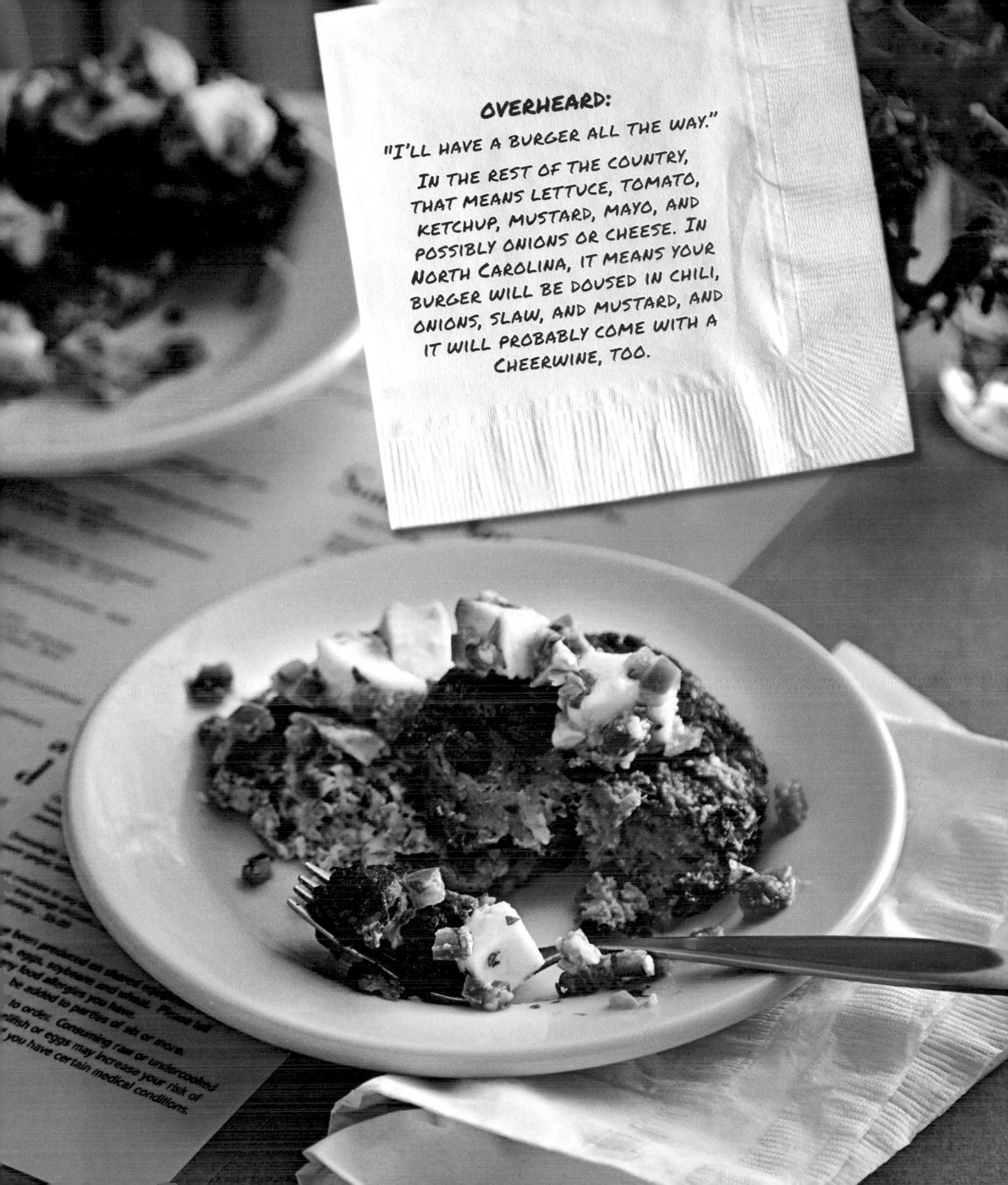

OVERHEARD:

"I'LL HAVE A BURGER ALL THE WAY."

IN THE REST OF THE COUNTRY, THAT MEANS LETTUCE, TOMATO, KETCHUP, MUSTARD, MAYO, AND POSSIBLY ONIONS OR CHEESE. IN NORTH CAROLINA, IT MEANS YOUR BURGER WILL BE DOUSED IN CHILI, ONIONS, SLAW, AND MUSTARD, AND IT WILL PROBABLY COME WITH A CHEERWINE, TOO.

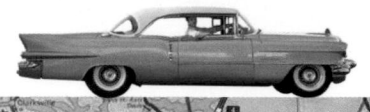

North Carolina bucket list

things to see and do (besides eat) here

1 Stroll the grounds of America's largest home, the **Biltmore Estate** in Asheville.

2 Stick your toes in the waters of the Atlantic along any of the stunning beaches of the **Outer Banks**.

3 Visit Charlotte's **Mint Museum**, which is housed in what was the original branch of the United States Mint and is now home to exceptional collections of American, contemporary, and European art.

4 Lower your handicap playing a round on what's considered golf architect Donald Ross's masterpiece, historic Pinehurst No. 2 at **Pinehurst Resort**.

5 Hike to the summit of **Chimney Rock** (or catch the elevator) for breathtaking panoramic views of the Carolinas *(pictured)*.

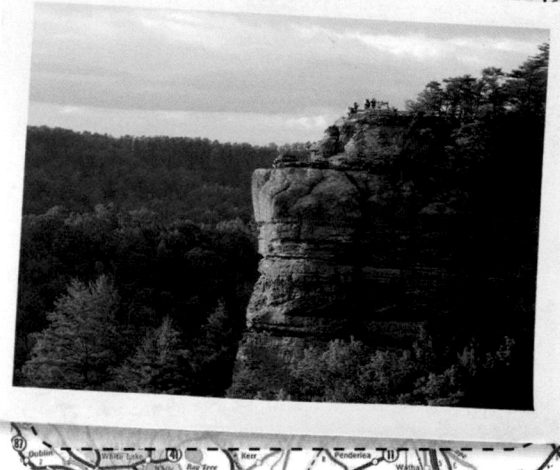

Spinach Potato Cakes

These little cakes are the perfect brunch side.

2	lb. red potatoes, peeled and cut into 2-inch pieces
1	tsp. olive oil
1½	tsp. minced fresh garlic
8	oz. fresh baby spinach
2	cups fine, dry breadcrumbs
1	cup (4 oz.) grated fresh Parmesan cheese
3	Tbsp. fresh lemon juice
½	tsp. table salt
½	tsp. freshly ground black pepper
2	dashes of hot sauce
2	large eggs, beaten
¼	cup olive oil

1. Cook potatoes in boiling water to cover 20 minutes or until tender. Drain. Cool completely. Cover and chill at least 1 hour.

2. Process potatoes in a food processor using a shredding disk. Transfer to a bowl.

3. Heat 1 tsp. olive oil in a large skillet over medium heat. Sauté garlic and half of spinach in hot oil 1 minute or until spinach begins to wilt. Add remaining spinach, and cook 2 minutes or until all spinach wilts. Drain. Cool spinach mixture slightly, and process in a food processor until smooth. Add to shredded potato. Stir in breadcrumbs and next 6 ingredients. Shape into 12 (3-inch) patties. Chill 30 minutes.

4. Preheat oven to 350°. Heat 1 Tbsp. olive oil in a large nonstick skillet over medium-high heat. Add 4 patties; fry 3 minutes on each side until browned and crisp. Drain on paper towels, and place on a baking sheet. Repeat procedure with remaining oil and patties.

5. Bake at 350° for 10 minutes or until crisp and thoroughly heated. **Makes: 6 servings**

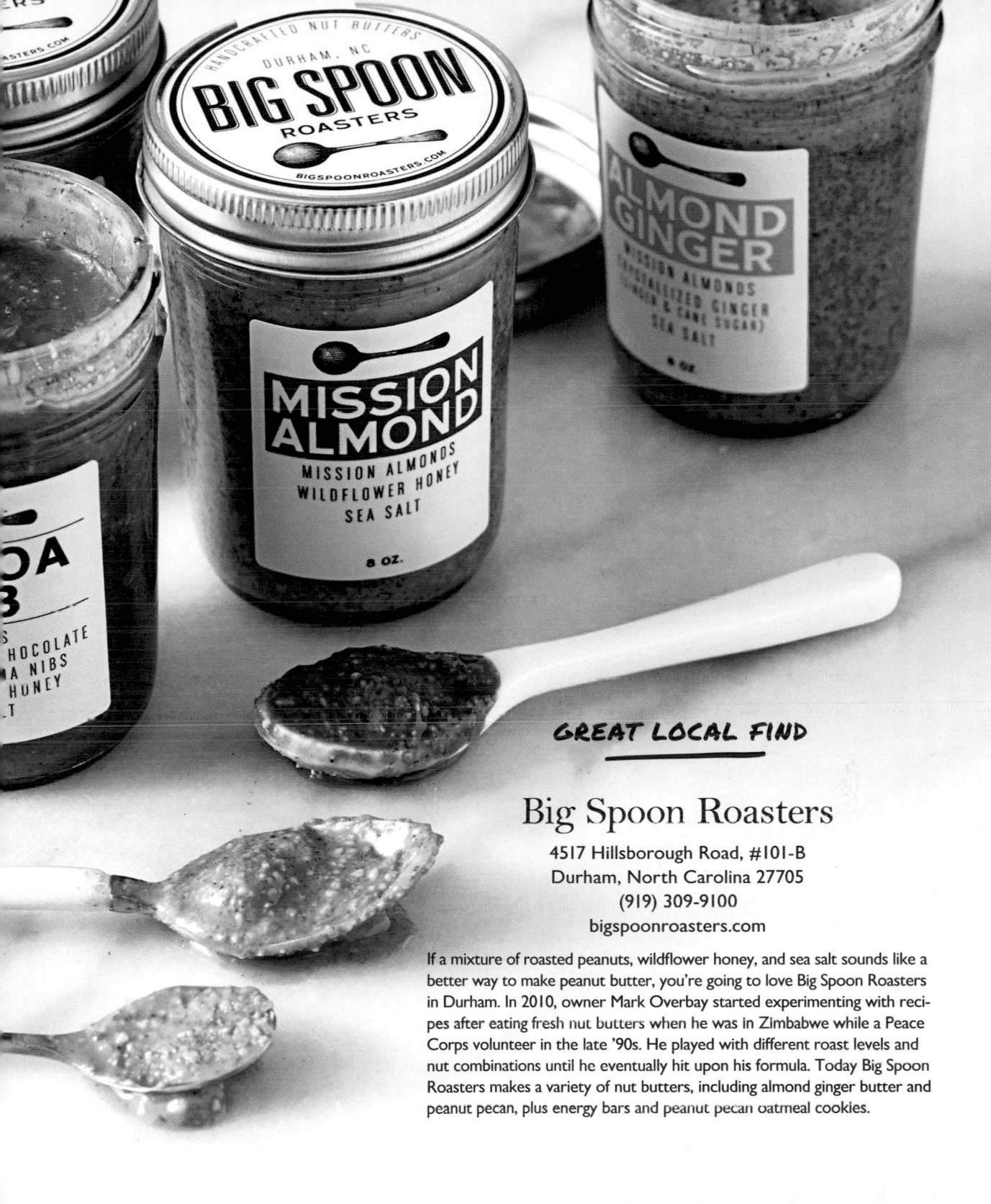

Big Spoon Roasters

4517 Hillsborough Road, #101-B
Durham, North Carolina 27705
(919) 309-9100
bigspoonroasters.com

If a mixture of roasted peanuts, wildflower honey, and sea salt sounds like a better way to make peanut butter, you're going to love Big Spoon Roasters in Durham. In 2010, owner Mark Overbay started experimenting with recipes after eating fresh nut butters when he was in Zimbabwe while a Peace Corps volunteer in the late '90s. He played with different roast levels and nut combinations until he eventually hit upon his formula. Today Big Spoon Roasters makes a variety of nut butters, including almond ginger butter and peanut pecan, plus energy bars and peanut pecan oatmeal cookies.

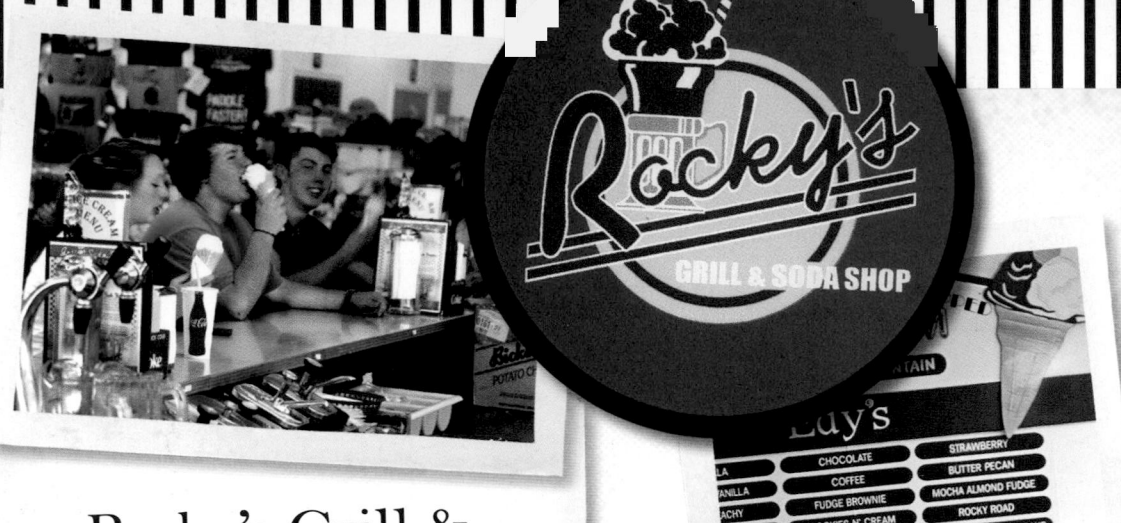

Rocky's Grill & Soda Shop

50 South Broad Street
Brevard, North Carolina 28712
(828) 877-5375
rockysnc.com

The Andrews Sisters topped the charts, a Cadillac cost $1,300, and FDR was in the White House. And in tiny Brevard, North Carolina, the original Varner's Drug Store opened in 1941 with a charming soda shop inside. Little has changed since then. Soda jerks still whip up rich frozen concoctions. Chili dogs and pimiento cheese sandwiches (with Mrs. Varner's original recipe) seduce even the most health-conscious. Current owner Dee Dee Perkins has carefully preserved Rocky's original Formica counters, chrome fixtures, and be-bop feel. "It's what every knock-off diner aspires to be." This is a family get-together restaurant," Dee Dee says. Slide into one of the red booths or hop on a bar stool and you can't help but feel a bit of nostalgia. The good news is you can take a piece of that home with you. D.D. Bullwinkel's gift shop sells hard candy, vintage toys, and outdoor equipment.

Mrs. Varner's Grilled Pimiento Cheese Sandwich

Why haven't I done this before? It's pure genius to grill a pimiento cheese.

- 2 (1.7-oz.) slices buttermilk bread
- ⅓ cup Mrs. Varner's Homemade Pimiento Cheese (facing page)
- 2 (¼-inch-thick) tomato slices
- 3 cooked hickory-smoked bacon slices
- 1 Tbsp. softened butter

1. Spread 1 bread slice with pimiento cheese. Top with tomato, bacon, and remaining bread slice. Spread sandwich on both sides with softened butter.
2. Heat a 10-inch nonstick skillet over medium-high heat. Add sandwich to pan; cook 1 to 2 minutes on each side or until golden brown.
Makes: 1 serving

Mrs. Varner's Homemade Pimiento Cheese

This is my favorite thing on Rocky's menu. It's a classic.

12 oz. sharp Cheddar cheese, shredded
6 oz. American cheese, shredded
1 (3-oz.) package cream cheese, softened
1 cup mayonnaise
2 tsp. lemon juice
1 (4-oz.) jar diced pimientos, drained

Combine first 3 ingredients in a bowl, stirring well. Stir in mayonnaise and remaining ingredients. Cover and chill until ready to serve. **Makes: 3½ cups**

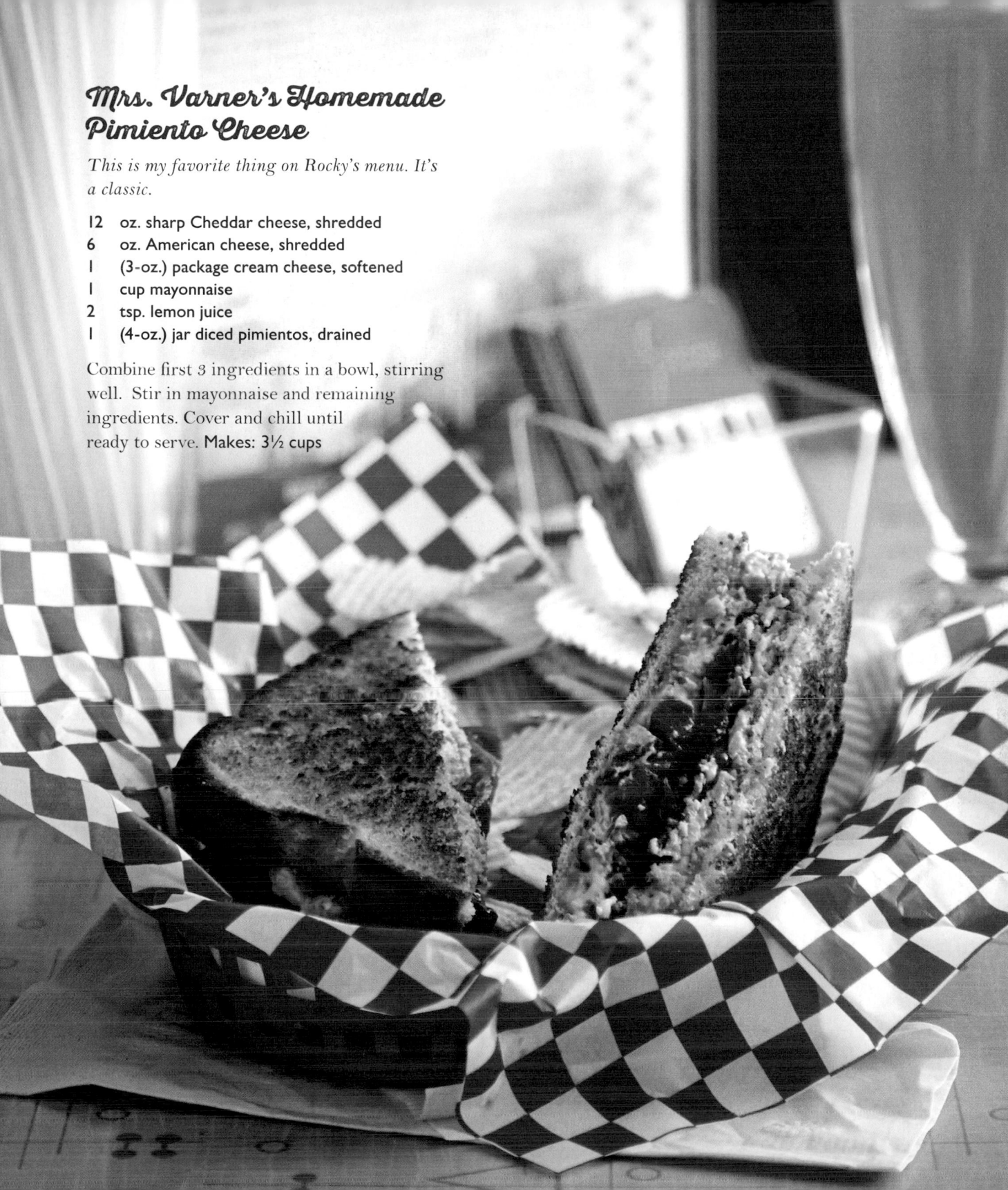

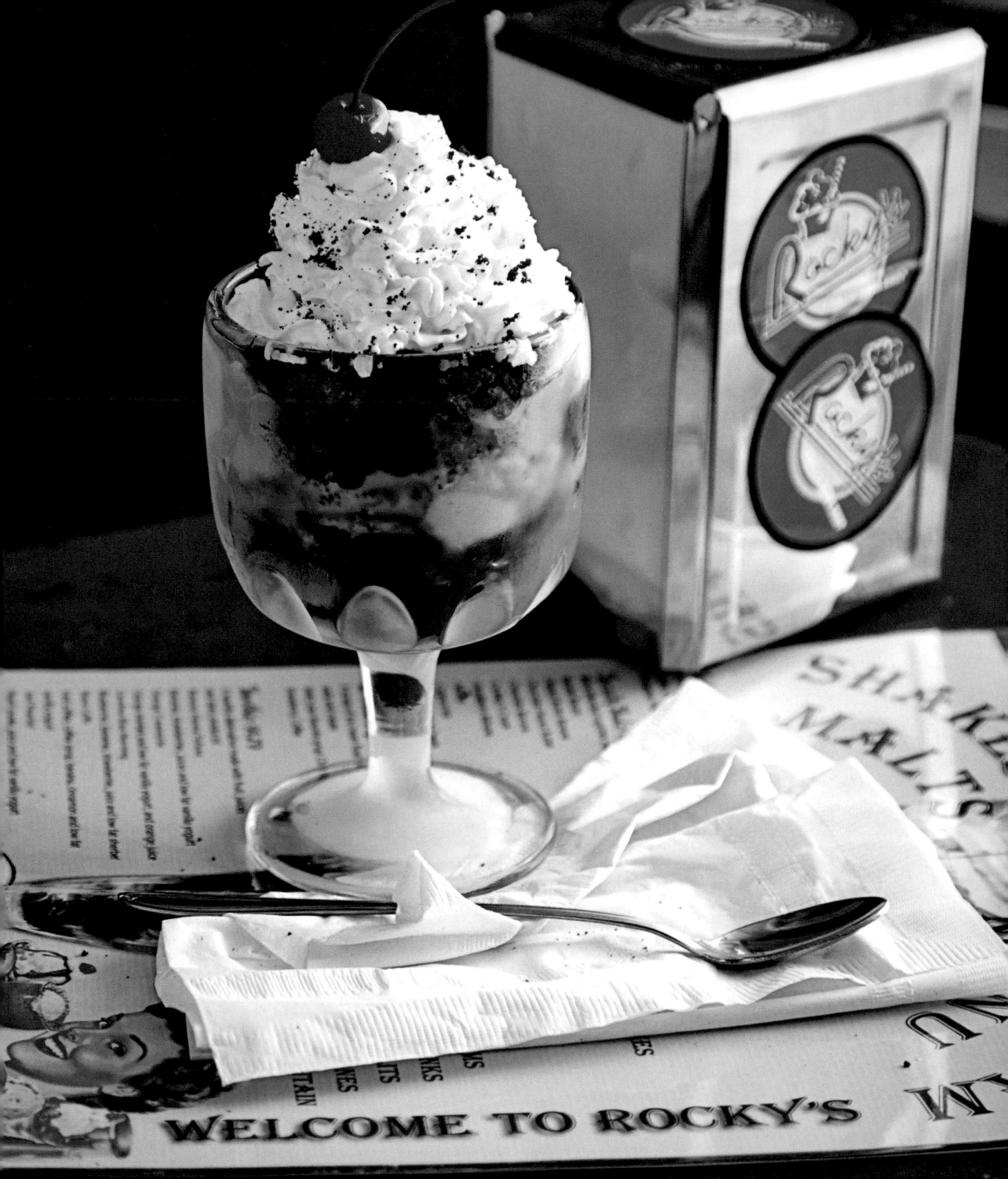

WELCOME TO ROCKY'S

French Broad River Sundae

The coffee sprinkles give this ice cream sundae its extra crunch.

⅓   cup store-bought hot fudge sauce
2   (½-cup) scoops coffee ice cream
½   cup chopped cream-filled chocolate sandwich cookies (4 cookies)
2¼   tsp. instant coffee granules, divided
Canned refrigerated instant whipped cream
1   maraschino cherry with stem

Place about 1 Tbsp. hot fudge sauce in bottom of a large glass goblet. Add 1 scoop coffee ice cream. Drizzle with 2 Tbsp. hot fudge sauce. Top with ¼ cup crumbled cookies; sprinkle with 1 tsp. coffee granules. Top with remaining scoop of ice cream. Drizzle with 2 Tbsp. hot fudge sauce; sprinkle with remaining ¼ cup crumbled cookies and 1 tsp. coffee granules. Top with whipped cream and cherry. Sprinkle with ¼ tsp. coffee granules. Serve immediately. **Makes: 1 serving**

SOUNDTRACK:

"GREEN EYES AND A HEART OF GOLD" BY THE LONE BELLOW

"WHEN MY TIME COMES" BY DAWES

"HEAD FULL OF DOUBT/ROAD FULL OF PROMISE" BY THE AVETT BROTHERS

"CORNBREAD AND BUTTERBEANS" BY CAROLINA CHOCOLATE DROPS

"AIN'T NO GRAVE" BY CROOKED STILL

Rocky's Chili Willy

4   kosher hot dogs
8   (1.6-oz.) hot dog buns
2   Tbsp. softened butter
2⅔   cups Rocky's Hot Dog Chili
Diced red onion

1. Grill hot dogs in a 10-inch nonstick skillet over medium heat 5 minutes or until hot and lightly browned, turning often.
2. Spread cut sides of buns with softened butter. Cook, cut sides down, in skillet over medium heat until toasted. Place hot dogs in buns, and top with Rocky's Hot Dog Chili. Sprinkle with diced onion. **Makes: 4 servings**

Variation: Rocky's Chili and Pimiento Cheese Dog Add 3 Tbsp. Mrs. Varner's Homemade Pimiento Cheese (page 145) to each Rocky's Chili Willy hot dog. Serve with deep-ridged potato chips and green tomato pickles.

Rocky's Hot Dog Chili

This chili has a bit of a kick, but won't send Grandma or small children running.

2   lb. ground chuck
2   Tbsp. finely chopped red onion
1⅔   cups ketchup
1½   Tbsp. paprika
1½   Tbsp. chili powder
¾   tsp. ground red pepper
1   tsp. ground cumin

Combine all ingredients in large saucepan. Cook over medium heat 25 minutes or until meat crumbles and sauce is thickened, stirring often. **Makes: 5¼ cups**

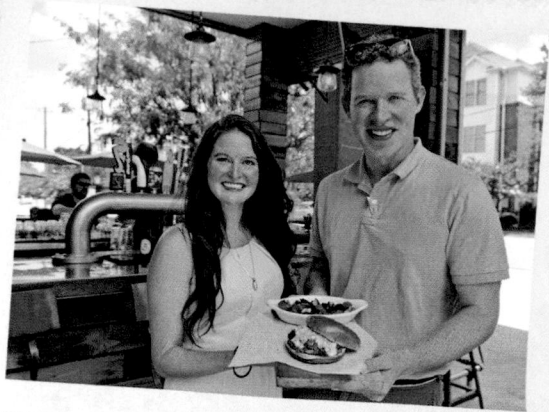

The Station

701 North Person Street
Raleigh, North Carolina 27604
(919) 977-1567
stationraleigh.com

The Station in Raleigh—so aptly named because it was once an Amoco station—now rocks a laid-back outdoor bar and a rooftop garden. Owner and Irishman Niall Hanley even encourages diners to bring their dogs—water bowls are provided outside and you can get a doggy bag if you can't finish your meal. But you won't be able to stop after one bite of The Station's spicy Sloppy Joe covered in cheese. Even though it's cool and casual here, they're serious about freshness. The fries, salad dressings, and condiments are all made in-house, and their cocktails are drinkable art. Fill 'er up.

Roasted Beet LT

2	(1¼-lb.) beets
8	oz. crème fraiche
¼	cup tightly packed, torn fresh tarragon leaves
2	Tbsp. fresh lime juice
½	tsp. lime zest
1	Tbsp. rice wine vinegar
⅛	tsp. table salt
⅛	tsp. freshly ground black pepper
8	(1½-oz.) slices sourdough bread, toasted
4	romaine lettuce leaves
1	large red tomato, cut into 8 thin slices

1. Preheat oven to 375°. Trim beet stems to 1 inch; gently wash, and place in an 11- x 7-inch baking dish. Add 2 cups water to dish.
2. Bake, covered, at 375° for 1 hour and 35 minutes or until tender. Drain and cool slightly (20 minutes). Peel beets, and cut into thin slices.
3. In a small bowl, combine crème fraiche, tarragon, and next 5 ingredients. Stir to combine.
4. Drizzle 1 Tbsp. tarragon crème fraiche evenly on 1 side of bread slices. Layer 1 lettuce leaf and 2 tomato slices on each of 4 bread slices; sprinkle with salt and pepper to taste. Layer 1 cup beet slices over tomato slices; top with remaining bread slices, crème fraiche side down. Cut sandwiches diagonally in half. Serve immediately.
Makes: 4 servings

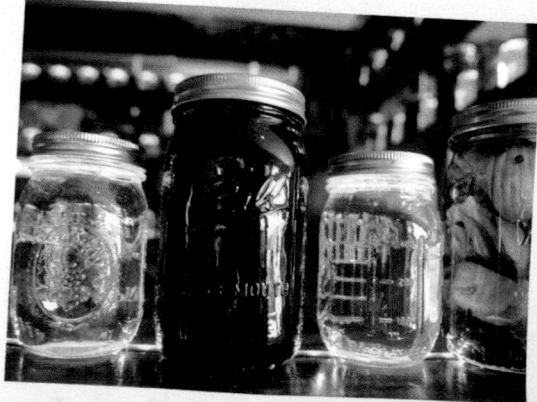

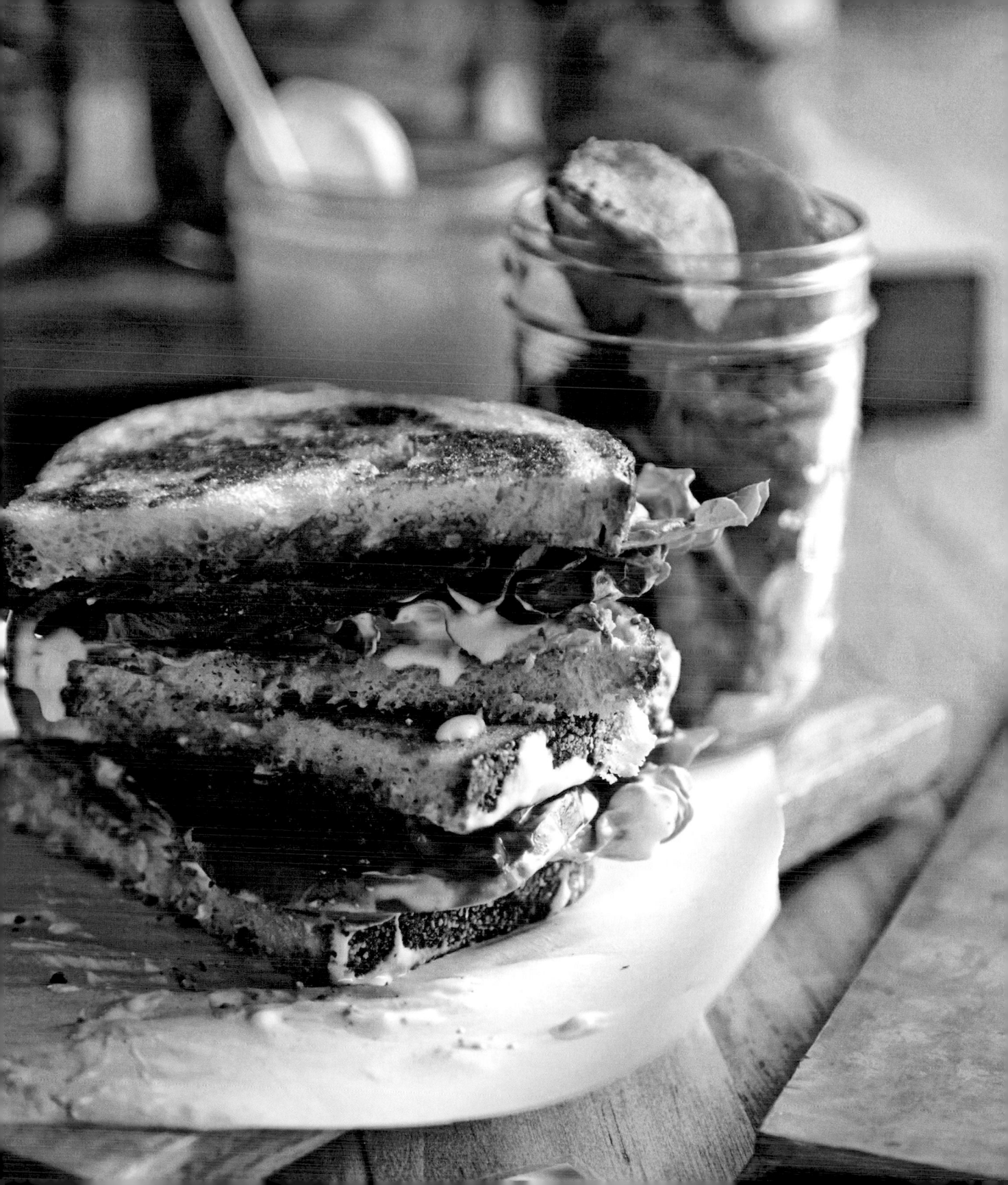

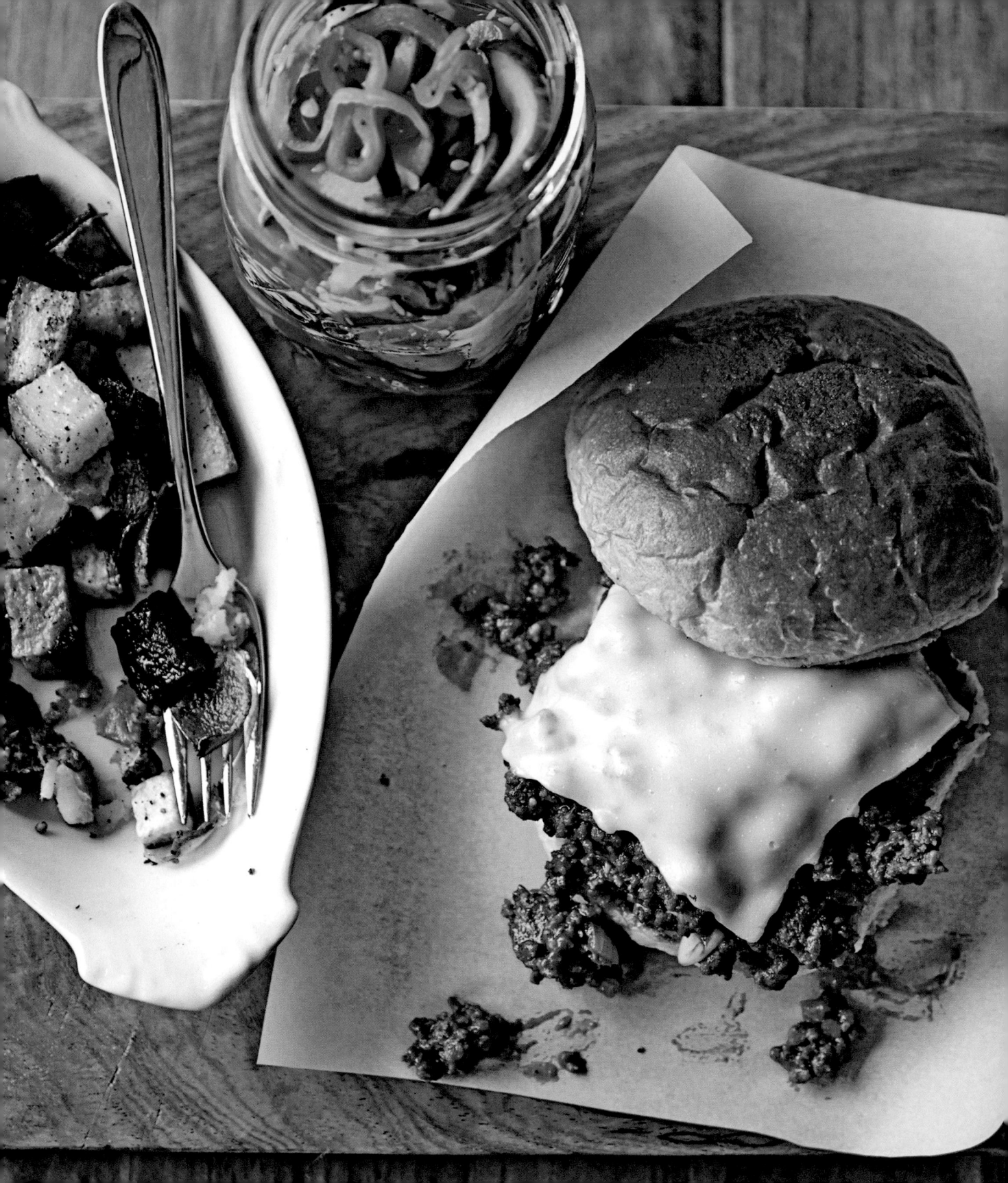

Sloppy Joe

2 lb. ground chuck
½ cup diced onion
1 cup ketchup
2 tsp. table salt
1 tsp. freshly ground pepper
2 tsp. Dijon mustard
1 small garlic clove, minced
4 (3¾-oz.) brioche buns
4 oz. hoop cheese, shredded

1. Cook beef and onion in a large cast-iron skillet over medium-high heat, stirring often, 6 minutes or until meat crumbles and is no longer pink; drain, reserving ¼ cup drippings. Return beef and reserved drippings to skillet. Stir in ketchup and next 4 ingredients. Bring to a simmer; remove from heat.

2. Spoon about 1 cup meat mixture on each bun bottom. Top evenly with cheese and bun tops.
Makes: 4 servings

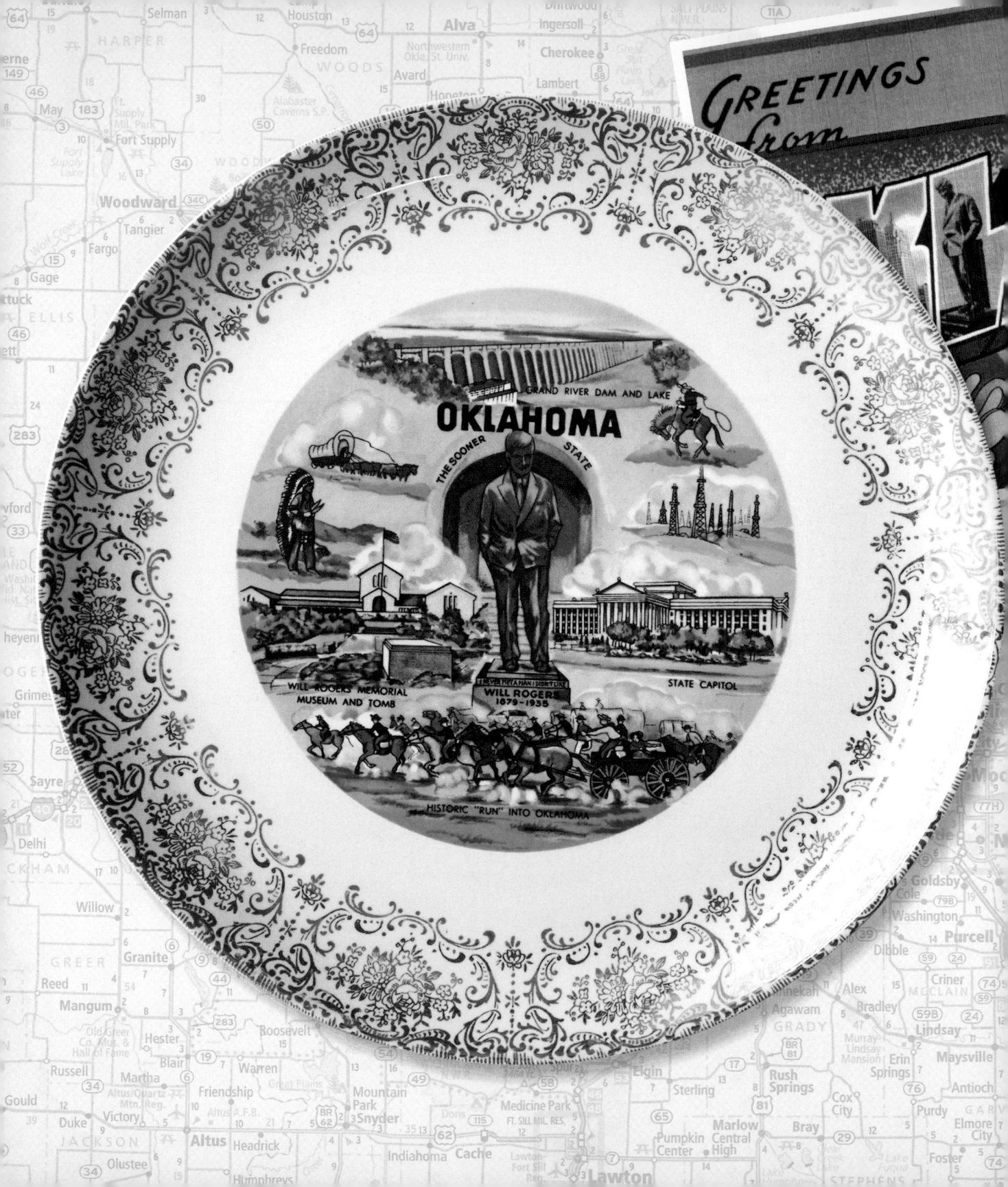

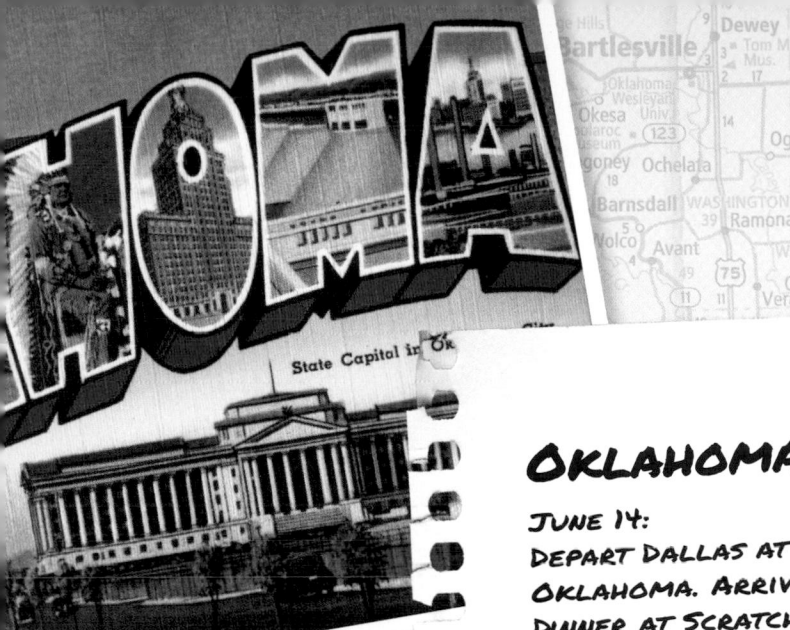

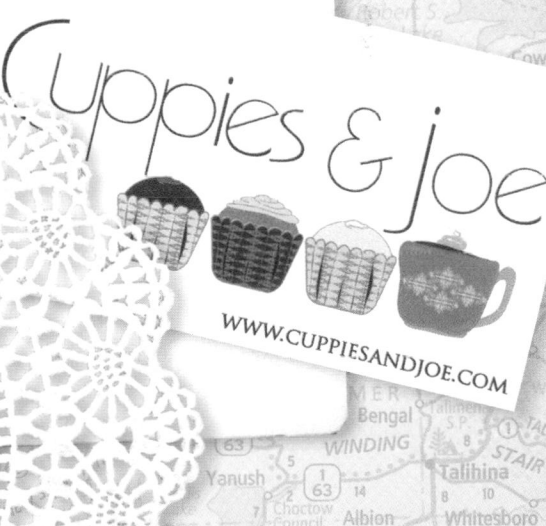

Oklahoma

June 14:
Depart Dallas at 9 A.M. for Norman, Oklahoma. Arrive Norman at 1 P.M. Dinner at Scratch Kitchen & Cocktails with owner Brady Sexton at 6 P.M. Spend the night.

June 15:
Breakfast at Syrup at 9 A.M. Drive to Oklahoma City for afternoon cupcakes and coffee at Cuppies & Joe. Spend the night.

June 16:
Depart Oklahoma City for Little Rock, Arkansas.

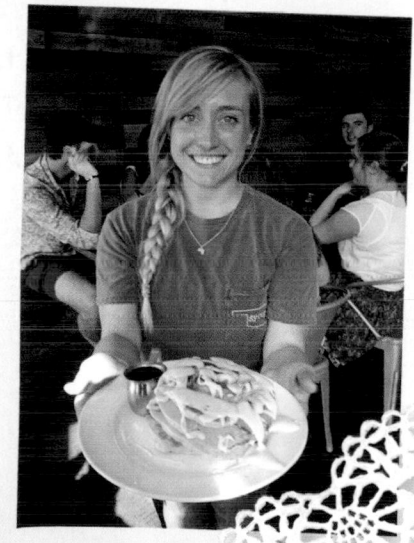

Cuppies & Joe

WWW.CUPPIESANDJOE.COM

syrup.

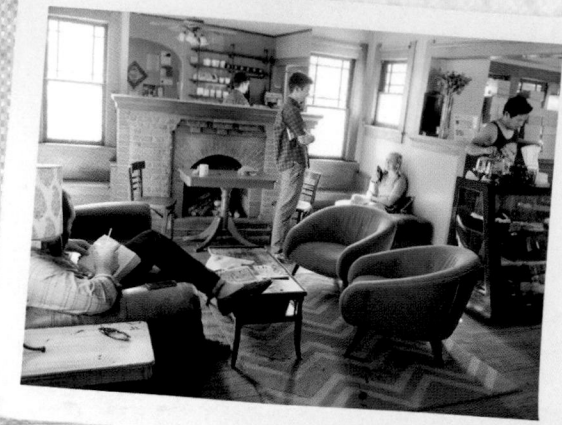

Cuppies & Joe

727 NW 23rd Street
Oklahoma City, Oklahoma 73103
(405) 528-2122
cuppiesandjoe.com

I found this lovely little bakery and java shop while wandering around Oklahoma City looking for a cup of coffee. The staff is as sweet as the cupcakes, which could explain why they've had so many proposals in this tiny cottage. Founded by the mother-daughter duo, Peggy Diefenderfer and Elizabeth Diefenderfer Fleming, Cuppies & Joe is located in a charming Arts & Crafts bungalow in Uptown 23rd District. So if it feels like you're sitting in a living room while you're scarfing down cupcakes and sipping coffee, well, you are. That's part of the appeal—everyone is made to feel at home with the Diefenderfers. ("Diefenderfer," by the way, is German for "rockin' cake lady.")

Salted Caramel-Chocolate Cupcakes

1   cup butter, softened
2   cups sugar
3   large eggs
2½ cups all-purpose flour
1   tsp. baking powder
½   tsp. baking soda
½   tsp. table salt
1   cup sour cream
2   tsp. Madagascar bourbon vanilla bean paste
Paper baking cups
Chocolate Buttercream Frosting
1   cup store-bought caramel sauce
Coarse sea salt

1. Preheat oven to 350°. Beat butter at medium speed with an electric mixer until creamy; gradually add sugar, and beat 2 minutes. Add eggs, 1 at a time, beating just until blended after each addition.

2. Combine flour, baking powder, baking soda, and salt; add to butter mixture alternately with sour cream, beginning and ending with flour mixture. Beat at low speed just until blended after each addition. Stir in vanilla bean paste.

3. Place paper baking cups in 2 (12-cup) muffin pans; spoon batter into cups, filling two-thirds full.

4. Bake at 350° for 20 minutes or until a wooden pick inserted in the centers comes out clean. Remove from pans to wire racks, and cool completely (about 30 minutes).

5. Insert metal tip no. 848 (large star tip) into a large decorating bag; fill with Chocolate Buttercream Frosting. Pipe frosting in a spiral on top of each cupcake. Drizzle each with caramel, and lightly sprinkle with coarse sea salt. **Makes:** 24 servings

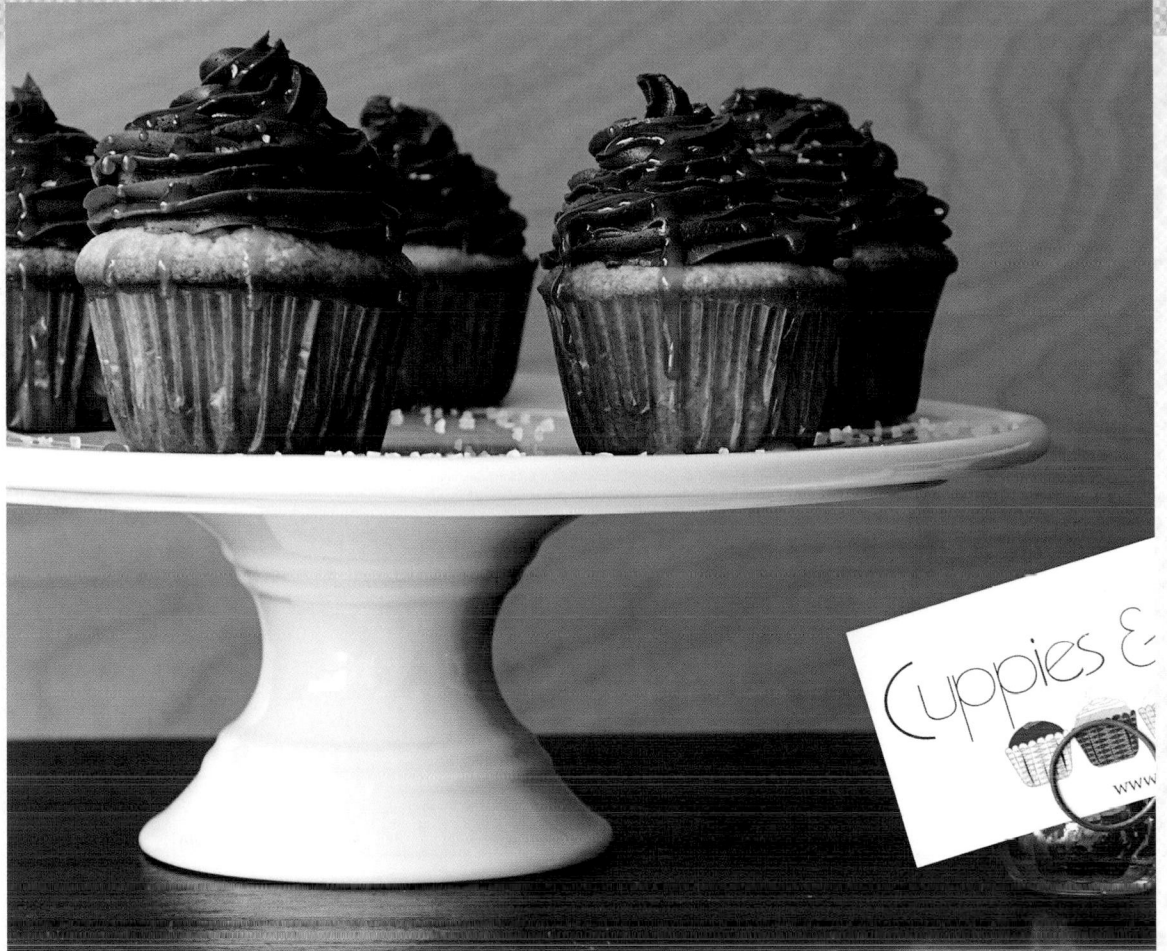

Chocolate Buttercream Frosting

1½ cups unsalted butter, softened
6 cups powdered sugar
¾ cup unsweetened cocoa
3 Tbsp. heavy cream
1½ tsp. vanilla extract

Beat butter at medium speed with an electric mixer until smooth. Gradually add powdered sugar and cocoa, beating at low speed until blended and smooth, scraping down sides of bowl as needed. Beat in cream and vanilla.
Makes: 4 cups

Joe Mamma

This refreshing summer coffee is not too sweet, but very frothy.

1½ cups half-and-half
¼ cup pure cane syrup
¼ cup brewed espresso

Combine all ingredients in a cocktail shaker. Cover with lid, and shake vigorously 30 seconds. Pour evenly into 2 ice-filled 1-pt. mason jars.
Makes: 2 servings
Note: We tested with Steen's Pure Cane Syrup.

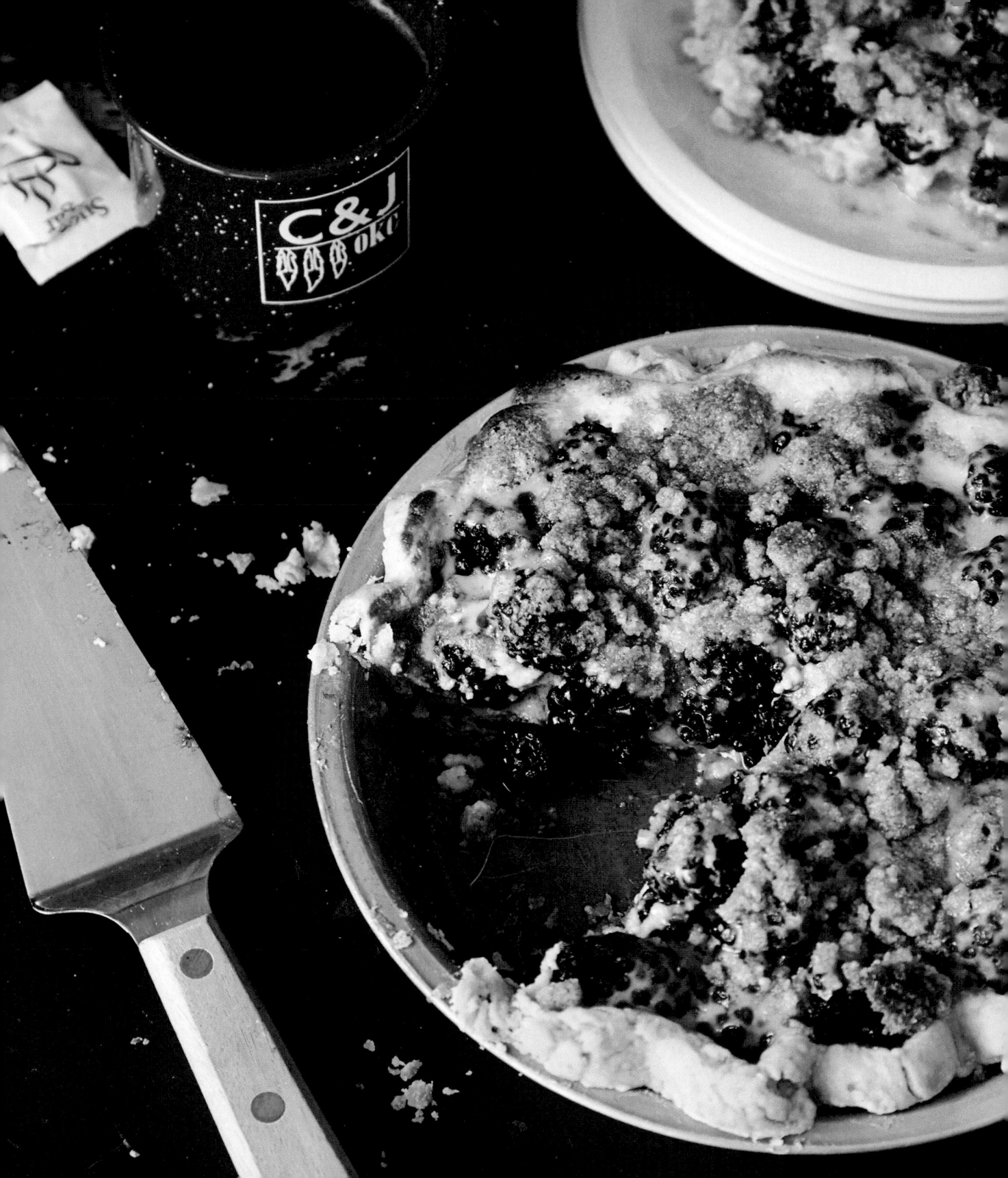

Blackberry Cream Pie

This is a rich, gooey bonanza of summer blackberries and flaky crust.

1	Cuppies & Joe's Piecrust
4	cups fresh blackberries
1	cup sour cream
1	cup sugar
3	Tbsp. all-purpose flour
1	large egg
2	Tbsp. butter
2	Tbsp. sugar
3	Tbsp. fine, dry breadcrumbs

1. Preheat oven to 375°. Fit piecrust into a 9-inch pie plate; fold edges under, and crimp. Prick bottom and sides with a fork. Bake 20 minutes or until light golden brown. Cool completely on a wire rack (about 30 minutes).
2. Place blackberries in crust. Combine sour cream, 1 cup sugar, flour, and egg, stirring well with a whisk; pour over blackberries, spreading evenly.
3. Place butter and 2 Tbsp. sugar in a small microwave-safe bowl. Cover and microwave at HIGH 30 seconds or until butter melts; stir to dissolve sugar. Stir in breadcrumbs. Sprinkle breadcrumb mixture over sour cream mixture.
4. Bake at 375° for 45 minutes or until top is golden brown and filling is puffed and set. Cool completely on a wire rack (about 2 hours).
Makes: 8 servings

Cuppies & Joe's Piecrust

3	cups all-purpose flour
1	tsp. table salt
1¼	cups shortening
1	large egg
1	Tbsp. white vinegar
¼	cup ice water

1. Whisk together flour and salt in a large bowl. Cut shortening into flour mixture with a pastry blender until shortening is the size of peas.
2. Whisk together egg, vinegar, and ice water in a small bowl. Add to flour mixture, stirring with a fork just until a soft dough forms.
3. Divide dough into thirds. Shape each portion into a flat disk (about 4 inches in diameter). If using immediately, roll into a 12-inch circle on a lightly floured surface.
4. If not using immediately, wrap each dough disk in plastic wrap. Place in a zip-top plastic freezer bag. Seal, label, and freeze up to 2 weeks. Thaw in refrigerator overnight. Roll out on a lightly floured surface, place in a 9-inch pie plate, and proceed with recipe. **Makes: 3 (9-inch) crusts**
Note: For ready-to-bake crusts, fit each pastry crust into a 9-inch pie plate; fold edges under, and crimp. Prick bottom and sides of crusts with a fork. Bake in a preheated 375° oven for 25 minutes or as directed.

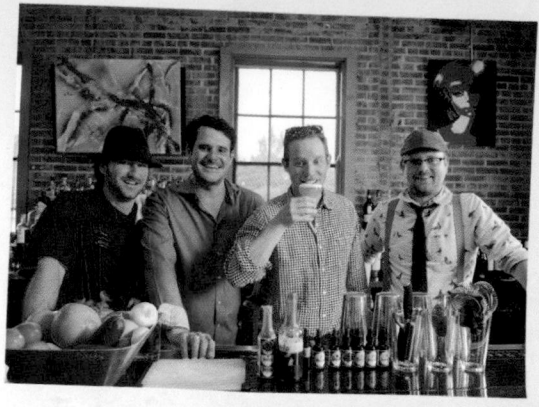

Scratch Kitchen & Cocktails

132 West Main
Norman, Oklahoma 73069
(405) 801-2900
scratchnorman.com

Housed in what used to be an old telephone switchboard building, Scratch's decor oozes cool sophistication. Edison bulbs illuminate the bar built by owner Brady Sexton. Inventive cocktails and a decadent menu are all crafted from, yes, scratch. When there's a sauce on the menu, it hasn't come from a bag or a powder—instead, the kitchen toils over it, reducing sauces for up to 12 hours. You can taste that difference in the pork chop. This double-bone monster weighs in at 16 ounces, and is marinated in herbs and served with a light apple compote. Or sample the strip steak, which is topped with a peppercorn sauce so tasty it made me want to lick the plate. Brady, a former oil and gasman, regards any artificial ingredients as the enemy. "There's a bar on the door to corn syrup and those fake sweeteners," he says.

Whiskey Smash

This quaff is tart and minty, but not too sweet. It's ideal for slow sipping on the front porch.

- ¼ cup bourbon
- 1½ Tbsp. fresh lemon juice
- 1½ Tbsp. Maple-Brown Sugar Syrup
- 5 to 7 fresh mint leaves
- 2 (3- x ½-inch) lemon peel strips
- 1 mint sprig

Combine first 5 ingredients in a cocktail shaker; fill shaker with ice. Cover with lid, and shake vigorously until thoroughly chilled (about 30 seconds). Pour through a fine wire-mesh strainer into a rocks glass filled with ice. Hold mint sprig in your hand; slap it with your other hand to awaken the oils. Place in drink. **Makes:** 1 serving
Note: We tested with Old Forester 90-proof Bourbon.

Maple-Brown Sugar Syrup

- 1 cup light brown sugar
- ¾ cup maple syrup

Bring 2 cups water to a simmer in a medium saucepan. Remove from heat; gradually add brown sugar, whisking until sugar dissolves. Whisk in syrup. Cool completely. Pour into a container; store, covered, in refrigerator up to 2 weeks. **Makes:** 2½ cups

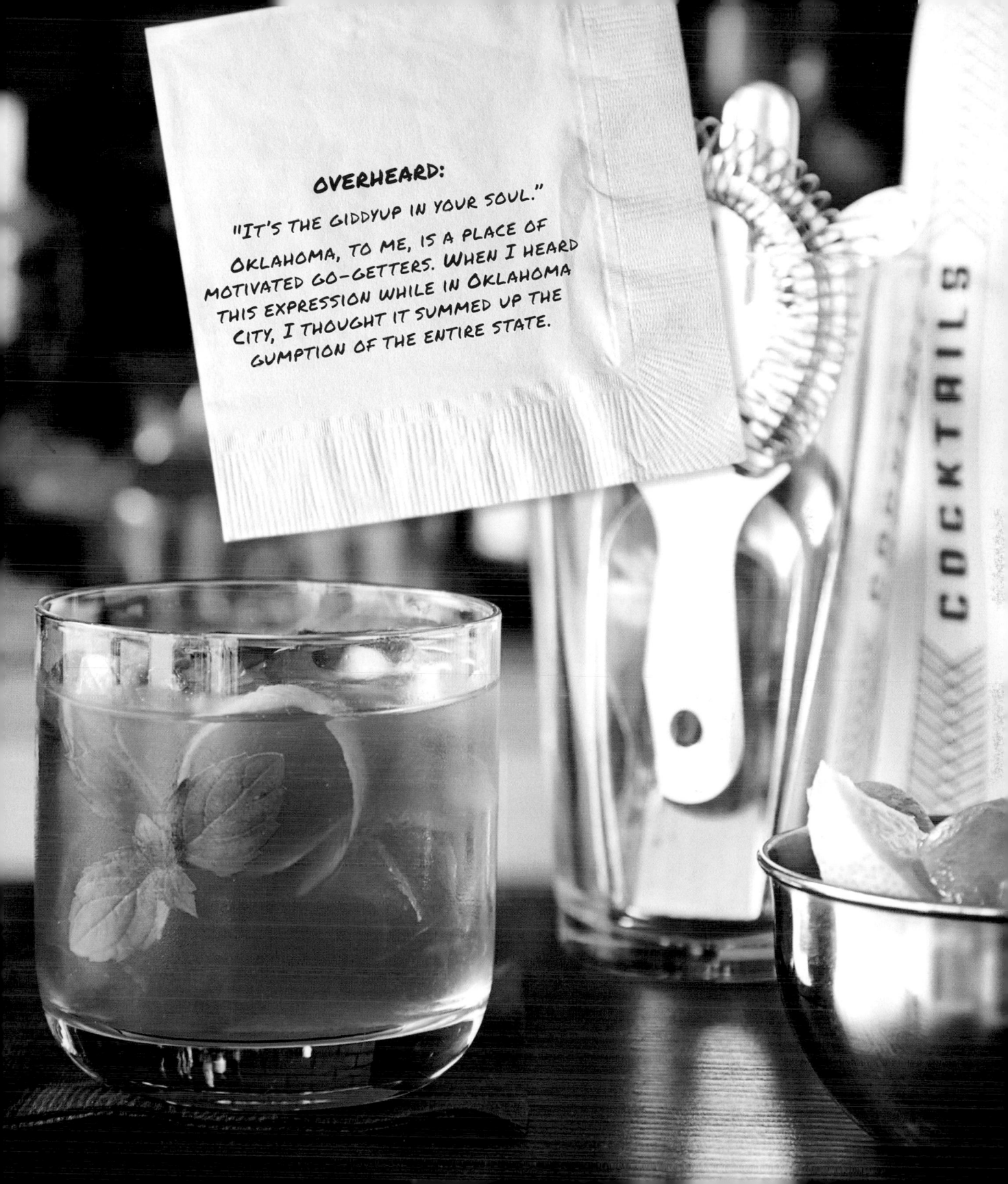

OVERHEARD:

"IT'S THE GIDDYUP IN YOUR SOUL." OKLAHOMA, TO ME, IS A PLACE OF MOTIVATED GO-GETTERS. WHEN I HEARD THIS EXPRESSION WHILE IN OKLAHOMA CITY, I THOUGHT IT SUMMED UP THE GUMPTION OF THE ENTIRE STATE.

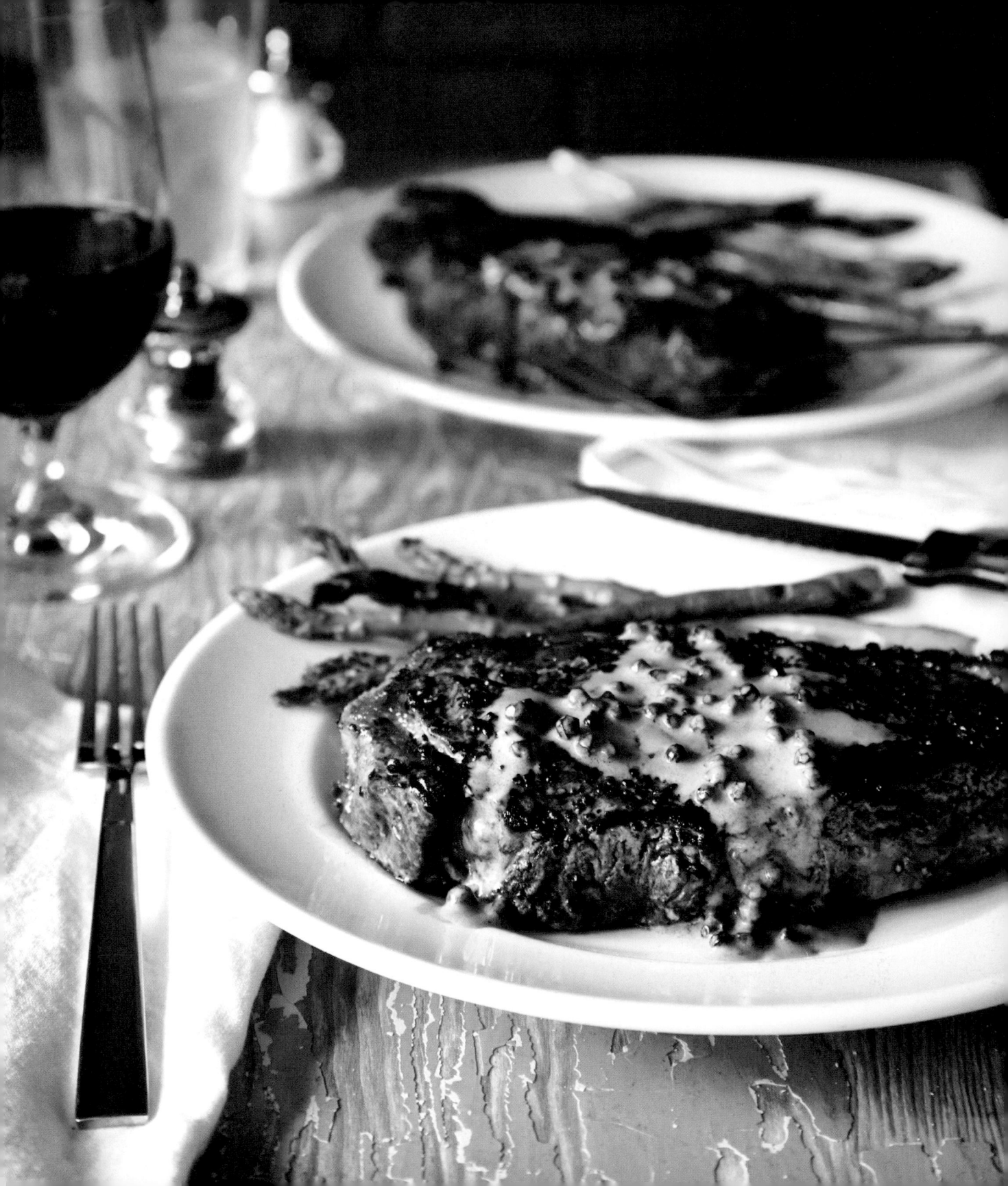

Steak au Poivre

This steak sauce is ridiculously rich without containing any fake thickeners. It's all work, but well worth it.

SAUCE

2	Tbsp. green peppercorns
½	cup white vinegar
1	Tbsp. butter
1	Tbsp. olive oil
1¼	lb. beef tenderloin trimmings, cut into ½-inch pieces
2	hickory-smoked bacon slices, cut crosswise into ½-inch pieces
2	cups chopped onion
1	cup chopped celery
1	cup chopped carrot
1	Tbsp. black peppercorns
3	garlic cloves, crushed
¼	cup tomato paste
1	bay leaf
1	cup dry white wine
1	cup brandy
2	qt. beef stock
1	cup heavy cream
1	Tbsp. cognac
1	tsp. lemon juice

STEAKS

4	(12-oz.) beef strip steaks (1 inch thick)
2	tsp. kosher salt
3	Tbsp. mixed whole peppercorns
1	Tbsp. coriander seeds
1	Tbsp. olive oil

1. Prepare Sauce: Combine green peppercorns, ½ cup white vinegar, and ½ cup water in a small saucepan. Bring to a boil; remove from heat, and let stand 1 hour until peppercorns sink to bottom of pan and are soft. Drain and reserve.

2. Heat butter and 1 Tbsp. olive oil in a large Dutch oven over medium-high heat until butter melts. Add beef trimmings. Cook 8 minutes or until dark brown. Stir and cook 5 minutes or until browned on all sides, stirring occasionally.

Add bacon; cook, stirring often, 5 minutes or until beginning to crisp.

3. Add onion and next 4 ingredients; cook, stirring often, 6 minutes or until vegetables are tender and onion is beginning to brown. Reduce heat to medium-low. Add tomato paste and bay leaf. Cook, stirring constantly, 1 minute or until tomato paste thickens and darkens in color.

4. Stir in white wine and brandy. Increase heat to medium-high; cook, uncovered, 10 minutes or until liquid almost evaporates.

5. Add beef stock. Bring to a boil; boil, uncovered, 1 hour and 10 minutes or until reduced by half. Pour mixture through a wire-mesh strainer lined with several layers of cheesecloth; discard solids. Wipe Dutch oven clean with a paper towel. Return 2 cups strained sauce to Dutch oven; add reserved green peppercorns. Bring to a boil; boil 15 minutes or until syrupy and reduced to 1 cup. Remove from heat; cover and set aside.

6. Prepare Steaks: Preheat oven to 400°. Sprinkle steaks on both sides with salt. Process peppercorn medley and coriander seeds in a coffee grinder until coarsely ground. Rub about 1 tsp. peppercorn mixture onto each side of steaks, reserving remaining 2 Tbsp. for another use.

7. Heat 1 Tbsp. olive oil in a 12-inch ovenproof skillet over medium-high heat. Place steaks, not touching each other, in skillet; cook 2 minutes or until well browned. Turn steaks over; place skillet in oven. Bake, uncovered, at 400° for 6 minutes or until a meat thermometer inserted in thickest part registers 140° (medium-rare). Transfer steaks to serving plates; let stand 3 minutes.

8. Meanwhile, stir heavy cream and cognac into sauce mixture. Cook, stirring gently, over low heat 1 minute or just until thoroughly heated. (Do not boil.) Remove from heat; stir in lemon juice. Serve sauce with steak. **Makes: 4 servings**
Note: Ask your butcher for trimmings from beef tenderloins that include some fat.

Moonshine Apple Pie

This tall, flaky pastry dish is full of apples, but it's the buttery goodness and filling that really make this dish shine.

PASTRY

2¼	cups unbleached all-purpose flour
1	Tbsp. sugar
1	tsp. table salt
¾	cup frozen unsalted butter
½	cup ice water

FILLING

1	cup firmly packed brown sugar
¼	cup all-purpose flour
1	Tbsp. ground cinnamon
¼	tsp. ground nutmeg
¼	tsp. ground allspice
½	cup salted butter, cut up
3	lb. Granny Smith apples (about 6 medium), peeled and thinly sliced
2	Tbsp. moonshine
1	large egg

Bottled cinnamon-sugar

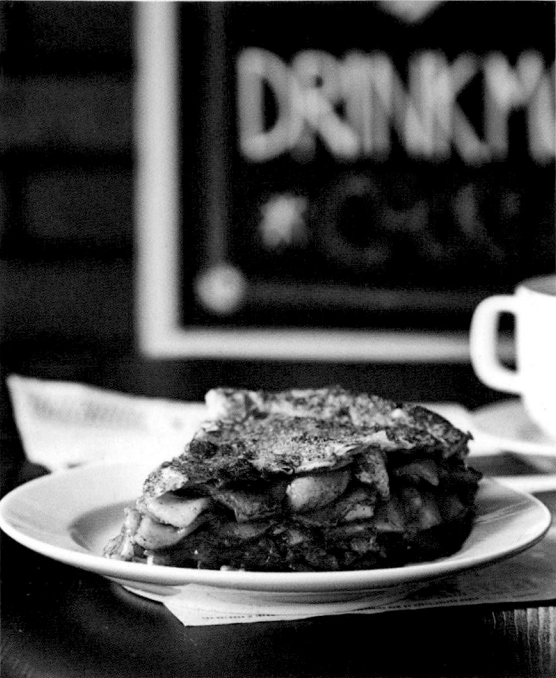

1. **Prepare Pastry:** Whisk together first 3 ingredients. Grate ¾ cup butter over flour mixture; stir with a fork. Add ice water, 1 Tbsp. at a time, stirring with a fork until a dough forms. Divide dough into 2 equal portions. Shape each portion into a ball. Roll 1 ball into an 11-inch circle on a floured surface; fit into a 9-inch pie plate. Fold edges under. Chill 30 minutes. Wrap remaining dough ball in plastic wrap; chill.

2. **Prepare Filling:** Preheat oven to 350°. Combine first 5 ingredients in a bowl. Add ½ cup butter to a large skillet; place over medium heat. Add apple slices; cook 10 minutes or until butter melts, stirring to coat slices as butter melts. Add brown sugar mixture and moonshine; cook, stirring constantly, 2 minutes or until brown sugar melts and mixture thickens. Remove from heat; set aside.

3. Line pastry with aluminum foil, and fill with pie weights or dried beans; bake at 350° for 20 minutes. Remove weights and foil, and bake 5 more minutes or until bottom is golden brown. Place on a wire rack to cool while preparing second pie crust.

4. Roll remaining dough ball into an 11-inch circle. Whisk together egg and 1 Tbsp. water in a small bowl. Brush egg wash onto edges of prebaked crust. Spoon pie filling into prebaked crust. Place dough circle over filling, pressing to adhere to bottom crust. Brush egg wash over top of pie; sprinkle with cinnamon-sugar. Cut slits in top of pie to allow steam to escape. Place pie on a baking sheet lined with foil.

5. Bake at 350° for 45 minutes or until crust is golden brown and filling is bubbly. Cool completely on a wire rack (about 1 hour). **Makes: 6 to 8 servings**

Note: We tested with Midnight Moon Moonshine.

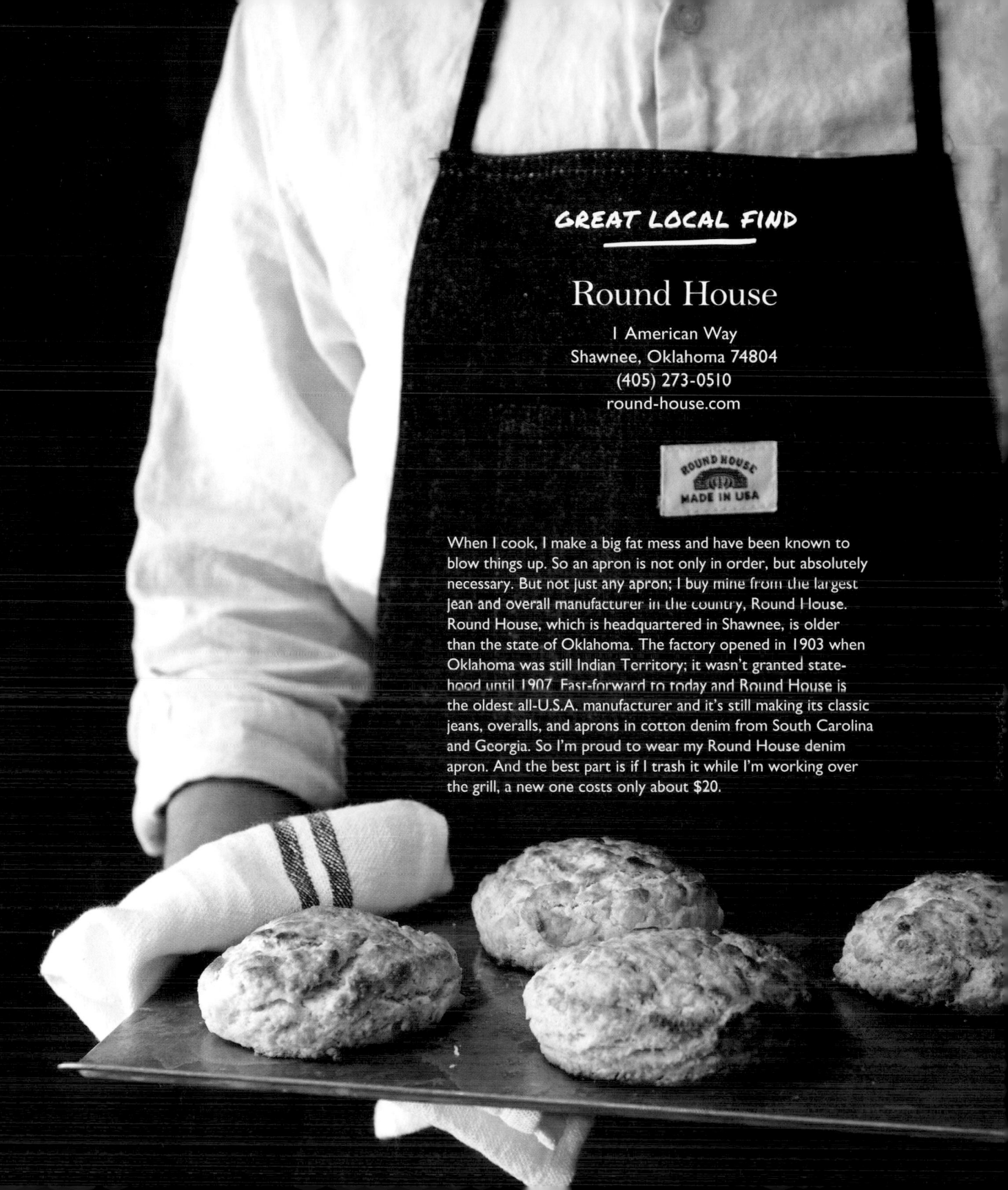

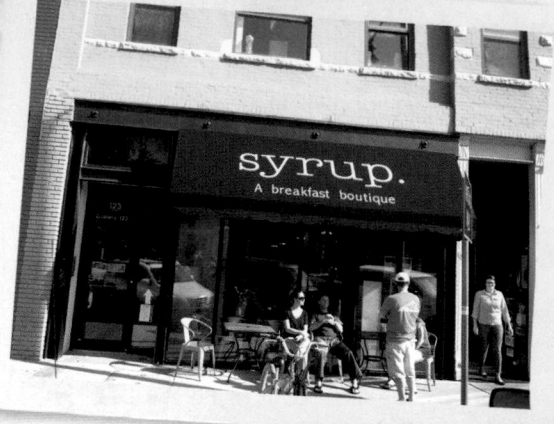

Syrup.

123 East Main Street
Norman, Oklahoma 73069
(405) 701-1143
syrupbreakfast.com

Few could stay in a bad mood at Syrup. Sunny yellow booths, rich coffee, and amazing breakfast selections will start any day out right. Even better, all of the profits from this sweet bistro go to charity. Owner Ashley Kennedy knew she wanted to go to South Africa when she was just 10 years old, and it's that passion that inspired the mission of Syrup. Well, that and good waffles. "I'm not a chef. I'm just a mother of four children who wanted a great breakfast," she says. And what a great breakfast she makes: Her cinnamon roll pancakes, pecan-smoked bacon, and amazing frittata won me over. But it's a South African dish, the "Morning Glory," (a waffle covered by eggs, sausage, bacon, and cheese), that really impressed.

Crunchy French Toast

The cornflake crust gives this French toast a crunchy texture that helps it stand up to a puddle of syrup.

4   large eggs
2   Tbsp. sugar
¾   tsp. ground cinnamon
½   tsp. vanilla extract
1/16 tsp. ground nutmeg
1   cup heavy cream
¾   cup half-and-half
4   cups cornflakes cereal, coarsely crushed
6   Tbsp. butter
8   (1.75-oz.) slices challah bread (about 1 inch thick)
Maple syrup

1. Whisk together first 5 ingredients in a large bowl. Whisk in cream and half-and-half. Place cornflake cereal in a shallow dish.
2. Melt 2 Tbsp. butter in a large nonstick skillet over medium heat. Dip 3 bread slices in egg mixture, turning to coat; dredge in crushed cereal. Cook coated slices in melted butter over medium heat 1 to 2 minutes on each side or until golden brown and egg is cooked in center.
3. Repeat procedure with remaining bread, egg mixture, cereal, and butter. Serve with maple syrup. **Makes: 4 servings**

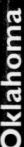

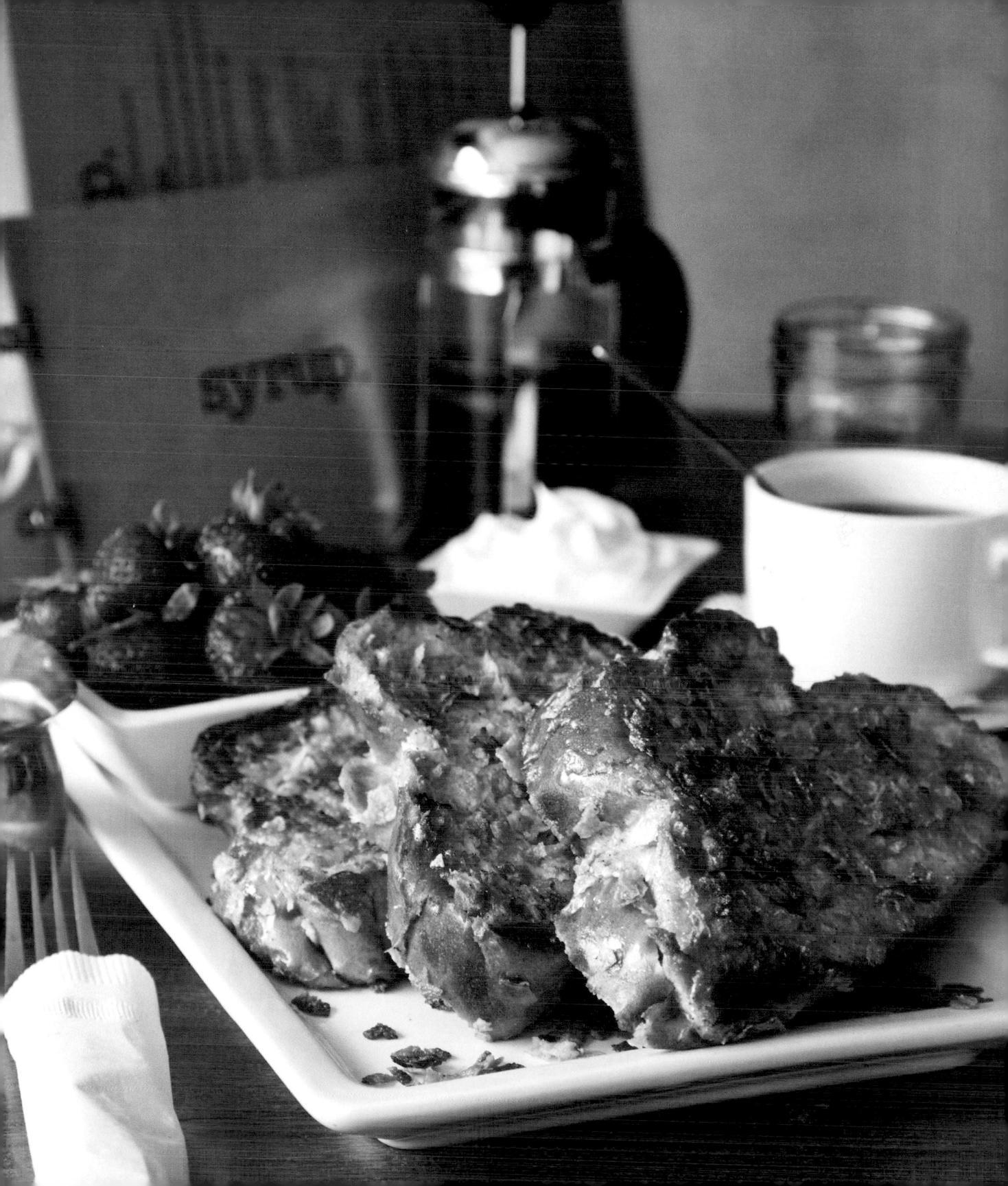

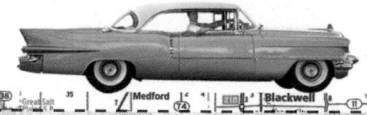

Oklahoma bucket list

things to see and do (besides eat) here

1 Take a tour along any of Oklahoma's 400 miles of **Route 66** *(pictured)*—the state has more surviving miles of the original route left than any other. Just be sure to pick up a Route 66 map before you head out, as state maps no longer include the early route.

2 Visit Frank Lloyd Wright's only skyscraper, **Price Tower**, in Bartlesville. The 19-story building opened in 1956 and is now listed as a National Historic Landmark.

3 Swing by historic **Stockyards City** in Oklahoma City to see some action—and by action we mean real cowboys working livestock at the largest cattle market in the world.

4 Travel back in time to 1903 touring the **Overholser Mansion**, considered Oklahoma City's first mansion and now listed on the National Register of Historic Places.

5 Catch a movie at one of the nation's coolest drive-ins: the **Winchester** in Oklahoma City.

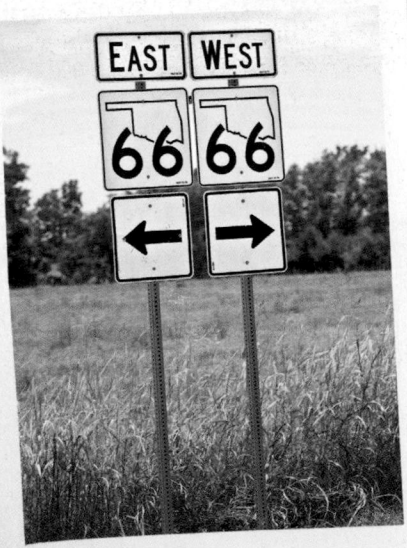

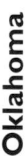

Stuffed "Frittata"

This hearty egg dish is packed with all kinds of morning goodness, but it's also perfect for brunch or one of my favorites, "brinner."

¼   cup butter
1   cup ¼-inch diced peeled potatoes
1   cup diced green bell pepper
1   cup diced onion
3   garlic cloves, minced
1   cup firmly packed fresh baby spinach, chopped
¾   cup chopped cooked applewood-smoked bacon (about 12 slices)
Vegetable cooking spray
10   large eggs
2   Tbsp. seasoned salt
1   cup milk
4   oz. Tillamook Cheddar cheese, shredded

1. Preheat oven to 350°. Melt butter in a large nonstick skillet over medium heat. Add potato and next 3 ingredients. Cook, stirring often, 8 minutes or until vegetables are tender. Stir in spinach and bacon. Remove from heat.

2. Lightly grease a 9-inch deep-dish pie plate with cooking spray. Transfer cooked mixture to prepared pie plate.

3. Whisk eggs and seasoned salt together in a separate bowl; whisk in milk. Pour egg mixture over vegetable mixture. Sprinkle with cheese.

4. Bake, uncovered, at 350° for 35 minutes or just until set and golden brown. Let stand 10 minutes before serving. **Makes: 8 servings**

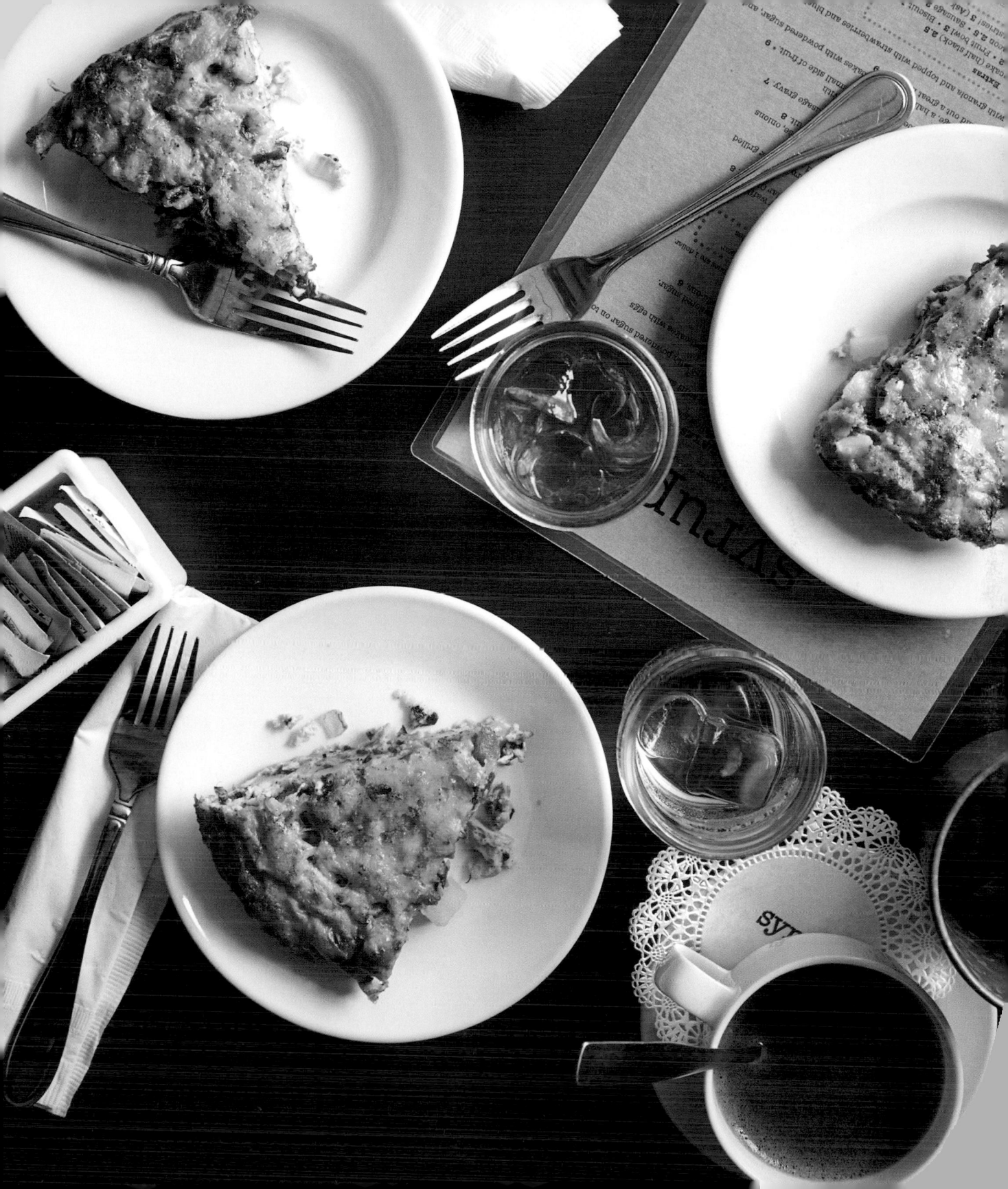

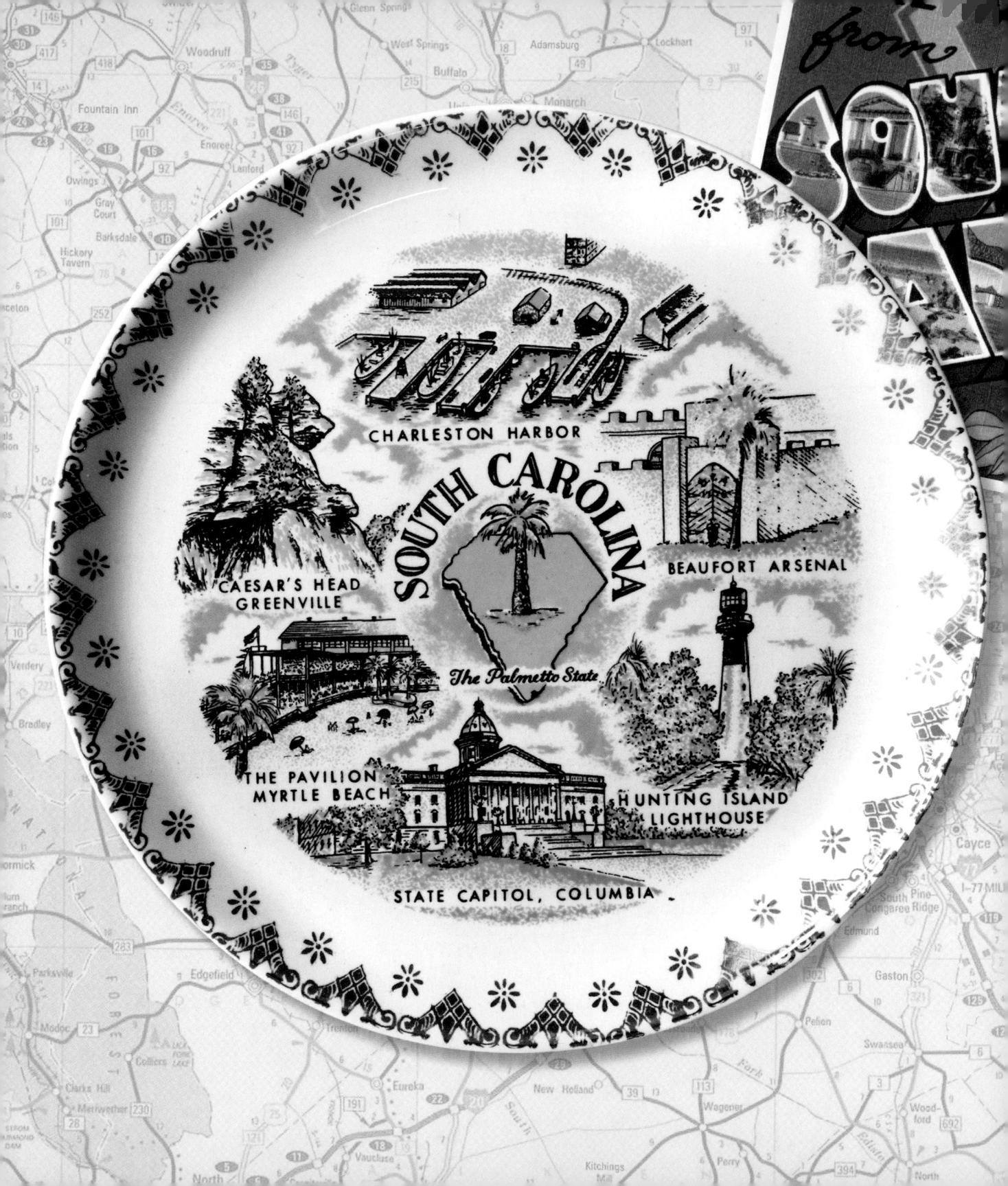

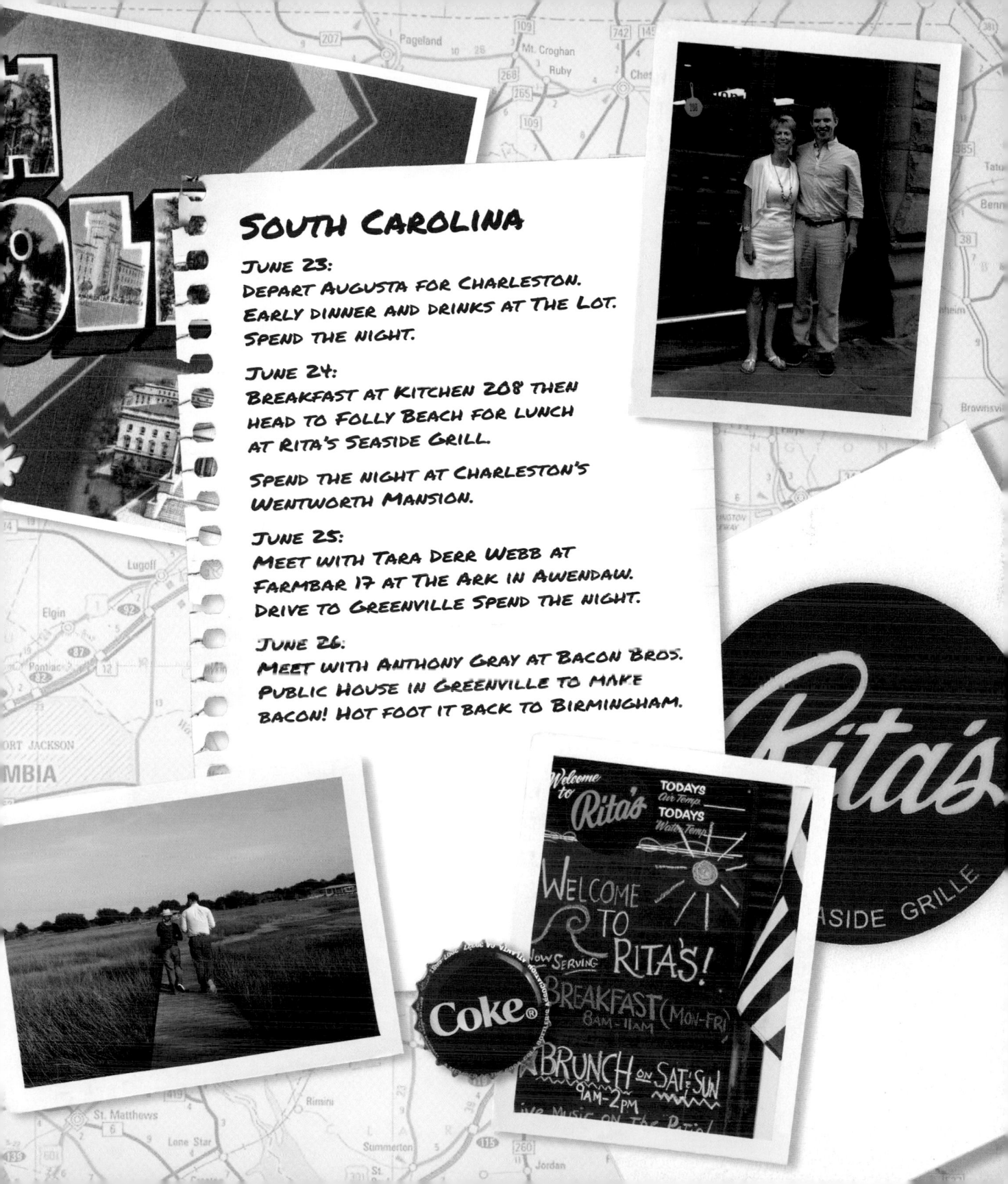

South Carolina

June 23:
Depart Augusta for Charleston. Early dinner and drinks at The Lot. Spend the night.

June 24:
Breakfast at Kitchen 208 then head to Folly Beach for lunch at Rita's Seaside Grill.

Spend the night at Charleston's Wentworth Mansion.

June 25:
Meet with Tara Derr Webb at Farmbar 17 at The Ark in Awendaw. Drive to Greenville Spend the night.

June 26:
Meet with Anthony Gray at Bacon Bros. Public House in Greenville to make bacon! Hot foot it back to Birmingham.

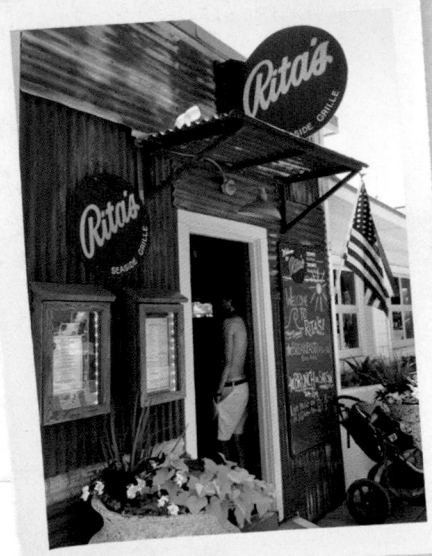

Rita's Seaside Grille

2 Center Street
Folly Beach, South Carolina 29439
(843) 588-2525
ritasseasidegrille.com

Don't dare call Folly Beach Charleston. Though it sits just minutes from the Holy City, Folly Beach has its own culture and vibe. Millionaires and surf bums get along with Southern ease, which makes this beach town one of my faves. Rita's Seaside Grill captures that same ethos with the best bar in town (the bar itself is covered with vintage surf shack stickers). Don't miss Rita's spicy blackened tuna nachos—try them with a house-squeezed watermelon margarita. The shrimp and grits are also a must. Then go work everything off body surfing in the Atlantic. The waves crash just steps away from Rita's doors.

Blackened Tuna Nachos with Watermelon Pico de Gallo

WATERMELON PICO DE GALLO

2   cups ¼-inch diced seedless watermelon
¼   cup ¼-inch diced red onion
¼   cup minced fresh cilantro
¼   cup minced fresh parsley
2   Tbsp. fresh lime juice
¼   tsp. table salt
¼   tsp. ground cumin

BLACKENED TUNA NACHOS

1   (1-lb.) tuna steak (1⅓ inches thick)
2   Tbsp. blackened redfish seasoning
2   Tbsp. canola oil, divided
1   cup very thin sweet onion strips (about ½ medium)
1   jalapeño pepper, seeded and minced
1   (15.5-oz.) can black beans, drained and rinsed
½   tsp. ground cumin
½   tsp. table salt
2   green onions, chopped
9   cups corn tortilla chips
1   lb. mild white Cheddar cheese, shredded

1. Prepare Watermelon Pico de Gallo: Combine all ingredients in a large bowl. Cover and chill 1 hour.
2. Prepare Blackened Tuna Nachos: Preheat oven to 350°. Sprinkle all sides of tuna with blackened redfish seasoning. Set aside.
3. Heat 1 Tbsp. oil in a large nonstick skillet over medium-high heat. Sauté onion and jalapeño pepper in hot oil 5 minutes or until softened. Stir in black beans and next 3 ingredients. Cook 2 minutes or until thoroughly heated.
4. Spread tortilla chips on a half sheet pan. Sprinkle with half of cheese. Spoon bean mixture evenly over top of cheese. Sprinkle with remaining half of cheese.
5. Wipe skillet clean; add remaining 1 Tbsp. oil, and heat over medium-high heat until hot. Add

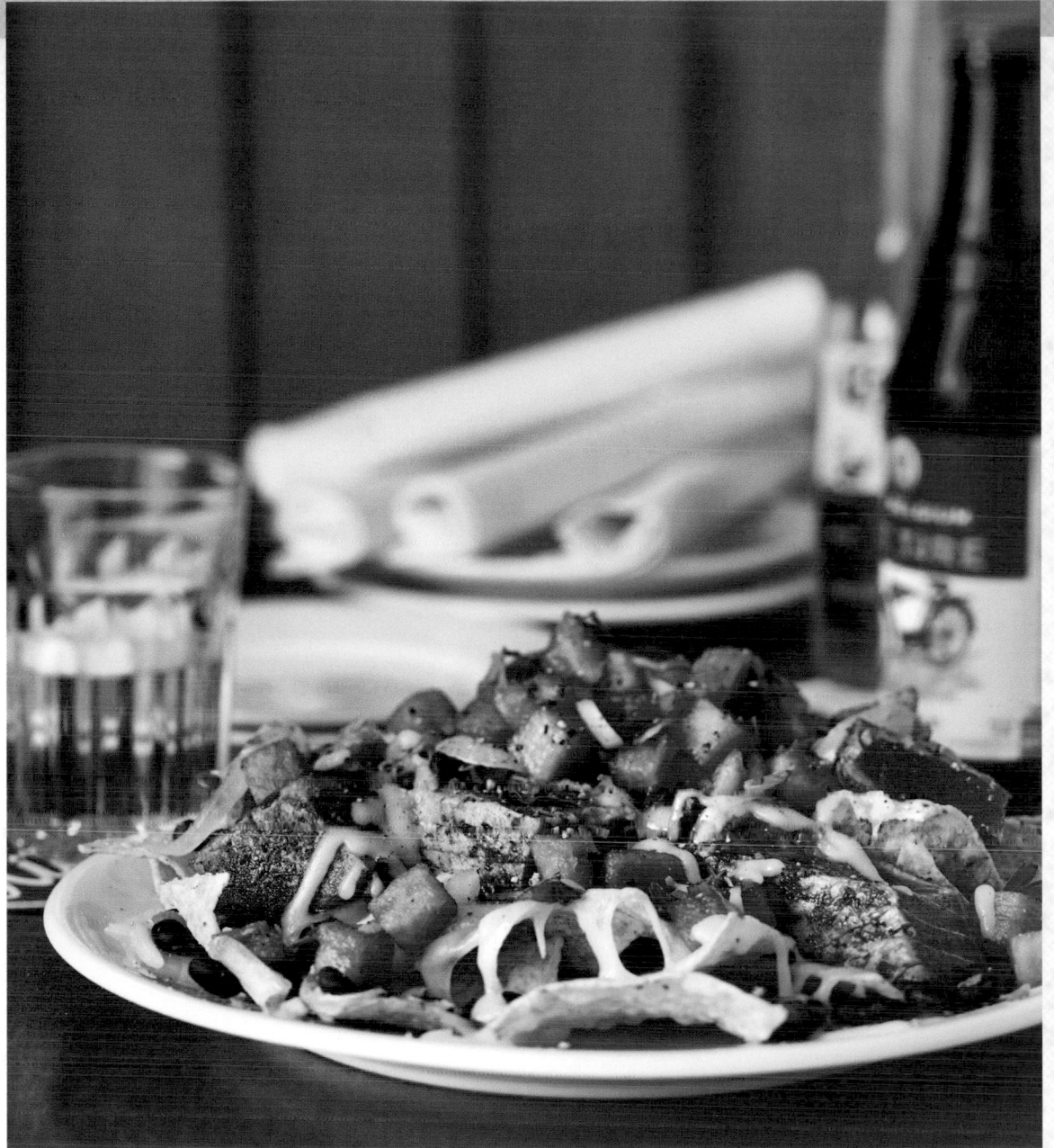

tuna steak, and sear on all sides, 4 minutes or to desired degree of doneness. Transfer to a cutting board; let stand 5 minutes.

6. Meanwhile, bake nachos at 350° for 7 minutes or until cheese melts. Remove from oven, and let stand 3 minutes. Cut tuna into thin slices; cut slices into 1-inch pieces, and arrange over top of nachos. Serve immediately with Watermelon Pico de Gallo. **Makes: 6 to 8 appetizer servings**

Shrimp and Grits

GRITS
2   cups milk
1   tsp. table salt
¼   tsp. freshly ground black pepper
1   cup uncooked stone-ground grits
2   Tbsp. unsalted butter
½   cup shredded mild Cheddar cheese

SHRIMP SAUCE
14   oz. peeled and deveined large shrimp (16 shrimp)
1   Tbsp. blackening seasoning
2   Tbsp. olive oil
½   cup dry white wine
1   cup heavy cream
½   cup chopped cooked bacon
1   cup finely diced vine-ripened tomato
½   cup sliced green onions (2 onions)

1. Prepare Grits: Bring first 3 ingredients and 2 cups water to a boil over medium-high heat in a medium saucepan. Slowly whisk in grits; cover, reduce heat, and simmer 25 minutes or until grits are tender and thickened, stirring often.
2. Add butter and cheese, whisking until butter and cheese melt. Cover and keep warm.
3. Meanwhile, prepare Shrimp Sauce: Pat shrimp dry with a paper towel. Toss together shrimp and blackening seasoning in a large bowl. Heat olive oil in a large skillet on medium-high heat; add shrimp, and cook 2 minutes on each side. Remove shrimp from skillet, and keep warm. Add white wine to skillet, stirring to loosen browned bits from bottom of skillet. Cook, uncovered, 1 minute or until wine is reduced by half. Add cream, bacon, and tomato; cook, stirring constantly, over medium-high heat 4 minutes or until thickened. Remove from heat; stir in shrimp. Spoon grits evenly into 4 bowls; top evenly with Shrimp Sauce. Sprinkle with green onions. Makes: 4 servings

Seafood Cobb Salad

8   oz. fresh crabmeat
5   cups firmly packed mixed salad greens
1   cup chopped cooked bacon
1   cup crumbled blue cheese
12   grape tomatoes, halved lengthwise
⅓   cup Seafood Cobb Salad Dressing
1   lb. cooked shrimp, peeled and deveined
6   hard-cooked eggs, peeled and halved

1. Pick crabmeat, removing any bits of shell.
2. Combine salad greens and next 3 ingredients in a large bowl; drizzle with Seafood Cobb Salad Dressing, and toss gently.
3. Divide greens mixture among 4 large salad bowls. Top with evenly with crabmeat, shrimp, and egg halves. Makes: 4 servings

Seafood Cobb Salad Dressing

2   Tbsp. white balsamic vinegar
¾   tsp. finely diced shallot
¾   tsp. finely chopped fresh parsley
¼   tsp. Dijon mustard
¼   tsp. honey
¼   tsp. table salt
Pinch of freshly ground black pepper
6   Tbsp. vegetable oil

Combine all ingredients, except oil, in a blender; process until pureed. Remove center piece of blender lid; secure blender lid on blender. With blender on, pour oil through center of lid in a thin stream; process until blended. Makes: ½ cup

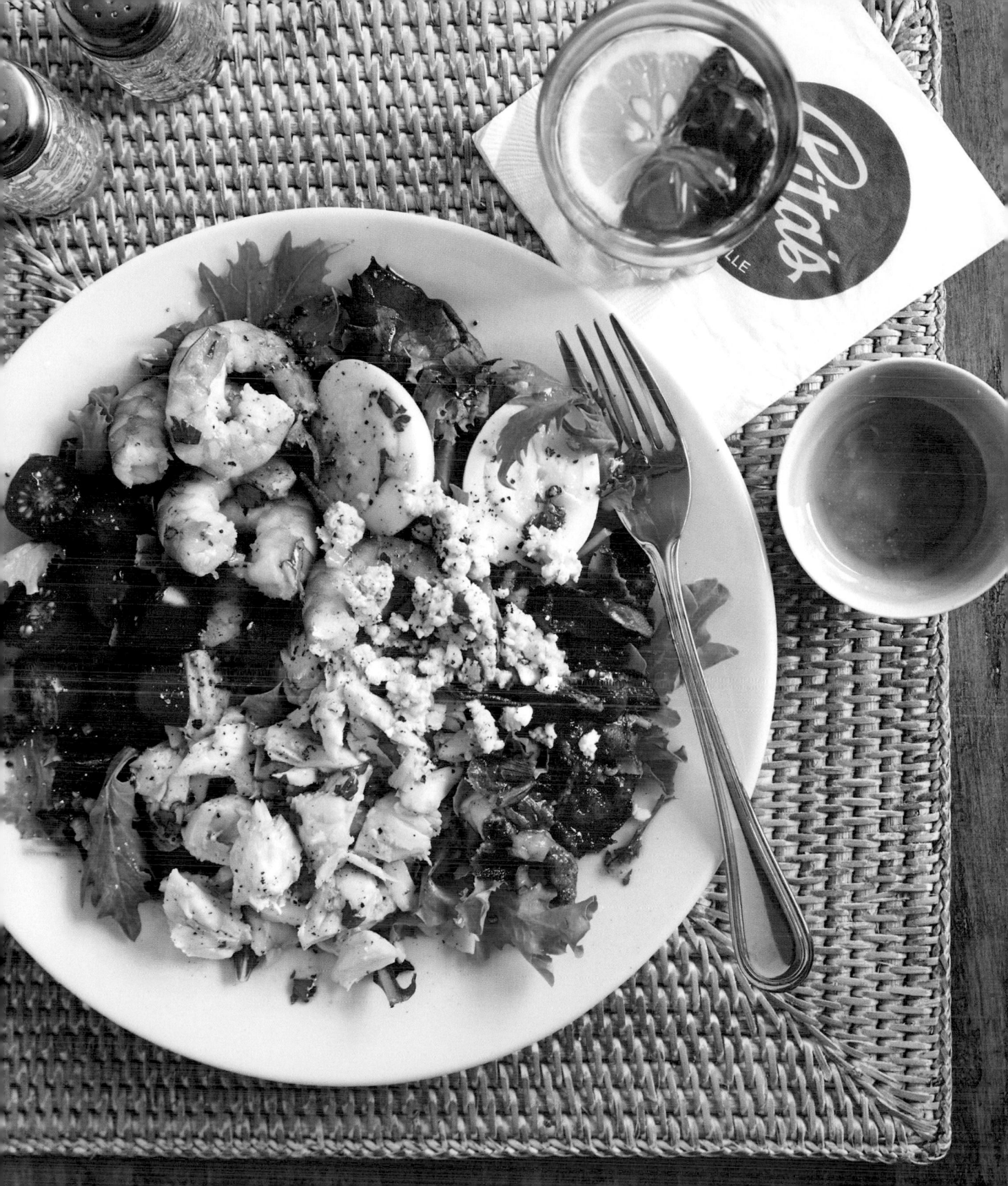

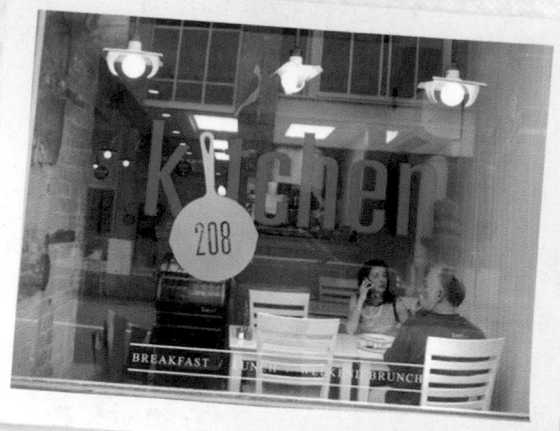

Kitchen 208

208 King Street
Charleston, South Carolina 29401
(843) 725-7208
kitchen208.com

Ah, breakfast. If you're a morning person, you'll adore this tucked-away gem on King Street in Charleston, and if you'd rather sleep in, go for the brunch. Kitchen 208's eggs, bacon, waffles, biscuits, and hot coffee represent the standard fare you'd expect from a spot that has a skillet for a logo. But once you read the menu carefully, you'll detect a distinct streak of humor. Take the "Bat Outta of Hell" sandwich: It's made with meatloaf and topped with braised collards. Besides giving a nod to some old school rockers, it's also delicious. I'll never look at plain meatloaf without wishing it had a hairdo of collards again.

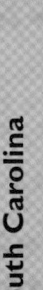

Bat Outta Hell

6 (2.1-oz.) unsliced sesame seed buns
6 Tbsp. softened butter
3 tsp. olive oil, divided
3 Tbsp. butter, divided
12 (3-oz.) slices Meatloaf (page 176)
2 cups warm well-drained Braised Collard Greens (page 176)
6 slices Gruyère cheese
1¼ cups Tomato Marmalade (page 177)
Long wooden picks
Garnish: pickled okra

1. Heat a large nonstick skillet over medium-high heat. Cut buns in half horizontally; spread cut sides of halves with softened butter, and cook, cut sides down, in 3 batches 1 to 2 minutes or until golden brown. Remove from skillet, and place 1 bun bottom on each of 6 plates.

2. Heat 1 tsp. olive oil and 1 Tbsp. butter in a large nonstick skillet over medium-high heat until butter melts; spread evenly over surface of skillet with a spatula. Place 4 meatloaf slices in skillet. Sear 2 minutes or until a golden brown crust forms. Turn slices over; spoon ⅓ cup warm collard greens on top of each of 2 meatloaf slices. Cook 1 minute or until meatloaf slices are warm, top each greens-topped meatloaf slice with 1 plain meatloaf slice.

3. Top each meatloaf-greens stack with 1 cheese slice. Cover and cook 2 minutes or until cheese begins to melt. Transfer stacks to 2 bun bottoms. Top each stack with 2 Tbsp. Tomato Marmalade and a bun top. Secure sandwiches with picks.

4. Repeat procedure twice with remaining buns, oil, butter, meatloaf slices, greens, cheese, and marmalade. **Makes: 6 servings**

Note: Greens should be drained in a wire-mesh strainer, pressing with the back of a spoon to remove as much moisture as possible before measuring.

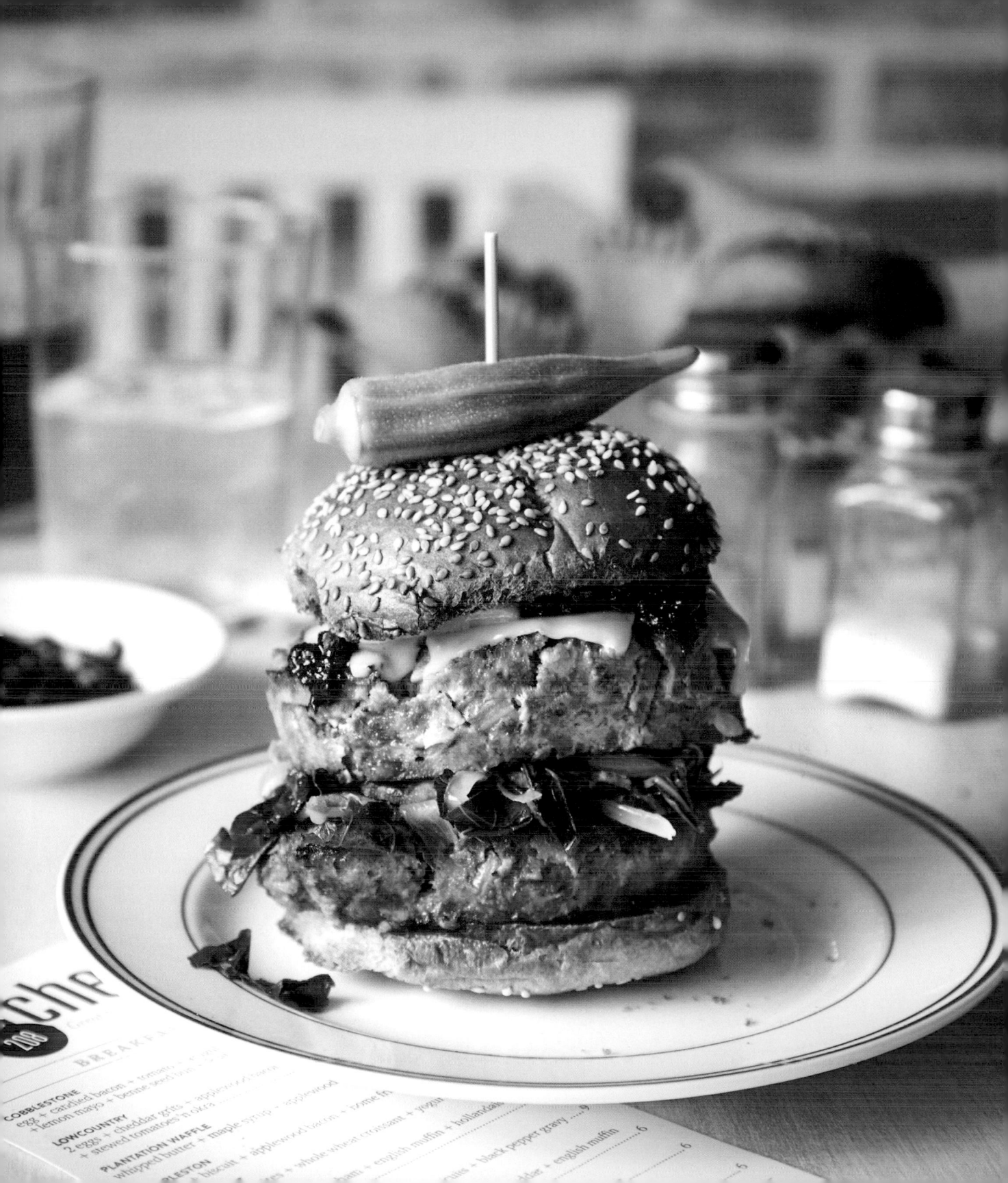

Meatloaf

1   lb. lean ground beef
1   lb. ground pork
1   cup fine, dry breadcrumbs
1   cup finely diced celery
¾   cup finely diced carrot
¾   cup finely diced onion
½   cup ketchup
1   Tbsp. kosher salt
1   Tbsp. granulated garlic
3   Tbsp. Worcestershire sauce
1½   tsp. cracked black pepper
1½   tsp. dried thyme
3   large eggs, beaten
Parchment paper

1. Preheat oven to 325°. Combine first 13 ingredients in a large mixing bowl. Blend well by hand.
2. Shape mixture into a 12½-inch log, 4 inches in diameter on a large piece of parchment paper. Roll log tightly in parchment paper; twist ends to tightly pack and seal mixture into roll. Roll in aluminum foil, twisting ends to tightly seal. Place wrapped log on a sheet pan lined with parchment paper.
3. Bake at 325° for 1 hour and 40 minutes or until a meat thermometer inserted through foil into center registers 160°.
4. Transfer wrapped log to a wire rack; cool 2 hours. Chill in refrigerator overnight.
5. Unwrap meatloaf; trim ends even with diameter of log. Cut remaining log into 12 equal slices. Makes: 12 servings

Braised Collard Greens

6   hickory-smoked bacon slices, cut crosswise into ½-inch pieces
2   cups julienne-cut onion
1   bunch fresh collard greens, large stems removed and coarsely chopped (14 cups chopped greens)
2   Tbsp. apple cider vinegar
1½   tsp. table salt
1½   Tbsp. hot sauce
½   tsp. sugar

1. Cook bacon in a Dutch oven over medium heat 4 minutes, stirring often, just until crisp. Add onion; cook, stirring constantly, 4 minutes or until tender. Gradually add greens, turning with tongs, until greens wilt and all greens are added. Reduce heat to medium-low; add vinegar and salt. Cover and cook 30 minutes or until tender, stirring occasionally.
2. Stir in hot sauce and sugar. Remove from heat. Transfer to a serving bowl. Serve with a slotted spoon. Makes: 4 to 6 servings

SOUNDTRACK:

"EVIL WOMAN"
BY THE ELECTRIC LIGHT ORCHESTRA

"40 DAY DREAM"
BY EDWARD SHARPE AND THE MAGNETIC ZEROS

"RYE WHISKEY"
BY THE PUNCH BROTHERS

"CAVALIER" BY SHOVELS + ROPE

Tomato Marmalade

5 lb. vine-ripened tomatoes
3 cups sugar
2 tsp. dried thyme
1 (3-inch) cinnamon stick
2 lemons

1. Cut out cores of tomatoes. Quarter tomatoes over a large bowl to catch juice; add quarters to bowl.

2. Process tomato quarters and any accumulated juices in food processor in 2 batches just until chopped. Add chopped tomato and juices to a large Dutch oven. Stir in sugar, thyme, and cinnamon stick.

3. Cut lemons in half. Squeeze juice on a reamer-style juicer to measure 3 Tbsp. juice, reserving pulp and removing seeds. Add lemon juice, pulp, and reamed lemon halves to tomato mixture.

4. Bring to a boil over medium-high heat. Reduce heat to medium, and cook, uncovered, 1 hour and 55 minutes or until mixture is very thick and reduced to 3½ cups, stirring often. Stir constantly during last 10 minutes of cooking. (Marmalade is thick enough when very little liquid, less than 2 Tbsp., bubbles to surface if left to simmer for a bit without stirring. Test readiness by placing a spoonful on a small plate; place in freezer for a couple of minutes or until cool. Hardly any juice should separate from the solid mound of mixture.) Remove from heat. Remove and discard lemon halves and cinnamon stick. Cool completely. Store, covered, in refrigerator. **Makes: 3½ cups**

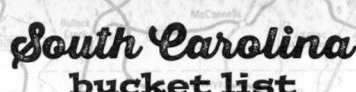

South Carolina
bucket list
things to see and do (besides eat) here

1. Everyone must, at some point, shop the many antiques, design, and clothing stores along **King Street** in Charleston.

2. History buffs should certainly check out the spot where the Civil War began, **Fort Sumter** in Charleston Harbor.

3. Learn to shag in **Myrtle Beach**, the unofficial home of the state dance.

4. Surf off **Folly Beach** *(pictured)*, a hangout for all kinds of South Carolinians for generations.

5. Pull over at **South of the Border** off I-95 in Hamer for campy kitsch that has no rival.

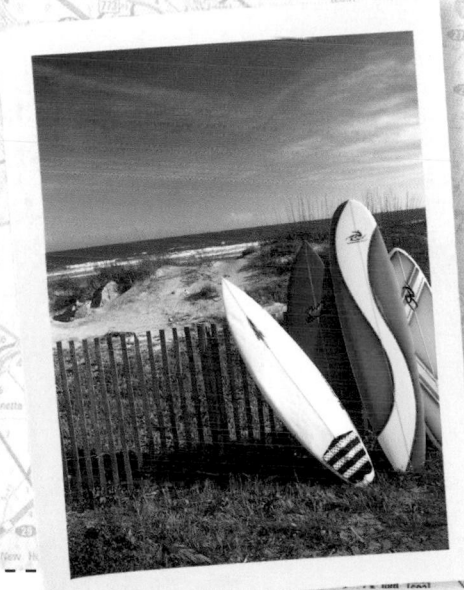

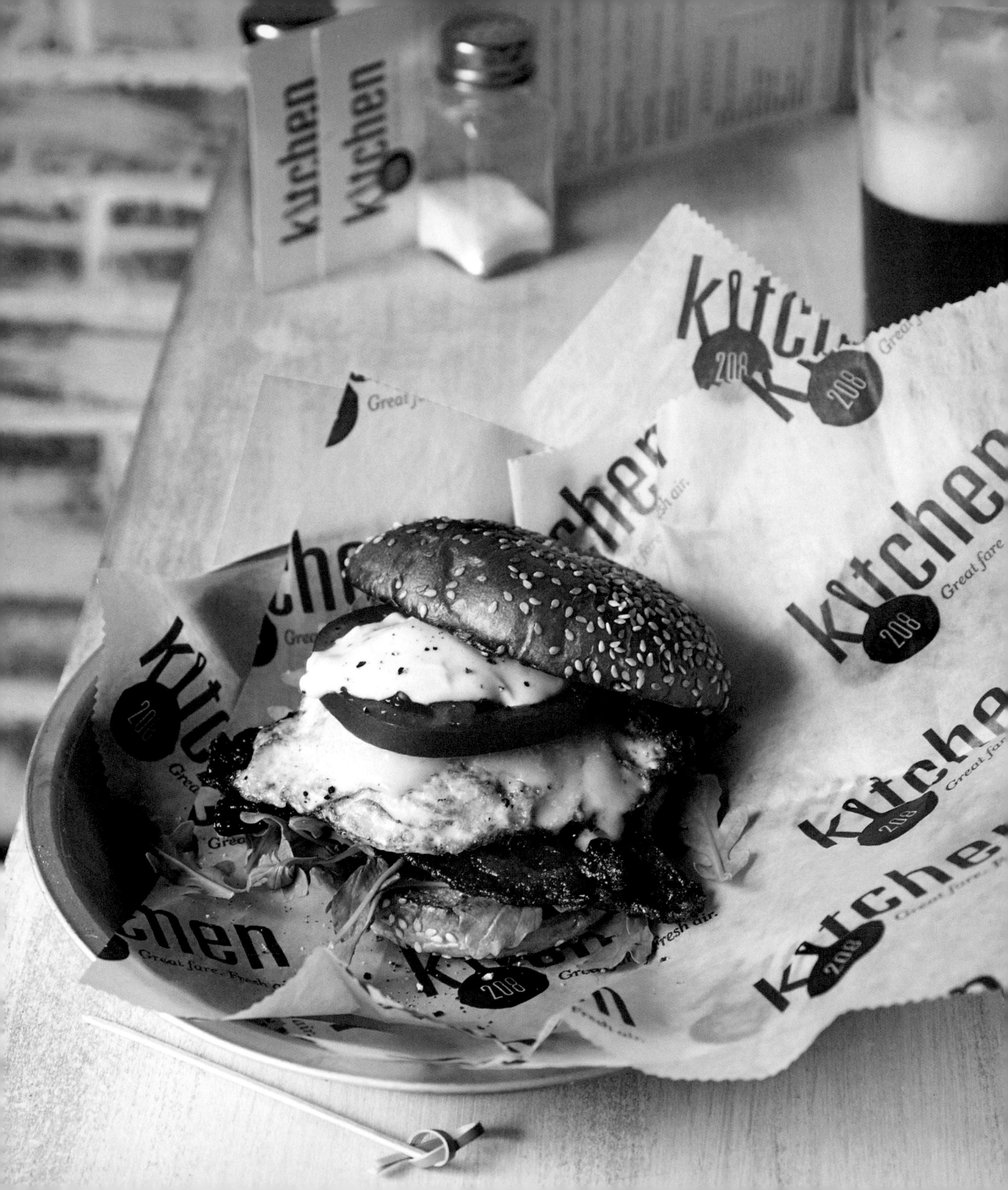

Cobblestone Sandwich

This is a hearty breakfast sandwich with a sophisticated edge (making it totally ok to eat a monster bacon, egg, and cheese sammie).

- 4 (2.1-oz.) sesame seed buns, unsliced
- 2 Tbsp. butter, softened
- 2 cups firmly packed fresh baby arugula
- 8 slices Candied Bacon
- 1 Tbsp. cold butter
- 4 large eggs
- 4 (0.75-oz.) slices Gruyère cheese
- 4 (½-inch-thick) slices vine-ripened tomatoes
- ¾ cup Lemon Aïoli

1. Cut buns in half horizontally; spread cut sides of buns evenly with 2 Tbsp. softened butter. Heat a large nonstick skillet over medium heat. Working with 2 buns at a time, place in skillet, cut side down. Cook 1 minute or until lightly toasted.
2. Place bun bottoms on individual plates. Top each with ½ cup arugula and 2 bacon slices.
3. Melt 1 Tbsp. cold butter in a large nonstick skillet over medium heat. Gently break eggs into hot skillet. Cook 2 minutes or until whites are almost set. Turn eggs over; cook 1 minute. Top each with 1 cheese slice. Remove from heat, cover, and let stand until cheese melts (about 2 minutes).
4. Place 1 cheese-topped egg, 1 tomato slice, and 3 Tbsp. Lemon Aïoli on top of bacon. Cover with bun tops. Serve immediately. **Makes: 4 servings**

Candied Bacon

- ½ cup sugar
- 8 thick-cut hickory-smoked bacon slices
- Vegetable cooking spray
- Parchment paper

1. Preheat oven to 350°. Place sugar in an 11-x 7-inch baking dish. Dredge bacon in sugar, shaking off excess.
2. Line a 15 x 10-inch jelly-roll pan with aluminum foil. Coat a wire rack with cooking spray. Set rack in prepared pan. Arrange bacon in a single layer on prepared rack.
3. Bake at 350° for 20 minutes or until golden brown and crisp. Cool completely on a work surface covered with parchment paper (about 20 minutes). **Makes: 4 servings**

Lemon Aïoli

- 4 large pasteurized egg yolks
- 1 tsp. lemon zest
- 3 Tbsp. fresh squeezed lemon juice (about 2 lemons)
- ½ tsp. table salt
- 1 cup canola oil

1. Combine egg yolks, lemon zest, lemon juice, salt, and 3 Tbsp. water in a blender; process until blended. Stop blender.
2. Remove center piece of blender lid; secure blender lid on blender. With blender on, pour oil through center of lid in a thin stream; process until thickened. Transfer to a container; cover and store in refrigerator for 2 weeks. **Makes: 1½ cups**

Quick Lemon Aïoli: Whisk together 1½ cups thick mayonnaise, 1 tsp. lemon zest, and 1½ Tbsp. lemon juice.

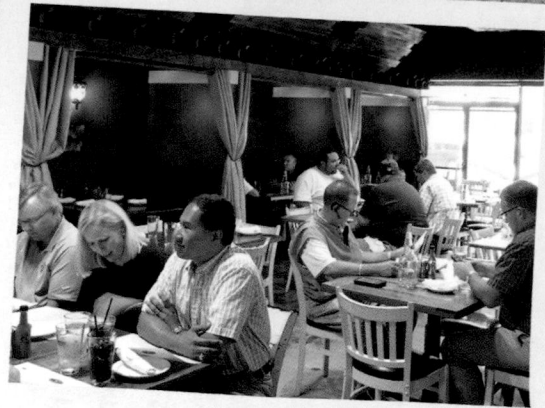

Bacon Bros. Public House

3620 Pelham Road
Greenville, South Carolina 29615
(864) 297-6000
baconbrospublichouse.com

Eat here and you'll know why God made the pig. Bacon Bros.' B.E.T. sandwich is on my last meal wish list. I haven't cried since my dog Gilbert died, but this sammie makes me want to weep (for joy). Sure, the recipe takes three days to make—so worth it. And if you think you know boiled peanuts, try these babies. Served warm, their saltiness is addictive, and they leave a lingering burn, which makes you thirsty. If you eat them at the bar at Bacon Bros., whiskey temptation of the Pappy and Four Roses awaits. Chef Anthony Gray is just a good Southern boy—he gets up every morning at 4 a.m. to butcher hogs, and that dedication to pork perfection lets me know he's headed to culinary greatness.

Boiled Peanuts

These aren't the salty boiled peanuts you buy from roadside stands. These have some fire!

- 5   lb. raw green peanuts
- 2   cups sliced Vidalia or other sweet onion
- 4   cups premium lager
- 1½   cups kosher salt
- 1   cup Worcestershire sauce
- ½   cup peeled garlic cloves (17 cloves)
- 6   Tbsp. hot sauce
- ¼   cup dried crushed red pepper
- 2½   jalapeño peppers, halved
- 2   bay leaves

Serve with: pickled jalapeño peppers

Combine first 10 ingredients and 4 qt. water in an 8- to 10-qt. Dutch oven or stockpot. Bring to a boil; reduce heat, cover, and simmer 4 hours or until peanuts are tender. Drain. Cool completely (1 hour). Remove and discard bay leaves. Serve with pickled jalapeño peppers. Store leftover peanuts in refrigerator. **Makes: 22½ cups**

Note: We tested with Pabst Blue Ribbon lager. You'll need about 2½ (12-oz.) bottles to measure 4 cups.

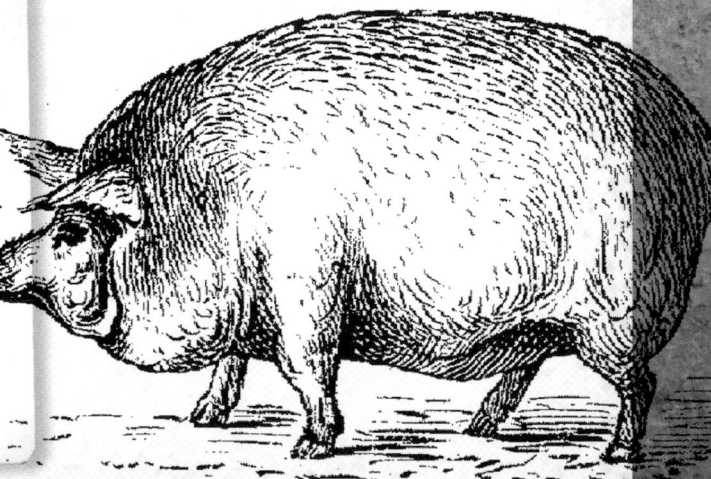

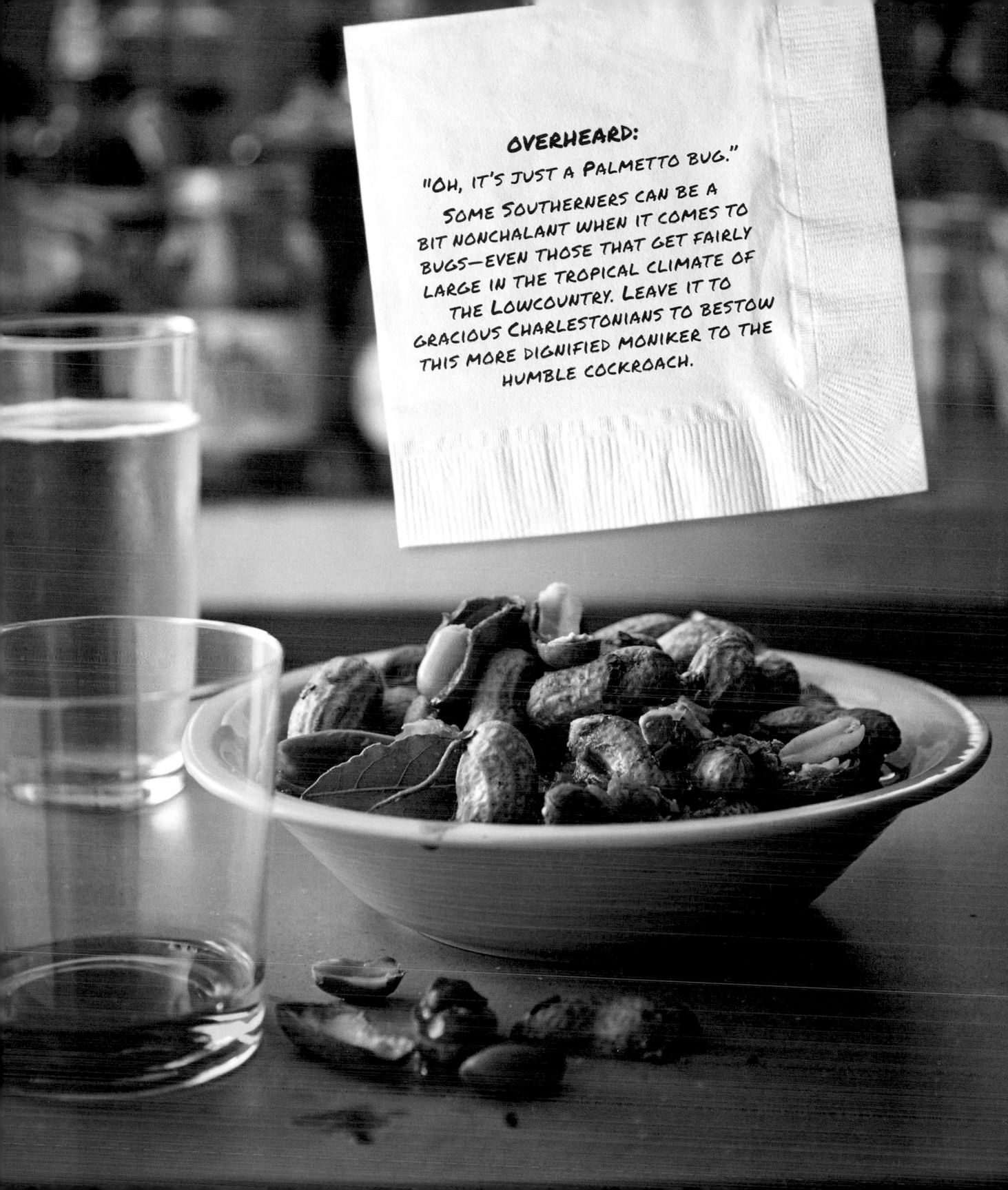

OVERHEARD:

"Oh, it's just a Palmetto bug."

Some Southerners can be a bit nonchalant when it comes to bugs—even those that get fairly large in the tropical climate of the Lowcountry. Leave it to gracious Charlestonians to bestow this more dignified moniker to the humble cockroach.

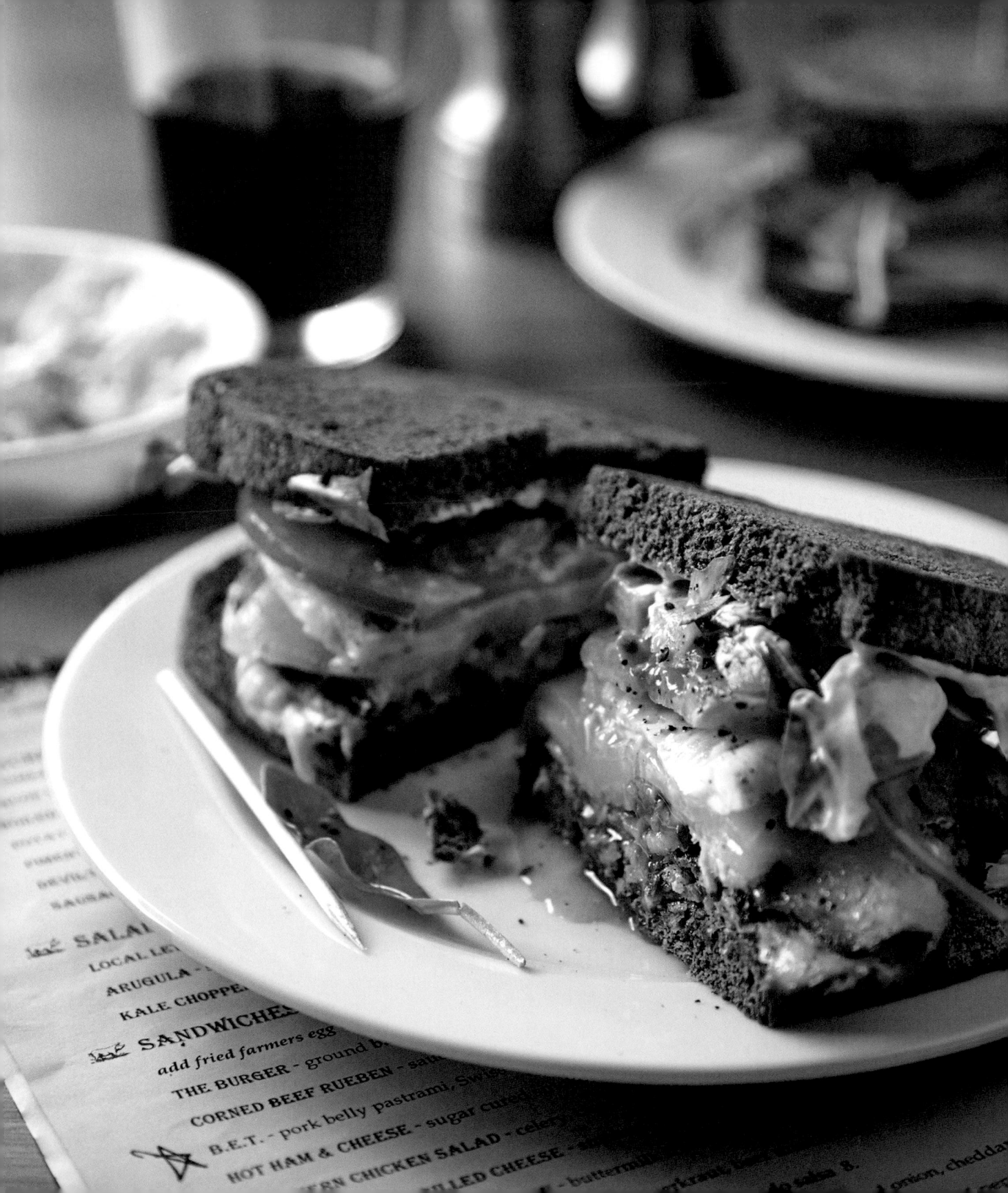

Pork Belly Sandwich

This may be my favorite sandwich in the world.

- 1 lb. thinly sliced Pork Belly
- 4 (1-oz.) slices Swiss cheese
- ¼ cup mayonnaise, divided
- 8 (1.1-oz.) slices pumpernickel bread, toasted
- 4 large eggs
- 8 thin yellow tomato slices
- 3 cups loosely packed arugula
- 2 tsp. lemon juice

1. Preheat oven to 175°. Place paper towels on a baking sheet; set aside. Cook Pork Belly slices, in 4 equal batches, in a large cast-iron skillet over medium-high heat 3 to 4 minutes or until edges are lightly crisp. Stack slices in each batch in skillet; place 1 cheese slice on top of each stack. Allow cheese to melt before removing stack from skillet. Transfer each stack to pre-pared baking sheet, and keep warm at 175° until all stacks are formed.

2. Spread 2 Tbsp. mayonnaise evenly on 1 side of 4 toast slices. Place 1 cheese-topped pork belly stack onto each toast slice, keep stacks and remaining toast slices warm in oven.

3. Drain drippings from skillet, reserving 3 Tbsp. drippings in skillet. Gently break eggs into hot drippings, and sprinkle with salt and pepper to taste. Cook 2 to 3 minutes on each side or to desired degree of doneness.

4. Place 1 egg on top of cheese on each stack. Top each with 2 tomato slices.

5. Toss arugula with lemon juice in a bowl. Remove sandwich stacks from oven. Divide arugula mixture evenly among servings. Spread remaining 2 Tbsp. mayonnaise on 1 side of remaining 4 toast slices, and place on sandwiches, mayonnaise sides down. Serve immediately. **Makes: 4 servings**

Pork Belly

- 6 Tbsp. coriander seeds
- 5 Tbsp. cracked black pepper, divided
- 5 Tbsp. kosher salt
- 3 Tbsp. turbinado sugar
- 4 large garlic cloves, minced and divided (2 Tbsp.)
- 1 (5.25-lb.) pork belly
- Hickory or cherry chunks

1. Place a small skillet over medium-high heat until hot; add coriander seeds, and cook, shaking pan often, 2 to 3 minutes or until toasted and fragrant. Crack seeds with a rolling pin or small cast-iron skillet.

2. Combine half of cracked coriander seeds, 2 Tbsp. cracked pepper, salt, turbinado sugar, and 1 Tbsp. garlic. Rub sugar mixture over surface of pork belly. Place in a large zip-top plastic freezer bag. Seal bag; marinate in refrigerator 3 days.

3. Soak wood chunks in water 2 hours. Prepare smoker according to manufacturer's directions, bringing internal temperature to 250° to 300°; maintain temperature for 15 to 20 minutes. Drain wood chunks, and place on coals.

4. Remove pork from bag; rinse with cold water, and pat dry with paper towels. Beginning at 1 short side, roll up pork, fat side out. Tie with kitchen string, securing at ¼-inch intervals; tie lengthwise in center.

5. Combine remaining 3 Tbsp. cracked pepper, remaining half of cracked coriander, and remaining 1 Tbsp. minced garlic. Rub over surface of pork.

6. Push coals toward 1 side of smoker. Place pork on lower cooking grate on opposite side from coals; cover with smoker lid. Maintain heat between 250° and 300° for 4 to 5 hours or until a meat thermometer inserted into center registers 180°. Remove pork from smoker. Cool pork completely (1 hour). Cover and chill overnight. Remove string, and cut into thin slices. **Makes: 20 servings**

The Lot

1977 Maybank Highway
Charleston, South Carolina 29412
(843) 225-0094
thelotcharleston.com

Music lovers and fans of bands like Shovels & Rope (one of my faves) know Charleston Pour House out on Maybank Highway. Carnegie Hall it ain't. But then, Carnegie Hall is a lousy spot to relax and have a beer on a Friday afternoon. In 2012, the owners opened The Lot next door. Since they share the same space, The Lot could have gone the way of bar food and popcorn. Instead, it's become a champion of local food. The only items the restaurant doesn't make in-house are the maple syrup and ketchup. I adore The Lot's steak, as well as any of the salads because they are so fresh. And if it's on the menu when you dine, order the Trotter Cake. It takes the staff 12 days to make, and this braised pork with sunny farm egg is best described as a sausage-barbecue hybrid. Still, whatever you call it, it's a must-try.

The Farmer's Pick

The restaurant changes up the ingredients for this salad based on what's fresh and in season. So you can build your own based on your favorite veggies or what's available locally.

- 2 ears fresh corn, husked and cut into 1-inch pieces
- 4 oz. green beans
- ¼ cup extra virgin olive oil
- 1 tsp. each fresh basil, fresh mint, fresh chives, fresh cilantro, fresh parsley, and fresh dill
- 1½ tsp. sea salt flakes
- 12 baby carrots, tops trimmed
- 4 radishes, quartered
- 2 pickling cucumbers (about ½ lb.), peeled and thinly sliced

Chili Aïoli (facing page)

1. Cook corn in boiling salted water to cover 1 minute; add green beans. Cook 2 minutes; drain. Plunge into ice water to stop the cooking process; drain.
2. Combine olive oil, herbs, and salt in a large bowl. Add carrots and next 2 ingredients; toss to coat. Divide vegetable mixture among 4 plates. Serve with Chili Aïoli. **Makes: 4 servings**

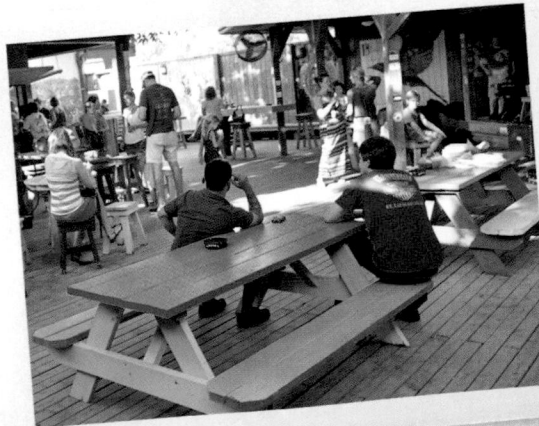

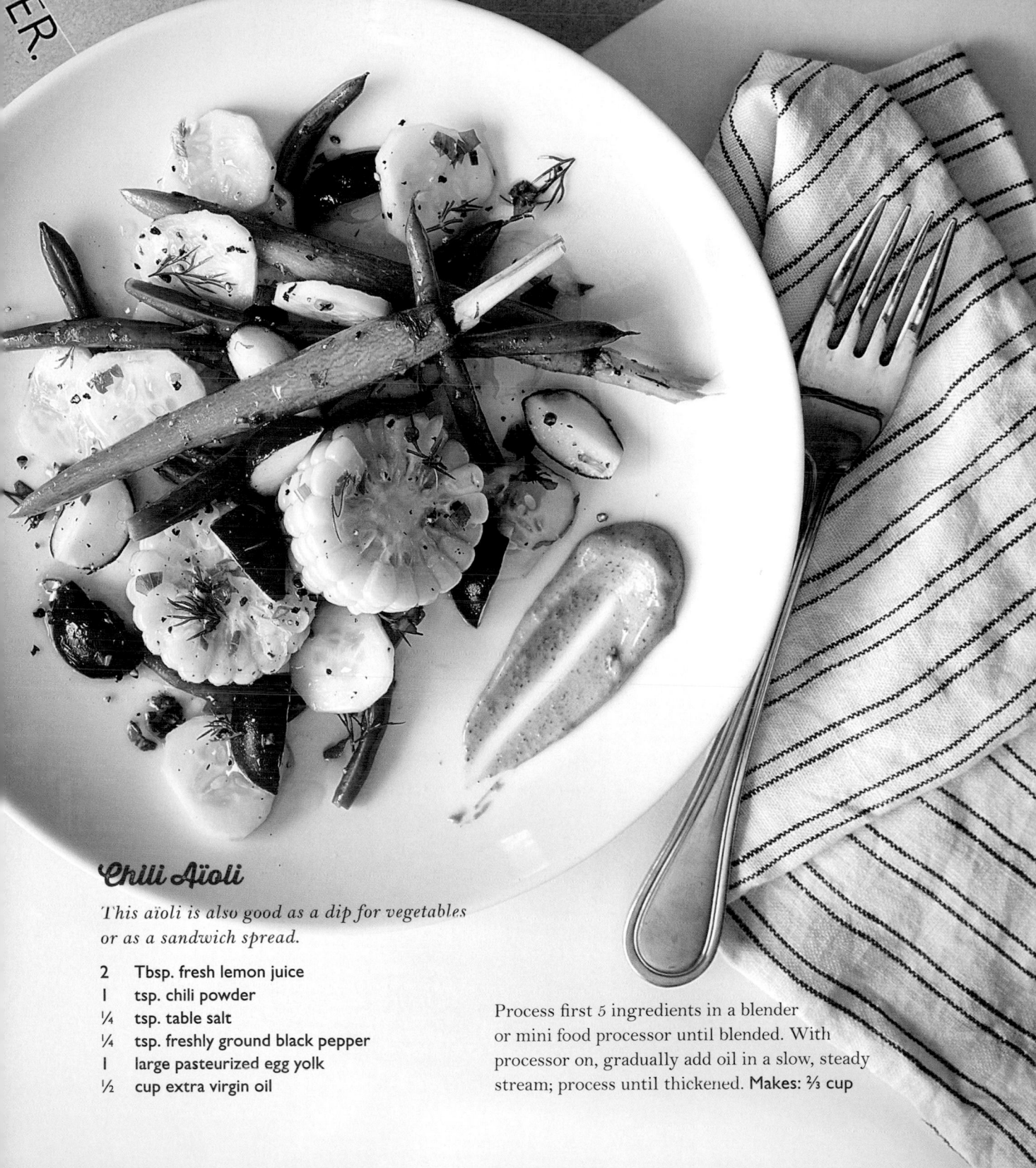

Chili Aïoli

This aïoli is also good as a dip for vegetables or as a sandwich spread.

2	Tbsp. fresh lemon juice
1	tsp. chili powder
¼	tsp. table salt
¼	tsp. freshly ground black pepper
1	large pasteurized egg yolk
½	cup extra virgin oil

Process first 5 ingredients in a blender or mini food processor until blended. With processor on, gradually add oil in a slow, steady stream; process until thickened. **Makes: ⅔ cup**

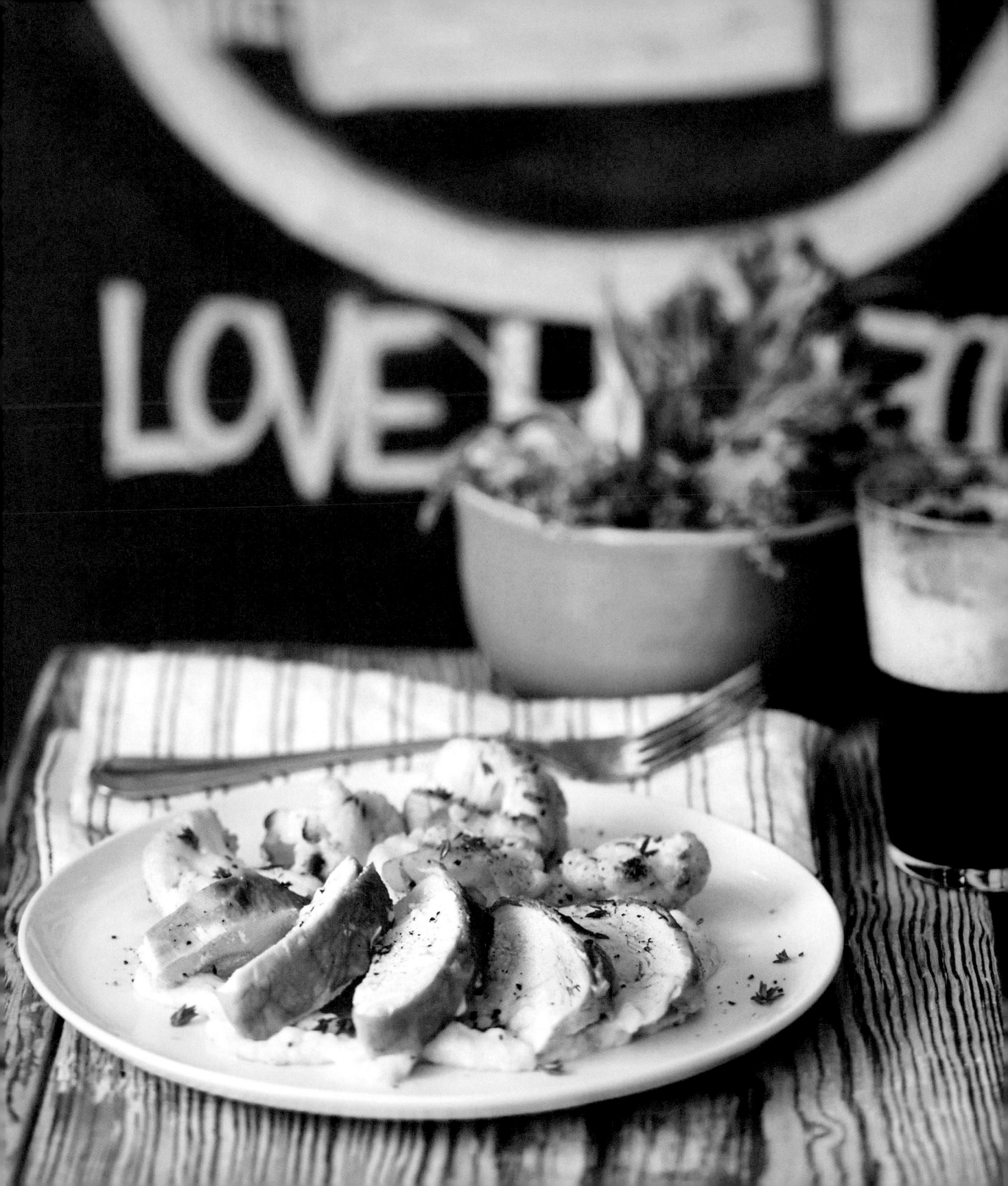

Smoked Chicken Breast

BRINE
- ½ cup table salt
- ¼ cup firmly packed light brown sugar
- 1½ Tbsp. fresh lemon juice
- 4 thyme sprigs

CHICKEN
- 2 (4-lb.) whole chickens
- 4 cups cherrywood chips
- Vegetable cooking spray

1. Prepare Brine: Bring all ingredients and 1 gal. water to a boil in a large Dutch oven, stirring until salt and sugar dissolve. Remove from heat; cool completely.

2. Prepare Chicken: Remove leg quarters and backs from chicken, and reserve for another use. Rinse breasts, and pat dry.

3. Place 1 chicken breast in each of 2 (2-gal.) zip-top plastic freezer bags. Add half of brine to each bag; seal bags. Chill overnight, turning bags occasionally.

4. Soak wood chips in water for 1 hour; drain.

5. Remove chicken from brine, discarding brine; drain and pat dry.

6. Light 1 side of grill, heating to 350° to 400° (medium-high) heat; leave other side unlit. Pierce the bottom of a 12- x 10-inch disposable aluminum foil pan several times with the tip of a knife. Place pan on lit side of grill; add 2 cup wood chips to pan. Place another disposable aluminum foil pan (do not pierce pan) on unlit side of grill. Pour 2 cups water in second pan. Let chips stand for 15 minutes or until smoking; reduce heat to medium-low. Maintain temperature at 275°.

7. Coat grill rack with cooking spray; place on grill. Place chicken, breast side up, on grill rack over foil pan on unlit side. Grill, covered with grill lid, for 2 hours or until a meat thermometer registers 165°. Replenish wood chips as needed. **Makes: 4 servings**

Grits

These grits taste like they contain cheese, even though they don't.

- ½ cup unsalted butter
- 1 tsp. table salt
- ½ tsp. freshly ground black pepper
- 3½ to 4 cups milk
- 1 cup uncooked stone-ground yellow grits
- 2 Tbsp. crème fraiche

Bring first 3 ingredients, 3 cups milk, and 1½ cups water to a boil in a large saucepan. Gradually add grits, whisking constantly. Reduce heat to low; cover and simmer 1 hour and 15 minutes or until grits are tender, stirring occasionally and adding remaining ½ to 1 cup milk as needed. Remove from heat; stir in crème fraiche. **Makes: 9 servings**

Cauliflower with Brown Butter

- 2 Tbsp. vegetable oil
- 1 large head cauliflower (about 1¾ lb.), cut into florets
- ¼ tsp. table salt
- ¼ tsp. freshly ground black pepper
- 2 Tbsp. butter
- 1 thyme sprig

1. Heat oil in a 10-inch cast-iron skillet over medium-high heat to smoke point. Add cauliflower florets to skillet in a single layer. Sprinkle with salt and pepper. Cook, without stirring or turning, 2 minutes or until browned on 1 side. Stir florets, and cook 2 minutes or until crisp-tender, stirring once. Transfer to a bowl.

2. Add butter and thyme to skillet, stirring to infuse thyme flavor into butter. Pour over cauliflower. Remove and discard thyme. Serve immediately. **Makes: 4 to 6 servings**

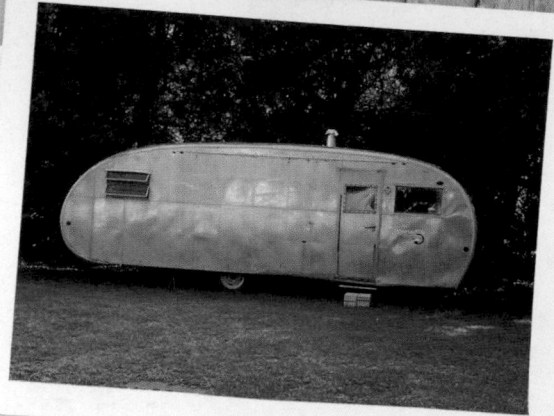

Farmbar 17
at The Ark

7259 Highway 17 North
Awendaw, South Carolina 29429
(323) 459-3156
thefarmbar26.com

When you get to the giant shipwrecked shrimp boat, you've made it to The Ark, my favorite gem in South Carolina. What started in a vintage Spartan trailer in Charleston has become a Lowcountry sensation for those with their foodie antennas raised. The Ark sits on U.S. 17 in what was a motel and general store. Chef and owner Tara Derr Webb pulls together the best of the Lowcountry's bounty to create culinary masterpieces, such as her Ridiculous Bacon Jam—a jam that is my jam. Though she's been in South Carolina for just a few years, her enthusiasm for local chefs and farmers has already made her retro Spartan trailer a must-stop detour. To taste the joy of simple Southern ingredients, make sure to try Tara's divine house-made butter, sprinkled with some local sea salt from nearby Bull's Bay.

Stoner Burger Part Deux

This is the famous burger that Tara began serving in downtown Charleston. People wait in line like crazy for this delicious bit of beef.

1	lb. ground chuck
½	lb. ground veal
1	Tbsp. coarsely chopped fresh thyme
¼	cup coarsely chopped pitted Niçoise olives
1	cup ricotta cheese
¼	tsp. sea salt
¼	tsp. freshly ground black pepper
4	(1-oz.) slices Cheddar cheese
4	(3.5-oz.) brioche buns, halved horizontally

Mayonnaise or aïoli

4   romaine lettuce leaves

Ridiculous Bacon Jam (page 190)

1. Combine first 5 ingredients in a large bowl, using hands. Shape meat mixture into 4 (1-inch-thick) patties.

2. Preheat grill to 350° to 400° (medium-high) heat. Sprinkle 1 side of patties with salt and pepper. Grill, covered with grill lid, 5 minutes on each side or until lightly charred and a meat thermometer registers 160°. Top each patty with 1 cheese slice during last 1 minute of cooking. Remove patties from grill, and let patties stand 5 minutes.

3. Spread cut sides of buns with desired amount of mayonnaise. Top with lettuce leaves, and place patties on bun bottoms. Top with desired amount of jam, and cover with bun tops. Serve immediately. **Makes: 4 servings**

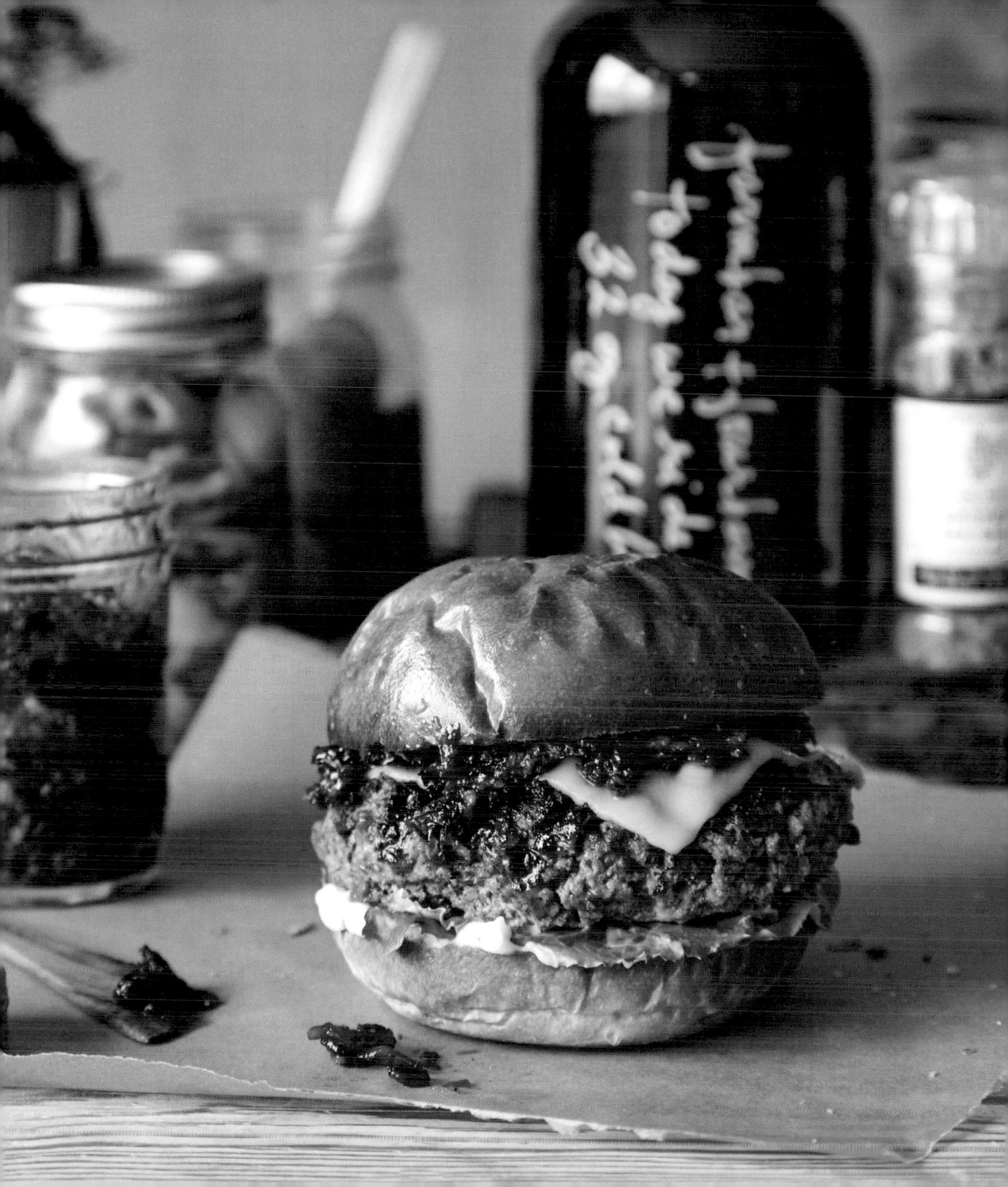

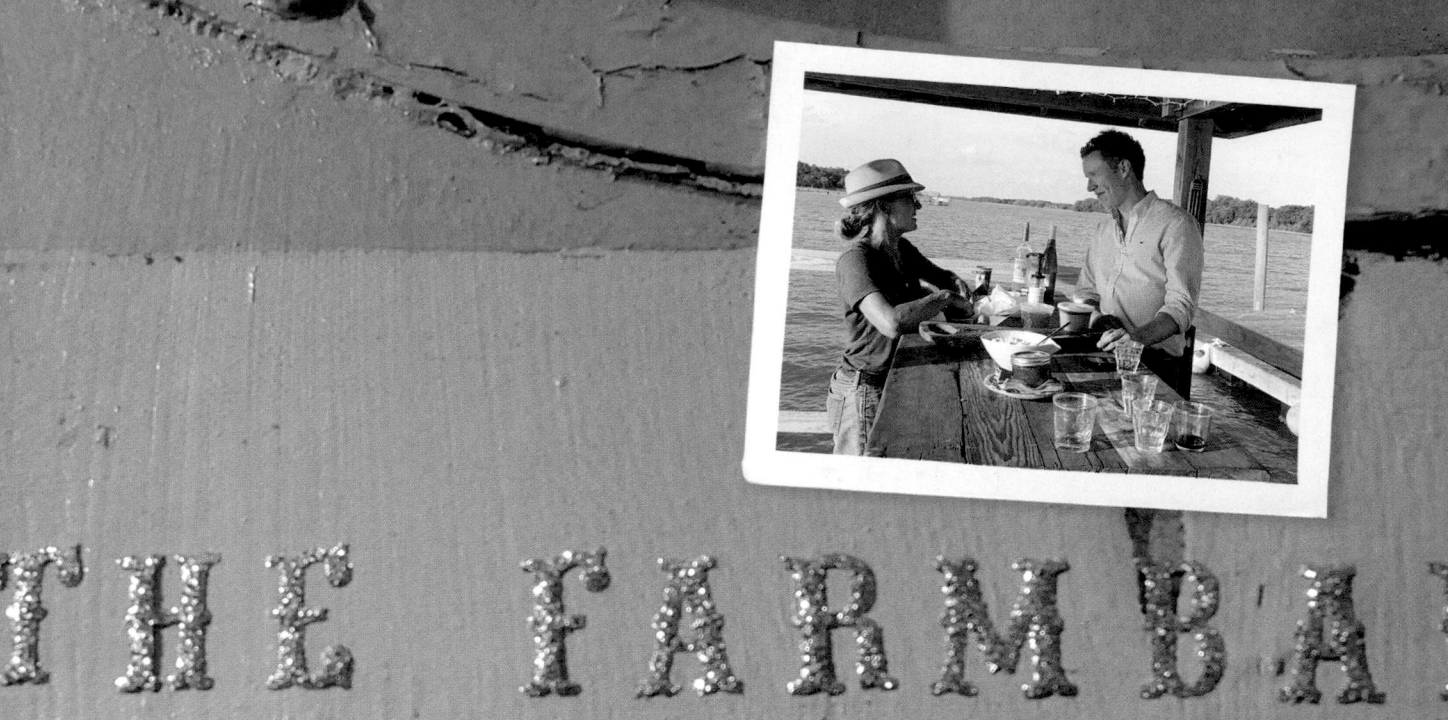

Ridiculous Bacon Jam

This bacon sauce combines my two favorite food groups: bacon and bourbon.

- ¼ cup currants
- ½ cup hot water
- 1½ lb. dry-cured bacon slices, cut crosswise into 1-inch pieces
- 1 cup coarsely chopped shallots (3 large shallots)
- 4 garlic cloves, coarsely chopped
- 1 tsp. coarsely ground black peppercorns
- ½ tsp. stone-ground mustard
- ½ tsp. ground ginger
- 1 bay leaf
- ½ cup bourbon
- ⅓ cup maple syrup
- ½ cup firmly packed dark brown sugar
- ¼ cup unfiltered apple cider vinegar

1. Combine currants and ½ cup hot water; let stand 10 minutes.

2. Cook bacon, in batches, in a large cast-iron skillet over medium heat until browned, but not crisp; drain, reserving 2 Tbsp. drippings in skillet.

3. Sauté shallots and garlic in hot drippings 5 minutes or until tender and translucent. Add peppercorns and next 3 ingredients; cook, stirring constantly, 1 minute. Add bourbon and maple syrup; bring to a boil, stirring to loosen browned bits from bottom of skillet. Stir in currants and soaking liquid, brown sugar, and vinegar; return to a boil. Add bacon; reduce heat to low, and simmer, uncovered, 12 minutes or until mixture is thickened and coats the back of a spoon, stirring occasionally. Remove from heat; cool slightly.

4. Remove and discard bay leaf. Pulse bacon mixture in a food processor until chunky, but still spreadable. Pour into hot, sterilized canning jars. Cover with lids; screw on bands. Cool completely (30 minutes). Store in refrigerator for 2 weeks.

Makes: 2½ cups

Note: We tested with Benton's Hickory-Smoked Country Bacon.

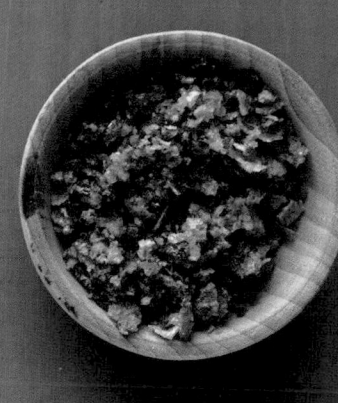

Bulls Bay Saltworks

P.O. Box No. 656
McClellanville, South Carolina 29458
bullsbaysaltworks.com

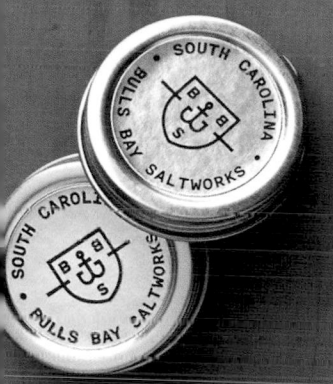

Taste the Carolina Flake salt from Bulls Bay and you'll never go back to table salt. This small-batch sea salt, completely devoid of table salt's metallic tang, perfectly seasons eggs, burgers, fries, popcorn—just about everything. Owners and homesteaders Rustin and Teresa Gooden source the salt just north of Charleston in Cape Romain, a protected Class 1 Wilderness Area (one of just 156 in the country). They use solar and wind power to dry out the seawater, leaving them with outstanding sea salt. Give the smoked sea salt a try, too—it's some of the best I've had.

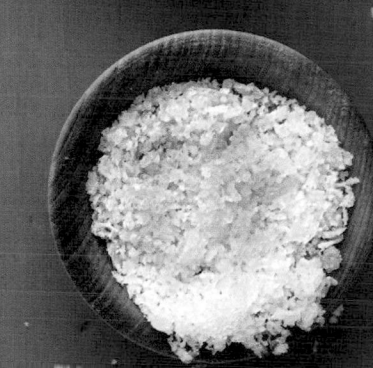

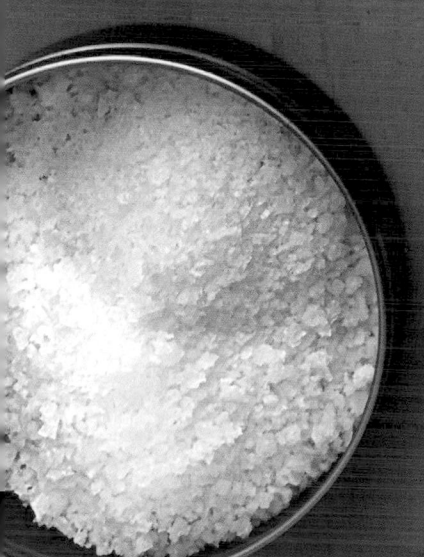

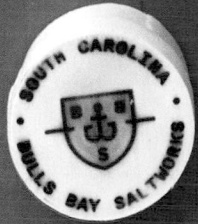

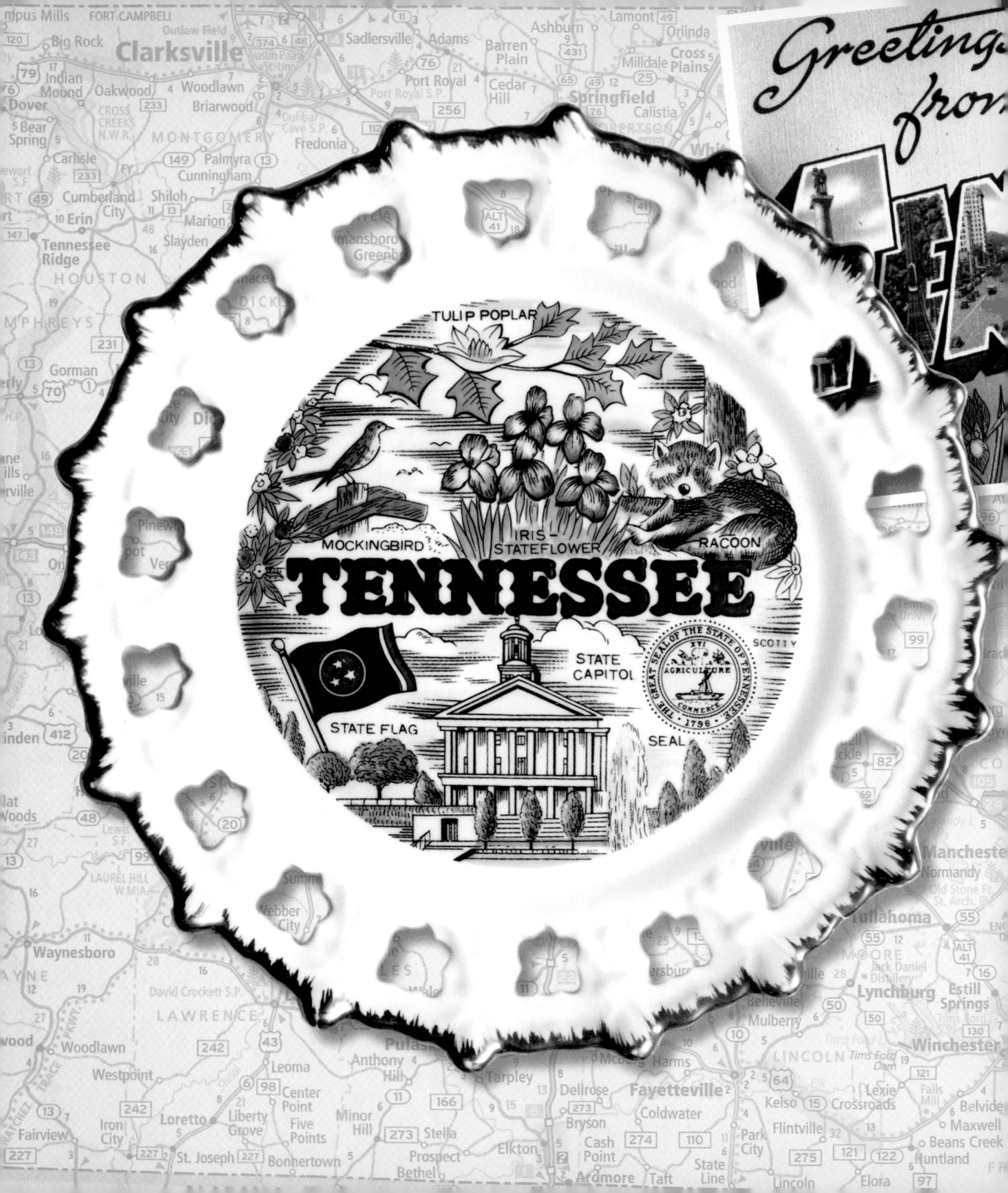

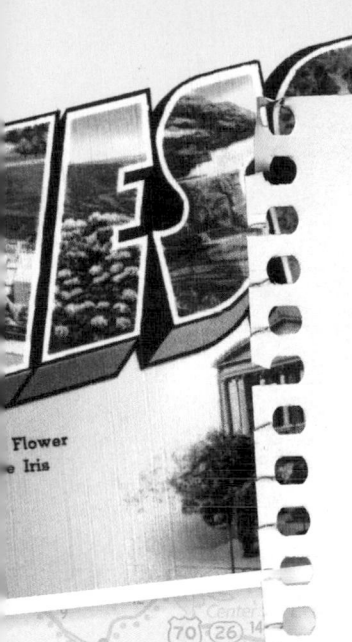

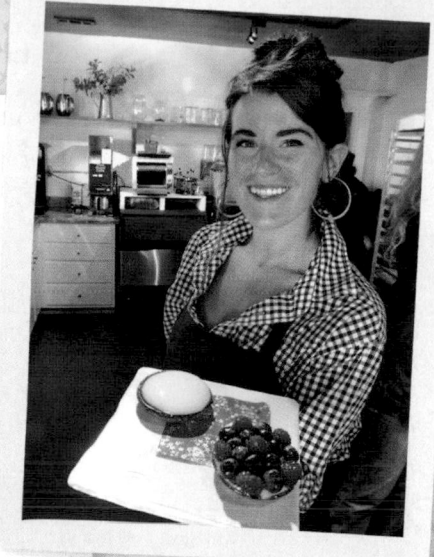

Tennessee

June 18:
Depart Scott, Arkansas at 6 p.m. for Memphis. Spend the night.

June 19:
Coffee and croissants at Tart in Memphis 9 a.m.
Return to Birmingham.

June 30:
Depart Birmingham at 8 a.m. for Nashville. Dinner and bowling at Pinewood Social. Bunk at Hutton.

July 1:
Up early for coffee at Barista Parlor in East Nashville.
Return to Birmingham.

July 7:
Depart Birmingham at 8 a.m. for Big Fatty's Catering Kitchen in Knoxville. Meet with Lisa Smith at 1 p.m.
Head to Roanoke, Virginia at 4 p.m.

August 7:
Check out Olive Bean Natural Grocery and Café in Signal Mountain on the way to Chattanooga, Tennessee. Spend the night in Chattanooga.

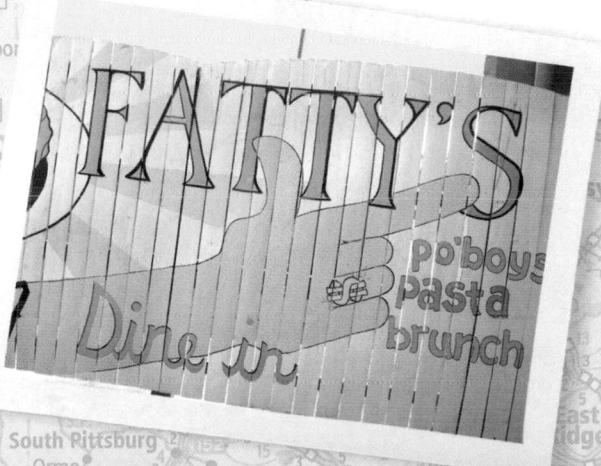

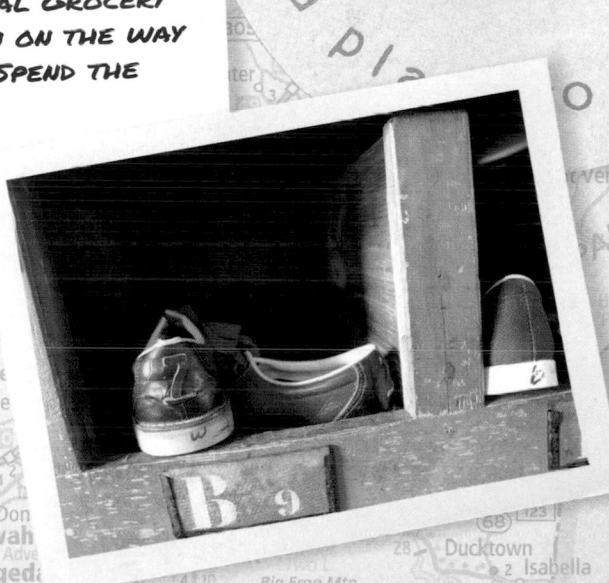

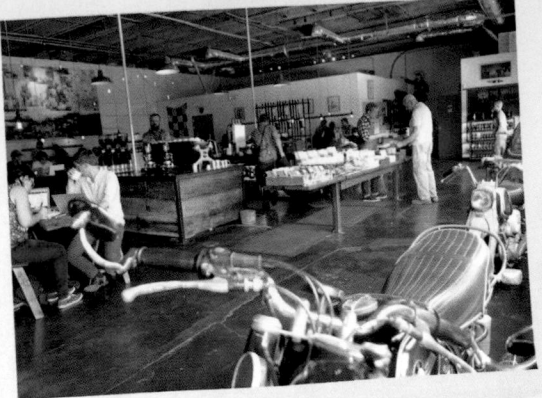

Barista Parlor

519B Gallatin Avenue
Nashville, Tennessee 37206
(615) 712-9766
baristaparlor.com

The U.S. Navy runs on two fuels: diesel and coffee. So I felt immediately at home seeing the giant anchor that marks this East Nashville coffee shop. But trust me, the coffee here is way better than the Navy's. There are some serious java wonks behind the counter at Barista Parlor. Sample the cold drip coffee, which lacks any bitter taste whatsoever. And oh, the espresso here. Hand-pulled to creamy perfection, espresso shots flow from a marvel of American design. In fact, the entire restaurant is a work of art, from the jaunty wooden table markers to the giant abstract Prussian sailing ship painting. You'll feel cool, and not at all like a third grader, eating the incredible Pop's Tart (with sprinkles) while listening to classic vinyl and sipping your favorite cup of joe. Like me, you'll want to drop anchor here all day.

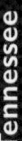

Salty Tennessee Whiskey Caramel

Deliciously mellow, this drink is neither too sweet nor too salty.

- 1 cup cold milk
- 3 Tbsp. brewed espresso, room temperature
- 2 Tbsp. Barista Parlor Caramel Sauce

Pour milk into a small bowl. Stir espresso and caramel sauce into milk, stirring 1 minute or until caramel dissolves, about 1 minute. Fill a 1-pt. wide-mouth canning jar with ice; pour milk mixture over ice, and serve immediately. **Makes:** 1 serving

Barista Parlor Caramel Sauce

- 1¾ cups sugar
- 1 tsp. white vinegar
- 1½ cups heavy cream
- 2½ Tbsp. bourbon
- ¼ tsp. table salt

1. Combine sugar, vinegar, and ¾ cup water in a 3-qt. saucepan. Bring to a boil; boil 11 minutes or until sugar melts and mixture turns a deep amber color. Remove from heat.
2. Combine cream, bourbon, and salt in a medium saucepan; bring to a boil. Remove from heat. Carefully pour hot cream mixture into caramel mixture, whisking constantly (mixture will bubble vigorously). Cook, stirring constantly, 1 minute or until sauce is thickened and smooth. Makes: 2 cups

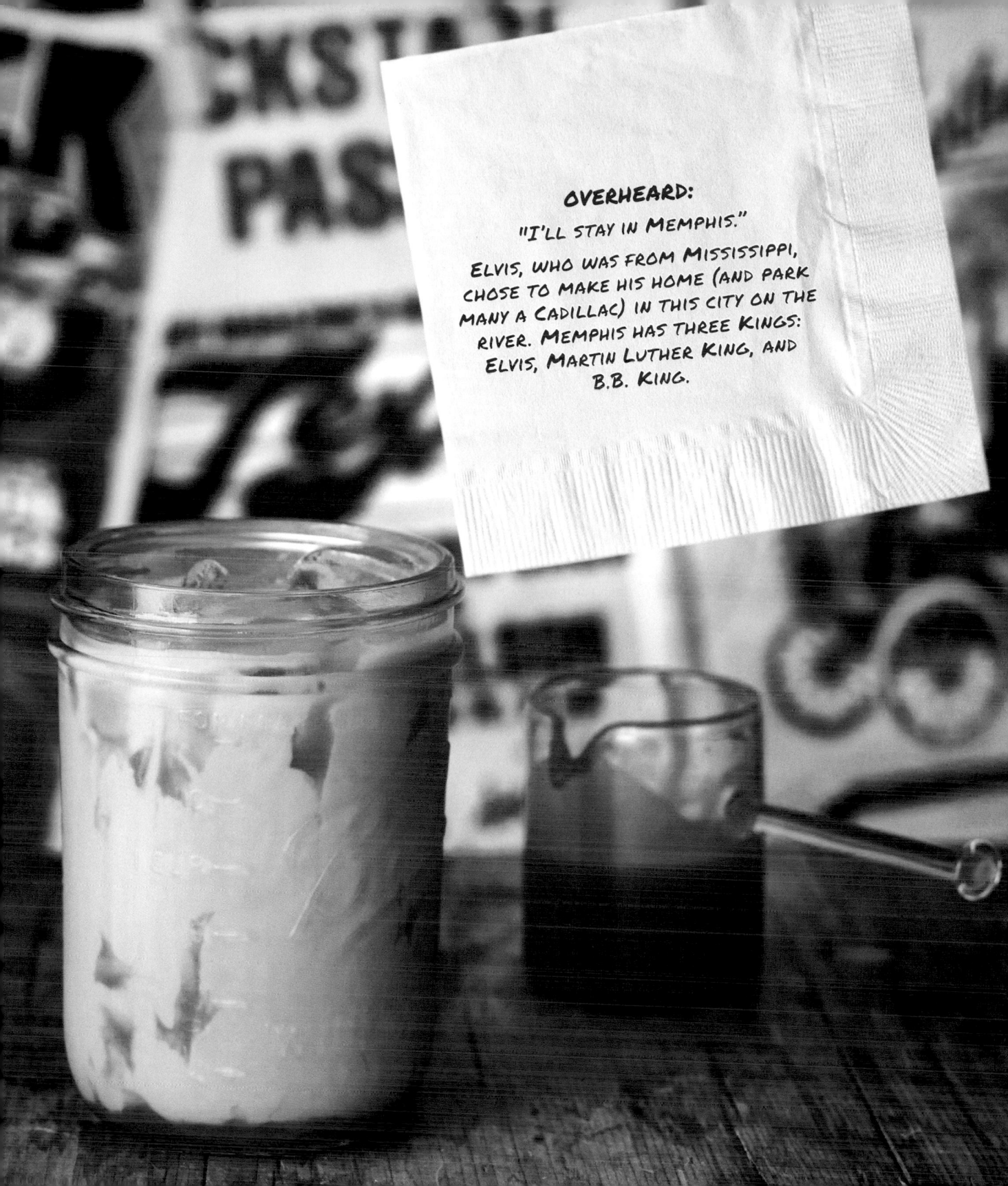

OVERHEARD:

"I'll stay in Memphis."

Elvis, who was from Mississippi, chose to make his home (and park many a Cadillac) in this city on the river. Memphis has three Kings: Elvis, Martin Luther King, and B.B. King.

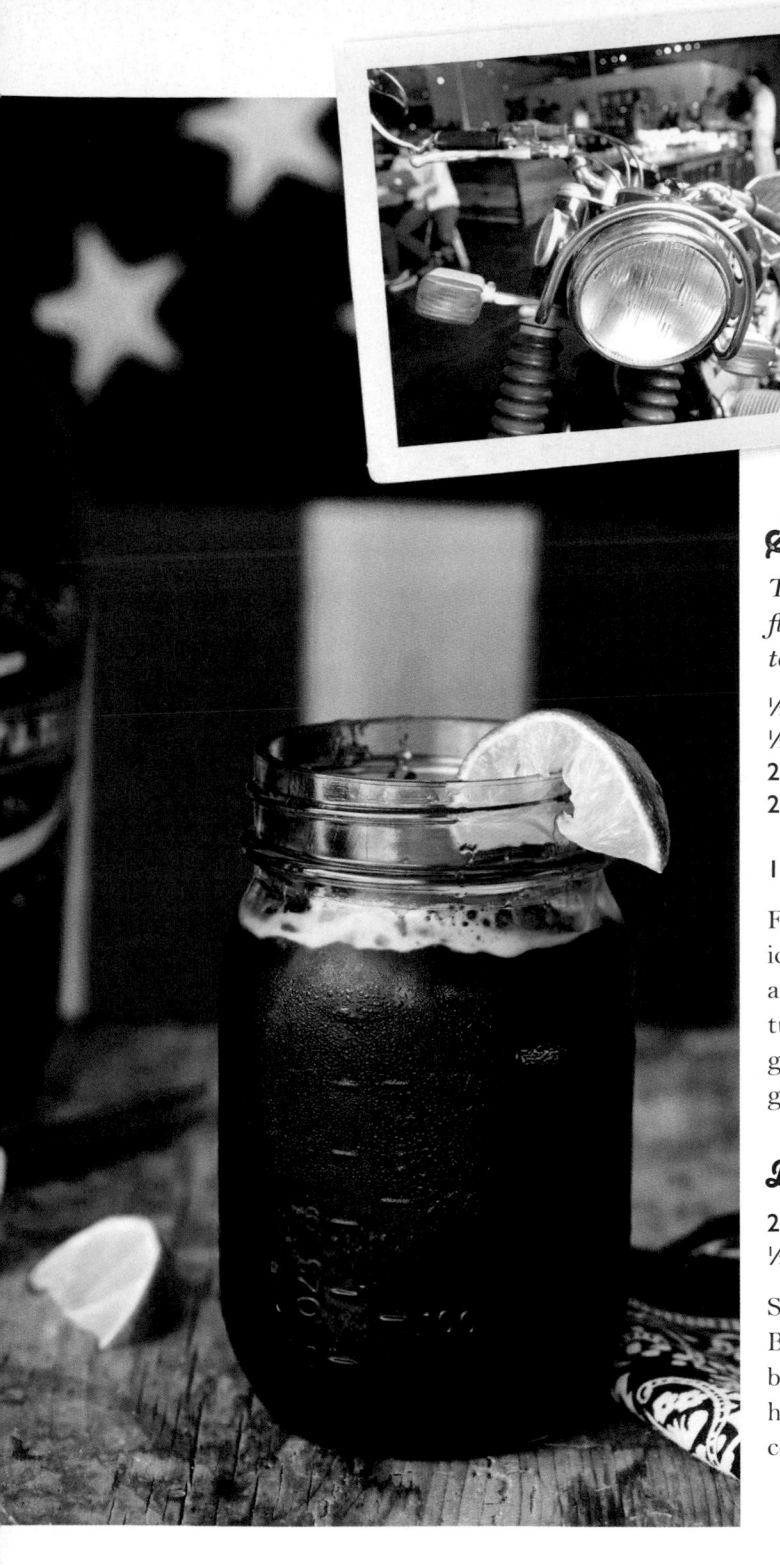

Shoeless Joe

This has an unusual bitter and sweet flavor that may take some getting used to, but ultimately it's pretty addictive.

- ½ cup club soda
- ½ cup Mexican cola soft drink
- 2 Tbsp. Black Cherry Simple Syrup
- 2 Tbsp. brewed espresso, cooled to room temperature
- 1 lime wedge

Fill a 1-pt. wide-mouth canning jar halfway with ice. Add club soda and cola. Stir together syrup and espresso in a shot glass; pour over cola mixture. Squeeze lime wedge over top of drink. Stir gently, and place squeezed lime wedge on edge of glass. Serve immediately. **Makes: 1 serving**

Black Cherry Simple Syrup

- 2 cups bottled black cherry juice
- ½ cup sugar

Stir together juice and sugar in a 2-qt. saucepan. Bring to a boil. Reduce heat to medium-high, and boil, uncovered, 15 minutes or until reduced by half. Remove from heat; cool completely. Store, covered, in refrigerator. **Makes: 1¼ cups**

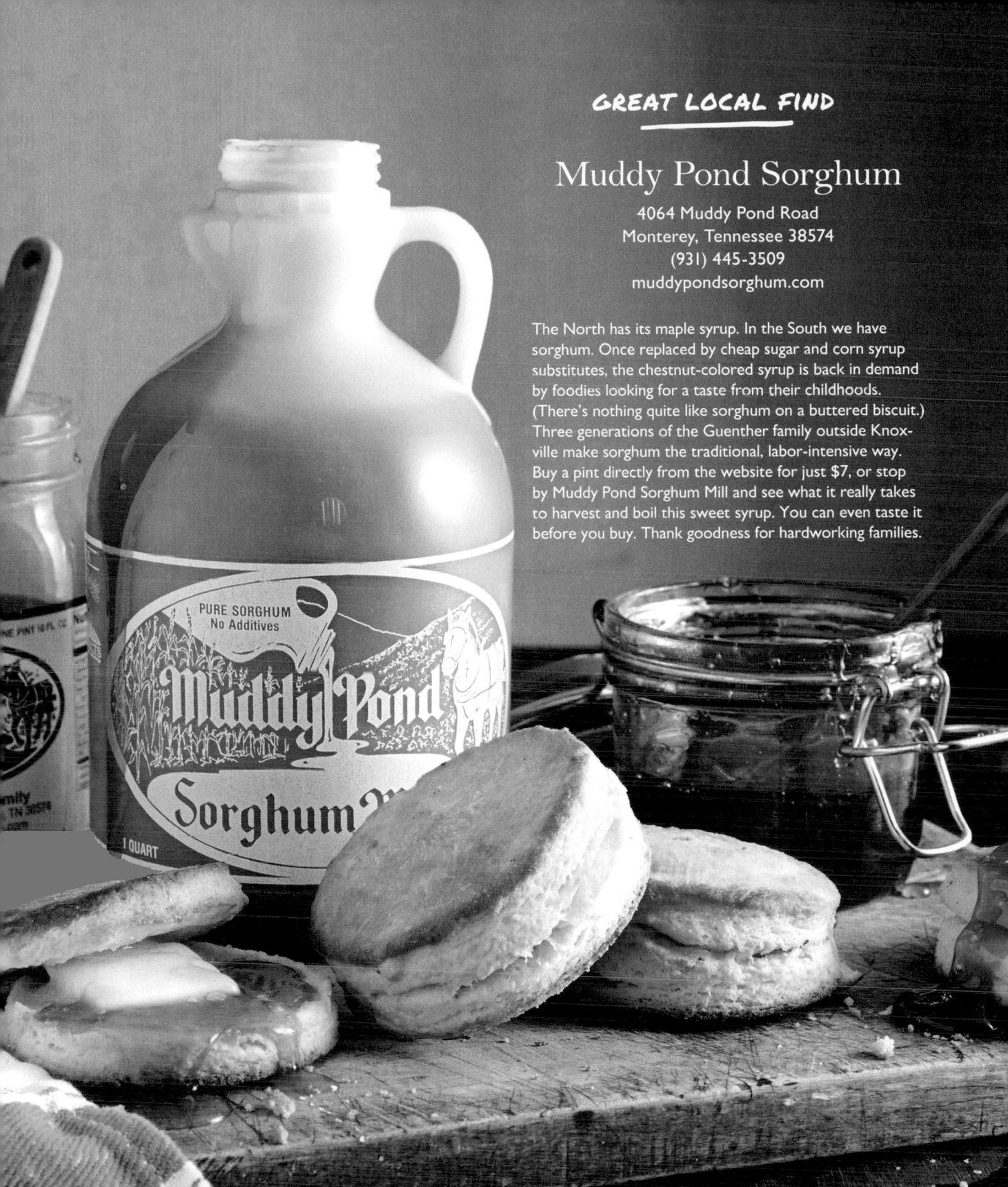

Muddy Pond Sorghum

4064 Muddy Pond Road
Monterey, Tennessee 38574
(931) 445-3509
muddypondsorghum.com

The North has its maple syrup. In the South we have sorghum. Once replaced by cheap sugar and corn syrup substitutes, the chestnut-colored syrup is back in demand by foodies looking for a taste from their childhoods. (There's nothing quite like sorghum on a buttered biscuit.) Three generations of the Guenther family outside Knoxville make sorghum the traditional, labor-intensive way. Buy a pint directly from the website for just $7, or stop by Muddy Pond Sorghum Mill and see what it really takes to harvest and boil this sweet syrup. You can even taste it before you buy. Thank goodness for hardworking families.

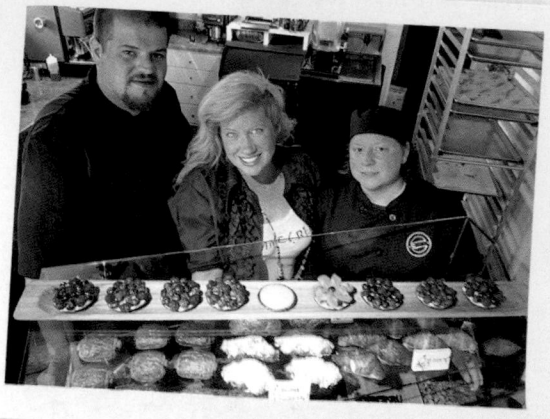

Tart

820 South Cooper Avenue
Memphis, Tennessee 38104
(901) 725-0091
tartmemphis.com

A rich cup of coffee and the perfect, buttery, flaky croissant... beautiful fresh tarts everywhere.... Am I in Paris? Non. If you think Memphis is all barbecue and burgers, think again. Tart puts a Southern twist on cafe culture. The staff here bakes all of the breads, makes every dish from scratch, uses local ingredients, and has captured the imagination of area artists. The house-made brioche is phenomenal. "It's a pain in the you-know-what, but worth it," Chef Abby Jestis says. "And if you use day-old brioche in the bread pudding, it's off the chain." This sassy restaurant in Memphis' Cooper-Young neighborhood proves there are no shortcuts to quality.

Poached Eggs in Brioche

This is decadent and the Tomato Hollandaise makes mastering this dish worthwhile.

4   brioche à tête or 4 (1-inch-thick) slices brioche loaf
4   oz. carved smoked fully cooked ham
1   tsp. white vinegar
4   large eggs
Tomato Hollandaise (page 200)
Garnish: chopped fresh basil

1. Preheat oven to 350°. Pull tops off brioches about 1 inch from top; carefully scoop out insides of bottoms, leaving a ½-inch-thick shell. (Cavities should be just large enough to fit a poached large egg.) Replace tops of brioche.
2. Place brioches and ham on a small baking sheet. Bake at 350° for 5 minutes or until warm.
3. Meanwhile, add water to depth of 3 inches in a large skillet. Bring to a boil; reduce heat, and maintain at a light simmer. Add white vinegar. Break eggs, and slip into water, 1 at a time, as close as possible to surface. Simmer 3 to 5 minutes or to desired degree of doneness. Remove with a slotted spoon.
4. Place ham in brioche shells. Top with poached eggs. Place each filled brioche on a plate, and spoon Tomato Hollandaise sauce over eggs. Serve each brioche with its top for dipping in egg. **Makes: 4 servings**
Note: If using sliced brioche loaf, cut out a whole in middle of bread large enough to hold a poached egg.

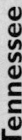

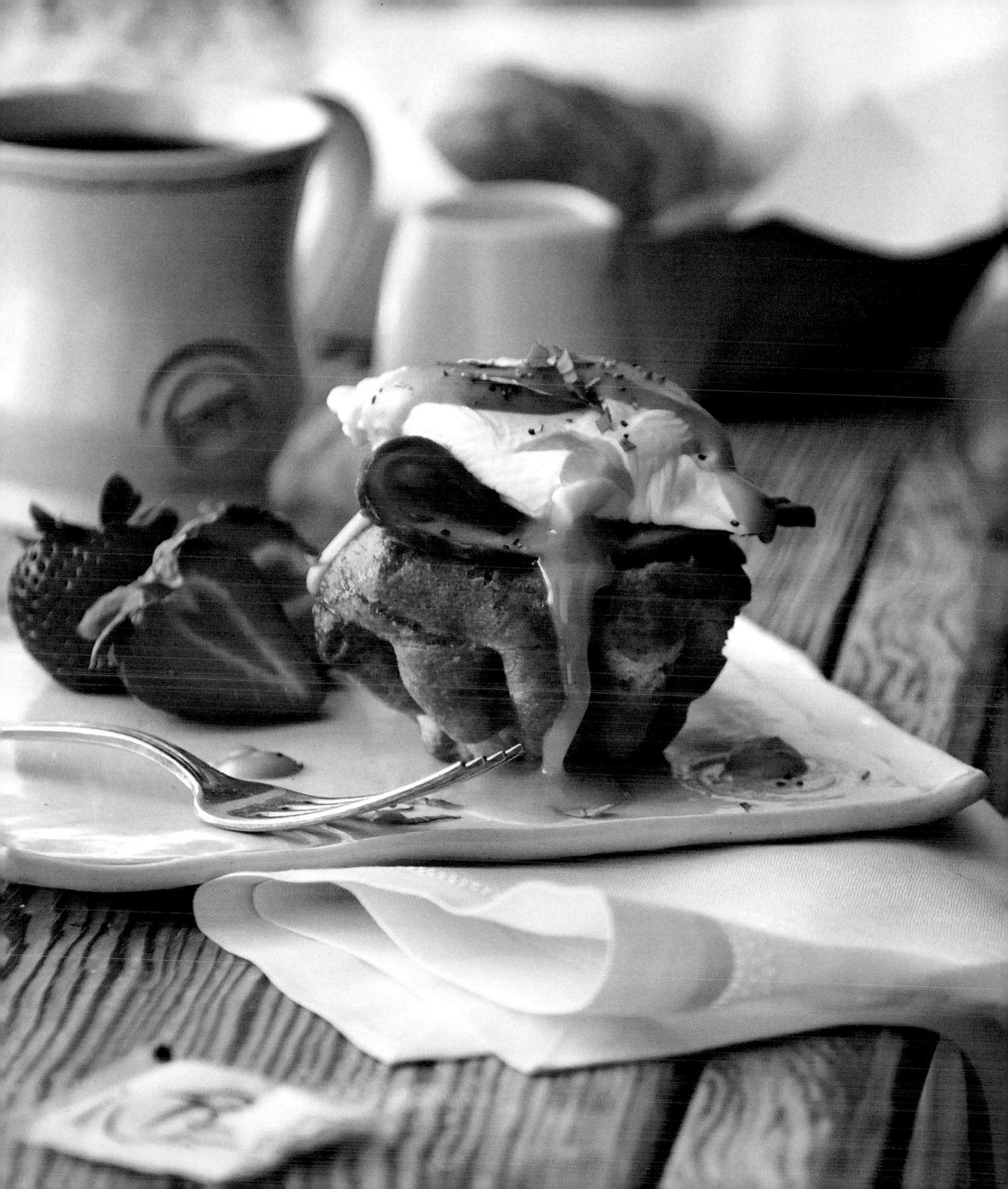

Tomato Hollandaise

½ cup butter
1 Tbsp. tomato paste
⅛ tsp. table salt
3 large egg yolks
1 Tbsp. minced fresh basil

1. Pour water to depth of 1 inch into bottom of a double boiler over medium heat; bring to a boil. Reduce heat to low, and simmer; place first 3 ingredients in top of double boiler over simmering water. Cook, stirring constantly, until butter melts.
2. Whisk egg yolks in a small bowl until thick and pale. Gradually whisk about half of hot butter mixture into yolks; add yolk mixture to remaining hot butter mixture, stirring constantly. Keep warm until ready to use. Stir in basil just before serving. **Makes: 4 servings**

Poached Pears with Greek Yogurt, Toasted Muesli, and Local Honey

This healthy and colorful dish is topped with crunchy house-made muesli.

2 cups Merlot
1 cup sugar
1 (3-inch) cinnamon stick
1 bay leaf
4 Bosc pears (1½ lb.), peeled and cored
1 cup Greek yogurt
1 cup Toasted Muesli
¼ cup honey

1. Stir first 4 ingredients and 2 cups water in a medium saucepan. Bring to a boil, stirring until sugar dissolves. Add pears. Bring to a boil; reduce heat, cover and simmer 20 minutes or until pears are tender. Cool. Remove pears from poaching liquid; cut into lengthwise slices.

2. Divide pear slices evenly among 4 shallow bowls. Top each serving with ¼ cup yogurt. Sprinkle each with ¼ cup Toasted Muesli, and drizzle with 1 Tbsp. honey. **Makes: 4 servings**

Toasted Muesli

Vegetable cooking spray
¼ cup honey
2 Tbsp. light molasses
1 Tbsp. vanilla extract
1 tsp. ground cinnamon
5 cups uncooked regular oats
2 cups chopped lightly toasted blanched hazelnuts
2 cups chopped lightly toasted almonds

1. Preheat oven to 325°. Lightly grease a half sheet pan with cooking spray. Stir together honey and next 3 ingredients in a 1-cup glass measuring cup.
2. Toss together oats and remaining ingredients in a large bowl. Pour honey mixture over oat mixture, and toss to coat well.
3. Spread mixture in prepared pan. Bake at 325° for 35 minutes, stirring every 10 minutes. Cool completely in pan. **Makes: 10½ cups**

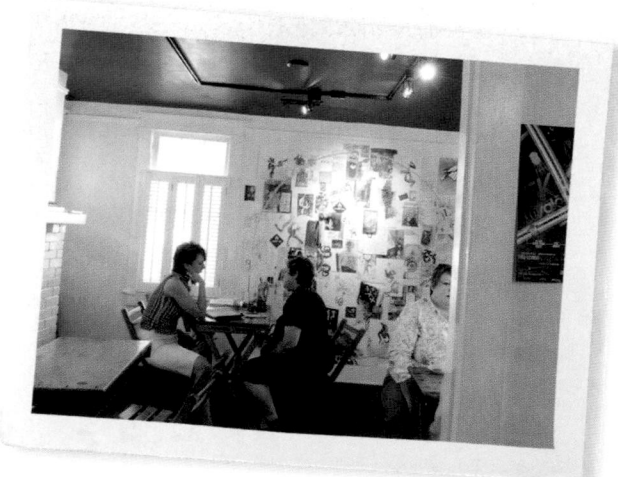

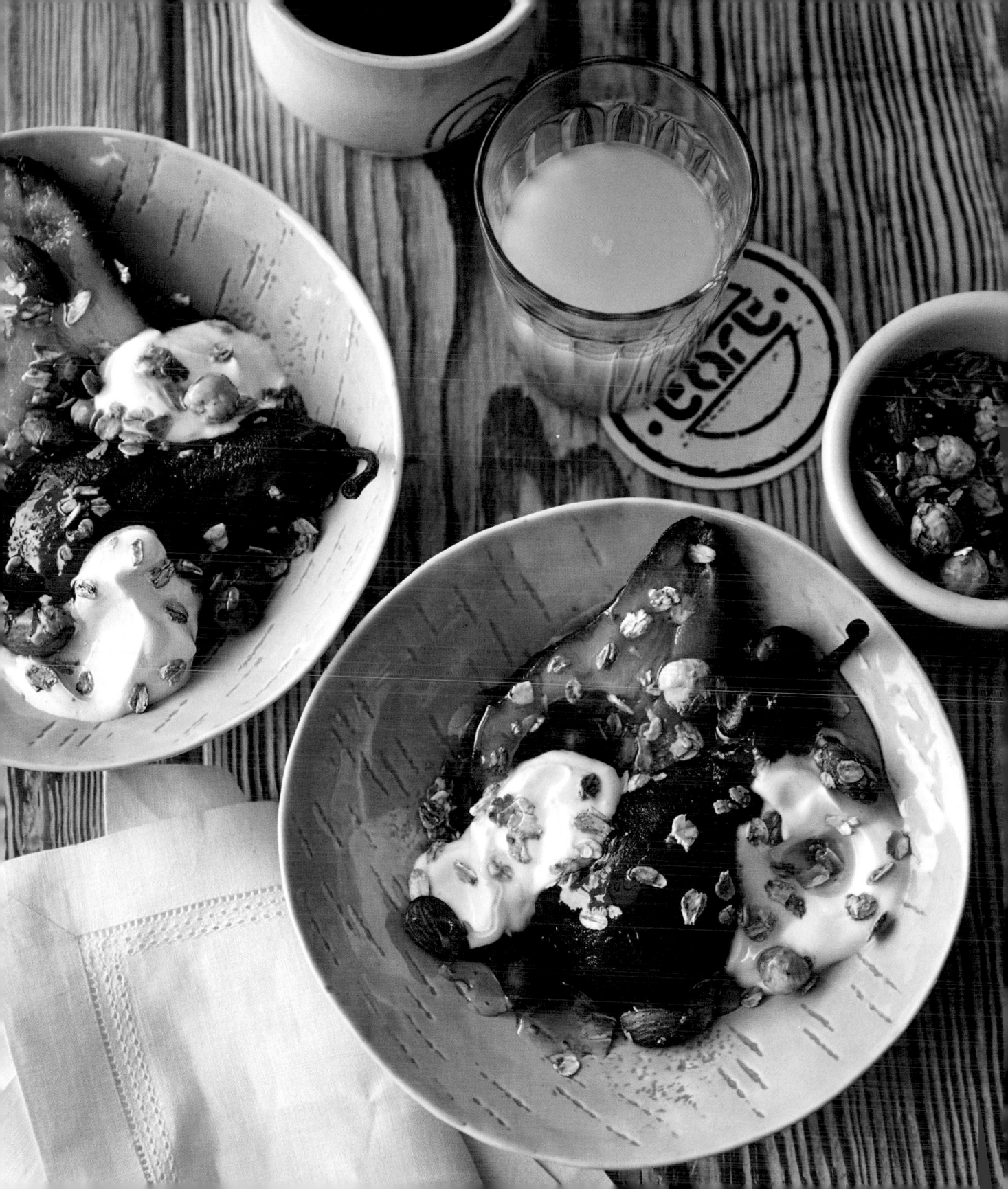

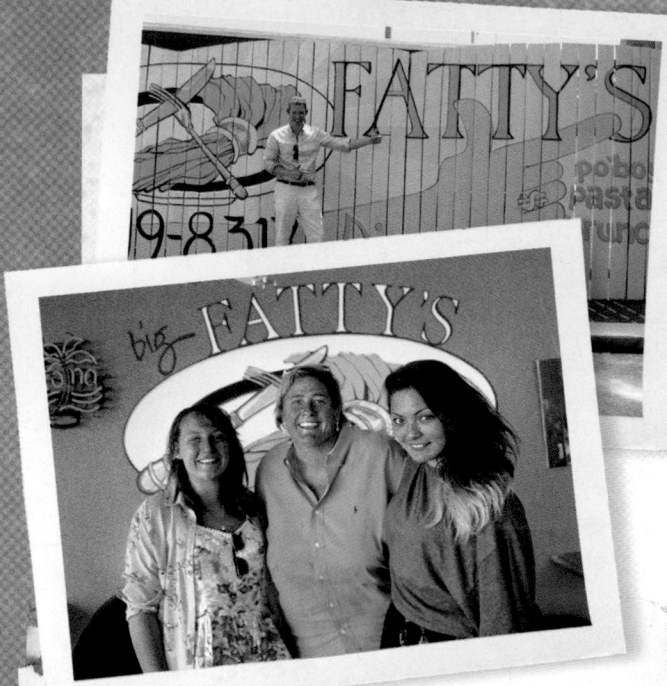

Big Fatty's Catering Kitchen

5005 Kingston Pike
Knoxville, Tennessee 37919
(865) 219-8317

*"I'm pimpin' food. I'm a food pimp,"
says my new BFF (best food friend) Lisa
Smith, who holds a degree from one of
the nation's finest culinary schools. But
don't assume her food is hoity-toity. "I
just cook what I like to eat," she says.
I like to eat what Lisa likes: She could
fry a dishrag and I'd eat it. Her shrimp
po' boy, crab-stuffed fried chicken, and
deep-fried cornbread made me consider
an industrial deep fryer for my kitchen.
Big Fatty's, as the name suggests, invites
diners to have fun. Everything here is a
little cheeky, including happy hour. Beers
are fifty cents "until someone pees." Yes,
that's printed right on the menu.*

Pulled Pork Crewban with Sweet Potato French Fries and Cranberry Mayonnaise

1	(3¼-lb.) boneless pork shoulder roast (Boston butt)
2	tsp. table salt
2	tsp. freshly ground black pepper
2	tsp. garlic powder
1	cup firmly packed light brown sugar
1	cup bottled barbecue sauce
6	hoagie rolls

Southern Coleslaw (page 204)
Deep-Fried Pickles (page 204)
Sweet Potato French Fries with Cranberry Mayonnaise (page 204)

1. Preheat oven to 300°. Trim excess fat from roast; place, fat side up, in a 9-inch square pan. Rub salt and next 2 ingredients over top of roast. Pat brown sugar over roast. Pour water to depth of 1 inch around roast. Cover pan tightly with aluminum foil.

2. Bake at 300° for 5½ hours or until very tender. Remove pan from oven. Transfer roast to a cutting board; let stand 5 minutes or until cool enough to handle. Remove fat from pork; place pork in a large bowl. Shred pork with 2 forks; stir in barbecue sauce.

3. Spoon about ¾ cup pork mixture onto bottom of each bun. Top each with ⅔ cup Southern Coleslaw, 8 Deep-Fried Pickles, and bun tops. Serve immediately with Sweet Potato French Fries with Cranberry Mayonnaise. **Makes: 6 servings**
Note: We tested with Sticky Fingers Memphis Original Barbecue Sauce.

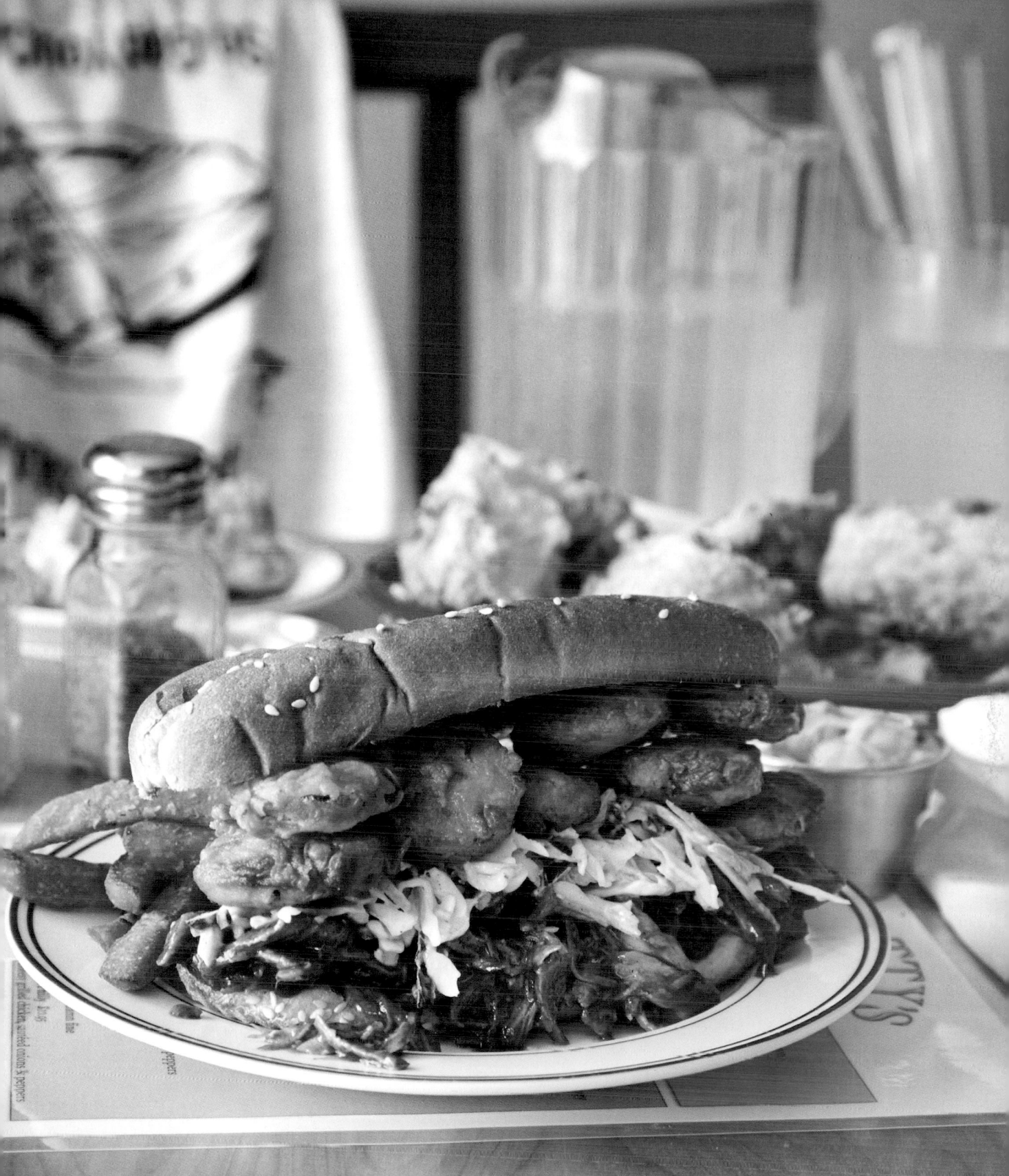

Southern Coleslaw

- ½ cup mayonnaise
- ¼ cup ketchup
- 1 Tbsp. sugar
- 2 Tbsp. bottled zesty Italian dressing
- 1 tsp. table salt
- 1 tsp. freshly ground black pepper
- 1 tsp. prepared horseradish
- 1 small garlic clove, minced
- 1 (16-oz.) package shredded coleslaw mix with carrots

Combine all ingredients except coleslaw mix, stirring well. Add coleslaw mix; stir until coated. Cover and chill. **Makes: 6 servings**

Deep-Fried Pickles

Canola oil
- ¾ cup all-purpose flour
- ¾ cup buttermilk
- 48 dill pickle chips

1. Pour oil into a skillet or medium saucepan to depth of 2 inches; heat to 350°.
2. Place flour in a shallow dish. Place buttermilk in a bowl. Dredge pickle chips in flour; dip in buttermilk. Dredge in flour, shaking off excess. Fry in hot oil 4 minutes, turning halfway through. Transfer to several layers of paper towels to drain using a slotted spoon. If desired, sprinkle with salt and pepper to taste. **Makes: 6 servings**

Sweet Potato French Fries with Cranberry Mayonnaise

CRANBERRY MAYONNAISE
- 2 cups mayonnaise
- ½ (14-oz.) can jellied cranberry sauce

SWEET POTATO FRENCH FRIES
Vegetable oil
- 1 (20-oz.) package frozen sweet potato French fries
- 2 Tbsp. vegetable oil
- 3 garlic cloves, minced
- ¼ cup crumbled blue cheese

1. Prepare Cranberry Mayonnaise: Stir together mayonnaise and cranberry sauce until blended.
2. Prepare Sweet Potato French Fries: Pour oil to depth of 3 inches in a Dutch oven; heat to 380°. Fry sweet potato French fries in hot oil 4 to 5 minutes. Drain on paper towels.
3. Heat 2 Tbsp. vegetable oil in a large skillet over medium-high heat. Add garlic; sauté 30 seconds or until tender. Add sweet potato fries. Toss well. Sprinkle with cheese. Serve immediately with Cranberry Mayonnaise. **Makes: 6 servings**

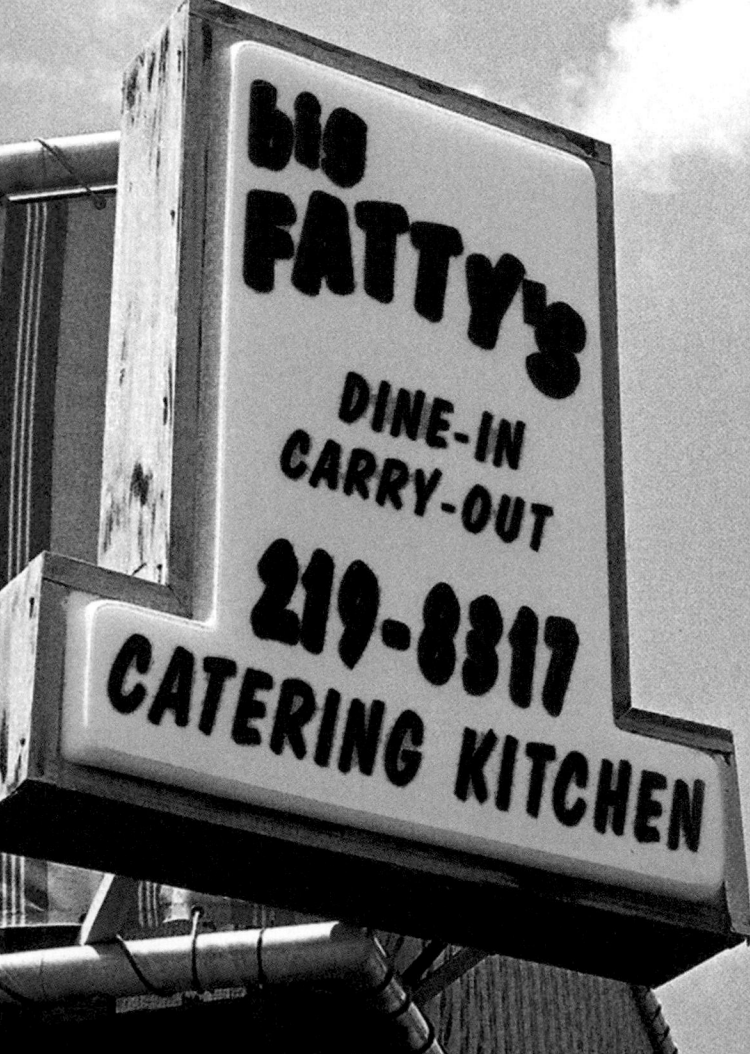

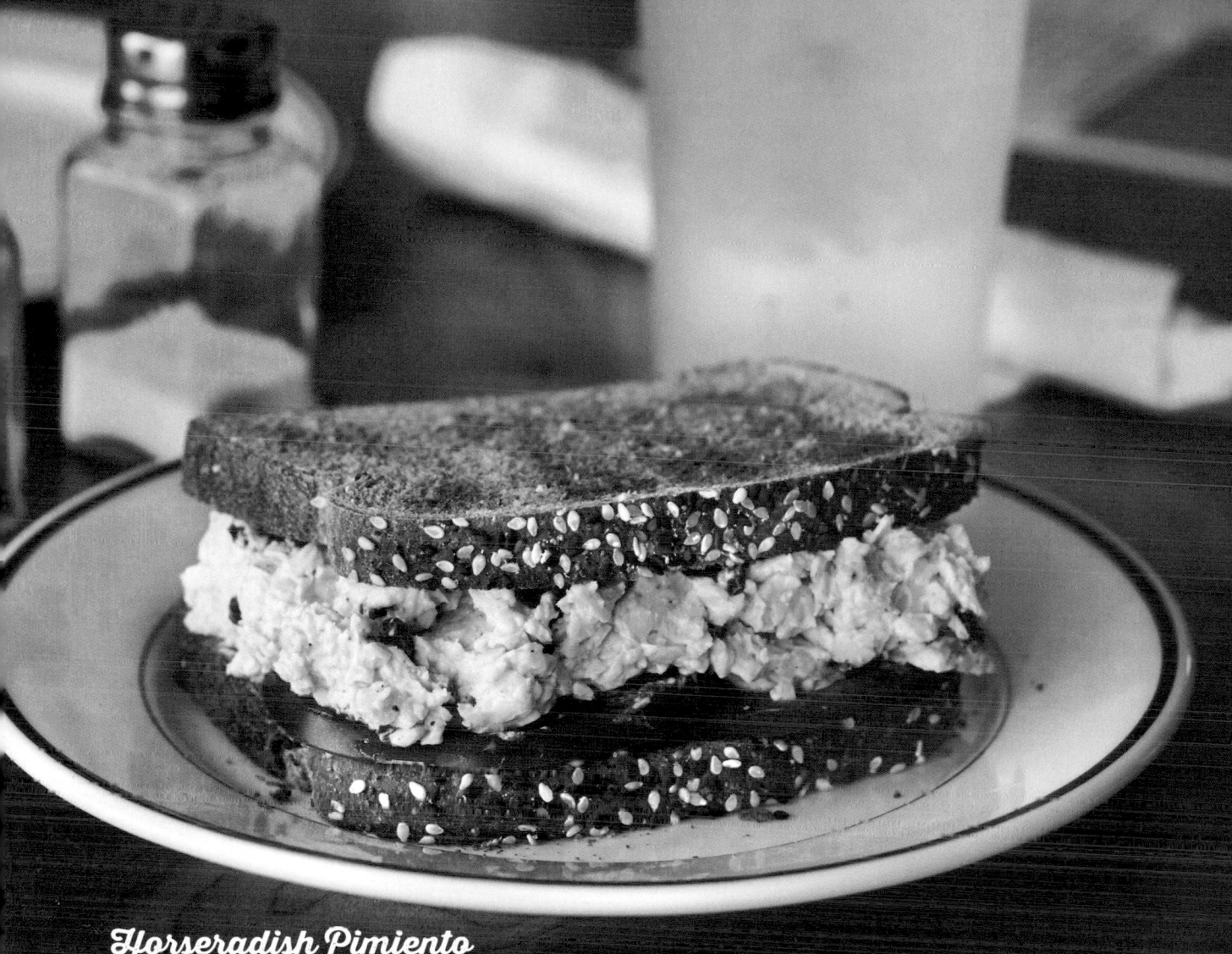

Horseradish Pimiento Cheese

1 (8-oz.) package processed cheese (such as Velveeta), cut into small cubes
1 (8-oz.) package cream cheese, softened
½ cup mayonnaise
2 Tbsp. prepared horseradish
1 tsp. freshly ground black pepper
½ tsp. table salt
½ tsp. minced fresh garlic
1 (16-oz.) block extra-sharp Cheddar cheese, shredded
1 (4-oz.) jar pimientos, undrained

1. Beat processed cheese and cream cheese at medium speed with an electric stand mixer until blended. Add mayonnaise and remaining ingredients. Beat until blended. Cover and chill.
Makes: 5 cups

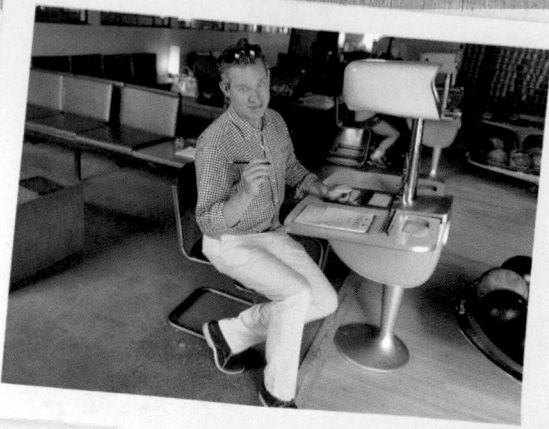

Pinewood Social

33 Peabody Street
Nashville, Tennessee 37210
(615) 751-8111
pinewoodsocial.com

This place makes me want to buy two-toned shoes, a hideous shirt, a pearlescent ball, and start my own bowling league. And I don't even like bowling. The vintage alley here, saved from a giant Midwest bowl-o-rama, wreaks hipster cool. Everything at Pinewood Social does: the copper bar, the setting in an old trolley warehouse, and the new-South menu. Even the tables are made from former bowling alley boards. Open all day, Pinewood Social makes an excellent spot to meet friends, write your novel, or have several of the "Bitter Wife" cocktails and do your best twinkle-toes-Fred-Flintstone impersonation. The menu is packed with addictive choices, such as the fried broccoli (which isn't battered) and the hot sweetbreads—both inventive twists on old favorites.

The Bitter Wife

This cocktail is fresh and sassy— not at all like a bitter wife.

1	Tbsp. golden syrup
3	Tbsp. gin
1½	Tbsp. lemon juice
1½	tsp. Batavia Arrack
2	dashes of Peychaud's bitters
¼	cup club soda

Orange peel strip

Combine golden syrup and 3 Tbsp. water in a small bowl, stirring until syrup dissolves. Combine gin, next 3 ingredients, and 1 Tbsp. syrup mixture in a cocktail shaker. Reserve remaining syrup mixture for another use. Fill shaker with ice; cover with lid, and shake vigorously until thoroughly chilled (about 20 seconds). Strain into a Collins glass filled with ice. Top with ¼ cup club soda. Twist orange peel, and add to glass. Serve immediately. **Makes: 1 serving**
Note: We tested with Lyle's Golden Syrup.

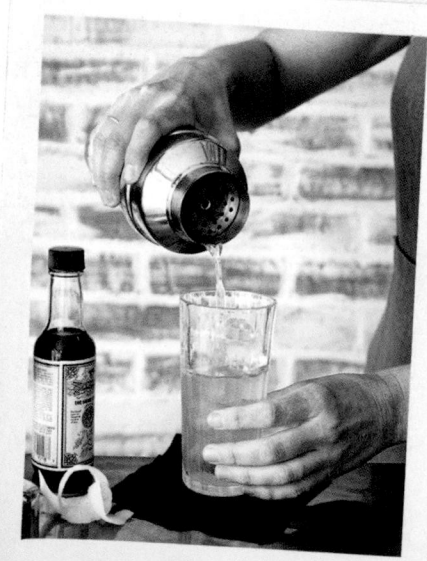

Peach Salad

PICKLED PEACHES

¾ cup sugar
1 cup white wine vinegar
1½ tsp. table salt
1½ tsp. black peppercorns
1 tsp. yellow mustard seeds
1 (3-inch) cinnamon stick
1 small star anise
3 large firm ripe peaches (1½ lb.), peeled, pitted, and cut into (½-inch) cubes

PEACH SALAD

2 unpeeled large peaches, pitted and quartered
¾ tsp. sea salt, divided
⅜ tsp. freshly ground black pepper, divided
2 Tbsp. olive oil, divided
4 cups loosely packed arugula
⅓ cup chopped pecans, toasted
½ tsp. minced fresh garlic
1 unpeeled peach, pitted, and cut into ⅛-inch-thick slices
1 (8-oz.) container Burrata

1. **Prepare Pickled Peaches:** Combine first 7 ingredients and 1 cup water in a medium saucepan. Bring to a boil, stirring until sugar dissolves. Place peaches in a medium bowl. Pour vinegar mixture over peaches. Let stand 1 hour or until cool. Cover and chill overnight.

2. **Prepare Peach Salad:** Preheat grill pan over medium-high heat. Sprinkle peach quarters with ¼ tsp. salt and ⅛ tsp. pepper; brush with 1 Tbsp. olive oil. Grill 3 minutes or just until grill marks appear. Remove peaches from pan, and set aside.

3. Toss together arugula, next 3 ingredients, ¾ cup pickled peaches, ¼ tsp. salt, ⅛ tsp. pepper, and remaining 1 Tbsp. olive oil in a large bowl. Reserve remaining pickled peaches for another use.

4. Place 3 dollops Burrata on each of 4 plates. Sprinkle with remaining ¼ tsp. salt and ⅛ tsp. pepper. Arrange 2 peach quarters on each plate. Top with arugula mixture. Serve immediately.

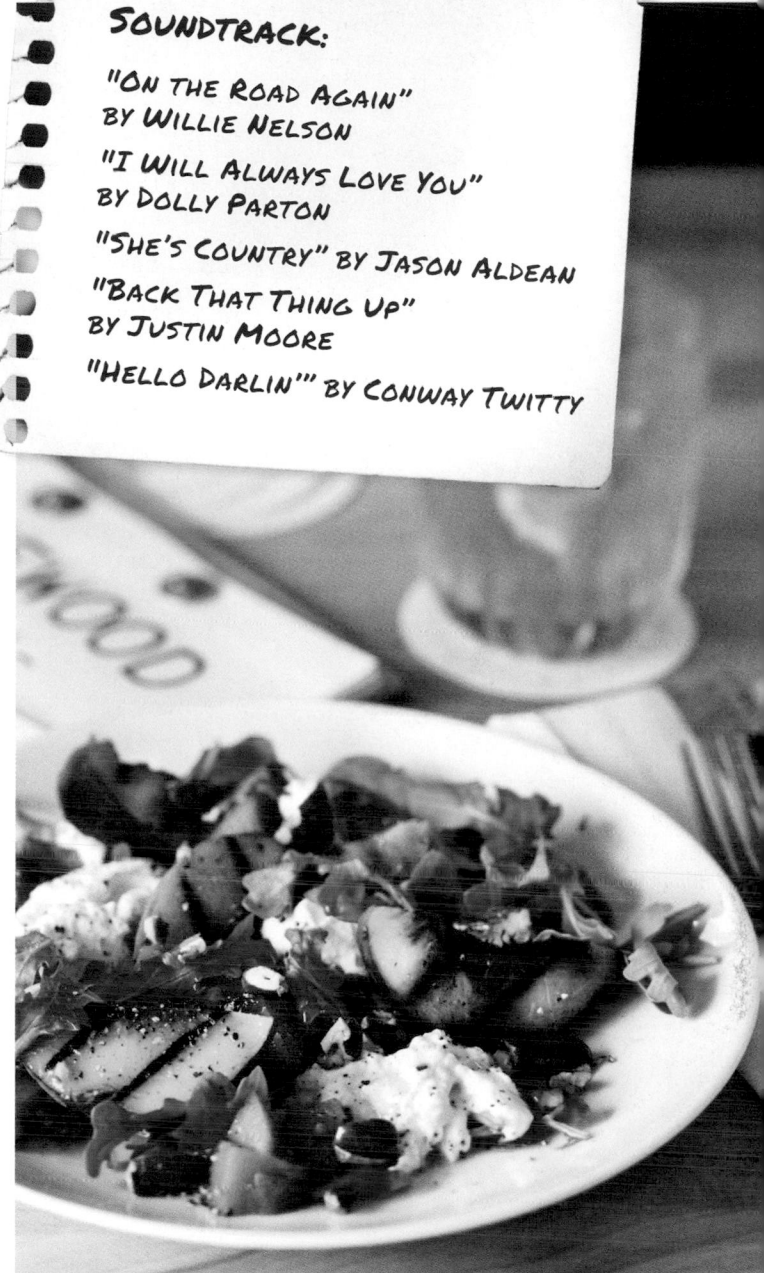

Makes: 4 servings

Note: Use a mandolin to cut fresh peach into ⅛-inch-thick slices.

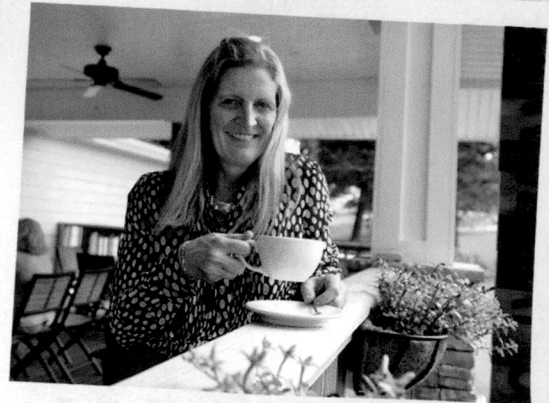

Olive Bean Natural Grocery and Cafe

1404 James Blvd.
Signal Mountain, Tennessee 37377
(423) 805-4888
olivebean.com

Climb up Signal Mountain and you will be rewarded at the summit. A cross between a farmers' market, general store, and urban bistro, Olive Bean is a haven for anyone seeking fresh, local, and delicious. Shannon, April, and Joseph Handy restored this quaint spot to its present-day beauty. Every tile, plank, and button on the leather banquette was installed by the Handy family, who certainly live up to their name. Excellent coffee and amazing produce abound, but tuck into the avocado smash or house-made crumpets. They taste delicious, and they're good for you. Lastly, the friendly staff makes you feel welcome as they serve up each dish with a smile.

Falafel

This baked falafel is much healthier than the traditional fried version.

1	cup dried chickpeas
2	garlic cloves
½	cup firmly packed fresh parsley leaves
1	small onion, quartered
1	medium carrot, cut into 1-inch pieces
½	red bell pepper, cut into 1-inch pieces
1	tsp. baking powder
¼	cup plain yogurt
1	Tbsp. ground cumin
1	tsp. kosher salt
1	tsp. freshly ground black pepper
½	tsp. dried crushed red pepper
Parchment paper	
¼	cup olive oil

1. Rinse and sort chickpeas according to package directions. Drain. Place chickpeas in a bowl. Cover with water 3 inches above peas; let soak 8 hours. Drain.

2. Preheat oven to 350°. With processor on, drop garlic through food chute; process until minced. Add chickpeas; process until consistency of coarse meal. Add parsley and next 3 ingredients. Process 20 to 30 seconds or until finely chopped, scraping down sides as needed.

3. Stir baking powder into yogurt. Add yogurt mixture, cumin, and next 3 ingredients to processor; process until blended. Shape chickpea mixture into 15 (1½-oz.) balls.

4. Place balls on a baking sheet lined with parchment paper. Bake at 350° for 40 minutes or until golden brown, brushing with olive oil every 10 minutes. **Makes: 5 servings**

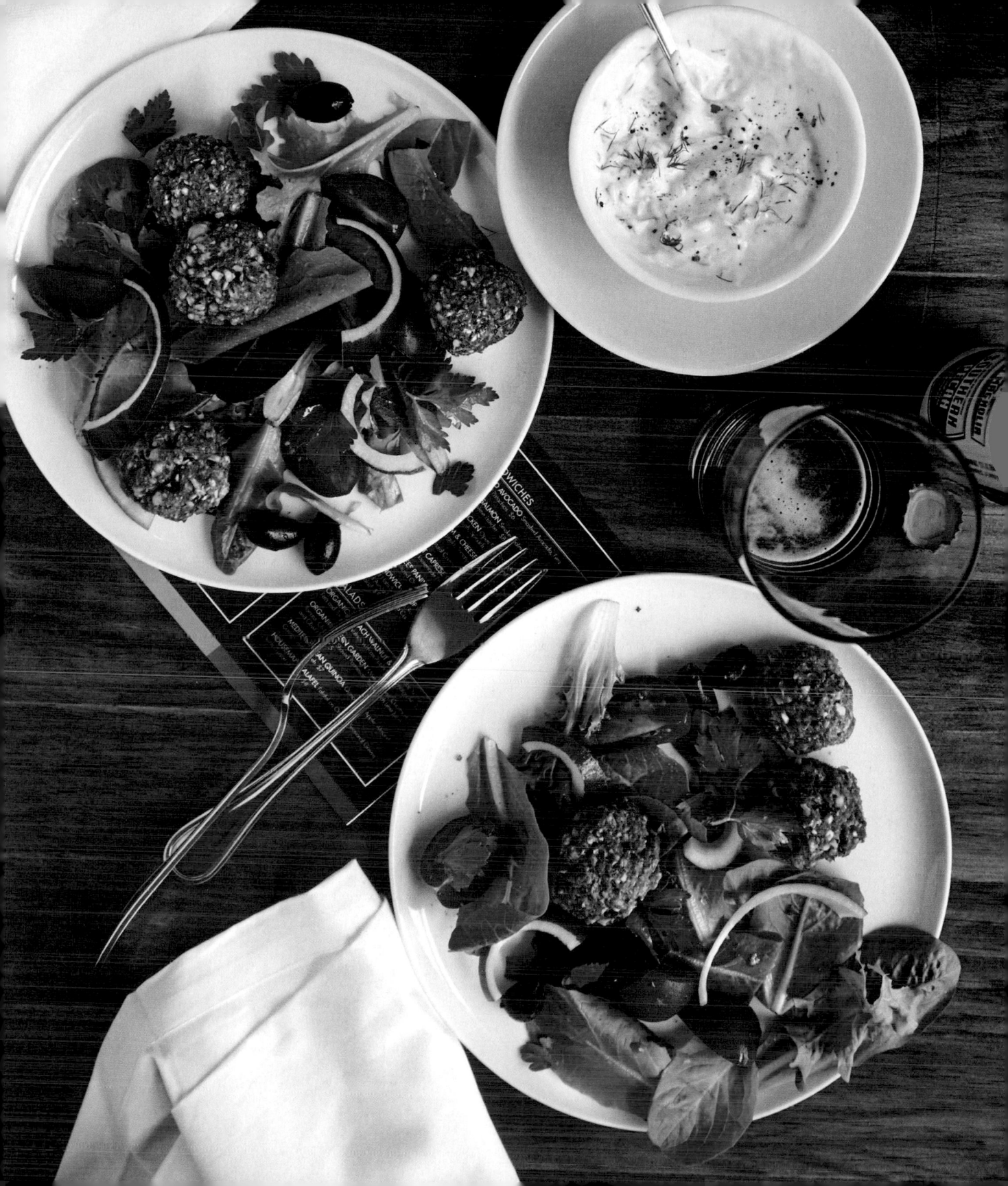

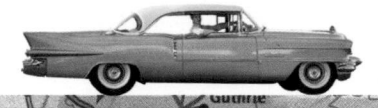

Tennessee bucket list

things to see and do (besides eat) here

❶ Attend a performance at the **Grand Ole Opry** in Nashville, or do some honky tonking on Lower Broadway.

❷ Tour Memphis from the back of a 1955 Cadillac with **American Dream Safaris** and visit Graceland, Sun Studios *(pictured)*, and Beale Street in style.

❸ Drop by the **Tennessee Aquarium** in Chattanooga to see the spot that kicked off the South's aquatic craze.

❹ Walk the haunting **Shiloh National Military Park,** which has preserved the historic sites of two 1862 Civil War battles for more than 120 years, making it the third oldest in the National Park system.

❺ Shop and enjoy a meal at **Hillsboro Village** near Vanderbilt University in Nashville, and then take in a film or live show at the Belcourt Theatre.

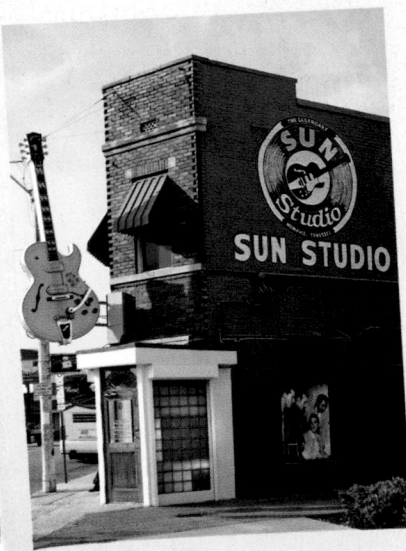

Tzatziki (*pictured on previous page*)

1   English cucumber, shredded
½   tsp. table salt, divided
1   cup sour cream
1   cup plain yogurt
⅓   cup olive oil
1   Tbsp. minced fresh dill
1   Tbsp. Champagne vinegar
1   garlic clove, minced

Combine cucumber and ¼ tsp. salt in a bowl; let stand 5 minutes; drain. Return cucumber to bowl. Stir in sour cream, next 5 ingredients, and remaining ¼ tsp. salt. Cover and chill 2 hours. **Note:** We tested with Stoneyfield Farms Organic Plain Yogurt. **Makes: 3 cups**

Crumpets

Serve these spongy cakes hot with butter or jam.

1   (¼-oz.) envelope active dry yeast
1½   cups warm water (100° to 110°)
1   cup warm milk (100° to 110°)
2½   cups all-purpose flour
1   cup whole wheat flour
1   tsp. table salt
1   tsp. baking powder
3   Tbsp. butter

1. Combine yeast and warm water in a bowl; let stand 5 minutes. Add milk and next 4 ingredients. Beat at medium speed with an electric mixer 2 minutes. Cover batter, and let stand 1 hour.
2. Melt 1½ tsp. butter per each of 3 batches in a large nonstick skillet over medium heat. Spoon about ½ cup batter in batches into 4 (3½-inch) buttered crumpet rings; cook 5 minutes or until edges begin to appear dry and bubbles begin to pop and create dimples. Remove rings; turn crumpets over, adding additional butter as needed. Cook 4 to 5 minutes or until firm and browned on other side. **Makes: 12 servings**

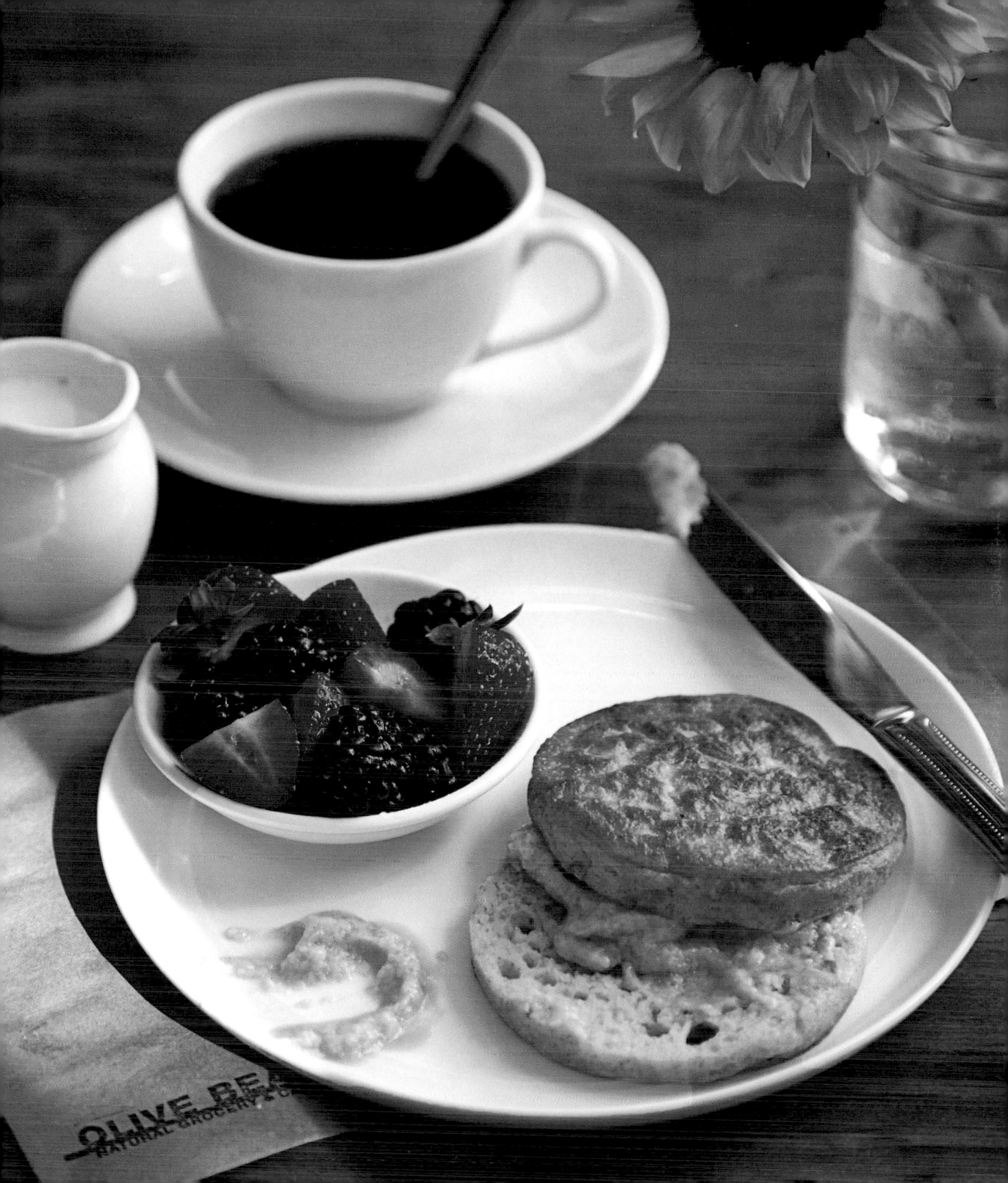

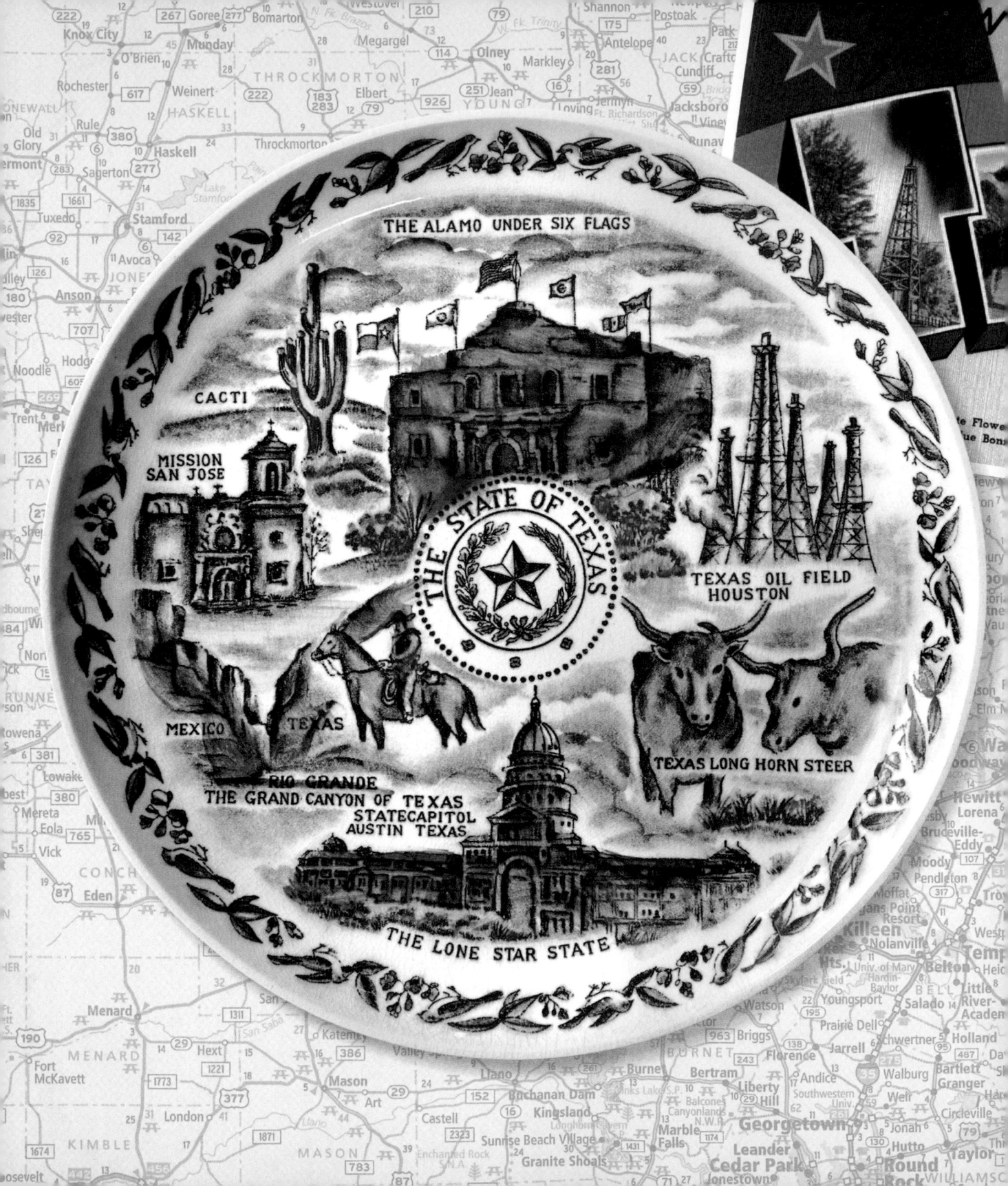

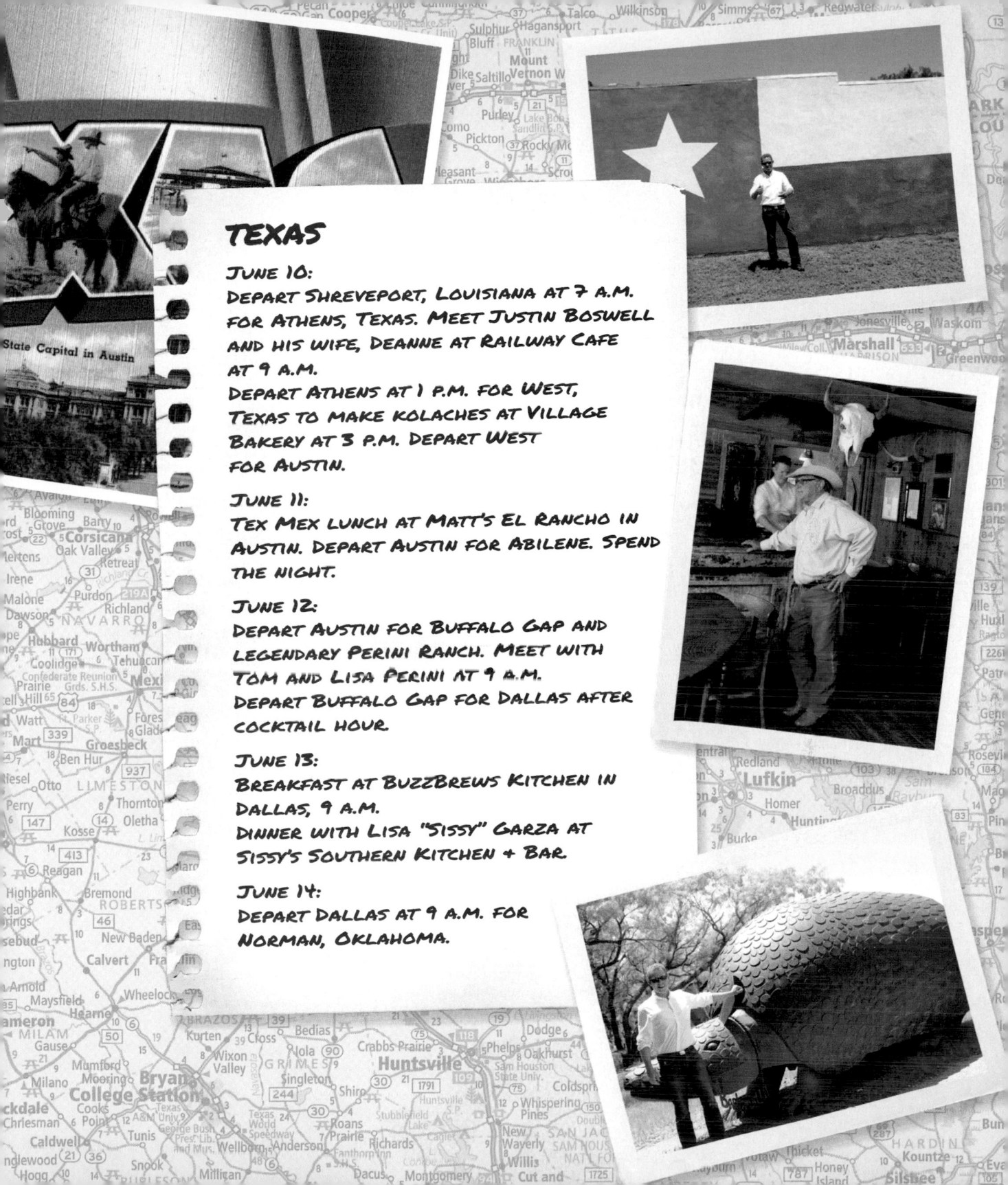

TEXAS

June 10:
Depart Shreveport, Louisiana at 7 a.m. for Athens, Texas. Meet Justin Boswell and his wife, Deanne at Railway Cafe at 9 a.m.
Depart Athens at 1 p.m. for West, Texas to make kolaches at Village Bakery at 3 p.m. Depart West for Austin.

June 11:
Tex Mex lunch at Matt's El Rancho in Austin. Depart Austin for Abilene. Spend the night.

June 12:
Depart Austin for Buffalo Gap and legendary Perini Ranch. Meet with Tom and Lisa Perini at 9 a.m.
Depart Buffalo Gap for Dallas after cocktail hour

June 13:
Breakfast at BuzzBrews Kitchen in Dallas, 9 a.m.
Dinner with Lisa "Sissy" Garza at Sissy's Southern Kitchen + Bar

June 14:
Depart Dallas at 9 a.m. for Norman, Oklahoma.

State Capital in Austin

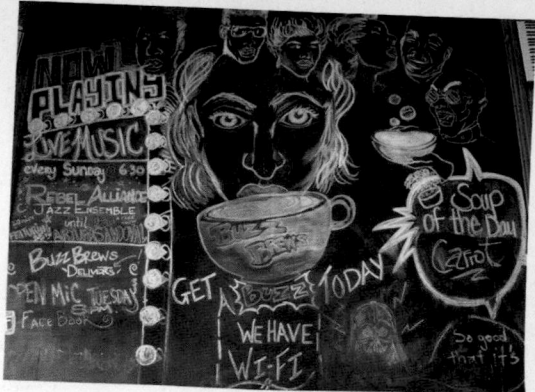

BuzzBrews

4154 North Central Expressway
Dallas, Texas 75204
(214) 826-7100
buzzbrews.com

My definition of a good day is when there's just 15 minutes between my last cup of coffee and my first cocktail. BuzzBrews in Dallas, which is open 24 hours, offers both awesome coffee and a great bar. Chef Ernest Belmore's menu is full of delicious comfort food and drinks. Even better, he and partner, Megan Estep, strive to make BuzzBrews an integral part of the community." The buzz in BuzzBrews doesn't refer to an alcohol or caffeine high," Ernest says. "The buzz you feel is doing something good for your community." The locally roasted java and large lattes will jump-start any early morning, and the food (especially the Bluto, my favorite) will satiate your hunger pangs, day or night. Don't miss anything with syrup—here they use only real maple syrup, a rarity in the restaurant business.

Bluto

8	oz. chorizo sausage, casings removed
2	Tbsp. Seasoning Oil (page 216)
¼	cup finely chopped onion
¼	cup chopped seeded plum tomato
2	Tbsp. minced seeded jalapeño peppers (about 1 large pepper)
3	hickory-smoked bacon slices, cooked and crumbled
3	large eggs
⅛	tsp. table salt
⅛	tsp. freshly ground black pepper
1½	tsp. butter
¾	cup (3 oz.) shredded Cheddar cheese

Chopped fresh cilantro
Accompaniments: Garlic Marbles (page 216), buttered toast, jelly

1. Brown chorizo in a medium skillet over medium-high heat, stirring often, 3 minutes or until meat crumbles and is no longer pink; drain well. Wipe skillet clean with paper towels. Heat skillet over medium-high heat. Add Seasoning Oil to skillet. Add chorizo, onion, and next 3 ingredients. Cook, without stirring, 1 minute; toss. Cook 1 minute. Remove from heat, and keep warm.

2. Whisk together eggs, salt, and pepper in a medium bowl. Melt butter in a 9-inch nonstick omelet pan over medium heat. Add egg mixture to omelet pan. As egg mixture starts to cook, gently lift edges of omelet with a spatula, and tilt pan so uncooked portion flows underneath. Cook 2 minutes or until almost set. Flip omelet over; cook 30 seconds (do not brown).

3. Transfer omelet to a plate. Sprinkle 1 side of omelet with ½ cup cheese and ¾ cup vegetable mixture; flip remaining side of omelet over filling. Top with remaining ¼ cup vegetable mixture, and sprinkle with remaining ¼ cup cheese. Sprinkle with cilantro. Serve immediately with accompaniments. **Makes: 1 serving**

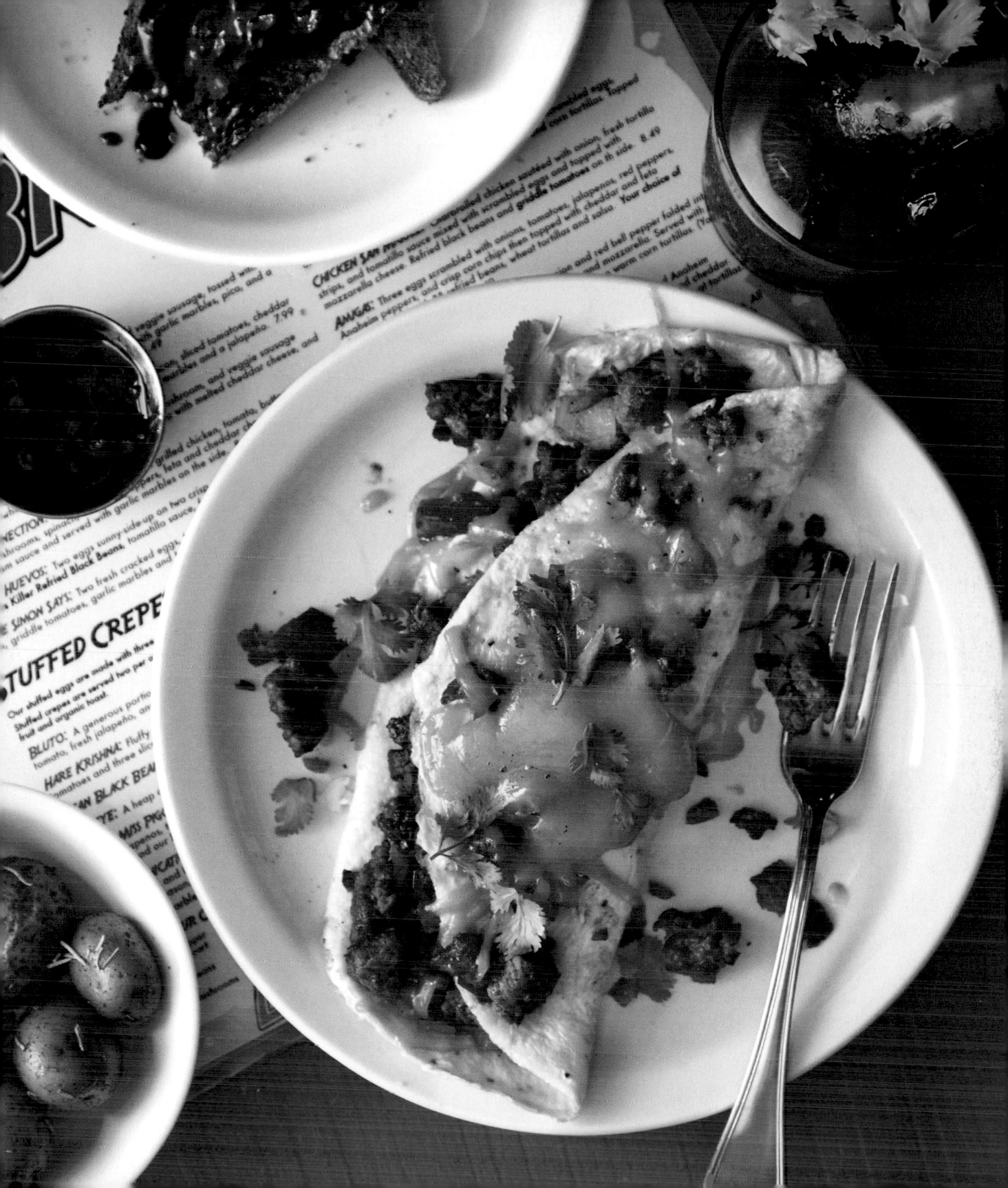

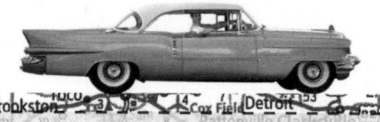

Texas bucket list

things to see and do (besides eat) here

1. Leave your mark in spray paint at Cadillac Ranch near Amarillo.

2. Check out the actual grassy knoll and The Sixth Floor Museum at Dealey Plaza in Dallas.

3. Rock out at the annual Austin City Limits Music Festival in the fall.

4. Go rafting down the Big Bend, or if adventure isn't your thing, plan a spring visit while bluebonnets are in bloom.

5. Visit the Texas State Fair (pictured) in Dallas, have a corn dog, and say howdy to Big Tex.

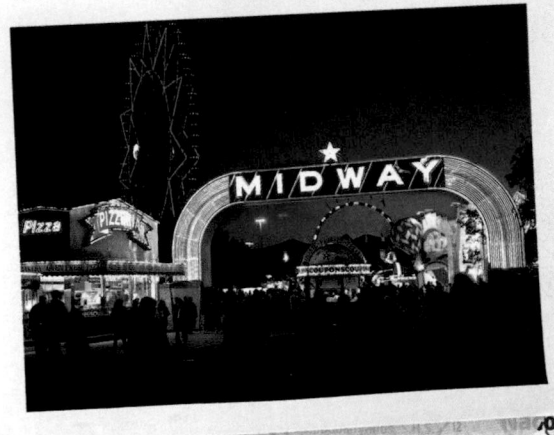

Garlic Marbles

These little potatoes are dusted with a savory powder that makes them hard to stop eating.

- 2½ cups cold water
- 1¼ lb. (1¼- to 1½-inch) yellow potatoes
- 1 (3-inch) rosemary sprig
- 1 small garlic clove, minced
- 1 tsp. table salt, divided
- ¼ tsp. onion powder
- ¼ tsp. dried oregano
- ¼ tsp. dried rosemary, crushed
- ¼ tsp. paprika
- ¼ tsp. ground red pepper
- ¼ tsp. ground allspice
- ½ tsp. Seasoning Oil
- ½ tsp. butter

1. Combine first 4 ingredients and ¾ tsp. salt in a large saucepan. Bring to a boil; reduce heat, and simmer, partially covered, 11 minutes or until potatoes are tender. Drain.

2. Combine onion powder, next 5 ingredients, and remaining ¼ tsp. salt in a small bowl. Place Seasoning Oil and butter in a large bowl; add hot potatoes; toss until butter melts and potatoes are coated. Sprinkle ½ tsp. spice mixture over potatoes, reserving remaining spice mixture for another use; toss until coated. **Makes: 4 servings**

Seasoning Oil

- ¾ cup canola oil
- 1 Tbsp. fresh lemon juice
- 1 Tbsp. dry white wine
- 2 tsp. minced red onion
- ⅛ tsp. table salt
- 5 garlic cloves, minced

Whisk together all ingredients. Cover and store in refrigerator. Stir before using. **Makes: 1 cup**

Hangover Soup

This spiced chicken soup has a kick and will make you sweat (if the Texas sun doesn't already).

HANGOVER SOUP

2   (8-oz.) chicken breasts
Canola oil
½   tsp. table salt
½   tsp. freshly ground black pepper
Vegetable cooking spray
2   (6-inch) corn tortillas, each cut into 8 strips
I   Tbsp. butter
I   Tbsp. olive oil
I   cup (4 oz.) shredded mozzarella cheese
Chopped fresh cilantro

SOUP BASE

½   tsp. table salt
½   tsp. granulated garlic
½   tsp. chicken base
⅛   tsp. ground white pepper
I½ tsp. olive oil
I   garlic clove, minced
½   cup pico de gallo
¼   cup chopped chayote squash*
¼   cup chopped unpeeled baking potato
⅔   cup canned crushed tomatoes
I   canned chipotle pepper in adobo sauce, drained and chopped
¼   cup frozen whole kernel corn, thawed
¼   cup chopped fresh cilantro

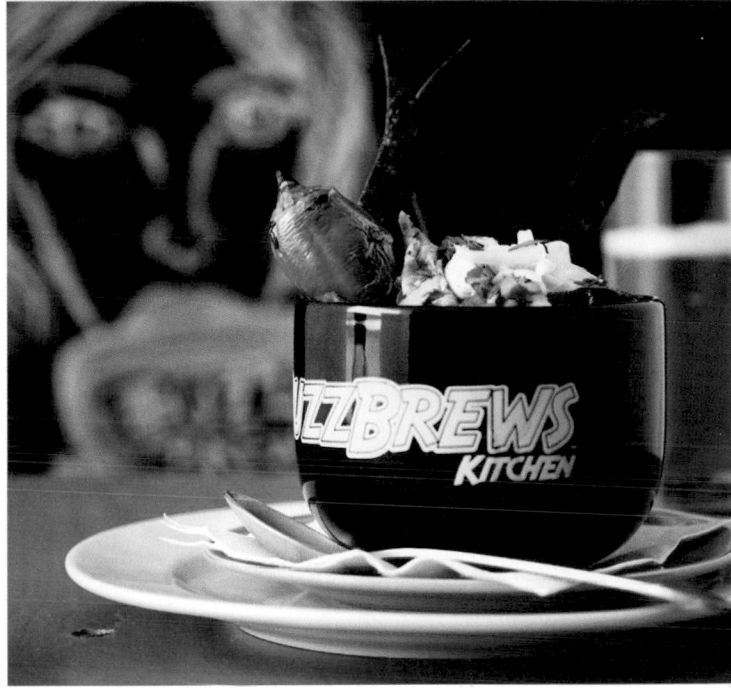

1. **Prepare Hangover Soup:** Preheat oven to 350°. Brush chicken with canola oil; sprinkle with salt and pepper. Line a baking sheet with aluminum foil. Coat foil with cooking spray. Place chicken on prepared pan. Bake at 350° for 30 minutes or until done. Let stand until cool enough to handle (about 20 minutes). Cut crosswise into 12 slices.
2. Pour canola oil to depth of ¼ inch into a medium skillet. Heat over medium-high heat until hot. Fry tortilla strips, in batches, 1 to 2 minutes or just until crisp and lightly browned, turning once. Drain on paper towels.
3. **Prepare Soup Base:** Combine first 4 ingredients and 2 cups water in a bowl, stirring until chicken base dissolves; set aside. Heat 1½ tsp. olive oil in a large saucepan over medium-high heat. Add garlic; sauté 30 seconds. Add pico de gallo; sauté 1 minute. Add squash and potato; sauté 2 minutes. Add tomatoes and chipotle pepper. Cook, stirring constantly, 2 minutes. Stir in reserved spice mixture. Bring to a boil; cover, reduce heat, and simmer 15 minutes or until potato is tender. Remove from heat; stir in corn and cilantro.
4. Meanwhile, heat butter and 1 Tbsp. olive oil in a large nonstick skillet until butter melts. Add chicken slices; cook 2 minutes or until thoroughly heated, turning once.
5. Ladle ¾ cup soup base into each of 4 (7-oz.) soup cups. Top each with 3 chicken slices and ¼ cup cheese. Sprinkle with cilantro. Place 4 tortilla strips in each bowl allowing tops to extend up out of cup. **Makes: 4 servings**
*Yellow squash may be substituted.

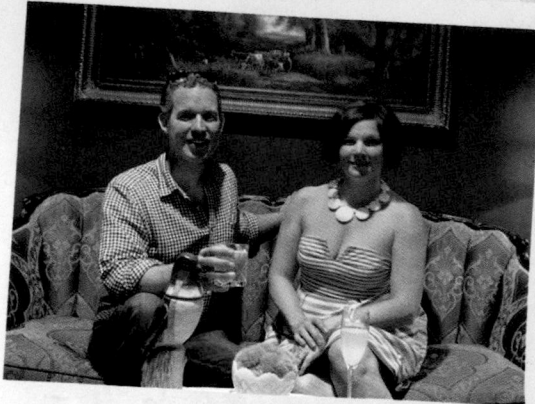

Sissy's Southern Kitchen & Bar

2929 North Henderson Avenue
Dallas, Texas 75206
(214) 827-9900
sissyssouthernkitchen.com

Some restaurants have the power to make a memory that lasts a lifetime, and Sissy's has that mojo. Owner Lisa "Sissy" Garza's obsession with details—her gorgeous brown and white Spode china, Waterford crystal, marble bar, and vintage chandeliers (saved from the original Neiman Marcus), come together to create what I'd call hip Southern gothic. Sissy's kitchen completes the effect by firing out endless plates of caviar-covered deviled eggs, pickled Gulf shrimp, roasted red snapper, and Texas quail on hoppin' John. And if you want a cocktail with your fried chicken, Sissy's bar is a creative wonderland. Try the Presbyterian Press or Sparkling Julep. And save room for dessert—her cookies and a milk punch are the best way to end to an evening.

Sissy's Pickled Gulf Shrimp

1	lb. peeled and deveined medium-size raw shrimp
½	cup blended olive oil
½	cup extra virgin olive oil
2	tsp. Old Bay seasoning
¾	tsp. garlic powder
¾	tsp. dried crushed red pepper
½	tsp. kosher salt
½	tsp. onion powder
¼	tsp. celery seed
⅛	tsp. ground allspice
2	garlic cloves, minced (about 1 Tbsp.)
1	cup halved grape tomatoes
1	cup finely julienned carrot
1	cup thin onion strips
½	cup fresh lemon juice (about 3 lemons)
½	cup coarsely chopped fresh parsley
⅓	cup sliced celery
15	bay leaves

1. Pour water to depth of 2 inches in a large saucepan; bring to a simmer. Add shrimp, and cook 1 minute or until shrimp turn pink; drain. Cool shrimp completely.
2. Combine shrimp, olive oils, and next 8 ingredients in a large bowl, tossing to evenly coat shrimp. Cover and marinate in refrigerator for 30 minutes.
3. Combine tomato and remaining ingredients; stir into shrimp mixture. Cover and marinate in refrigerator 3 hours. Remove and discard bay leaves before serving. **Makes: 4 servings**

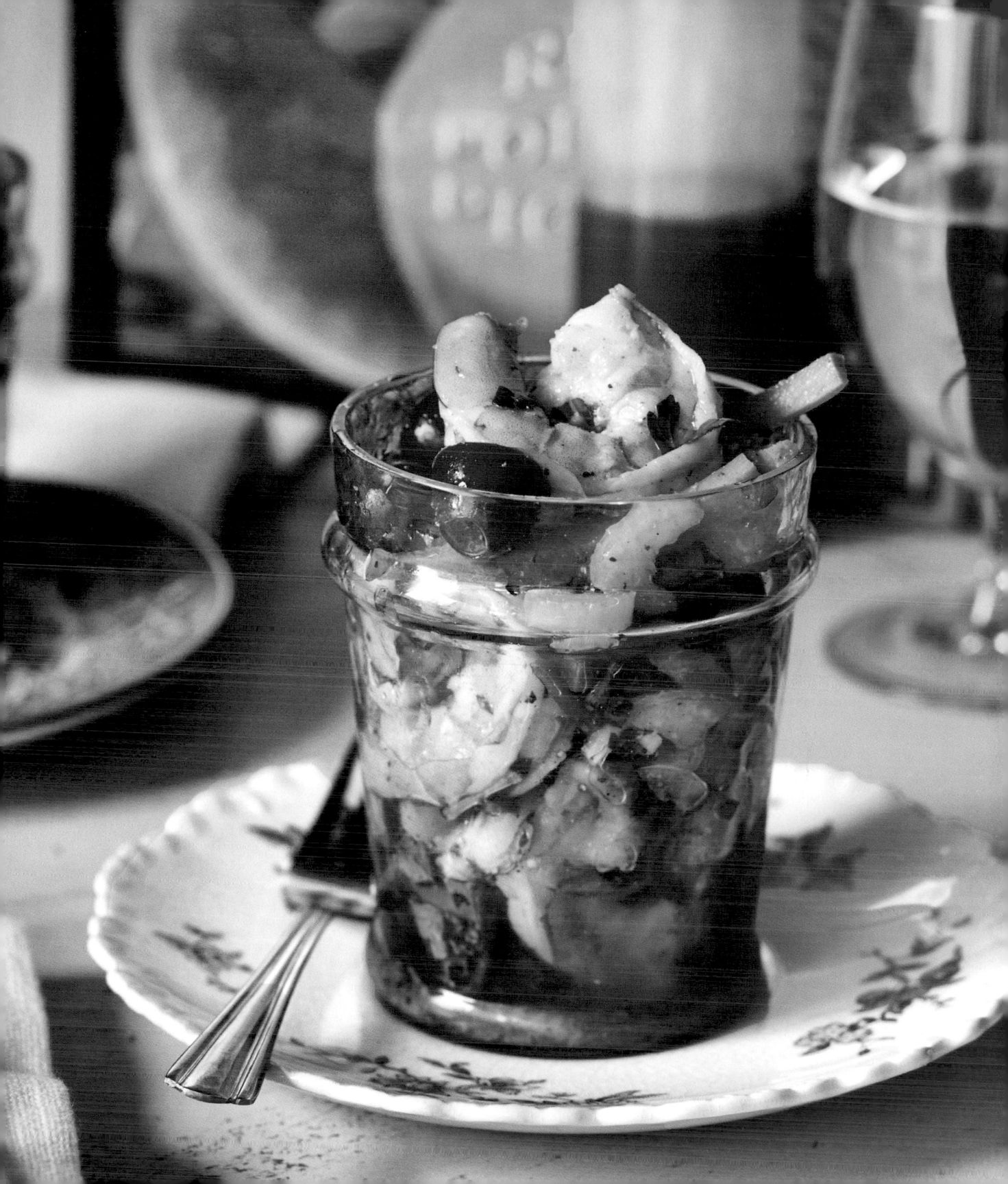

Sissy's Cast Iron Quail with Hoppin' John

STEEN'S SYRUP GLAZE

2 Tbsp. shortening
2 Tbsp. all-purpose flour
¼ cup finely chopped onion
5 Tbsp. Steen's pure cane syrup*
3 Tbsp. Worcestershire sauce
½ garlic clove
½ tsp. juniper berries
½ bay leaf

HOPPIN' JOHN

1¼ cups frozen black-eyed peas
1½ tsp. butter
1½ tsp. blended olive oil
½ cup diced onion
¼ cup (¼-inch) diced red bell pepper
¼ cup (¼-inch) diced green bell pepper
¼ cup (¼-inch) diced celery
1 garlic clove, minced
2 Tbsp. dark roux from Steen's Syrup Glaze
1¼ cups chicken stock
¾ cup diced andouille sausage
½ bay leaf
2 Tbsp. butter
5 cups cold cooked long-grain rice (cooked without salt)
½ tsp. table salt
¼ tsp. freshly ground black pepper

QUAIL

8 (4½-oz.) quail, dressed
½ tsp. table salt
¼ tsp. freshly ground black pepper
1½ Tbsp. blended olive oil
¼ cup thinly sliced green onions (2 small onions)
4 tsp. finely diced red bell pepper

1. Prepare Steen's Syrup Glaze: Heat shortening over high heat until melted. Stir in flour; reduce heat to medium. Cook, stirring constantly with a wooden spoon, 5 minutes or until roux is milk chocolate brown. Add onion; cook, stirring constantly, 4 minutes or until onion caramelizes and roux turns dark chocolate brown. Remove from heat; cool 2 minutes.

2. Reserve 2 Tbsp. roux for later use. Add syrup and remaining 4 ingredients to remaining 1 Tbsp. roux. Bring to a simmer, and cook 4 minutes or until mixture is thickened and saucy, stirring constantly. Remove from heat; pour through a fine wire-mesh strainer into a bowl. Discard solids. Cover and keep warm.

3. Prepare Hoppin' John: Combine peas and 3 cups water in a medium saucepan. Bring to a boil; reduce heat, cover, and simmer 25 minutes or until tender. Drain and set aside.

4. Heat 1½ tsp. butter and 1½ tsp. oil in a medium saucepan over medium-high heat until butter melts. Add onion and next 4 ingredients; sauté 5 minutes or until tender. Whisk in reserved 2 Tbsp. roux until blended. Whisk in stock. Bring to a simmer; cook, uncovered, 10 minutes or until thickened, stirring occasionally.

5. Add sausage, bay leaf, and peas. Return to a boil; reduce heat, and simmer, uncovered, 5 minutes. Remove from heat; discard bay leaf.

6. Melt 2 Tbsp. butter in a Dutch oven. Add pea mixture, rice, salt, and pepper. Toss lightly with a fork. Cook over medium heat 3 minutes or until thoroughly heated.

7. Prepare Quail: Preheat oven to 450°. Sprinkle quail evenly with salt and pepper. Heat 1½ Tbsp. blended oil in a cast-iron skillet over medium-high heat. Add quail; cook 3 minutes on each side or until browned. Place skillet in oven, and bake, uncovered, at 450° for 6 minutes; drizzle quail with glaze. Bake 2 more minutes or until a meat thermometer inserted in breast registers 160°.

8. Divide Hoppin' John mixture among 4 plates. Place 2 quail on each plate. Sprinkle with green onions and red bell pepper. **Makes: 4 servings**
*Light molasses may be substituted.

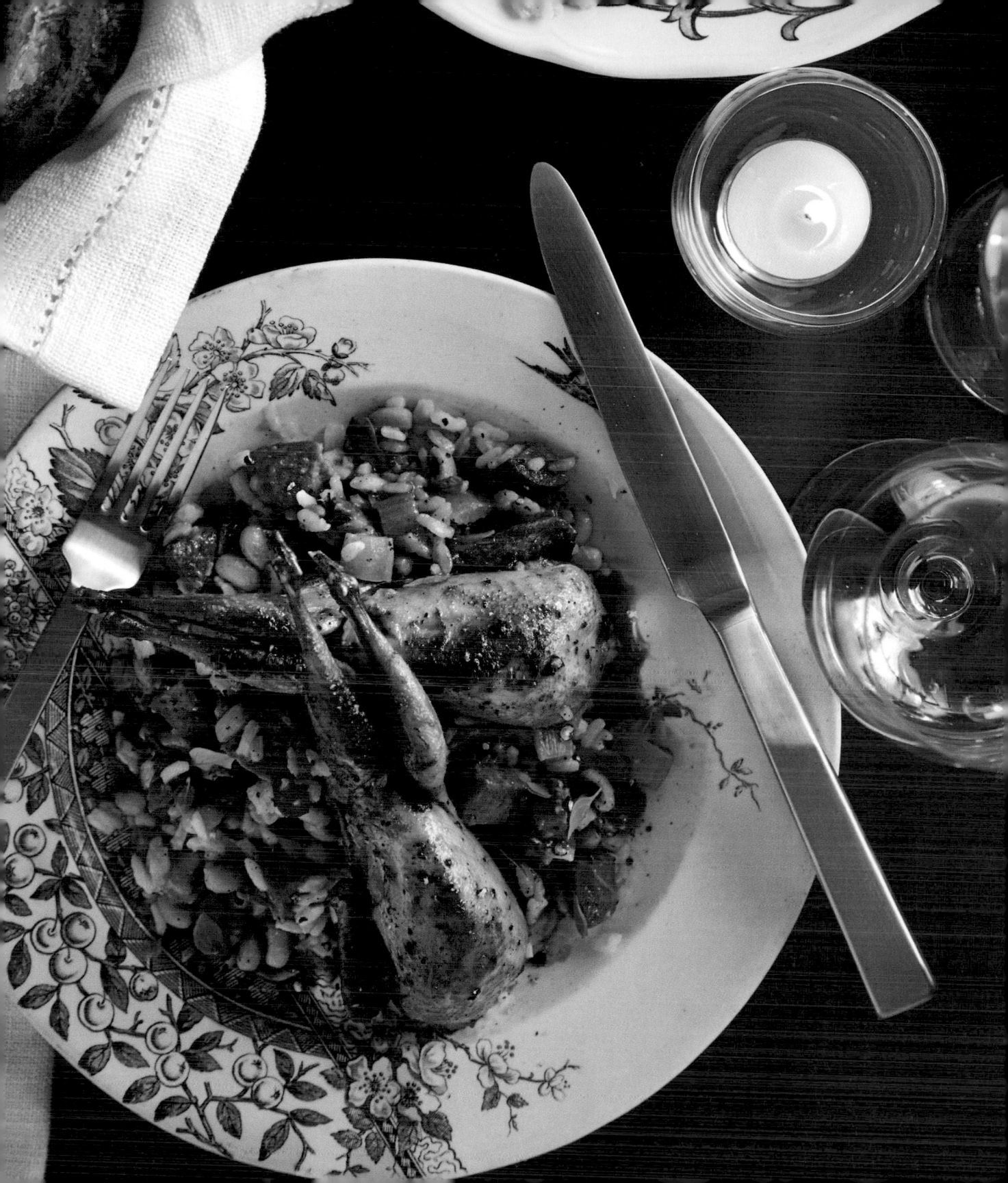

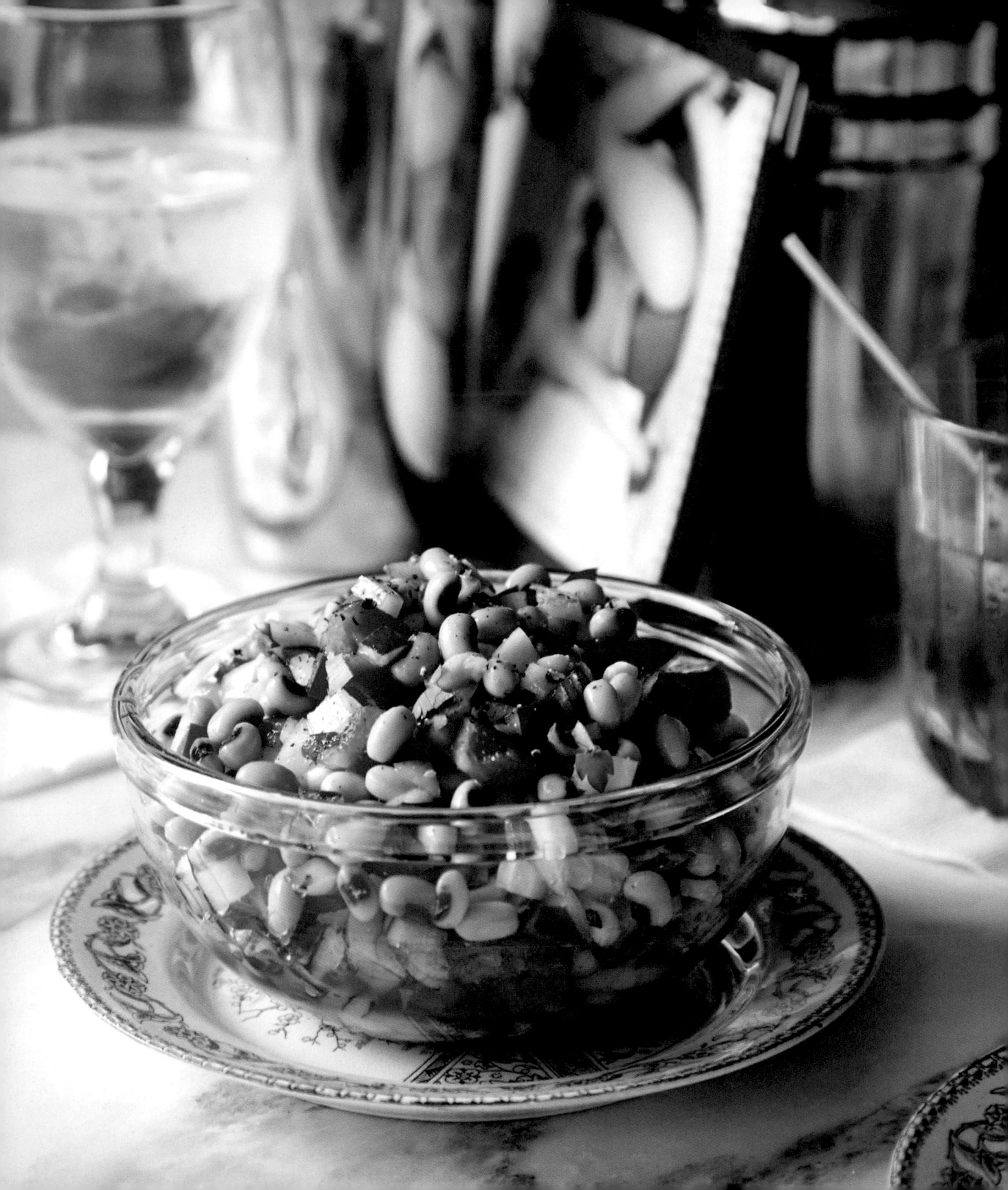

Texas Caviar Field Pea Salad

- 2 cups fresh black-eyed peas
- ½ cup extra virgin olive oil
- 2 Tbsp. red wine vinegar
- 1½ tsp. kosher salt
- 1 tsp. Louisiana hot sauce
- ½ tsp. freshly ground black pepper
- 2 garlic cloves, minced
- 1 cup finely chopped red bell pepper
- ½ cup finely diced yellow onion
- ½ cup diced red onion
- ⅓ cup finely chopped fresh flat-leaf parsley

1. Bring peas and 4 cups water to a boil in a 3-qt. saucepan; reduce heat, cover, and simmer 20 minutes or until tender. Drain. Plunge peas into ice water to stop the cooking process; drain.

2. Combine olive oil and next 5 ingredients in a large bowl, stirring well. Add peas, bell pepper, and remaining ingredients; toss well. Serve immediately, or cover and marinate in refrigerator overnight. Salad may be made up to 5 days ahead.

Makes: 6 servings

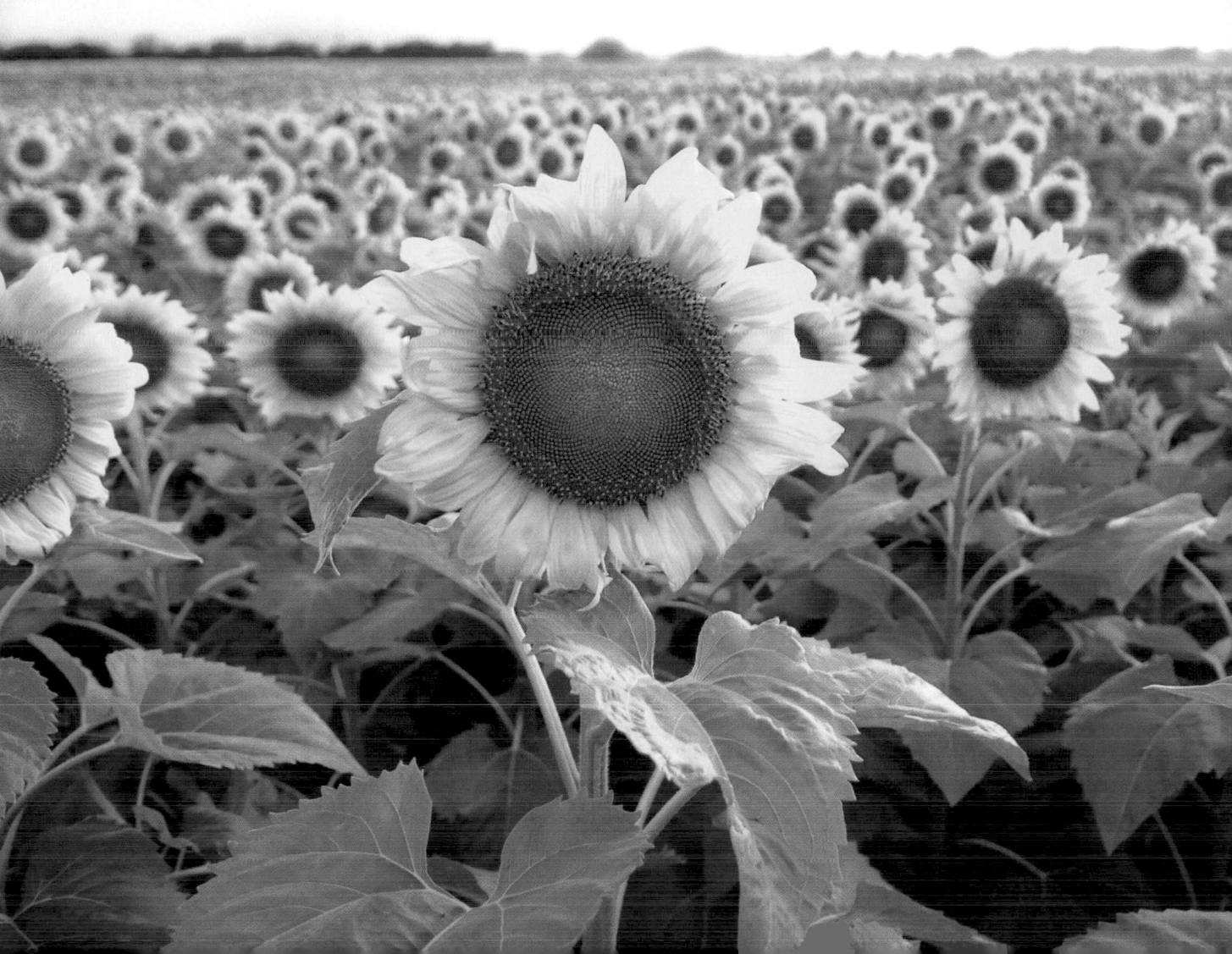

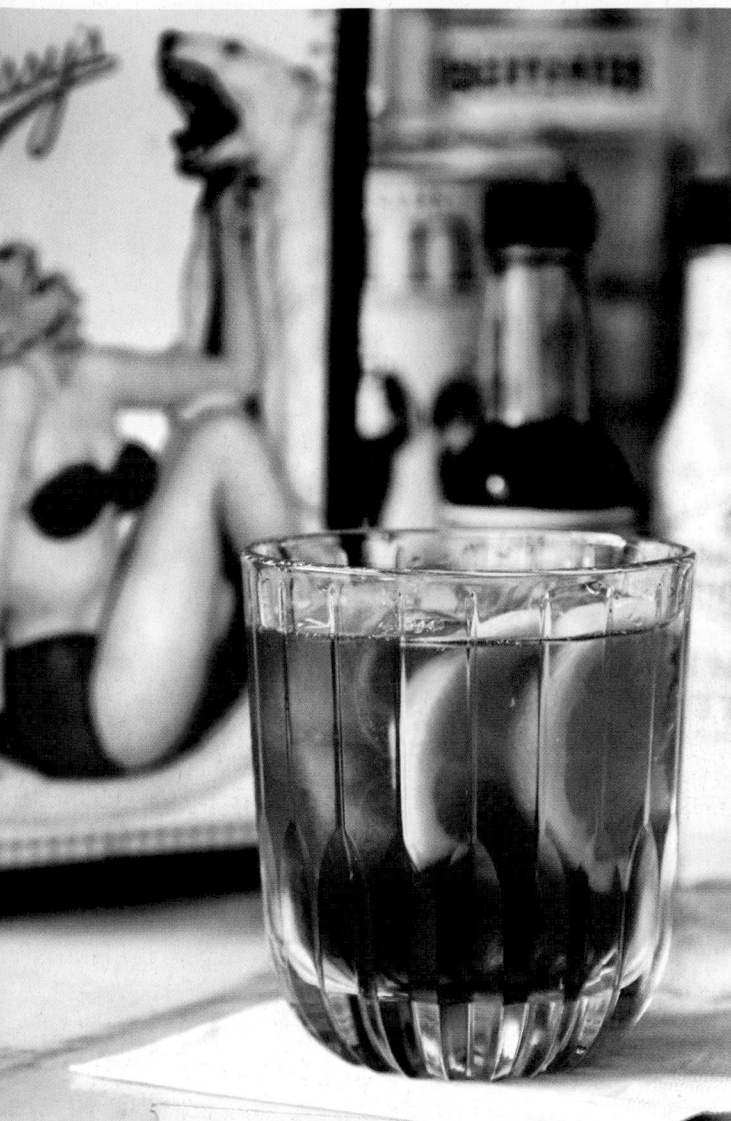

Oven-Roasted Collard Greens

These roasted collards are a far cry from the boiled variety.

- 1½ tsp. kosher salt
- 1 tsp. freshly ground black pepper
- ¼ tsp. dried crushed red pepper
- ⅔ cup extra virgin olive oil, divided
- 1¼ cups vertically sliced onion
- 5 garlic cloves, minced
- 2 lb. collard greens, washed, trimmed, and coarsely chopped (2 bunches)

1. Preheat oven to 500°. Combine first 3 ingredients in a small bowl.
2. Heat ⅓ cup oil in a large heavy roasting pan in preheated oven 2 minutes. (Watch closely and don't let it smoke.) Add onion and garlic. Bake at 500° for 10 minutes or until beginning to brown, stirring every 5 minutes.
3. Add greens; sprinkle with salt mixture, and drizzle with remaining ⅓ cup oil, tossing well with tongs. Bake at 500° for 20 minutes or until greens are tender, stirring twice. **Makes: 4 servings**

Presbyterian Press

This simple bourbon cocktail is as austere as a Presbyterian sermon, but absolutely satisfying because it's not too sweet or too strong.

- ¼ cup bourbon
- 6 Tbsp. ginger ale, chilled
- Garnish: lemon wedge

Pour bourbon over ice in an old-fashioned glass. Add ginger ale; stir gently. **Makes: 1 serving**
Note: We tested with Baker's Bourbon and Fever Tree Ginger Ale.

SOUNDTRACK:

"TEXAS RUBY" BY A.J. CROCE
"RAISED ON IT" BY SAM HUNT
"DALLAS" BY JOHNNY WINTER
"SHE'S LIKE TEXAS" BY JOSH ABBOTT BAND
"THAT'S RIGHT (YOU'RE NOT FROM TEXAS)" BY LYLE LOVETT

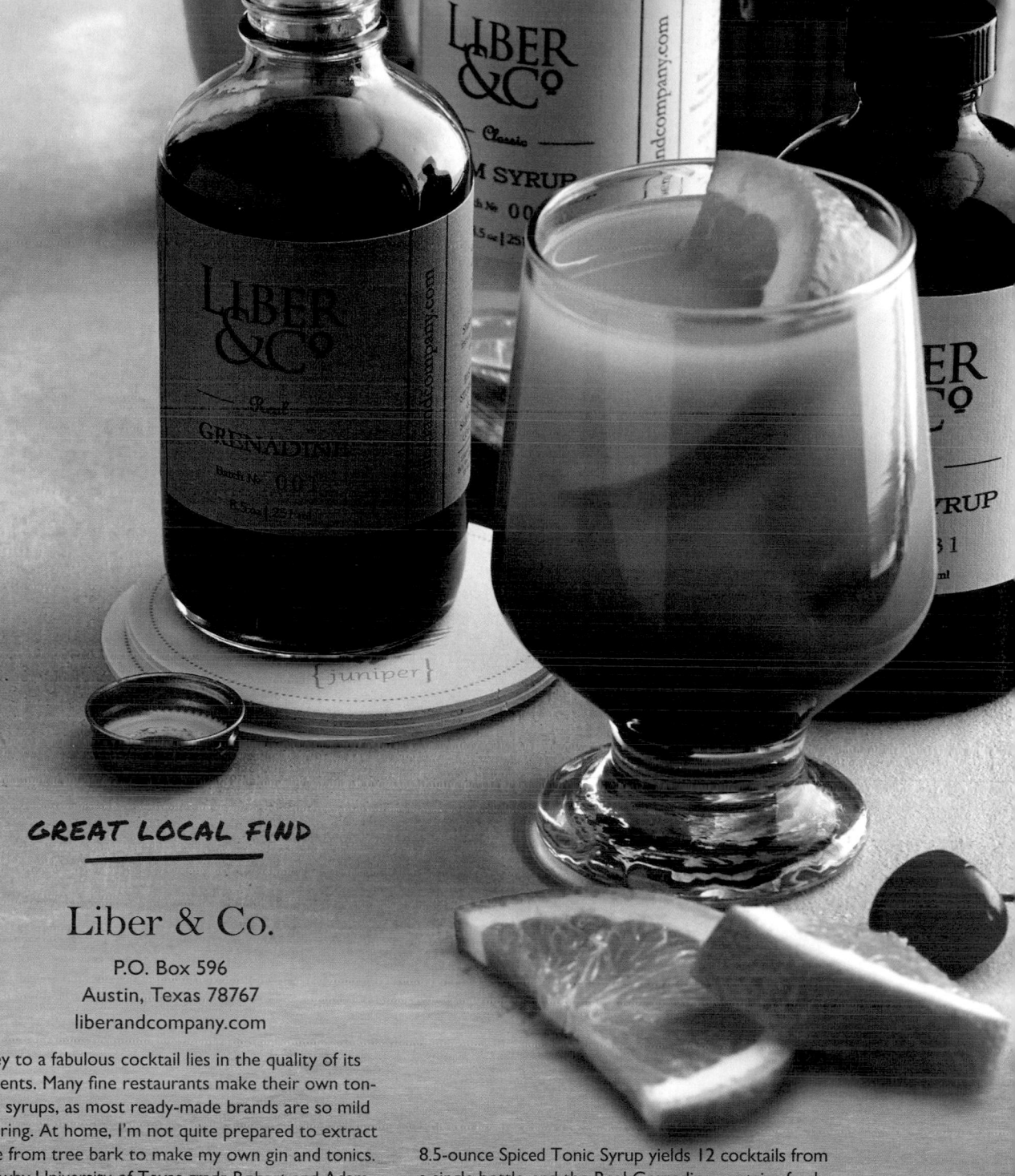

GREAT LOCAL FIND

Liber & Co.

P.O. Box 596
Austin, Texas 78767
liberandcompany.com

The key to a fabulous cocktail lies in the quality of its ingredients. Many fine restaurants make their own tonics and syrups, as most ready-made brands are so mild and boring. At home, I'm not quite prepared to extract quinine from tree bark to make my own gin and tonics. That's why University of Texas grads Robert and Adam Higginbotham and Chris Harrison concocted Liber & Co. Their goal: to provide the best ingredients to create craft cocktails at home. And they succeeded—Liber & Co.'s

8.5-ounce Spiced Tonic Syrup yields 12 cocktails from a single bottle, and the Real Grenadine contains fresh pomegranate juice, pure cane sugar, and orange blossom water—a stark contrast to today's ruby-red substitutes, which are mostly corn syrup and red dye.

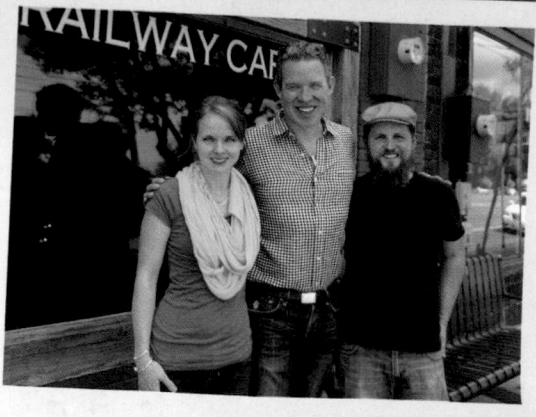

Railway Cafe

210 North Palestine Street
Athens, Texas 75751
(903) 264-7245
railwaycafe.net

This super stylish restaurant sits about an hour outside of Dallas, but boasts the cool feel of San Francisco or Austin. Chef Justin Boswell and his wife, Deanne, were high school sweethearts (and the king and queen of prom) in Athens who ventured off to bigger cities for culinary training. But the lure of their hometown eventually brought them back to Athens." It was the faces on the parents and grandparents whenever we left that brought us home," Deanne says. Now the couple sees delight on the hometown faces at Railway Cafe as they bite into the delicious fare that has put a twist on Texas classics. I flipped for the Gouda mac and cheese, homemade ice cream, and roasted chicken quesadilla. Now the sound of a lonesome train whistle will get my mouth watering.

Roasted Chicken Quesadillas

Chicken anchors the zesty, cheesy filling in these to-die-for quesadillas. Roast your own chicken or save time and buy a rotisserie chicken from the deli.

- 1 (8-oz.) package shredded sharp Cheddar cheese
- 1 (8-oz.) smoked Gouda cheese round, shredded
- 1 (8-oz.) block pepper Jack cheese, shredded
- 6 Tbsp. unsalted butter, softened
- 12 (10-inch) flour tortillas
- 6 cups Roasted Chicken (facing page)*
- 1½ cups Cilantro Cream (facing page)
- ¾ cup Pico de Gallo (facing page)
- ½ head romaine lettuce, chiffonade

1. Preheat oven to 175°. Combine first 3 ingredients in a large bowl. Spread about 1½ tsp. butter on 1 side of each tortilla. Place 1 tortilla, buttered side down, in a large nonstick skillet. Place ½ cup chicken and ½ cup cheese mixture on 1 half of tortilla. Fold tortilla over filling. Move quesadilla to 1 side of skillet, keeping straight side in center of skillet. Add another tortilla, buttered side down, to opposite side of pan, overlapping first quesadilla. Fill and fold. (Straight sides will meet in center of pan.)
2. Cook over medium-high heat 1 to 2 minutes on each side or until cheese melts. Repeat procedure with remaining tortillas, chicken, and cheese. (Keep quesadillas warm in oven at 175° until all quesadillas are cooked.) Cut each quesadilla into 4 wedges. Serve hot with Cilantro Cream, Pico de Gallo, and lettuce.

Makes: 12 servings

*Deli-roasted chicken may be substituted.

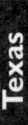

Roasted Chicken

1 (3½- to 4-lb.) whole chicken
1 tsp. table salt, divided
1 Tbsp. canola oil
1 tsp. paprika
½ tsp. dried thyme

1. Preheat oven to 375°. Remove giblets and neck, and rinse chicken with cold water. Drain cavity well; pat dry. Sprinkle cavity with ½ tsp. salt. Tie ends of legs together with string; tuck wing tips under. Place chicken on a roasting rack, breast side up; brush entire bird with canola oil; sprinkle with paprika, thyme, and remaining ½ tsp. salt. Bake at 375° for 20 minutes.
2. Reduce oven temperature to 325°, and bake for 1 hour and 45 minutes or until a meat thermometer inserted into thickest portion of thigh registers 165°. Remove from oven; let stand 15 minutes. **Makes: 4 servings**

Cilantro Cream

2 cups sour cream
2 cups coarsely chopped fresh cilantro (1 bunch)
½ cup buttermilk
½ tsp. table salt
2 garlic cloves, coarsely chopped
1 green onion, coarsely chopped
1 jalapeño pepper, stem removed, halved, and seeded

Process all ingredients in a blender until smooth. Pour into a bowl. Cover and chill. Store, covered, up to 3 days in refrigerator. **Makes: 3 cups**

Pico de Gallo

3 cups finely chopped tomato (1½ lb.)
1 cup chopped onion
½ cup chopped fresh cilantro
¼ cup diced seeded jalapeño pepper (1 pepper)
¼ cup fresh lime juice (about 3 limes)
½ tsp. table salt
¼ tsp. freshly ground black pepper

Combine all ingredients in a medium bowl, stirring well. Chill.
Makes: 4 cups

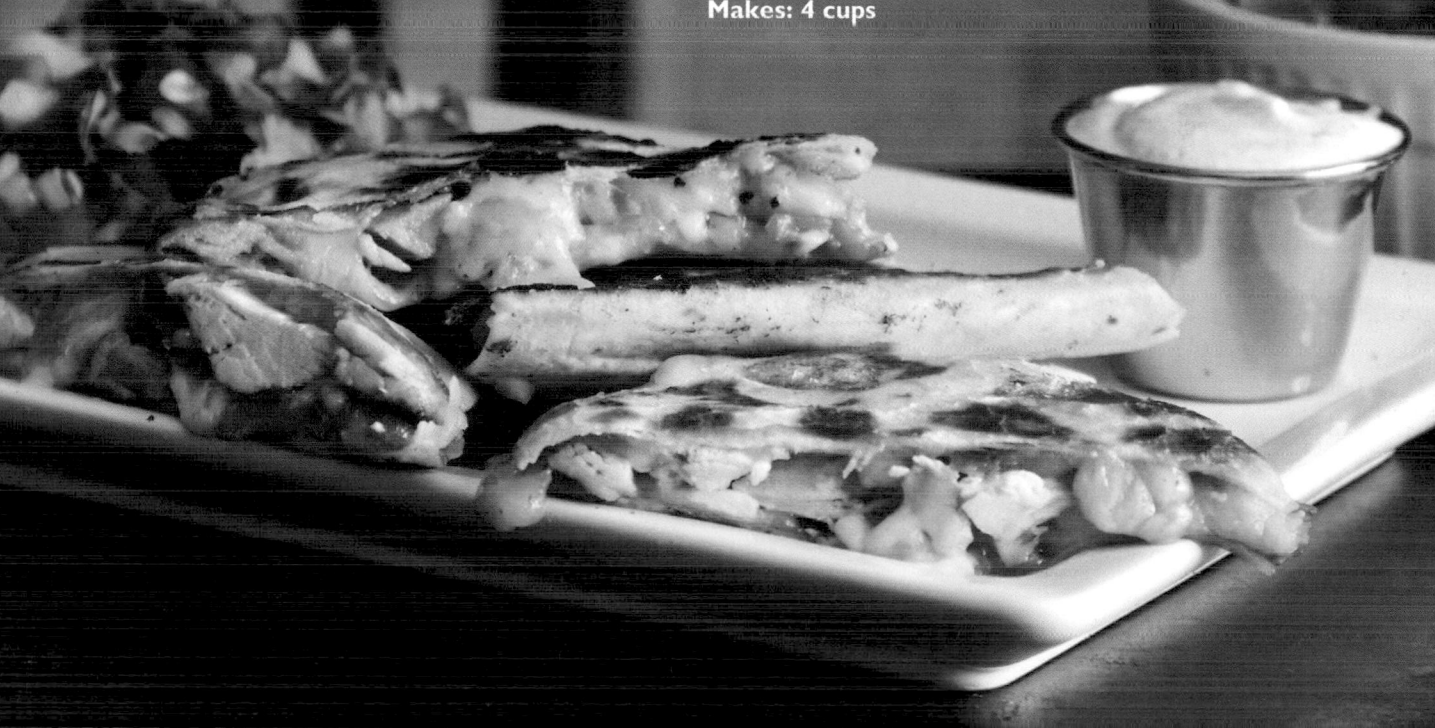

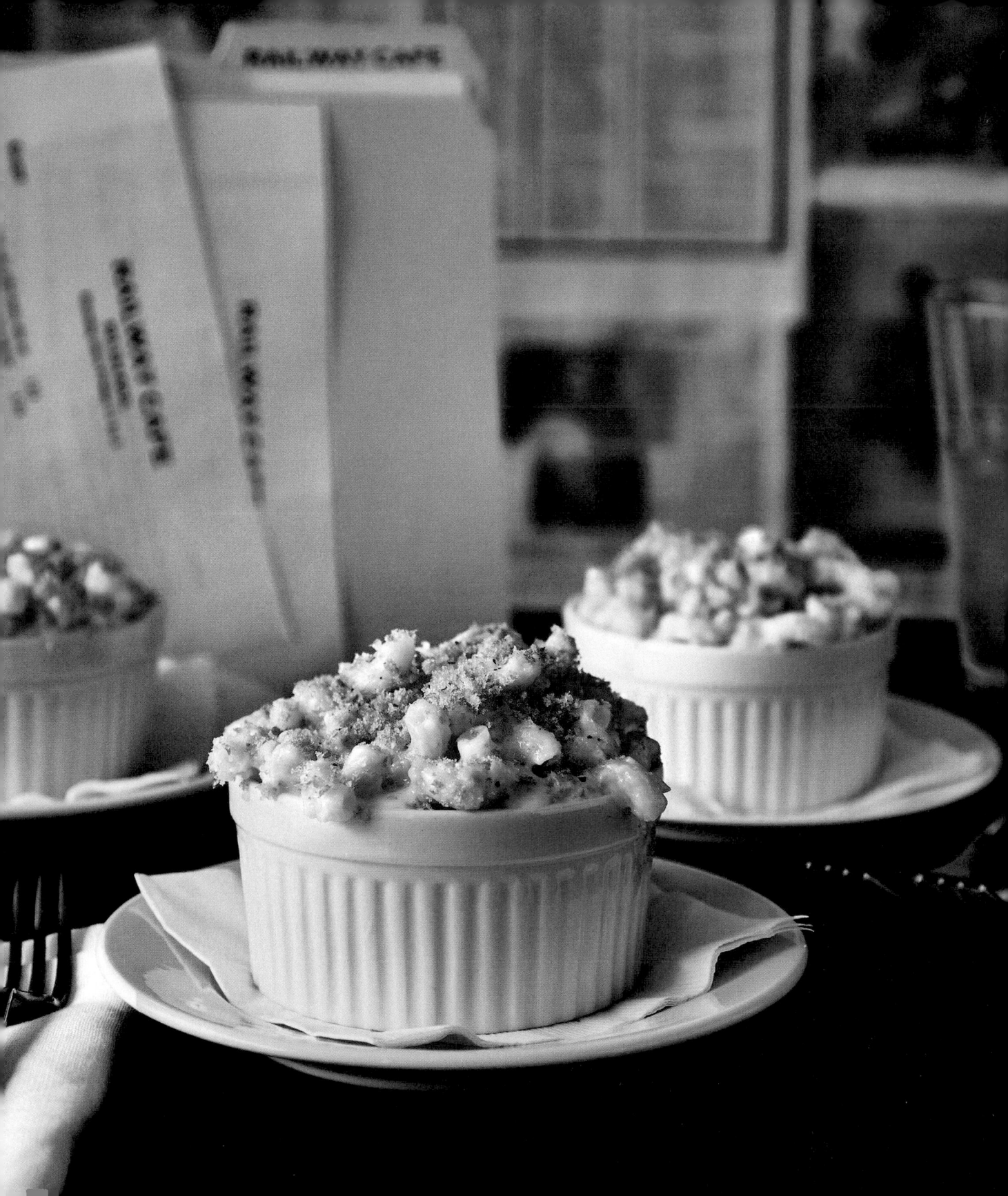

Mac and Cheese

The creaminess of the smoked Gouda balances the sharpness of the white Cheddar. The breadcrumbs on top add a nice crunch.

2	cups uncooked elbow macaroni
½	cup unsalted butter
½	cup all-purpose flour
2¼	cups milk, divided
½	tsp. table salt
½	tsp. freshly ground black pepper
4	oz. white Cheddar cheese, shredded
4	oz. smoked Gouda cheese, shredded
I	cup soft, fresh breadcrumbs

Vegetable cooking spray

1. Cook pasta according to package directions; drain.

2. Preheat oven to 375°. Melt butter in a 3-qt. heavy saucepan over low heat; whisk in flour until smooth. Cook 1 minute, whisking constantly. Gradually whisk in 2 cups milk; cook over medium heat, whisking constantly, until mixture is thickened and bubbly. Stir in salt and pepper.

3. Add cheeses; cook, stirring constantly, 2 minutes or until cheese melts. Stir in pasta and remaining ¼ cup milk

4. Spoon macaroni mixture into 6 (8-oz.) lightly greased ovenproof ramekins or custard cups. Top evenly with breadcrumbs. Coat tops of breadcrumbs with cooking spray. Bake, uncovered, at 375° for 15 minutes or until browned. **Makes: 6 servings**

Mexican Vanilla Crème Brûlée

The Mexican vanilla gives the crème brûlée a rounded, more natural flavor.

I	qt. heavy cream
9	large egg yolks
I	large egg
I	cup sugar
2	Tbsp. Mexican vanilla extract
I	tsp. kosher salt
½	cup sugar

1. Preheat oven to 350°. Bring cream to a simmer in a 3-qt. saucepan over medium heat; remove from heat.

2. Whisk together egg yolks and next 4 ingredients in a large bowl. Gradually whisk in hot cream. Pour mixture through a fine wire-mesh strainer into another bowl.

3. Set 8 (6-oz.) ramekins or custard cups in a large roasting pan. Ladle custard mixture into cups. (Cups will be almost full.) Pull out oven rack, and carefully set pan on rack. Add hot tap water (about 115°) to pan to depth of 1 inch. Lay a large piece of aluminum foil on top of cups to loosely cover. Carefully slide rack back into oven

4. Bake at 350° for 30 to 35 minutes or until set (a sharp knife inserted off center should come out clean). Remove ramekins from water bath; place on a wire rack. Cool completely (about 30 minutes). Cover and chill at least 2 hours.

5. Gently blot any moisture that collected on top of custards during chilling with a paper towel. Sprinkle 1 tsp. sugar on top of each custard. Caramelize sugar until golden using a kitchen torch, holding torch 1 to 2 inches from sugar and moving torch back and forth. Sprinkle each custard with 1 tsp. sugar; repeat caramelizing procedure heating to a deeper golden color. Sprinkle each custard with 1 tsp. sugar; repeat caramelizing procedure heating to a deep amber color. Serve immediately. **Makes: 8 servings**

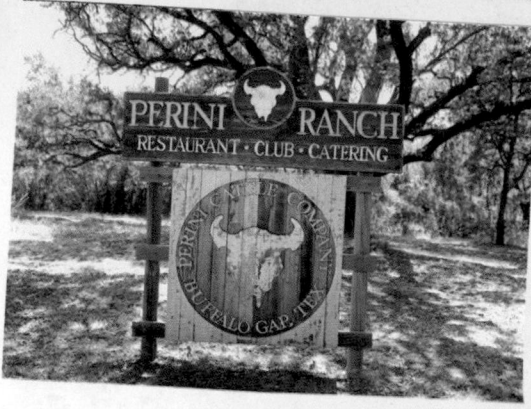

Perini Ranch

3002 Highway 89
Buffalo Gap, Texas 79508
(325) 572-3339
periniranch.com

Nestled in a mesquite forest, down a dirt road, and surrounded by roaming longhorns, Perini Ranch defines what it means to be a Texas steak house. The old tin roof, bullet holes in the bar (yep, they're real), cowboy hats hanging from antlers, and pure Texas fare—it's all as authentic as Tom and Lisa Perini. No Hollywood decorator styled this place, which isn't close to anywhere, but has a loyal following nonetheless. Hell, they just got air conditioning in 2013. Yet Perini Ranch is a concept now copied by every wannabe steak house in America." You can't just hang a Texas star and be Texas", Tom says. The real stars are the fresh food and cocktails. Both are a cut above and made me understand why people drive all the way to Buffalo Gap to eat here.

Zucchini Perini

They may have only come up with this dish because it rhymed with their last names, but who cares, it's delish.

- ½ lb. ground chuck
- ½ lb. hot Italian sausage, casings removed
- 2¼ cups chopped onion (1 large onion)
- 1 (28-oz.) can whole tomatoes
- 2 tsp. dried oregano
- ½ tsp. freshly ground black pepper
- ¼ tsp. garlic powder
- 1 (8-oz.) can tomato sauce
- 1 (6-oz.) can tomato paste
- ½ tsp. table salt, divided
- 1 Tbsp. olive oil
- 5 cups (¼-inch) zucchini slices
- 1 cup (4 oz.) freshly grated Parmesan cheese

1. Preheat oven to 350°. Cook first 3 ingredients in a large ovenproof skillet over medium-high heat, stirring often, 6 to 8 minutes or until meat crumbles and is no longer pink. Drain and return to skillet.
2. Coarsely chop tomatoes in can using scissors; drain and add to meat mixture. Stir in oregano, next 4 ingredients, and ¼ tsp. salt. Bring to a boil; reduce heat, and simmer, uncovered, 5 minutes.
3. Meanwhile, heat olive oil in a large skillet over medium-high heat. Add zucchini and remaining ¼ tsp. salt; cook 4 minutes or until zucchini is crisp-tender, stirring often. Stir zucchini into meat sauce. Sprinkle with cheese.
4. Bake, uncovered, at 350° for 20 minutes or until cheese melts and is beginning to brown.
Makes: 10 servings

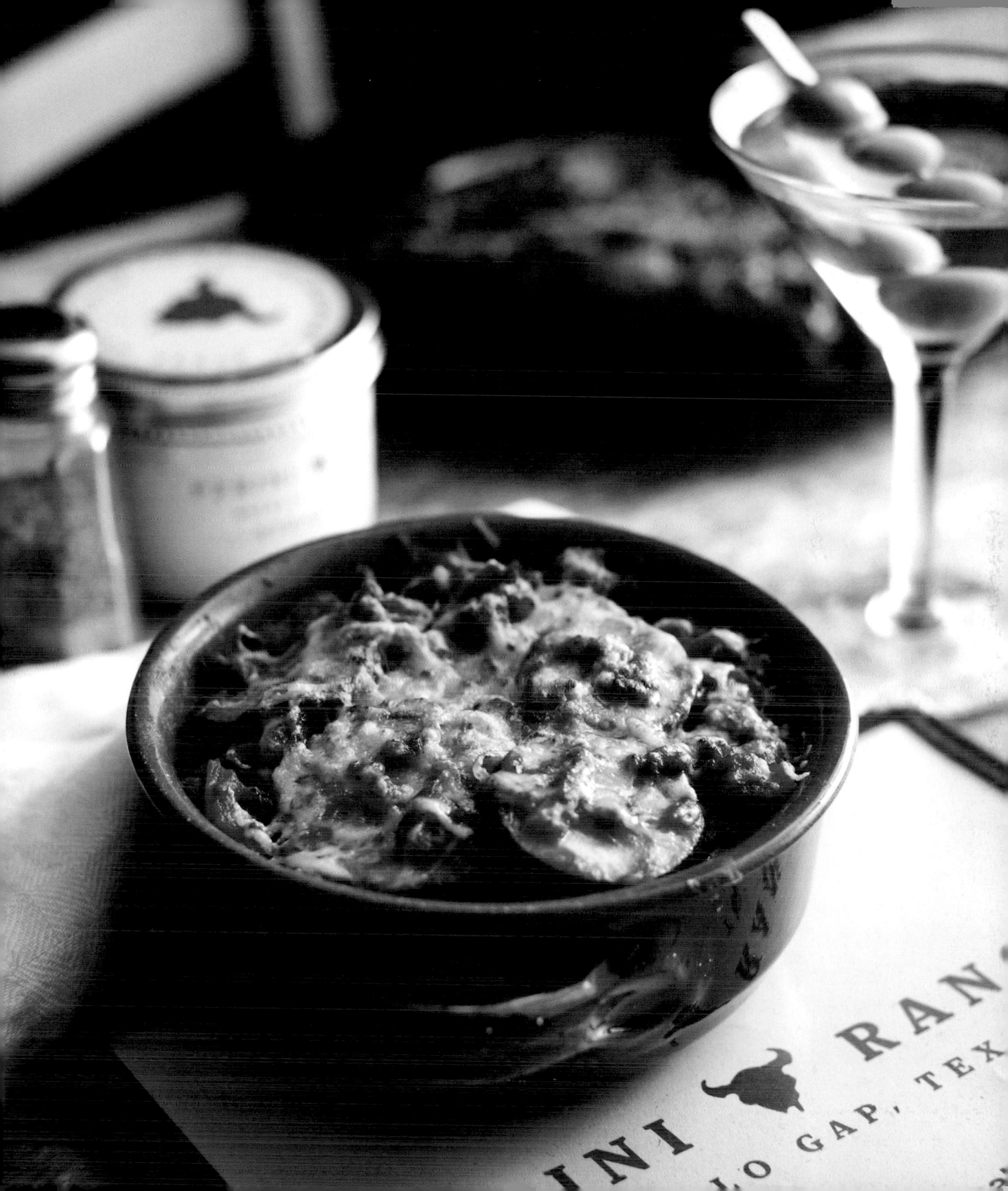

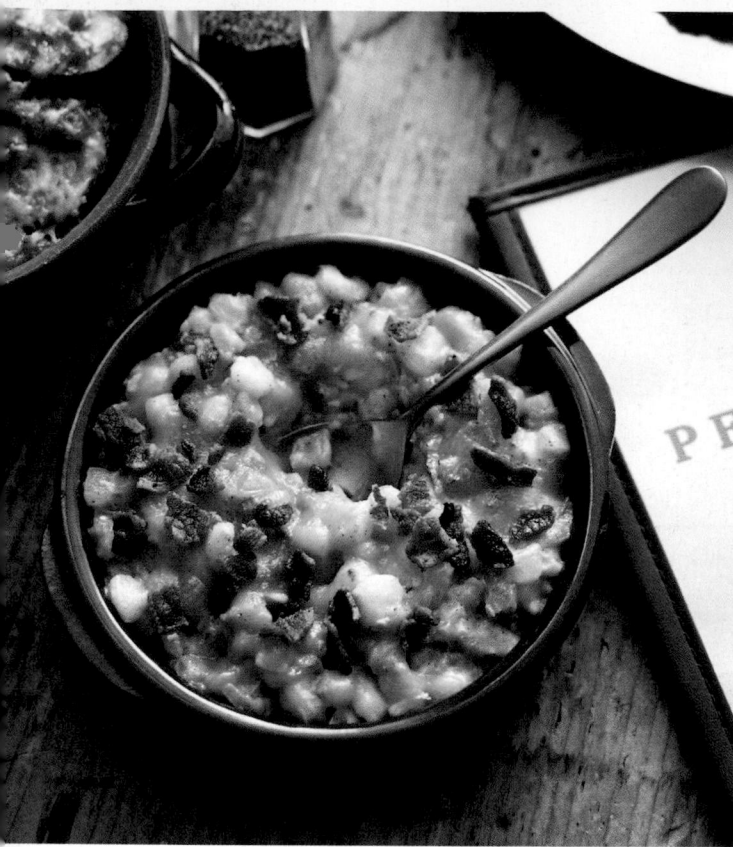

Bread Pudding with Whiskey Sauce

This bread pudding is a ranch favorite, and it still holds the texture of the bread, which is key.

BREAD PUDDING

Vegetable cooking spray
2   large eggs
2½ cups milk
1   cup sugar
2   Tbsp. butter, melted
1   Tbsp. Mexican vanilla extract
5   cups (1-inch) sourdough bread cubes (about 8 oz.)
½   cup chopped pecans

WHISKEY SAUCE

½   cup sugar
½   cup butter
½   cup whipping cream
¼   cup sour mash whiskey

1. Preheat oven to 325°. **Prepare Bread Pudding:** Lightly grease an 8-inch square (2-qt.) baking dish with cooking spray. Whisk eggs in a large bowl. Whisk in milk and next 3 ingredients.
2. Place bread cubes in prepared dish; sprinkle with pecans. Pour milk mixture over bread mixture, pressing gently to submerge all bread in liquid.
3. Bake, uncovered, at 325° for 1 hour or until puffed, lightly browned, and set.
4. Cool in dish on a wire rack 15 minutes or until warm.
5. **Prepare Whiskey Sauce:** Combine all ingredients in a medium saucepan. Bring to a simmer, stirring constantly, over medium heat. Simmer 1 minute or until sugar dissolves. Serve sauce with bread pudding. **Makes: 6 servings**
Note: We tested with Jack Daniel's Tennessee Sour Mash Whiskey.

Green Chile Hominy

4   (15-oz.) cans white hominy
10 hickory-smoked bacon slices
1   cup chopped onion
2   (4.5-oz.) cans chopped green chiles, undrained
1   Tbsp. pickled jalapeño pepper juice
2   cups (8 oz.) shredded Cheddar cheese

1. Drain hominy, reserving ½ cup liquid. Cook bacon in 2 batches in a skillet until crisp, about 6 minutes; remove bacon, reserving 2 Tbsp. drippings in skillet. Crumble bacon.
2. Sauté onion in hot drippings 5 minutes or until tender. Stir in hominy liquid, green chiles, jalapeño juice, and half of bacon. Bring to a simmer; stir in hominy. Add cheese, stirring until melted. Top with remaining half of bacon. **Makes: 14 servings**

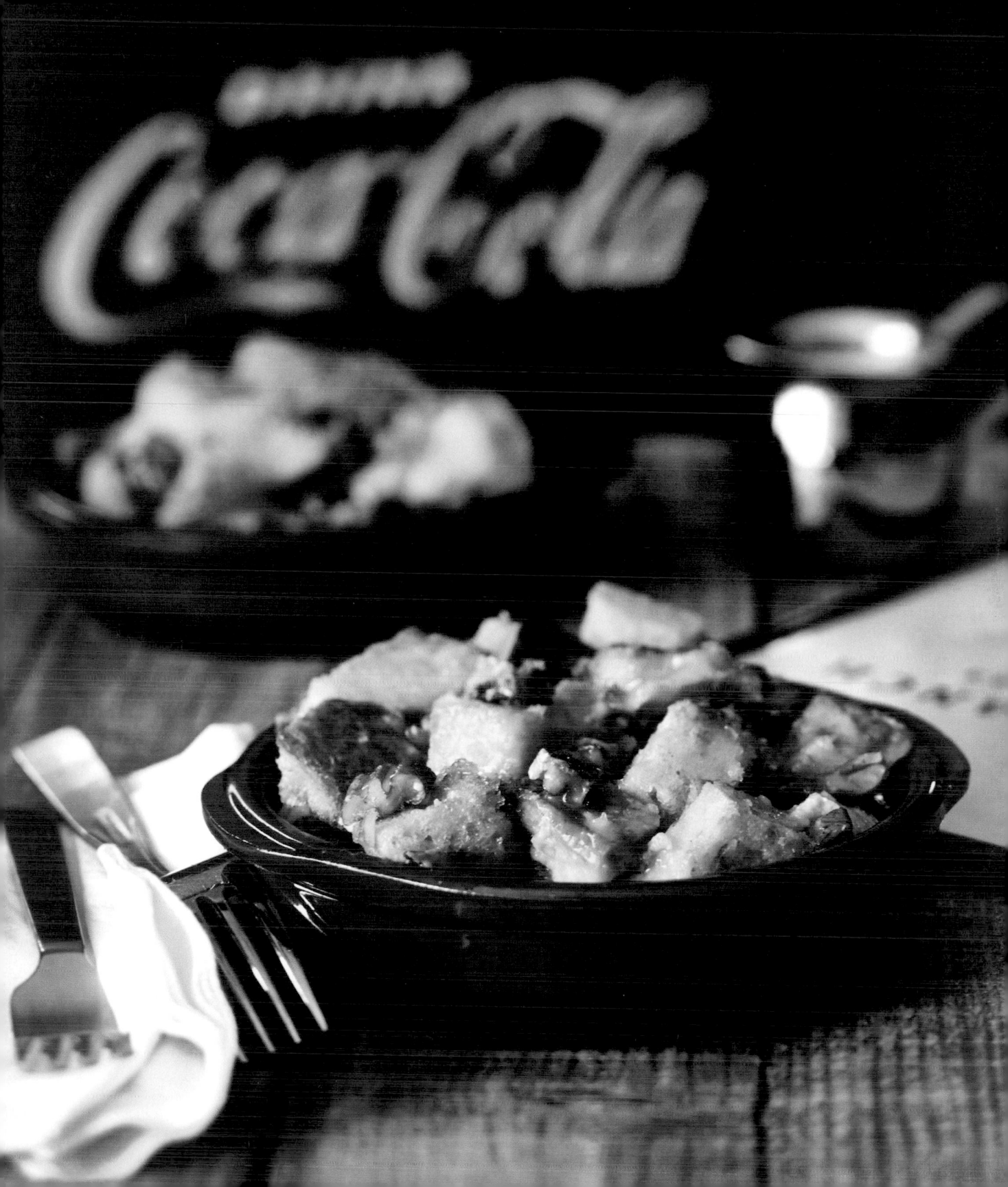

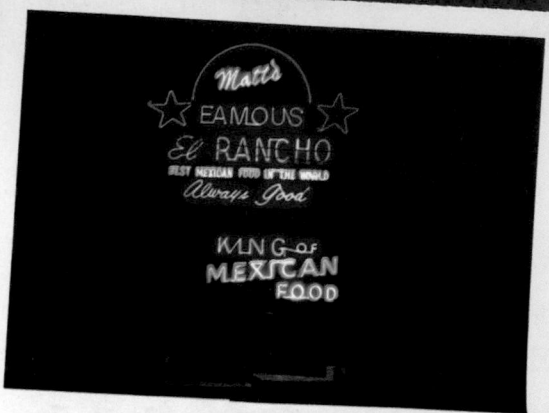

Matt's El Rancho

2613 South Lamar Blvd.
Austin, Texas 78704
(512) 462-9333
mattselrancho.com

When Matt Martinez opened El Rancho in 1952, Austin was home to just a handful of Mexican restaurants. So in order to promote his El Rancho, the Olympian and former prizefighter took his logoed matchbooks to the valets at the city's best hotels. Soon everyone from pop stars to presidents was eating his chile rellenos, house-ground corn tortillas, and fresh-squeezed margaritas. LBJ had the chile rellenos shipped to the White House. Everything here is made with such love and care by Matt's three daughters, Gloria Reyna, Cecilia Muela, and Cathy Kreitz, who maintain his passion for cooking from scratch. El Rancho grinds the corn for and fries more than 500,000 tortillas a month. From shrimp quesadillas and traditional nachos to flan and pralines, everything at this Austin institution is superb.

Matt's El Rancho Chile Relleno

MEAT FILLING

1	lb. ground chuck
¼	cup finely chopped sweet onion
3	Tbsp. finely chopped celery
1	Tbsp. finely chopped green bell pepper
2	tsp. ground cumin
1½	tsp. granulated garlic
1	tsp. table salt
½	tsp. freshly ground black pepper

RELLENOS

Vegetable oil
6	fresh poblano peppers (about 1½ lb.)
2	cups all-purpose flour
½	tsp. table salt
¼	tsp. freshly ground black pepper
2	cups buttermilk

Vegetable cooking spray
Ranchero Sauce (facing page)
2	cups (8 oz.) shredded American cheese
¼	cup raisins
¼	cup chopped pecans

1. **Prepare Meat Filling:** Cook all ingredients in a large skillet over medium heat, stirring often, 7 minutes or until meat crumbles and is no longer pink. Drain. Keep warm.

2. **Prepare Rellenos:** Preheat oven to 375°. Pour oil to depth of 2 inches in a Dutch oven; heat oil to 375°. Wash peppers and dry thoroughly. Cook peppers, in batches, in hot oil, turning often, 3 to 5 minutes, or until blistered. Remove peppers from oil with a slotted spoon, and wrap in a damp cloth. Let stand 10 minutes. (Reduce heat to low while peppers stand.) Remove skins from peppers; cut a lengthwise slit in each pepper, keeping stems intact. Remove seeds and membranes.

3. Heat oil to 375°. Combine flour, salt, and pepper in a shallow dish. Place buttermilk in a bowl. Dredge peppers in flour mixture. Dip in buttermilk; dredge in flour mixture, shaking off excess.

Fry peppers, in 2 batches, 1 to 2 minutes on each side or until golden brown. Drain on paper towels.

4. Lightly grease a 13 x 9-inch baking dish with cooking spray. Open peppers, and arrange in prepared dish. Spoon about ½ cup meat mixture into each pepper. Top with Ranchero Sauce; sprinkle with cheese.

5. Bake, uncovered, at 375° for 8 minutes or until cheese begins to melt. Sprinkle with raisins and pecans; bake 1 to 2 more minutes or until cheese begins to bubble. Serve immediately. **Makes:** 6 servings

Ranchero Sauce

If you prefer your salsa hot, substitute jalapeños for the bell pepper in this simple, tasty recipe.

1	Tbsp. cornstarch
1½	tsp. table salt
1	tsp. granulated garlic
1	tsp. ground cumin
1	tsp. chopped fresh oregano
¼	tsp. freshly ground black pepper
2	Tbsp. olive oil
1	cup finely chopped onion
½	cup finely chopped celery
½	cup finely chopped green bell pepper
2	cups canned beef broth
1	(14½-oz.) can cut whole tomatoes, coarsely chopped

1. Combine first 6 ingredients in a small bowl, stirring until cornstarch is blended.

2. Heat oil in a 2-qt. saucepan over medium-high heat. Add onion, celery, and bell pepper. Sauté 3 minutes. Stir in cornstarch mixture. Add broth and tomatoes.

3. Bring to a boil; reduce heat to low, and simmer 20 minutes, stirring occasionally. **Makes: 3 cups**

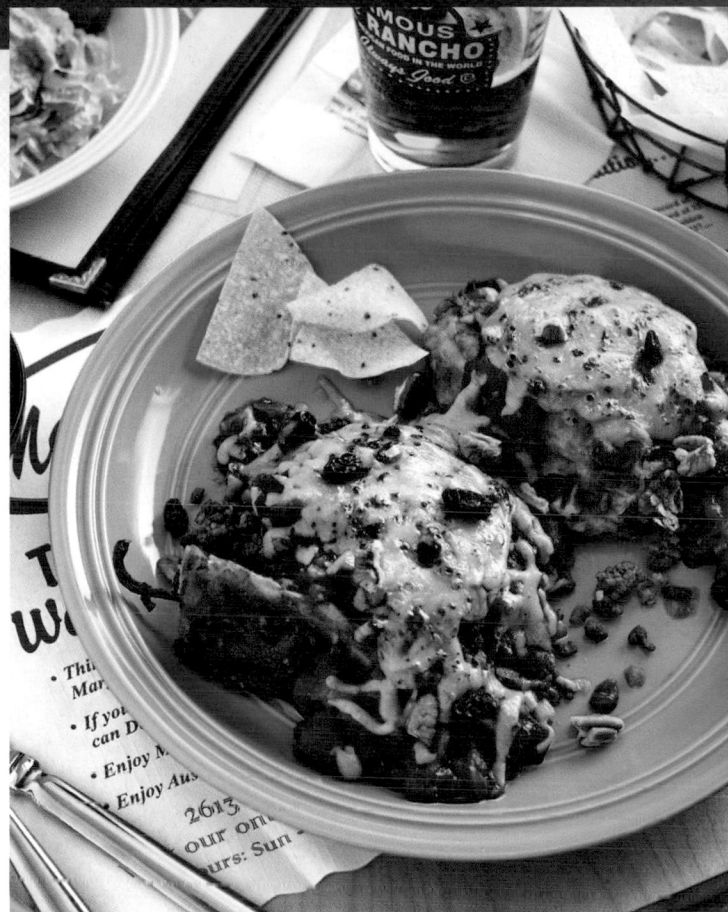

Matt's El Rancho Guacamole

1	garlic clove, peeled
1	tsp. table salt
3	Tbsp. lemon juice
3	Tbsp. canola oil
4	ripe avocados, halved
1	cup chopped tomato

1. Place peeled garlic clove on a cutting board with salt. Smash garlic and salt together using flat side of a knife to make a paste. Transfer garlic paste to a medium bowl. Add lemon juice and next 2 ingredients; mash with a potato masher to desired consistency.

2. Stir in tomato, and serve immediately. **Makes: 2 cups**

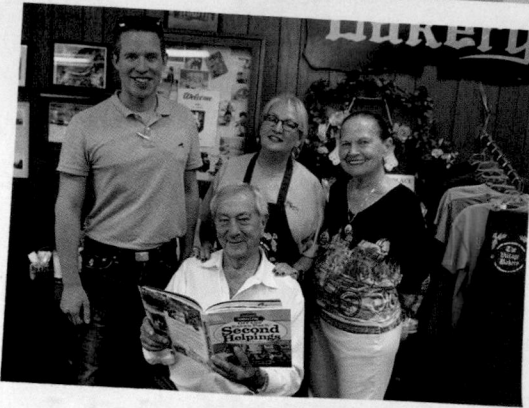

The Village Bakery

113 East Oak Street
West, Texas 76691
(254) 826-5151

The Czechoslovakian kolache is like a little pillow from the oven. Many places sell them up and down the interstate, but if you want perfection, head to the hamlet of West. Here, Village Bakery has been making kolaches the same since 1952. The recipe is the secret formula of Wendel Montgomery, who kicked off the kolache craze in Texas. Thanks to Wendel, the kolache is now as Texas as a pair of cowboy boots. His daughter, Mimi Montgomery Irwin, upholds the traditions at Village Bakery and showed me how to prepare hand-formed apricot, poppy seed, and cherry kolaches. This bakery also created the now-famous klobasniki, which is the same dough but filled with sausage (never call it a "sausage kolache"). Don't expect perfection from your first batch—as the Czechs say, Bez práce nejsou kolache, (without work there are no kolaches).

Kolache

DOUGH

1	(¼-oz.) envelope active dry yeast
¼	cup warm water (100° to 110°)
¾	cup milk
½	cup butter, cut into small pieces
¼	cup sugar
1	tsp. table salt
4¼	cups all-purpose flour
2	large eggs

Garnish: sifted powdered sugar

APRICOT FILLING

2	cups coarsely chopped dried apricots
⅓	cup sugar
1	Tbsp. butter
½	tsp. ground nutmeg
1	Tbsp. cornstarch

POSIPKA TOPPING

¾	cup sugar
6	Tbsp. all-purpose flour
¾	tsp. ground cinnamon
1½	Tbsp. butter, melted

1. Prepare Dough: In a bowl, dissolve yeast in warm water (100° to 110°).

2. In a 2-qt. saucepan, heat milk, butter, sugar, and salt to 115° to 120° over medium heat, stirring until butter almost melts. Remove from heat, and cool slightly. Combine milk mixture and 2 cups flour, stirring with a wooden spoon. Add yeast mixture and eggs, beating well. Stir in 2 cups flour.

3. Turn out onto a lightly floured surface. Knead in enough of the remaining flour (about ¼ cup) to make a soft dough. Continue kneading until smooth and elastic (2 minutes). Shape into a ball. Place dough in a lightly greased bowl, turn once to grease surface. Cover and let rise in a warm place (80° to 85°), free from drafts (about 1 hour), or until doubled in bulk.

4. Meanwhile, prepare Apricot Filling: Combine apricots and 3 cups water in a 2-qt. saucepan.

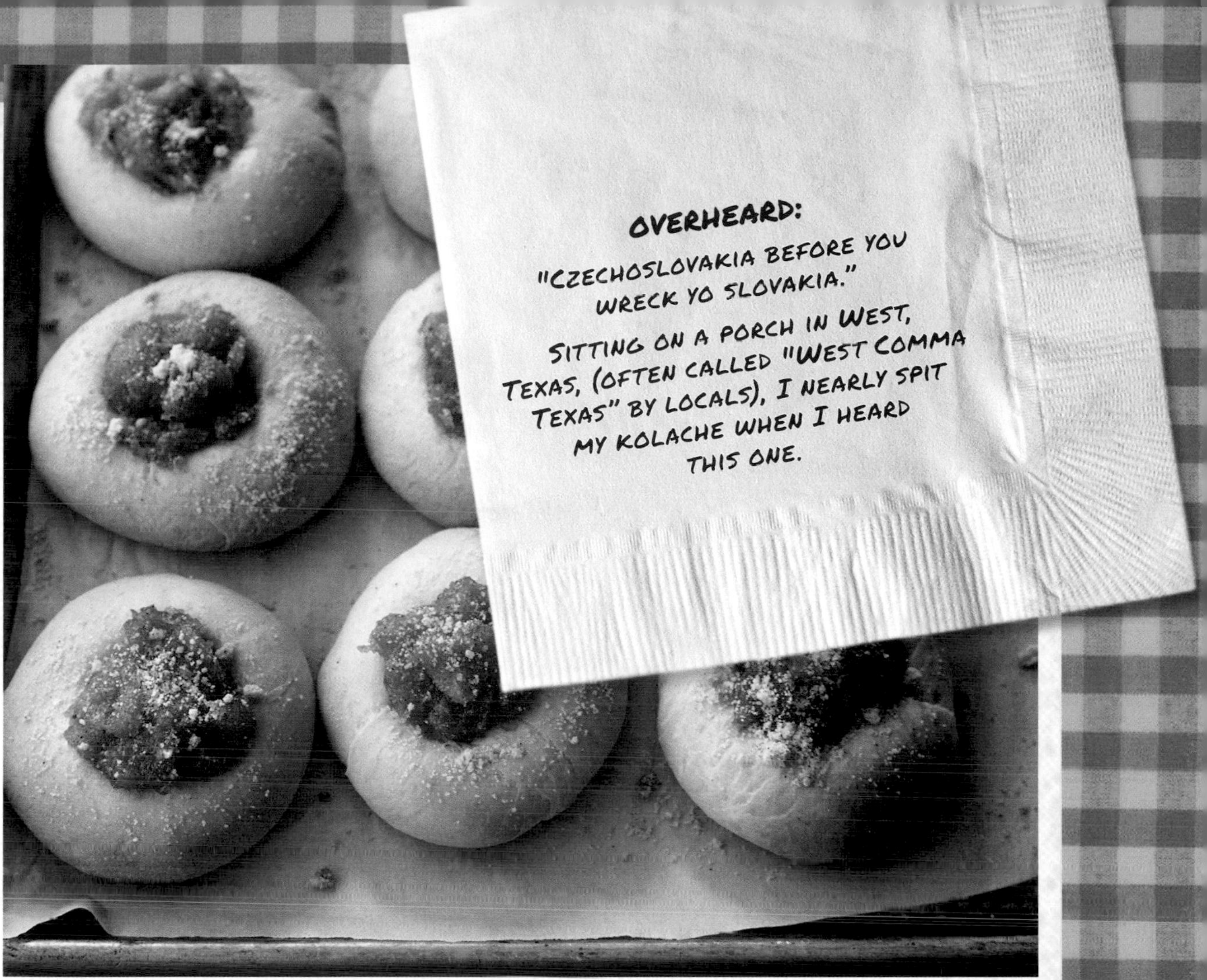

OVERHEARD:

"CZECHOSLOVAKIA BEFORE YOU WRECK YO SLOVAKIA."

SITTING ON A PORCH IN WEST, TEXAS, (OFTEN CALLED "WEST COMMA TEXAS" BY LOCALS), I NEARLY SPIT MY KOLACHE WHEN I HEARD THIS ONE.

Bring to a boil; cover, reduce heat, and simmer 10 minutes. Drain. Return apricots to saucepan. Add ⅓ cup sugar, 1 Tbsp. butter, and nutmeg. Cook over medium heat 2 minutes or until butter melts and sugar dissolves, mashing apricots with a fork. Combine cornstarch and 3 Tbsp. water. Stir cornstarch mixture into apricot mixture. Cook 1 minute or until thickened and clear. Cool 10 minutes.

5. **Prepare Posipka Topping:** Combine all ingredients until mixture resembles coarse meal.

6. Punch dough down; turn out onto a lightly floured surface. Divide dough into 2 portions. Cover; let stand 10 minutes.

7. Shape each portion into 9 balls. Place 3 inches apart on greased baking sheets. Flatten each ball into a 3-inch circle. Cover; let rise in warm place (80° to 85°) until doubled in bulk (about 45 minutes).

8. Preheat oven to 375°. With your fingers, make a 1-inch indentation in the center of each circle. Spoon 1 heaping Tbsp. filling evenly into each indentation. Sprinkle topping on tops of kolaches.

9. Bake at 375° for 15 to 18 minutes or until golden brown. Transfer to a wire rack; cool completely (about 30 minutes). **Makes: 18 servings**

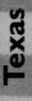

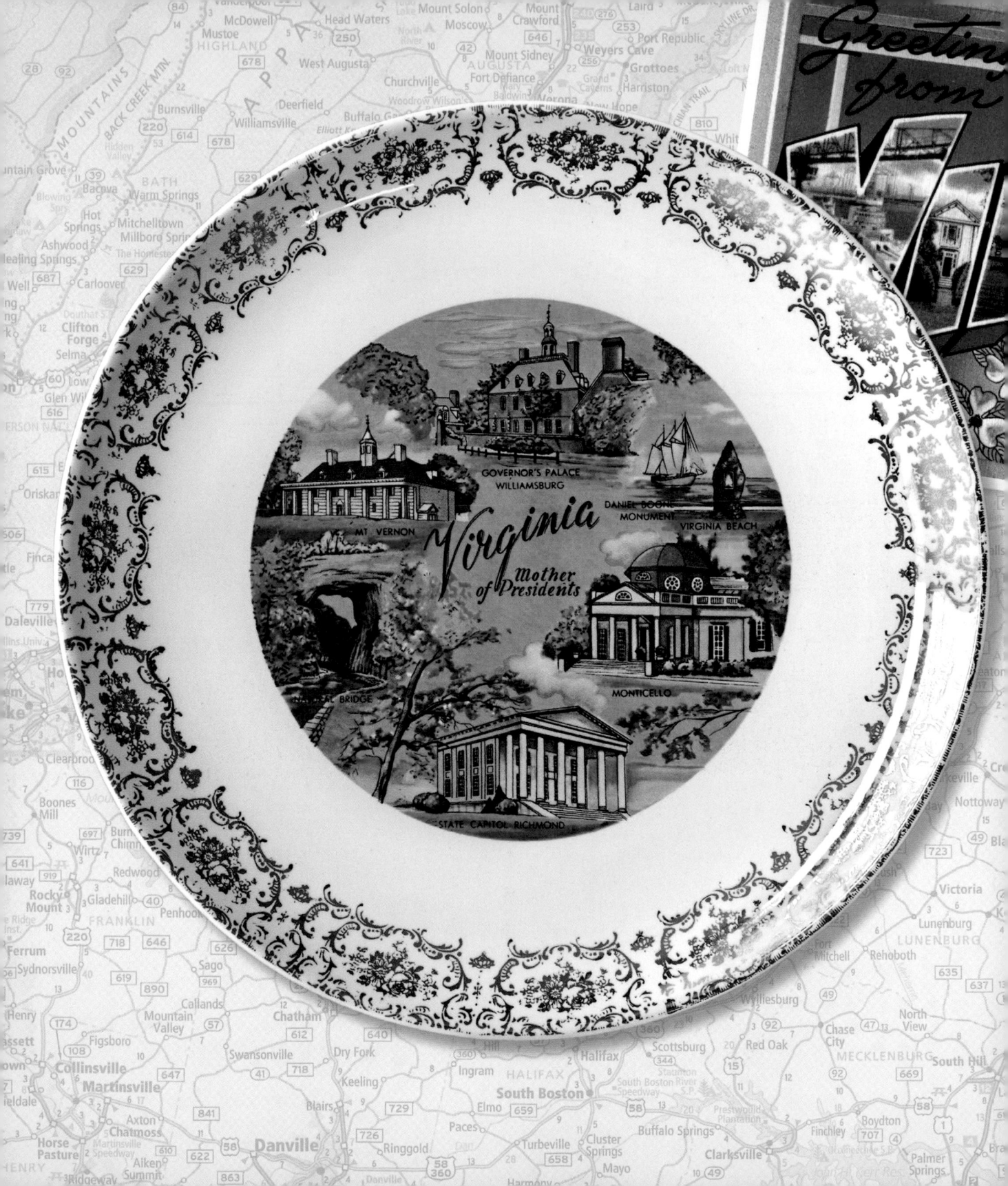

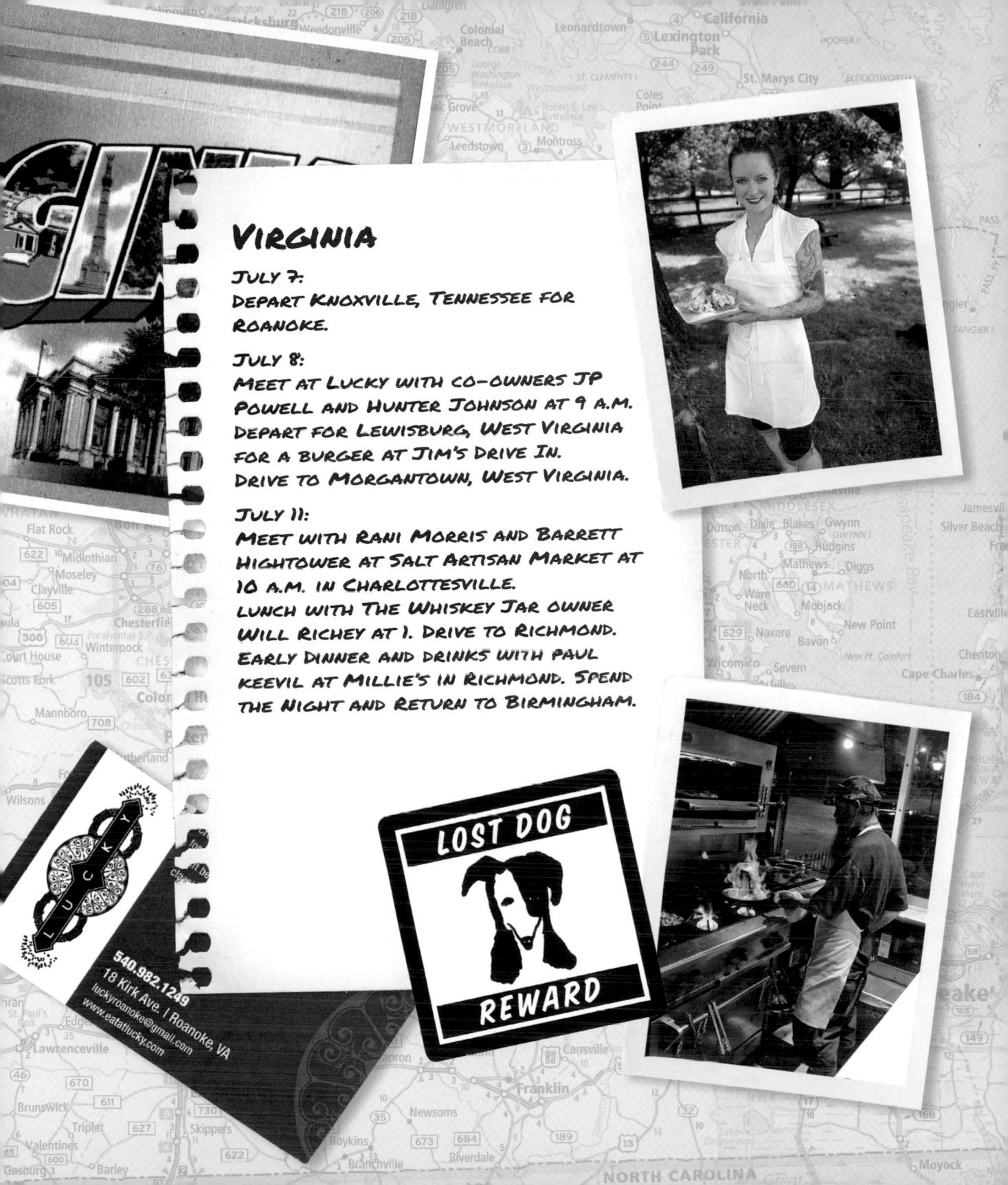

Virginia

July 7:
Depart Knoxville, Tennessee for Roanoke.

July 8:
Meet at Lucky with co-owners JP Powell and Hunter Johnson at 9 a.m. Depart for Lewisburg, West Virginia for a burger at Jim's Drive In. Drive to Morgantown, West Virginia.

July 11:
Meet with Rani Morris and Barrett Hightower at Salt Artisan Market at 10 a.m. in Charlottesville. Lunch with The Whiskey Jar owner Will Richey at 1. Drive to Richmond. Early dinner and drinks with Paul Keevil at Millie's in Richmond. Spend the night and return to Birmingham.

540.982.1249
18 Kirk Ave. | Roanoke, VA
luckyroanoke@gmail.com
www.eatatlucky.com

LOST DOG

REWARD

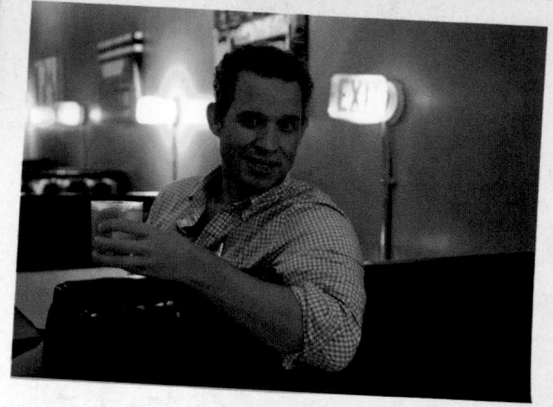

Lucky

18 Kirk Avenue SW
Roanoke, Virginia 24011
(540) 982-1249
eatatlucky.com

Musicians and Lucky co-owners JP Powell and Hunter Johnson took design inspiration for the restaurant from spots they'd visited across the country while touring. The result—an edgy place that features raised booths, flattering lighting, and a bar with more bourbon than even I can drink. Chef Jeff Farmer brings a menu with a rock-and-roll edge—think dishes like decadent duck pâté, savory octopus and chili salad, and enormous lamb shanks. Hunter mans the bar, and his cocktails, like the Strawberry Cucumber Smash (a mixture of gin, strawberry, balsamic vinegar, and bitters), are outrageous. "The important thing in life is to keep making music," he says. Fortunately, he has a team that makes music for your ears and mouth.

Border Spring's Chicken Fried Lamb Shank with Pickled Mustard Seeds and Baked Beans

PICKLED MUSTARD SEEDS

½ cup yellow mustard seeds
½ cup white vinegar
¼ cup sugar
1½ tsp. kosher salt

LAMB

4 (1-lb.) lamb shanks
2 tsp. table salt
Olive oil
1 (2-inch) rosemary sprig
1 (2-inch) thyme sprig
1 (2-inch) marjoram sprig
1 small garlic clove, smashed
Canola oil
1¼ cups all-purpose flour
1 tsp. herbes de Provence
1 tsp. smoked paprika
¼ tsp. sea salt
Baked Beans (facing page)

1. **Prepare Pickled Mustard Seeds:** Place mustard seeds in a medium bowl. Bring vinegar, sugar, kosher salt, and 1 cup water to a boil in a small nonreactive saucepan. Pour over mustard seeds. Cool completely (about 1 hour and 30 minutes). Cover and chill overnight.
2. **Prepare Lamb:** Rub each lamb shank with ½ tsp. table salt. Place in a bowl. Cover and chill overnight. Rinse and pat dry.
3. Preheat oven to 325°. Place lamb in a 5-qt. cast-iron Dutch oven. Cover lamb completely with olive oil. Add rosemary sprig and next 3 ingredients. Bake, covered, at 325° for 3 hours or until fork-tender. Cool completely in oil in Dutch oven (about 3 hours).
4. Pour canola oil to depth of 2½ inches in a Dutch oven; heat to 350°. Combine flour and

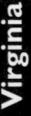

next 3 ingredients in a shallow dish. Remove lamb from oil, patting lightly with paper towels to remove excess oil. Dredge in flour mixture, shaking off excess. Fry, in batches, in hot canola oil 2 to 3 minutes or until light brown. Drain on paper towels. **Makes: 4 servings**

Baked Beans

These sweet baked beans may look like something out of a can but taste far from mass produced.

- 1⅓ cups dried navy beans
- 2 thick hickory-smoked bacon slices, cut crosswise into ½-inch pieces
- ½ cup chopped onion
- 1 large garlic clove, minced
- 2 Tbsp. canola oil
- 1 Tbsp. bourbon
- 1 (8-oz.) can tomato sauce
- ¼ cup firmly packed dark brown sugar
- 1 Tbsp. apple cider vinegar
- 1 tsp. table salt
- ½ tsp. mustard seeds
- ¼ tsp. smoked paprika
- 1½ tsp. Dijon mustard
- ½ tsp. chipotle chile powder

1. Rinse and sort beans according to package directions. Place beans in a 4-qt. saucepan. Cover with water 2 inches above beans; let soak 8 hours. Drain.

2. Return beans to saucepan. Cover with water 2 inches above beans. Bring to a boil; cover, reduce heat, and simmer 50 minutes or until tender, but not softened. Drain. Pour into a greased 8-inch baking dish.

3. While beans cook, sauté bacon, onion, and garlic in hot oil in a 2-qt. saucepan over medium-high heat 5 minutes or until onion is tender. Remove from heat; stir in bourbon. Cook 1 minute or until liquid is almost evaporated.

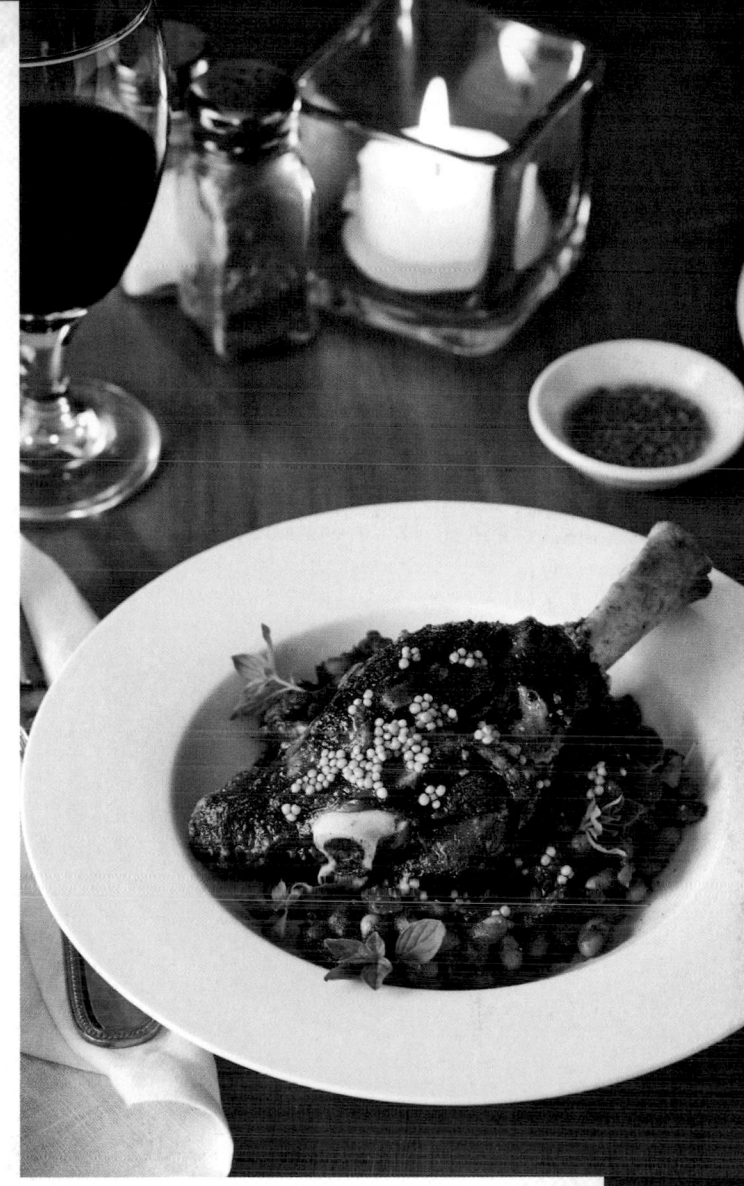

Stir in tomato sauce and next 7 ingredients. Bring to a simmer; cover and cook 15 minutes, stirring occasionally.

4. Preheat oven to 375°. Stir sauce and ⅓ cup water into beans in baking dish. Bake, covered, at 375° for 40 minutes or until beans are tender, stirring once. **Makes: 4 to 5 servings**

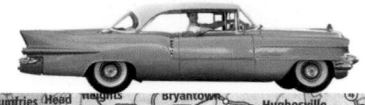

Virginia
bucket list

*things to see and do
(besides eat) here*

❶ Go train spotting in Roanoke at the Virginia Museum of Transportation.

❷ Drive along the historic James River, which is home to a large number of plantations listed in the National Register of Historic Places, including the Berkeley Plantation, site of the first official Thanksgiving in 1619.

❸ Walk Monument Avenue in Richmond, not only for its monuments, but also for its astounding collection of mansions built in the early 20th century.

❹ Soak in the genius that was Thomas Jefferson's while touring his home, Monticello *(pictured)*, in Charlottesville.

❺ Pay your respects to our nation's heroes at Arlington National Cemetery, a majestic spot to see the price of freedom.

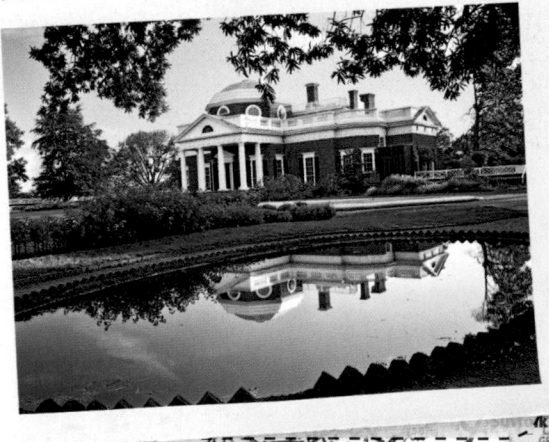

Duck Liver Pâté

SPICE MIX

14 white peppercorns

7 whole allspice

5 whole cloves

2 bay leaves, broken in pieces

PÂTÉ

Shortening

9 oz. lard

1½ cups finely chopped onion

2½ tsp. table salt, divided

1½ lb. duck livers, trimmed

⅓ cup brandy

3 large eggs

¾ cup whipping cream

Accompaniments: French bread baguette slices, cornichons, Dijon mustard, sweet onion chutney

1. Prepare Spice Mix: Process spices in a coffee mill or blender until finely ground.

2. Prepare Pâté: Lightly grease (with shortening) 4 (5¾- x 3¼-inch) loaf pans. Line pans with plastic wrap, allowing 2 inches to extend over sides.

3. Melt lard in a large skillet over medium heat. Add onion and 1 tsp. salt. Cook, stirring constantly, 4 minutes or until onion is very tender. Remove from heat; cool 40 minutes.

4. Preheat oven to 350°. Rinse livers, and pat dry with paper towels. Process livers, spices, brandy, eggs, and remaining salt in a food processor until smooth. With processor running, slowly add onion mixture, processing until smooth. Add cream; process until blended.

5. Pour mixture into pans. Fold plastic wrap over top; cover with foil. Set pans in a large roasting pan. Add hot water halfway up sides of pans.

6. Bake at 350° for 1 hour and 20 minutes or until a meat thermometer inserted in center registers 165°. Transfer pans to a wire rack. Cool completely (90 minutes). Chill 8 hours.

7. Lift pâté from pans. Slice and serve with accompaniments. **Makes: 20 servings**

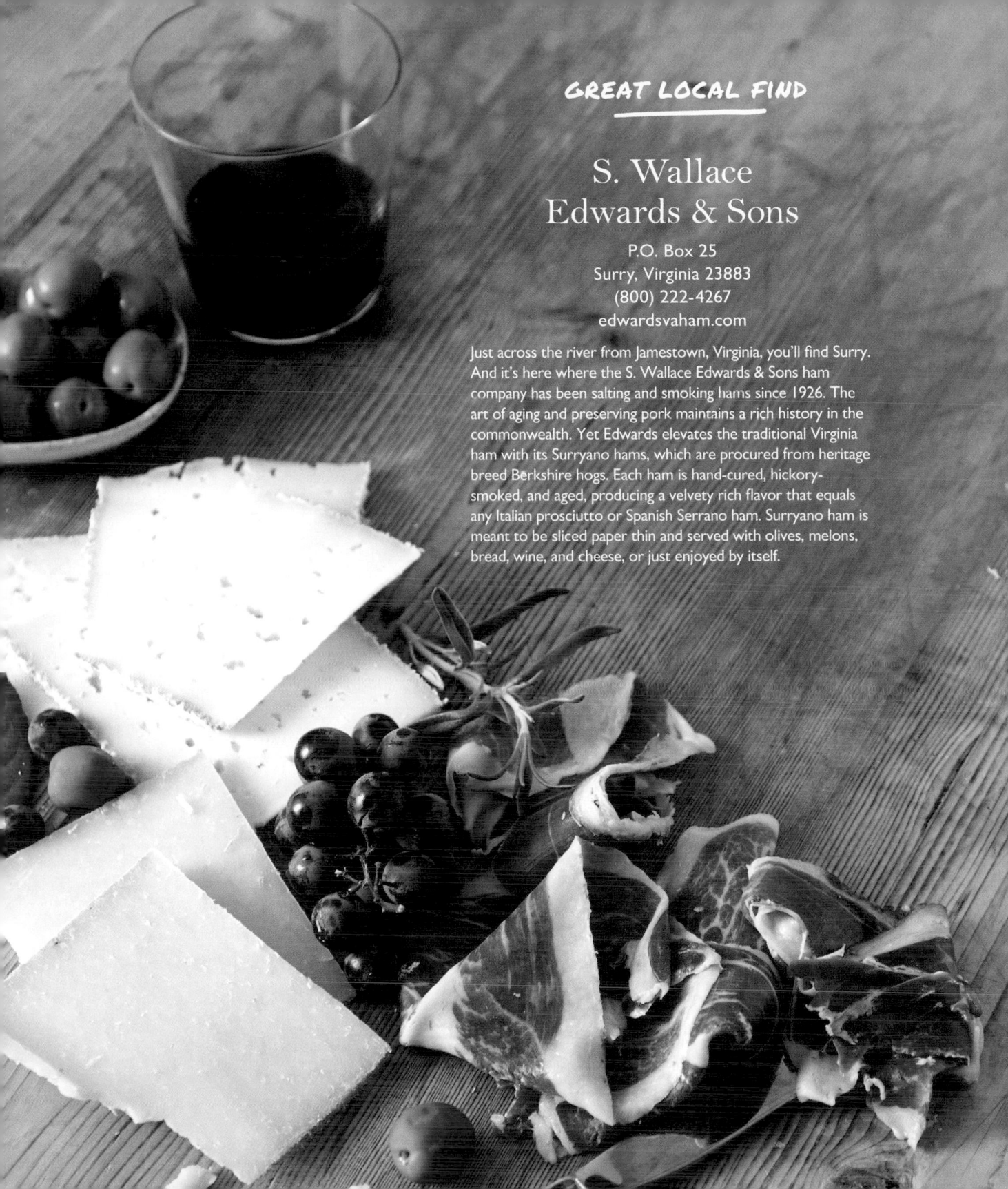

S. Wallace Edwards & Sons

P.O. Box 25
Surry, Virginia 23883
(800) 222-4267
edwardsvaham.com

Just across the river from Jamestown, Virginia, you'll find Surry. And it's here where the S. Wallace Edwards & Sons ham company has been salting and smoking hams since 1926. The art of aging and preserving pork maintains a rich history in the commonwealth. Yet Edwards elevates the traditional Virginia ham with its Surryano hams, which are procured from heritage breed Berkshire hogs. Each ham is hand-cured, hickory-smoked, and aged, producing a velvety rich flavor that equals any Italian prosciutto or Spanish Serrano ham. Surryano ham is meant to be sliced paper thin and served with olives, melons, bread, wine, and cheese, or just enjoyed by itself.

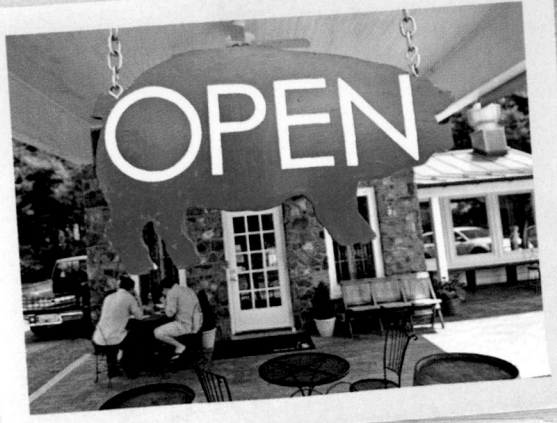

Salt Artisan Market

1330 Thomas Jefferson Parkway
Charlottesville, Virginia 22902
(434) 270-2072
saltcville.com

Wind up past Monticello, through the
lush vineyards that surround Thomas
Jefferson's home and you'll come upon
this 1920s service station tucked into the
bend of the road. Renovated by partners
Rani Morris and Barrett Hightower (and
Barrett's grandmother, who painted seven
coats of red on the screen door), this
little station makes for one of the most
charming spots in Virginia. Guests come
for simple picnic provisions (cheeses,
local sausages, chips, and chocolate),
but are often surprised by Rani's menu.
From her chicken salad to the amazing
Local Soul (a tofu sandwich), Rani's
food exudes passion and energy. Don't
miss her twist on the classic croque
monsieur. It's made with salty Virginia
ham and local cheese, both of which
make it unforgettable. And ask for an
off-menu item known as "the cookie."
Just trust me.

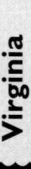
Rosemary Spiced Cashews

*This perfect appetizer whips up quickly for
those unexpected drop-in guests. These make
an excellent snack served with cheese and
wine, especially Virginian Viognier.*

1   lb. whole raw cashews
1   Tbsp. minced fresh rosemary
3   Tbsp. butter, melted
2   tsp. kosher salt
3   Tbsp. light brown sugar
⅛   tsp. ground red pepper

1. Preheat oven to 350°. Bake cashews in a single
layer in a shallow pan 10 minutes or until lightly
toasted and fragrant, stirring halfway through.
Transfer to a large bowl. Add rosemary and
remaining ingredients; toss well.
2. Return cashew mixture to pan. Bake cashews
in a single layer 8 more minutes or until toasted,
stirring halfway through. Remove from oven;
stir. Cool completely in pan on a wire rack
(30 minutes). **Makes: 4 cups**

White Chocolate-Dipped Lime Macaroons

*My favorite cookie? A macaroon. Salt's recipe
puts a delicious twist on this classic cookie.*

2   large eggs
½   cup sugar
1   tsp. lime zest
½   tsp. vanilla extract
⅛   tsp. table salt
3   cups sweetened flaked coconut
Parchment paper
4   oz. white chocolate, chopped

1. Preheat oven to 350°. Whisk together first 5
ingredients. Fold in coconut. Drop by rounded
tablespoonfuls, 1½ inches apart, onto a large
baking sheet lined with parchment paper.

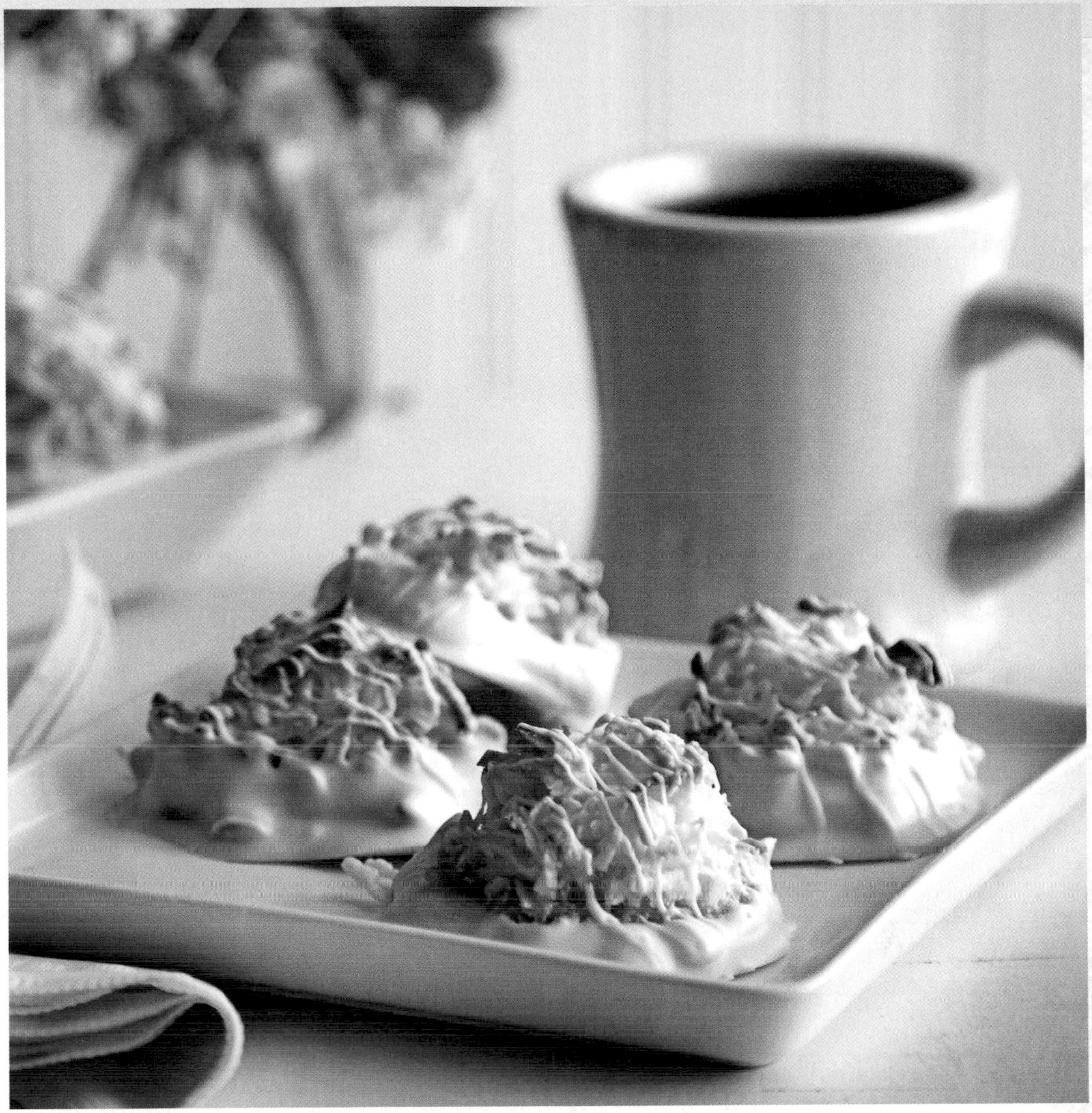

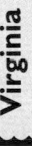

2. Bake at 350° for 18 to 20 minutes or until lightly browned. Cool 2 minutes on pans. Transfer to wire racks. Cool completely (20 minutes).
3. Place chocolate in a medium-size microwave-safe bowl. Microwave at HIGH 1 minute or until melted; stir every 30 seconds until smooth. Dip bottoms of cooled macaroons in melted chocolate. Place on a parchment paper-lined baking sheet.
4. Spoon remaining chocolate into a 1-qt. zip-top plastic freezer bag. Snip 1 corner of bag to make a tiny hole (about ⅛ inch in diameter). Squirt chocolate in a zigzag pattern over tops of cookies. Chill 20 minutes or until chocolate is firm. **Makes: 20 servings**

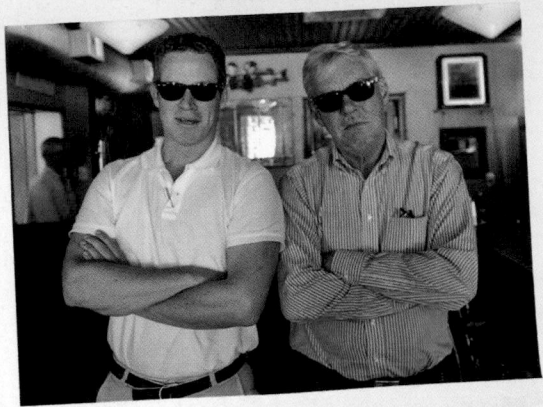

SOUNDTRACK:

"I WILL ALWAYS LOVE YOU" BY TIDEWATER

"YEAH, YEAH, YEAH" BY MY RADIO

"COME GET IT BAE" BY PHARRELL WILLIAMS

"SAME OLD TRAIN" BY MERLE HAGGARD

"SWEET VIRGINIA" BY THE ROLLING STONES

Millie's

2603 East Main Street
Richmond, Virginia 23223
(804) 643-5512
milliesdiner.com

I've lost a lot of time here. It could be the excellent bar or cozy booths. Maybe it's the music you can select from the chrome tabletop jukeboxes. More than likely, however, it's because of Paul Keevil, the former Brit rocker and world traveler who founded Millie's in L.A. and brought it to Richmond in 1989. Paul has no doubt talked many others into just one more drink. And then there's the food. Millie's brunch is a Richmond institution that serves up dishes such as the "Devil's Mess," a hot combo of chorizo, avocado, and melted white Cheddar. At dinner, try the pork loin or rockfish, both could be served in a high-end restaurant rather than this neighborhood eatery. When asked about that attention to quality, Paul says simply, "It's easier to do it the right way." Well said.

Virginia Crab Salad with Avocado and Citrus

This simple salad is sweet and creamy, tart and delicious.

1	lb. fresh lump crabmeat, drained
½	cup mayonnaise
3	Tbsp. finely chopped fresh flat-leaf parsley
¼	tsp. table salt
¼	tsp. freshly ground black pepper
¼	tsp. lemon zest
¼	tsp. lime zest
2	tsp. fresh lemon juice
2	tsp. fresh lime juice
1	head Bibb lettuce
1	avocado, halved and thinly sliced
1	orange, sectioned

Garnishes: dash of extra virgin olive oil and microgreens

1. Pick crabmeat, removing any bits of shell. Stir together mayonnaise and next 7 ingredients in a large bowl. Gently fold in crabmeat.
2. Place 1 lettuce leaf on each of 6 plates. Scoop ½ cup crab salad onto lettuce leaf. Top evenly with avocado slices and orange sections. **Makes: 6 servings**

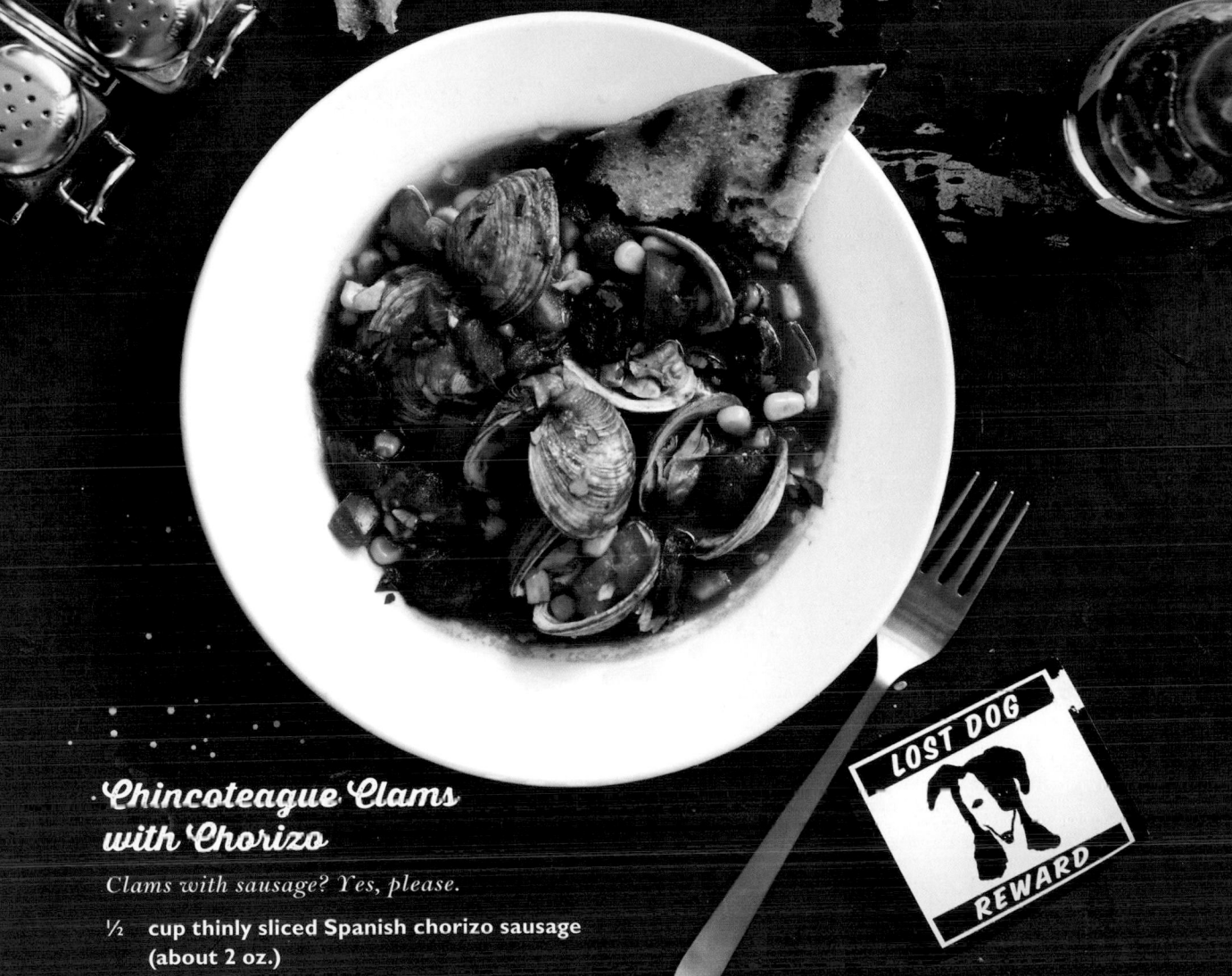

Chincoteague Clams with Chorizo

Clams with sausage? Yes, please.

½ cup thinly sliced Spanish chorizo sausage (about 2 oz.)
1 Tbsp. diced shallots
2 garlic cloves, minced
1¼ cups fresh corn kernels (2 ears)
1¼ cups diced tomato
1½ tsp. smoked paprika
Pinch of ground saffron (optional)
1 cup dry white wine
24 little neck clams in shells, scrubbed
Chopped fresh flat-leaf parsley
Dash of extra virgin olive oil
Crusty French bread

1. Cook chorizo in a 4-qt. saucepan 1 to 2 minutes or until browned, stirring occasionally. Add shallots and garlic; sauté 30 seconds. Add corn, next 2 ingredients, and, if desired, saffron; sauté 2 minutes.

2. Stir in wine. Cook, uncovered, over high heat 2 minutes. Add clams; cover and cook 4 minutes or until clams open. Place clams in a serving bowl; discard unopened clams. Cook broth, uncovered, 1 minute.

3. Pour broth over clams. Sprinkle with parsley and olive oil. Serve immediately with crusty French bread. **Makes: 2 servings**

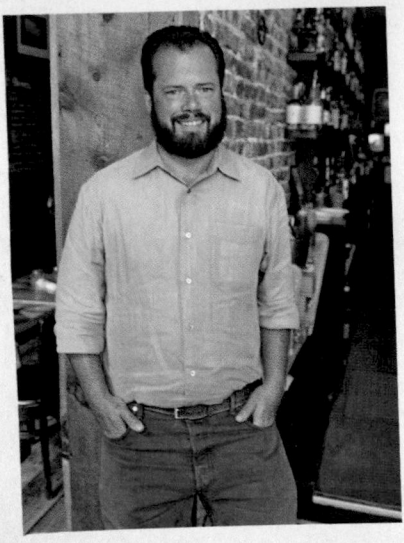

The Whiskey Jar

227 West Main Street
Charlottesville, Virginia 22902
(434) 202-1549
thewhiskeyjarcville.com

Heart-pine floors and tables, brick walls, and a vast collection of brown liquor give this tucked-away spot a cozy vibe. It's the kind of place where you linger over a cocktail and watch the people wander Charlottesville's brick-lined mall. Gobble up a bowl of Tomato Okra Stew or scarf down a tomato sandwich and you'll know why The Whiskey Jar is so popular. "I just like using simple, fresh ingredients," says owner Will Richey. Will sure knows fresh: He drives to the restaurant daily from his nearby farm. His inspiration comes from the North Carolina side of his family, so you'll see a lot of Tarheel influences on the menu. But one Virginia classic you can't miss is baker Rachel Pennington's cobbler.

Tomato Okra Stew

A medley of fiery seasonings makes this some of the smokiest stew I've ever tried.

Hickory wood chunks
6¼ lb. plum tomatoes, halved lengthwise
2 Tbsp. extra virgin olive oil
2 cups chopped onion
1 lb. okra, sliced
2 Tbsp. cane syrup
½ tsp. dried crushed red pepper
½ tsp. Cajun seasoning
2 tsp. each minced fresh parsley, thyme, and chives

1. Soak wood chunks in water 1 hour. Prepare smoker according to manufacturer's directions, bringing internal temperature to 200°; maintain temperature for 15 to 20 minutes.
2. Drain wood chunks, and place on coals. Place tomatoes on upper cooking grate; cover with smoker lid.
3. Smoke tomato slices, maintaining temperature inside smoker at 200°, for 1 hour and 30 minutes.
4. Heat oil in a large saucepan over medium heat. Add onion; cook, covered, 2 minutes, stirring occasionally. Add okra; cook, covered, 4 minutes, stirring often. Add smoked tomatoes, cane syrup, red pepper, Cajun seasoning, and ¾ cup water. Bring to a boil; cover, reduce heat, and simmer 40 minutes or until okra is tender, stirring occasionally. Stir in fresh herbs, salt and pepper to taste, and ½ cup water. **Makes: 10 servings**
Note: We tested with Emeril's Cajun Seasoning.

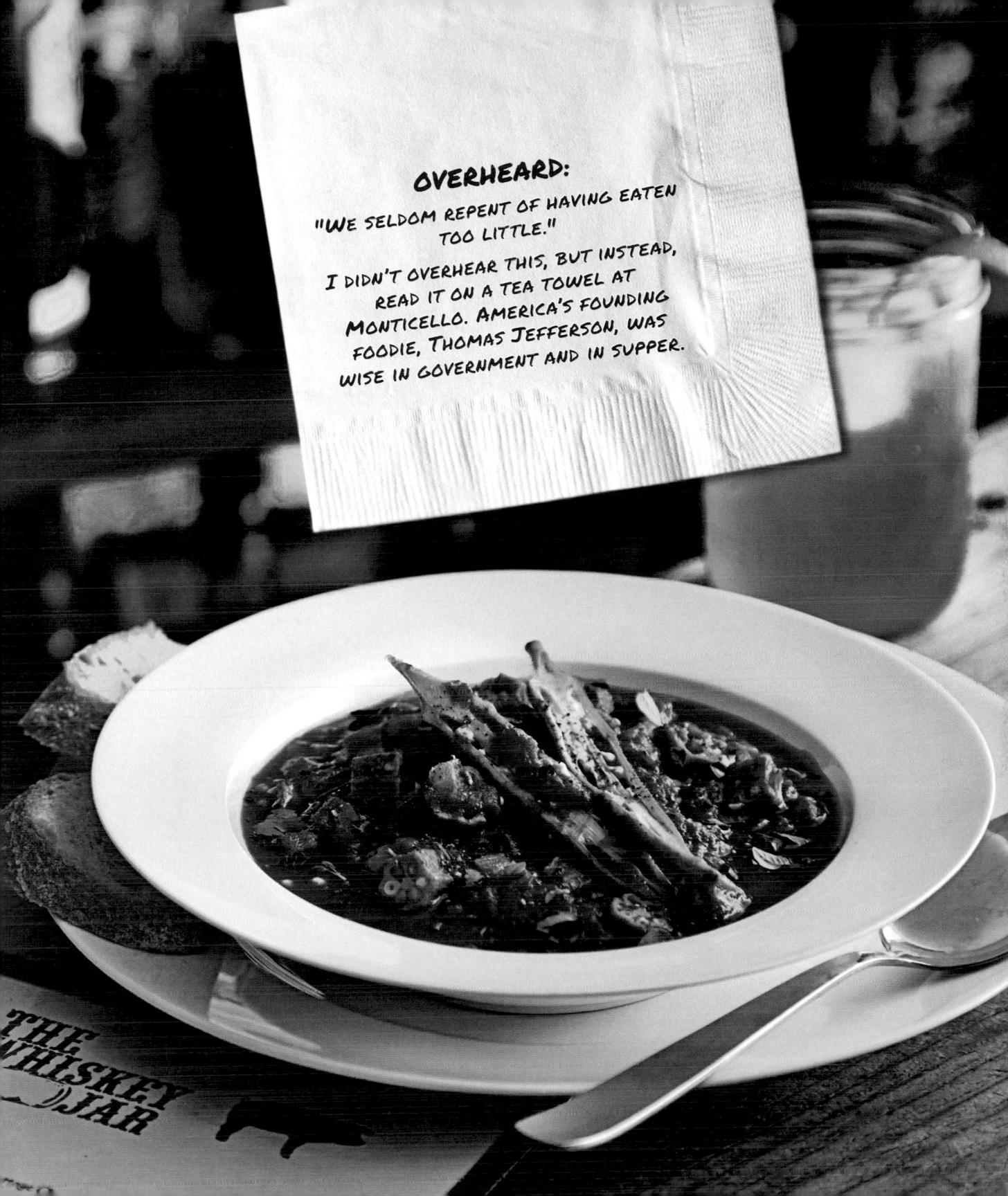

THE WHISKEY JAR

Biscuit and Tomato Bread Salad

This is a great use for old biscuits.

3   cups (½-inch) diced onion (about 2 medium)
2   tsp. fennel seeds
2   tsp. fresh thyme leaves
4   garlic cloves, coarsely chopped
2   bay leaves
1¾ cups extra virgin oil, divided
¾   tsp. table salt, divided
¾   tsp. freshly ground black pepper, divided
4   day-old (3-inch) biscuits, cut into 1-inch cubes
6   cups mixed salad greens
8   medium tomatoes (3 lb.), cut into 1-inch pieces
4   tsp. red wine vinegar
Chopped fresh basil
Chopped fresh parsley
Garnish: mixed sprouts

1. Combine first 5 ingredients, all of the oil except 1 Tbsp., ¼ tsp. salt, and ¼ tsp. pepper in a 1-qt. saucepan. Bring to a simmer over medium-low heat; cook 40 minutes or until onion is very soft. Cool to room temperature (1 hour). Discard bay leaves.
2. Preheat oven to 350°. Place biscuit cubes in a bowl; drizzle with remaining 1 Tbsp. olive oil, and sprinkle with remaining ½ tsp. salt and ½ tsp. pepper, tossing well. Spread cubes in a single layer on a small baking sheet. Bake at 350° for 15 minutes or until crisp and golden brown.
3. Place 1½ cups salad greens in each of 4 large shallow bowls. Place tomato in a large bowl. Spoon ½ cup onion mixture over tomato; toss well. Add biscuit croutons; toss gently. Spoon tomato mixture evenly over greens in each bowl. Drizzle each salad with 1 tsp. red wine vinegar. Sprinkle with desired amount of basil and parsley. **Makes: 4 servings**

Roasted Trout and Summer Vegetables

2   (13-oz.) whole dressed rainbow trout
2½ Tbsp. olive oil, divided
¾   tsp. table salt, divided
⅜   tsp. freshly ground black pepper, divided
1   large shallot, thinly sliced and separated into rings
1   lemon, thinly sliced
2   fresh thyme sprigs
Vegetable cooking spray
1   Tbsp. butter
⅔   cup sliced yellow squash
⅔   cup sliced zucchini
5   oz. fresh green beans, trimmed and cut into 1-inch pieces
Garnish: lemon wedges and fresh thyme leaves

1. Preheat broiler with oven rack 6 inches from heat. Brush cavities and outsides of both fish with 1½ Tbsp. oil; sprinkle cavities and outsides evenly with ½ tsp. salt and ¼ tsp. pepper. Divide shallot rings, lemon slices, and thyme sprigs between cavities in both fish.
2. Place fish on a rack coated with cooking spray in a broiler pan lined with aluminum foil. Broil 3 minutes on each side or until skin begins to crisp; reduce oven temperature to 450°, and bake 3 minutes or until fish flakes with a fork.
3. Heat butter and remaining 1 Tbsp. oil in a large nonstick skillet over medium-high heat until butter melts. Add vegetables; sauté 4 minutes or until browned but crisp-tender. Sprinkle with remaining ¼ tsp. salt and remaining ⅛ tsp. pepper. Serve vegetables with fish. **Makes: 2 servings**

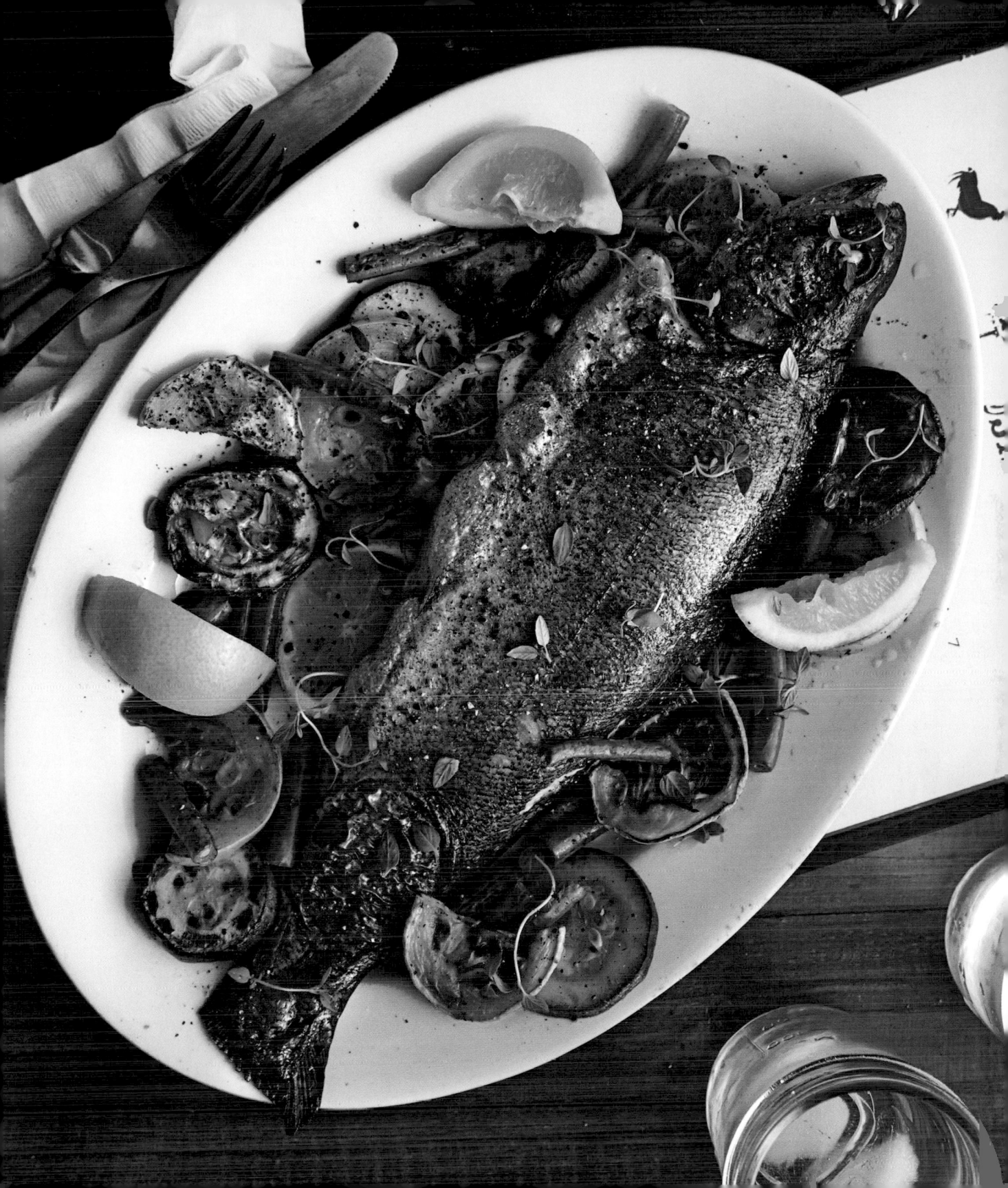

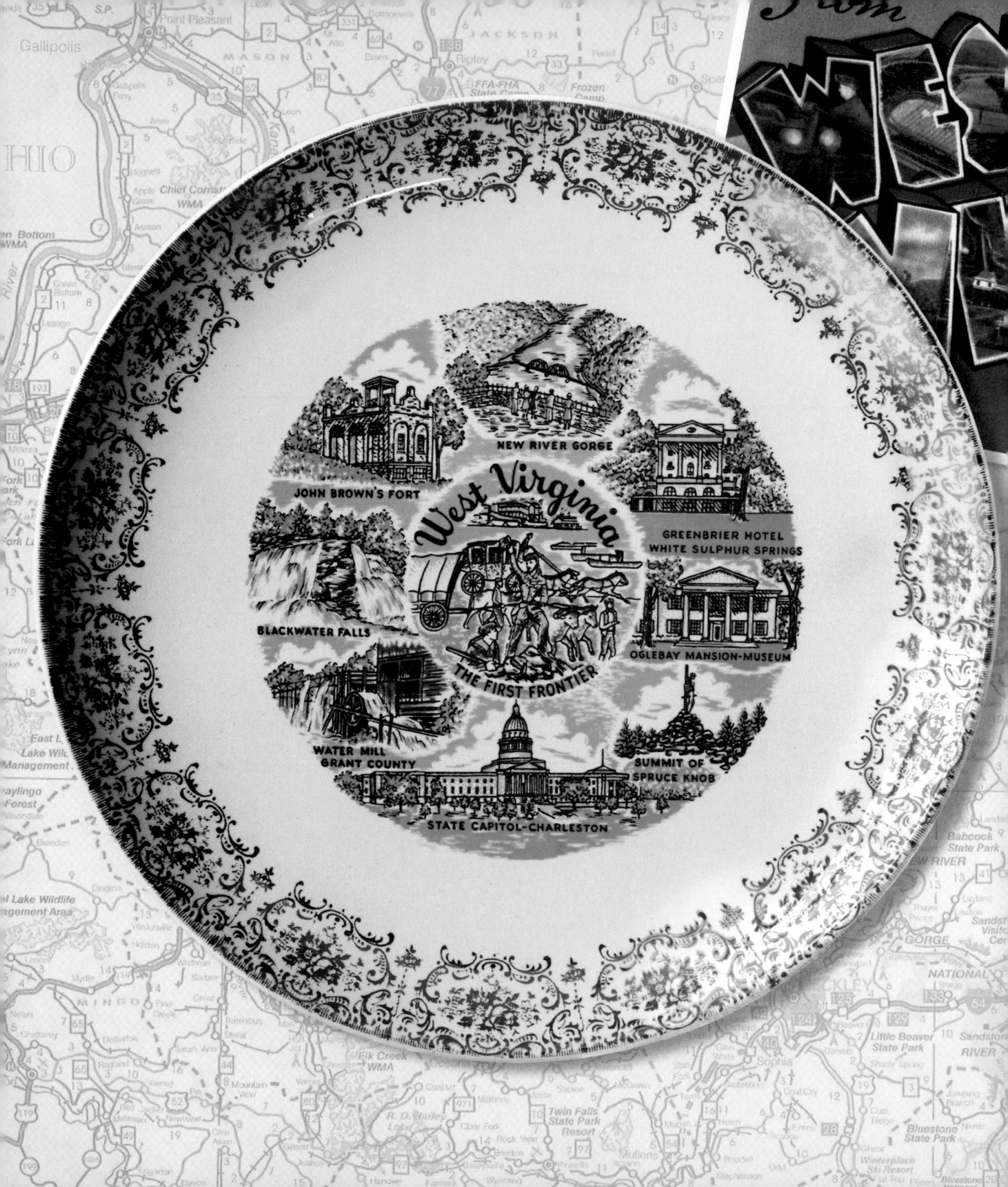

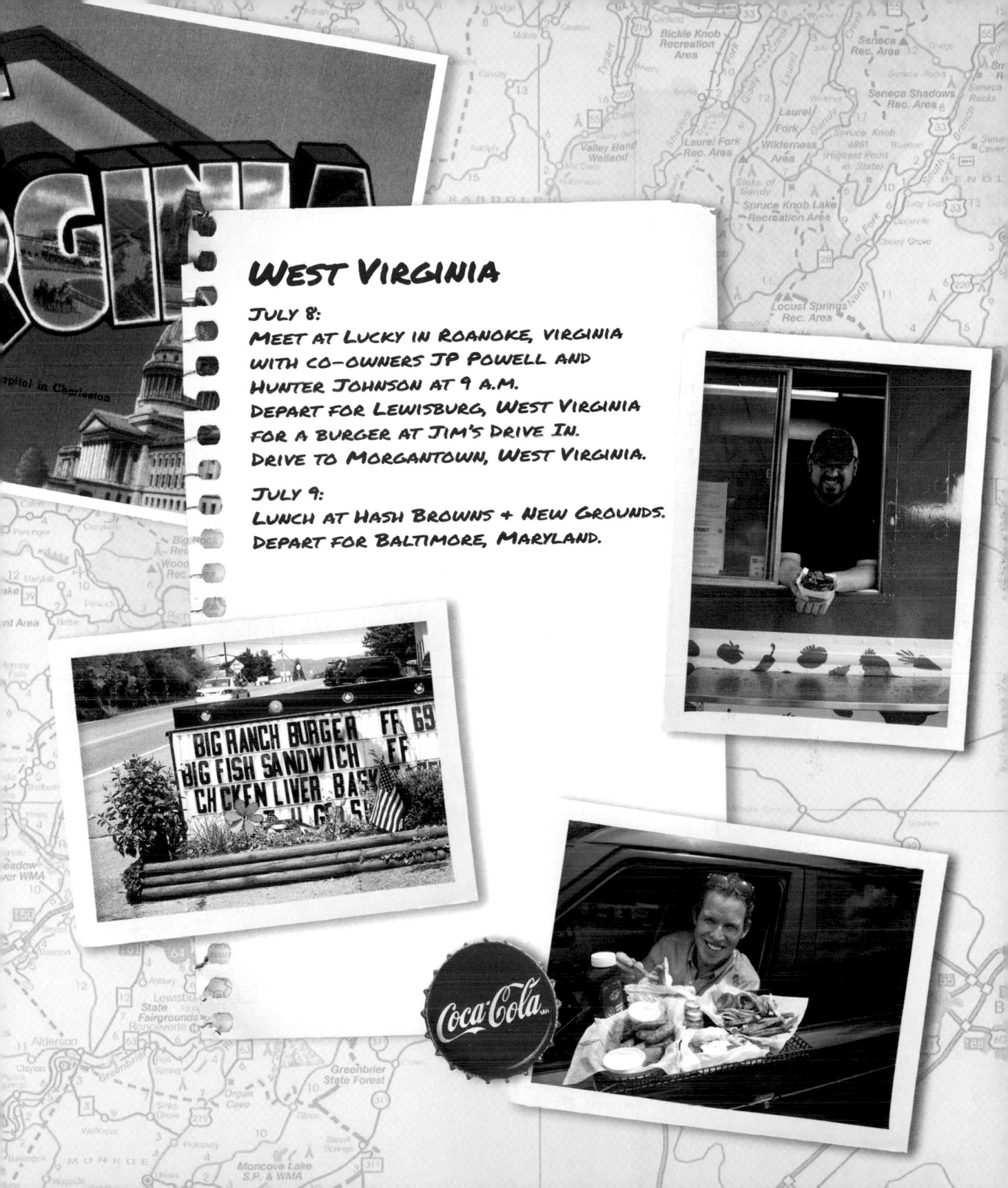

West Virginia

July 8:
Meet at Lucky in Roanoke, Virginia with co-owners JP Powell and Hunter Johnson at 9 a.m.
Depart for Lewisburg, West Virginia for a burger at Jim's Drive In.
Drive to Morgantown, West Virginia.

July 9:
Lunch at Hash Browns + New Grounds.
Depart for Baltimore, Maryland.

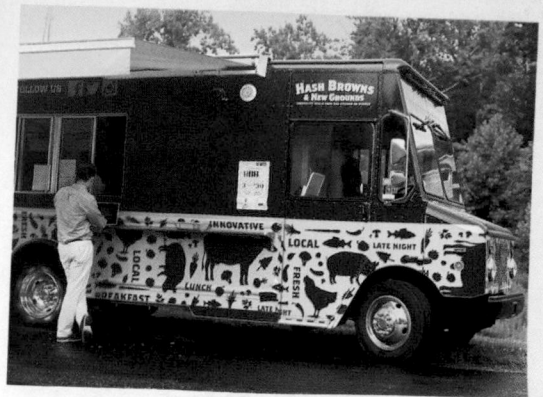

Hash Browns & New Grounds

625 North Street
Morgantown, West Virginia 26505
(304) 641-1215

You'd think a state with as many pick-ups as West Virginia would have more trucks of the food variety. Not so. "I'm the third food truck in the state, but hoping that West Virginia embraces the concept," says Hash Browns & New Grounds chef and owner Cody Thrasher. His Thrasher Taco is filled with barbecue chicken, mango, and kiwi, and is like a luau in your mouth. And his jalapeño gnocchi mac and cheese is so addictive, you'll regret tomorrow how much of this stuff you can't stop eating today. Best of all, his prices are embarrassingly cheap. "Every day I feature something on a stick—and it's just a buck," Cody says. To track Cody and his food truck, follow him on Twitter @ThrasherHBNG.

Thrasher Taco

This food truck specialty is a hearty mixture of spicy chicken and fresh fruit salsa.

BARBECUE CHICKEN AND SAUCE

2 garlic bulbs
¼ cup olive oil, divided
6 chicken leg quarters (6½ lb.)
1½ cups chopped onion
½ cup minced shallots
1½ cups ketchup
½ cup apple cider vinegar
1½ cups hot sauce
1 cup firmly packed light brown sugar
½ cup granulated sugar
½ cup Turkish red pepper flakes
½ cup light molasses
3 Tbsp. garlic powder
3 Tbsp. onion powder
2 Tbsp. kosher salt
16 (6-inch) corn tortillas
Kiwi-Mango Salsa (facing page)
Sesame Aïoli (facing page)
Sliced green onions (optional)

1. Prepare Barbecue Chicken and Sauce: Preheat oven to 425°. Cut off pointed end of garlic; place garlic on a piece of aluminum foil, and drizzle with 2 Tbsp. oil. Fold foil to seal.

2. Bake at 425° for 30 minutes; cool 30 minutes.

3. Reduce oven temperature to 400°. Heat remaining 2 Tbsp. oil in a large nonstick skillet over medium heat. Cook chicken quarters in hot oil, in 3 batches, 3 minutes on each side or until browned. Transfer chicken to a large roasting pan, reserving drippings in skillet. Squeeze pulp from garlic bulbs. Add garlic, onion, and shallots to drippings in skillet; sauté 5 minutes or until onion is tender. Stir in ketchup and apple cider vinegar, stirring to loosen browned bits from bottom of pan. Remove from heat.

4. Process hot sauce and next 7 ingredients in a blender; stir into ketchup mixture in skillet.

Remove and discard skin from chicken; return chicken, skinned side up, to baking pan. Pour sauce mixture over chicken. Cover with aluminum foil, and bake at 400° for 1½ hours or until chicken is very tender.

5. Remove chicken from sauce, reserving 1 cup sauce. Store remaining sauce in refrigerator, and reserve for another use. Cool chicken 15 minutes. Remove chicken from bones, and place in a bowl; discard bones. Skim fat from reserved sauce. Coarsely chop chicken.

6. Combine chicken and reserved 1 cup sauce in a large nonstick skillet. Cook over high heat 2 minutes or until slightly caramelized, stirring once.

7. Spoon ⅓ cup chicken mixture into each tortilla. Top each taco with 2 Tbsp. Kiwi-Mango Salsa and desired amount of Sesame Aïoli. Sprinkle with green onions, if desired. Serve immediately.
Makes: 8 servings
Note: We tested with Crystal Hot Sauce.

Kiwi-Mango Salsa

1½	Tbsp. minced fresh cilantro
1	Tbsp. fresh lime juice
1	Tbsp. white vinegar
1½	tsp. minced fresh ginger
1	tsp. sugar
1	tsp. tequila
½	tsp. kosher salt
⅓	cup finely chopped red onion
2	large kiwifruit, peeled and cut into ¼-inch cubes
1	large mango, peeled and cut into ¼-inch cubes

Stir together first 7 ingredients in a medium bowl. Add onion and remaining ingredients; toss gently. Cover and chill at least 8 hours or up to 18 hours. Makes: 8 servings

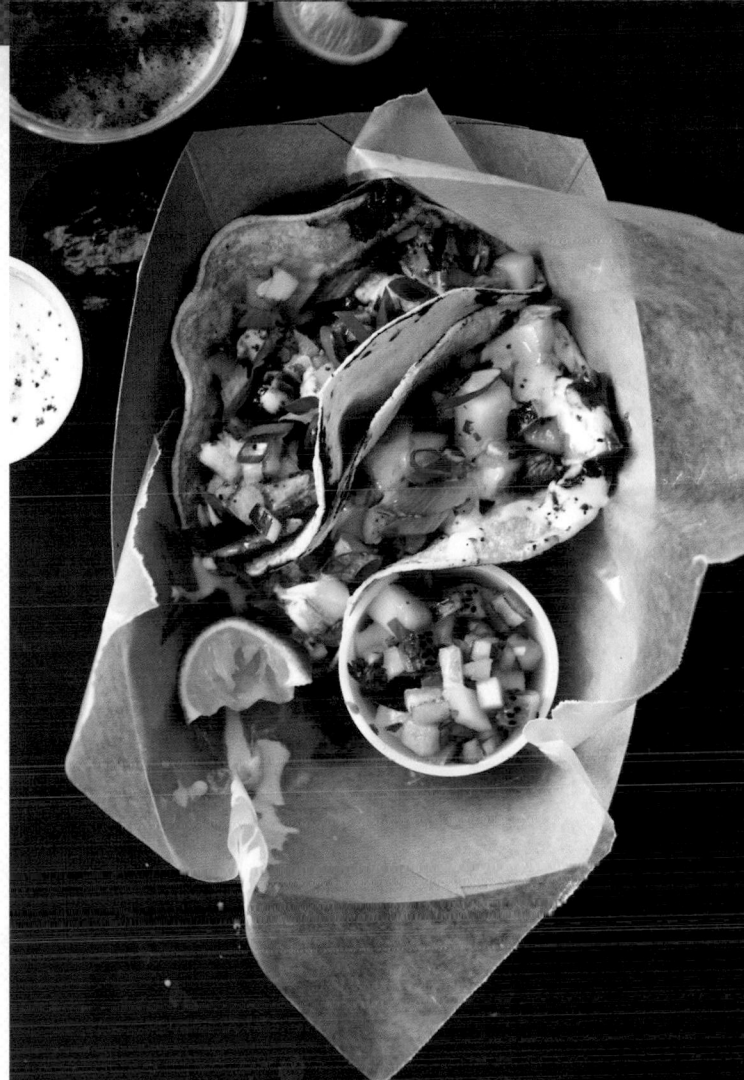

Sesame Aïoli

½	cup mayonnaise
¼	cup buttermilk
1½	tsp. dark sesame oil
1	tsp. Asian hot chili sauce (such as Sriracha)
1	tsp. honey
⅛	tsp. table salt
⅛	tsp. freshly ground black pepper

Whisk together all ingredients in a small bowl. Cover and chill 8 hours. Makes: about ¾ cup

Jalapeño Gnocchi Mac & Cheese

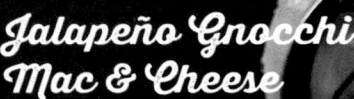

This creamy twist on mac and cheese really packs a punch.

- **3**   **Tbsp. butter, divided**
- **2**   **cups panko (Japanese breadcrumbs)**
- **2**   **(16-oz.) packages vacuum-packed gnocchi**
- **½**   **cup coarsely chopped seeded jalapeños (3 large)**
- **⅓**   **cup finely chopped shallots**
- **2**   **cups half-and-half**
- **1**   **(16-oz.) package processed cheese (such as Velveeta), cubed**
- **6½**   **oz. whole pepperoni sausage, diced**
- **Hot sauce (optional)**

1. Melt 2 Tbsp. butter in a medium skillet over medium-high heat. Add panko; cook, shaking pan often, 2 minutes or until toasted. Remove from heat.

2. Cook gnocchi according to package directions. Drain.

3. Meanwhile, melt remaining 1 Tbsp. butter in a Dutch oven over medium heat. Add jalapeños and shallots; sauté 4 to 5 minutes or until tender. Add half-and-half; bring to a simmer. Add cheese. Cook, stirring constantly, 5 minutes or until smooth. Stir in gnocchi and pepperoni. Cook, stirring constantly, 3 minutes or until thoroughly heated.

4. Spoon 1 cup cheese mixture into each of 8 bowls. Sprinkle each serving with ¼ cup crumb mixture. Serve with hot sauce, if desired.
Makes: 8 servings

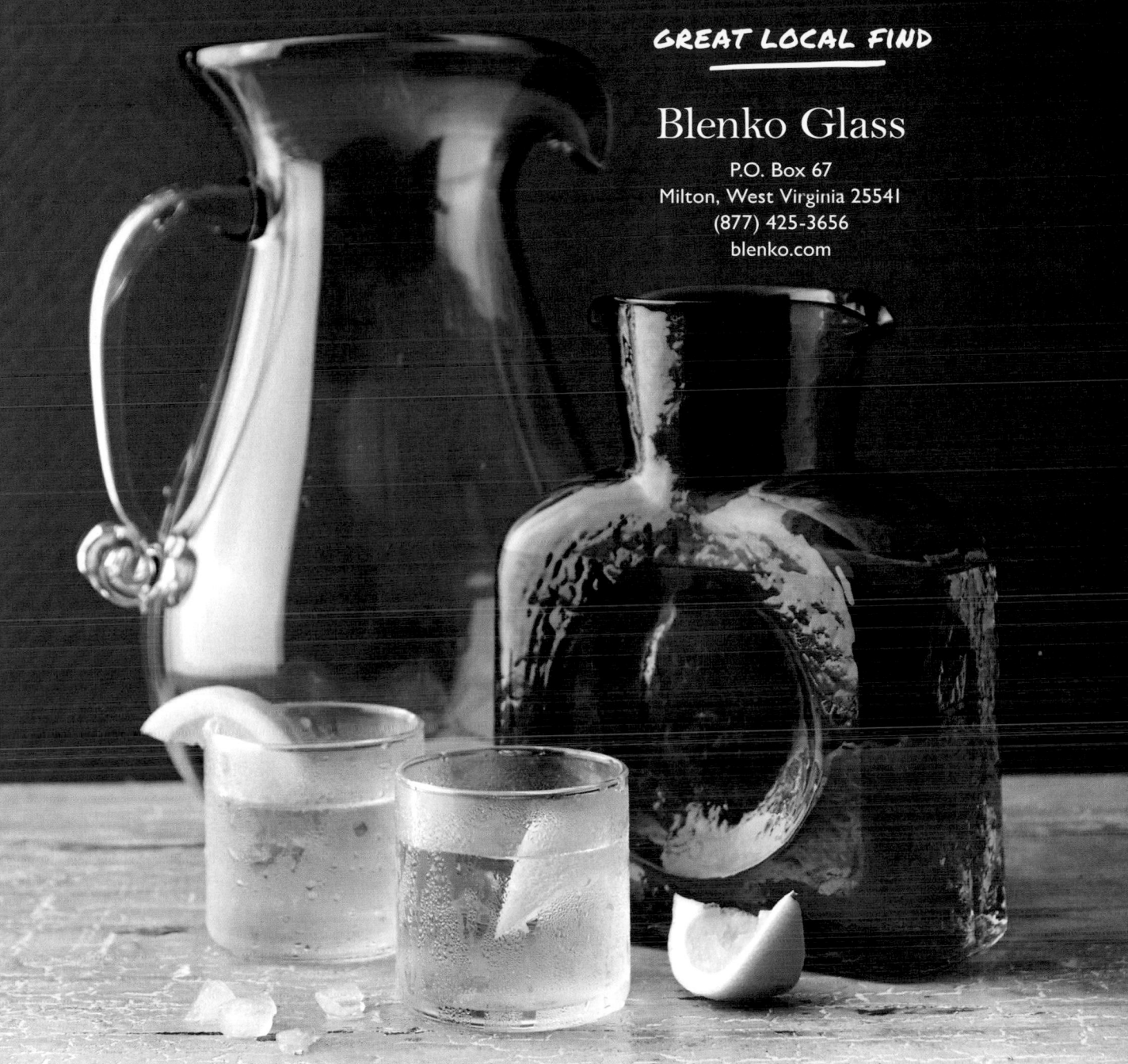

Glass is an ancient and reliable material. It doesn't leach toxins or melt in the sun like some plastics. It doesn't pollute our oceans, or leave any aftertastes when you use it to store your leftovers. That is why I think glass makes the best vessel for foods and drinks. Plus, it's beautiful and can last for lifetimes. For years, I've made stained glass windows using Blenko Glass from West Virginia. But the company also makes gorgeous glass bowls, pitchers, and limited-edition pieces. Check out the 384 water bottle, a masterpiece of color and functionality. Like Coca-Cola from the bottle, water tastes better when served from one of these sculptural pieces.

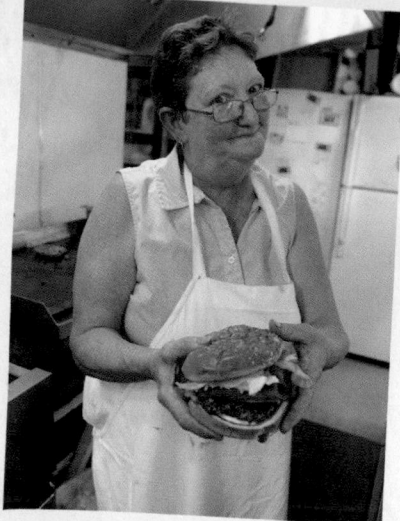

Jim's Drive In

Route 60 W, West Washington Street
Lewisburg, West Virginia 24901
(304) 645-2590

Some of the waitresses at this classic drive-in have worked here for more than 40 years. In fact, Jim's Drive In owner Katherine Massie waitressed for the restaurant in the 1960s. You can see her pay stub (a whopping $9.37) in the foyer if you get out of your car. Jim's still uses trays that hang in your car window, and they carry quite a load. The restaurant's Ranch Burger starts with a half-pound of ground chuck and is finished with red onion and grilled ham. It puts the average cheeseburger to shame. Jim's features barbecue sandwiches wrapped in wax paper. Deceptively simple and delicious, the barbecue is a snap to make if you can keep an eye on a boiling pot. Otherwise, take a cruise to Jim's Drive In, park with your sweetie, and try out the amazing service for yourself.

Kathy's Barbecue

Owner Kathy Massie usually tops this sweet and savory barbecue sandwich with coleslaw.

1	(5¼-lb.) bone-in pork shoulder (Boston butt), trimmed
2	cups ketchup
⅓	cup firmly packed light brown sugar
1	tsp. table salt
10	hamburger buns

1. Combine pork and water to cover in a large Dutch oven or stockpot. Bring to a boil; reduce heat, cover, and simmer 3 hours or until very tender; drain. Let stand until cool enough to handle.

2. Remove and discard bone and fat; pull meat apart into large pieces by hand. Transfer pork to a large bowl; stir in ketchup, brown sugar, and salt. Serve warm in buns. **Makes: 10 servings**

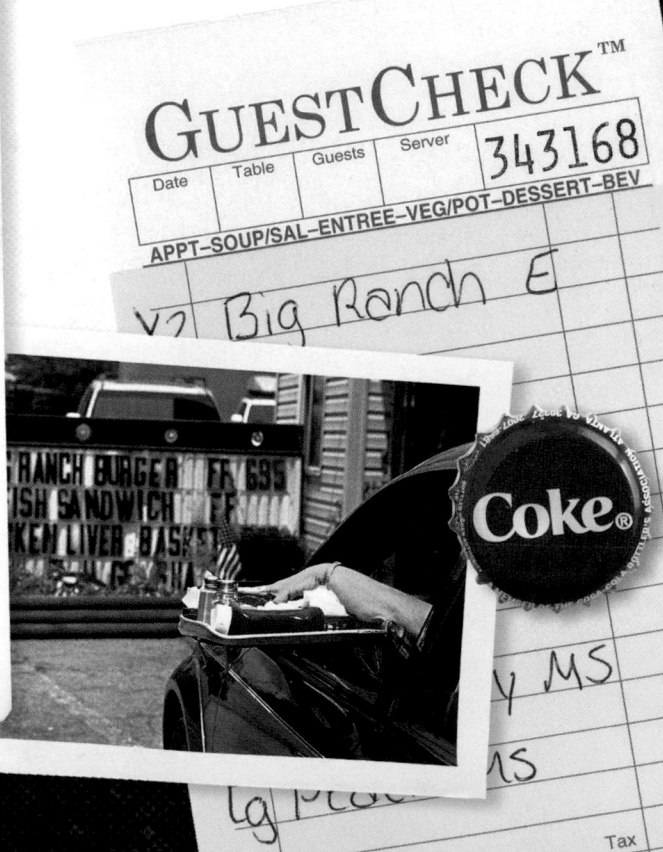

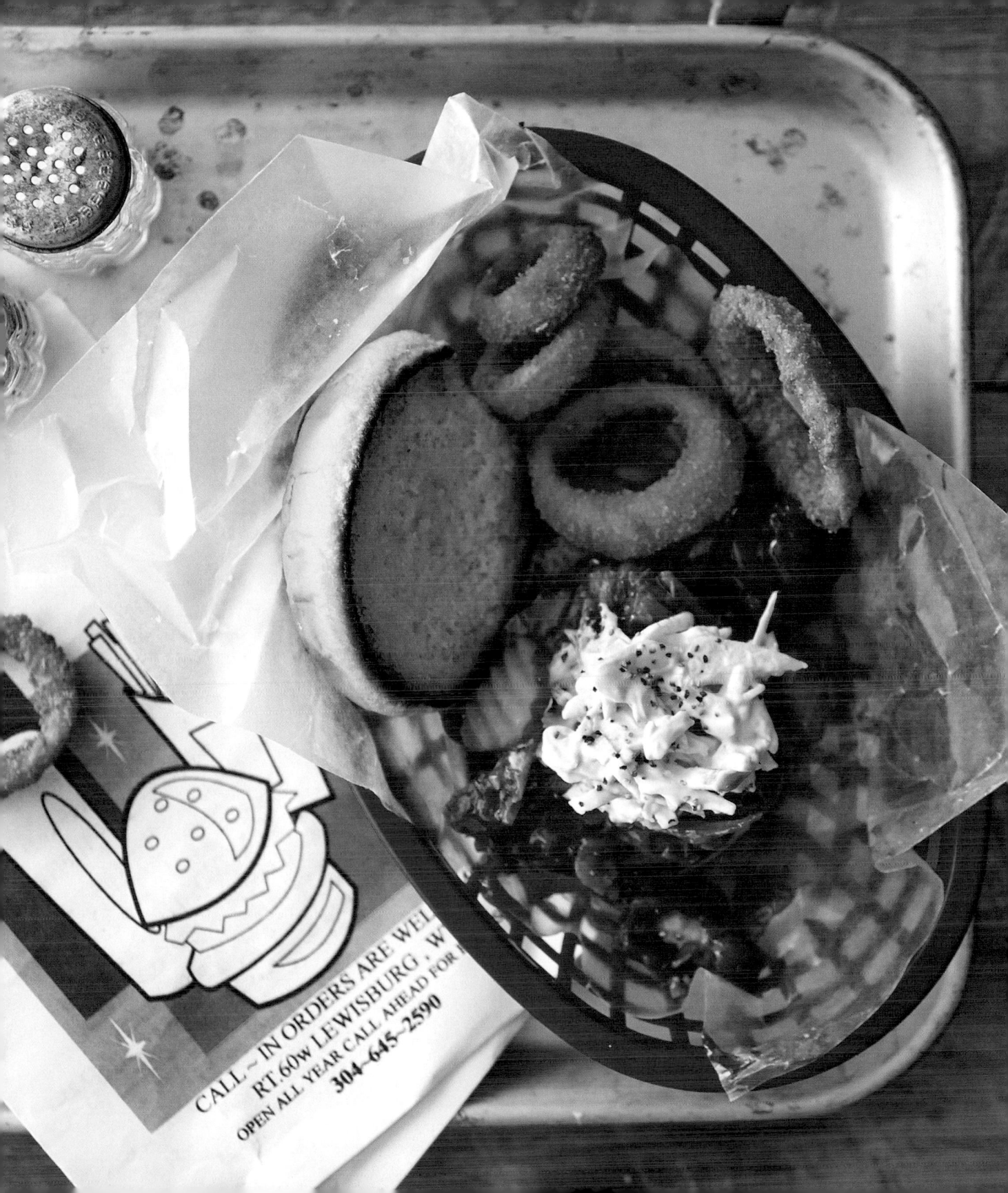

CALL – IN ORDERS ARE WEL
RT.60w LEWISBURG . W
OPEN ALL YEAR CALL AHEAD FOR
304-645-2590

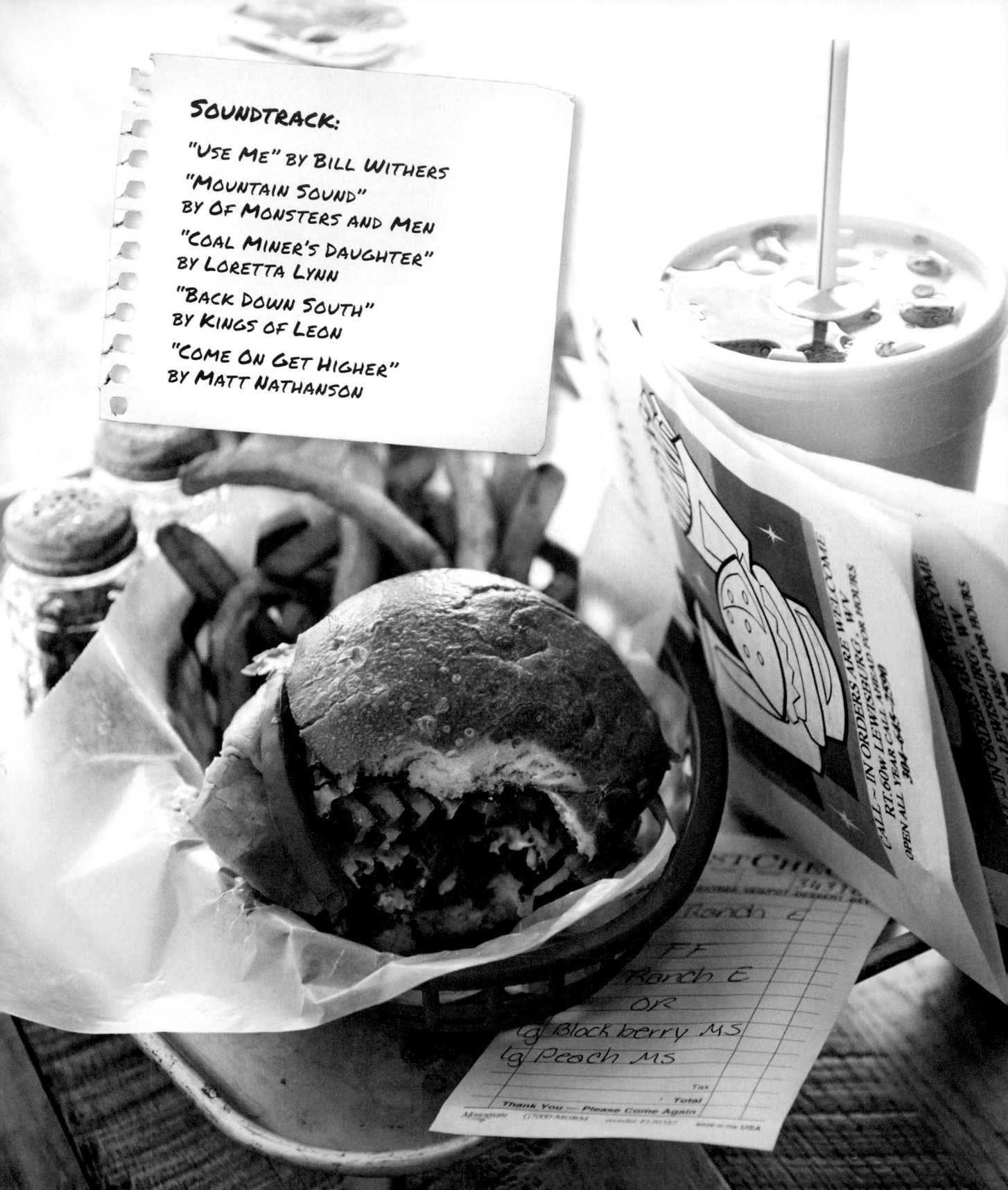

Ranch Burger

Slightly spicy, Jim's famous Ranch Burger is garnished with ham instead of bacon.

½	lb. ground chuck
¼	tsp. table salt
¼	tsp. freshly ground black pepper
1	Tbsp. butter, softened
1	(3-oz.) hamburger bun
1½	Tbsp. mayonnaise
1½	tsp. vegetable oil
2	slices processed American cheese
2	oz. thinly sliced ham
4	sweet pickle slices
2	Tbsp. pickled sliced jalapeños (optional)
1	thin tomato slice
1	thin red onion slice
1	iceberg lettuce leaf

Wax paper

1. Shape beef into a 5-inch patty, about ¾ inch thick; sprinkle both sides with salt and pepper. Spread butter on cut sides of bun. Heat a medium cast-iron skillet over medium-high heat. Add bun halves to skillet, cut sides down. Cook 1 to 2 minutes or until toasted. Transfer to a plate; spread mayonnaise on cut sides of toasted bun.

2. Heat oil in skillet; add beef patty. Cook 4 minutes on each side for medium or until desired degree of doneness. Top patty with cheese during last minute of cooking; place on bun bottom. Add ham to skillet; cook 1 to 2 minutes or until lightly browned, turning once.

3. Top patty with pickle slices and, if desired, jalapeño slices. Layer ham, tomato slice, onion slice, and lettuce on sandwich. Cover with bun top. Wrap sandwich in wax paper. Let stand 2 minutes before serving. **Makes: 1 serving**

West Virginia bucket list
things to see and do (besides eat) here

1 Try your hand at fly-fishing, archery, or even falconry at **The Greenbrier** in White Sulphur Springs.

2 Take a drive over the **New River Gorge Bridge** *(pictured)*, one of the world's longest steel single-span arch bridges on Route 19 near Fayetteville.

3 Stroll through the historic section of **Harpers Ferry**, one of the most fought-over spots of the Civil War.

4 Shop the gorgeous artisan Appalachian crafts and art at **Tamarack** in Beckley.

5 Hop aboard the **Durbin & Greenbrier Valley Railroad** for a vintage railcar excursion and see the Appalachian scenery from the tracks.

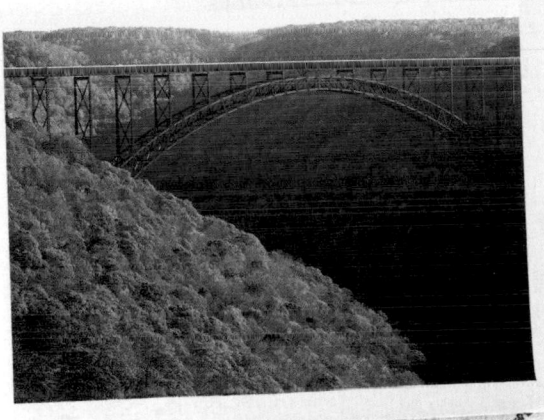

Where to Rest and Recharge

I know, I know—a lot of penny pinchers say, "Oh, you're only going to sleep there" as an excuse to brown-bag their accommodations. Don't make that mistake. A hotel can make or break your vacation. Like most people, I've stayed in some hotels that I'd rather forget; places where I've thrown a towel down before I've taken off my shoes and socks; places that still have the dreaded bedspread, and quite possibly haven't washed it since the first Bush administration.

The problem is, it's hard to spot these hotels on the Internet. Every hotel looks wonderful online. The Internet, with its pretty pictures, can make the Buckatunna Best Western look comparable to New York's Waldorf Astoria. Then you get there and find out your room is as big as a can of tuna. Not good.

The good news is I've stayed in all of the hotels listed here, and they are all excellent, in vastly different ways. Some are inns, some are resorts. Some cost $100 a night. Others can soar to ten times that amount. Yet each is special and speaks to its community. That's important. In our age, we can motor from one end of the country to another, and every interstate hotel looks vaguely the same. Not these—each is different, each is special, and each will leave you with a memory worth the price.

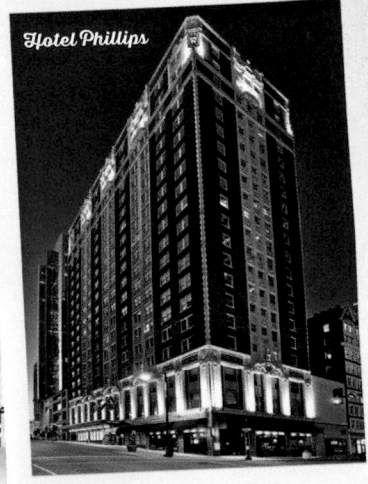

Alabama

The Tutwiler Hotel
2021 Park Place
Birmingham, Alabama 35203
(205) 322-2100
hamptoninn.hilton.com $

The Tutwiler Hotel is a name long associated with the Magic City, and it remains the most lauded historic hotel in Birmingham (it's listed as a National Historic Landmark). Today, you can stay at many new luxury and mid-luxury hotels in Alabama's largest city, but none boast the architectural beauty of the Tutwiler. Best of all, the hotel is now a Hampton Inn, which means excellent service and cleanliness at a modest price point.

Arkansas

Inn at the Mill
3906 Johnson Mill Blvd.
Springdale, Arkansas 72762
(479) 443-1800
innatthemill.com $

Not only can you eat a superb meal here, but Inn at the Mill also sports 46 gorgeous guest rooms on an absolutely stunning property. With rates starting below $100, the value here is well worth the drive. Large rooms and an incredible staff round out the experience. The Mill is close to a number of Arkansas attractions, including the University of Arkansas, the Walton Arts Center, and the gorgeous Ozarks.

Florida

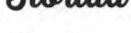

One Ocean Resort & Spa
1 Ocean Blvd.
Atlantic Beach, Florida 32233
(904) 249-7402
oneoceanresort.com $$$$

South Florida is known for its resorts ranging from the Biltmore Hotel in Miami to The Breakers in Palm Beach. But northern Florida's One Ocean Resort & Spa gives those grande dames a run for their money. Finished in 2008, this posh boutique resort boasts the elegance of a Ritz-Carlton but the intimacy of a smaller property. With an impressive art collection, spa, and location on the beach, One Ocean makes a superb spot to hang out and get creative.

Georgia

Mansion on Forsyth Park
700 Drayton Street
Savannah, Georgia 31401
(912) 238-5158
mansiononforsythpark.com $$

Gorgeous is the only way to describe this Victorian mansion. The vast art collection, luxurious appointments, outstanding restaurant, and excellent location make this one of my favorite spots in the state. Not only does the hotel have a killer spa, but its restaurant, 700 Drayton, is also worth the splurge. Note that during wedding season, this place gets covered up with parties galore, which may be a good thing if your crasher skills are up to the task.

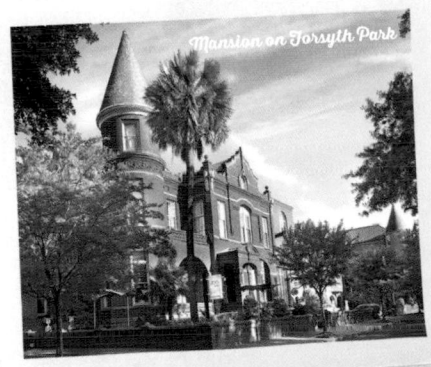

Price Guide: *Hotel rates vary by season, day of the week, and events in town. Still, on average, for each dollar symbol listed, assume about $100 per night for a double-occupancy room. Want a bargain? Ask for off-season dates, check for discounts, and join the hotel's e-mail list. Often the best rates go to the most loyal customers.*

Kentucky

Gratz Park Inn
120 West Second Street
Lexington, Kentucky 40507
(859) 231-1777
gratzparkinn.com $$

I'm a dog person, so I love that I can take my furry buddy to this historic hotel. Leave it to horse country to have such a generous pet policy at one of the city's finest hotels. From the comfortable lobby to the spacious and well-appointed rooms, the Gratz Park Inn doesn't nickel and dime guests to death. Don't you hate it when you have to pay $14.99 a night for WI-FI in a hotel that already charges a hefty room premium? None of that here. Both parking and Internet are free at this lovely spot.

Louisiana

Windsor Court Hotel
300 Gravier Street
New Orleans, Louisiana 70130
(504) 523-6000
windsorcourthotel.com $

New Orleans is a French town. So what is a hotel bearing the most English of all names doing here? That's NOLA, a mixture of just about everywhere and everything. And the Windsor Court, befitting its name, pampers its guests in regal style. Huge rooms, an incredible wine selection, a lobby with pressed papers hanging on wooden rods, a museum-quality art collection, and a location just steps from the French Quarter make the Windsor Court one of the finest places to lie your head in the Big Easy.

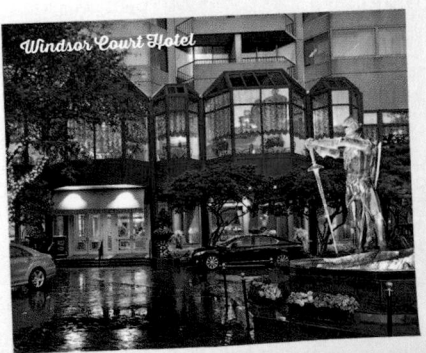

Maryland

Robert Morris Inn
314 North Morris Street
Oxford, Maryland 21654
(410) 226-5111
robertmorrisinn.com $

Named for the financier of the American Revolution, the Robert Morris Inn remains steeped in history. It's located in tiny Oxford, one of Maryland's oldest towns, right next to one of the oldest ferries on this continent. Step inside and you'll feel like you've stepped back in time 400 years. The slate floors, wide-plank walls, and 300-year-old main staircase are worn like a loved walking stick. Things are crooked here and there and you won't find modern amenities—if you want pay-per-view, head to a hotel in Easton. Yet for charm and a warm welcome, this is where to be.

Missouri

Hotel Phillips
106 West 12th Street
Kansas City, Missouri 64105
(877) 704-5341
hotelphillips.com $$

When it comes to classic cars and posh hotels, I love the Art Deco period. And there's just something about pulling up next to the welcoming awning of this Kansas City belle that makes one feel, well, glamorous. The Hotel Phillips has a formal exterior but oddly relaxed feel—like a woman in a ball gown who has slipped off her high heels. Step into the swanky lobby, grab a drink at the bar, and head upstairs to the Crystal Ballroom to admire the Jazz Age details. Or simply make for your room—most defy old-hotel style with wild colors and cool textiles. It's all part of the Phillips' charm.

North Carolina

Proximity Hotel
704 Green Valley Road
Greensboro, North Carolina 27408
(336) 379-8200
proximityhotel.com $$$

Walk into the Proximity Hotel and you'll probably notice the striking lobby and the modern decor. But what you may not realize is that this hotel is the first certified LEED Platinum by the U.S. Green Building Council in the United States. With its 100 solar rooftop panels that heat the hotel's water to elevators that actually generate electricity, the Proximity stands as one of the most eco-conscious hotels in the country.

Oklahoma

Skirvin Hilton Hotel
One Park Avenue
Oklahoma City, Oklahoma 73102
(405) 272-3040
skirvinhilton.com $$

For more than a century, the Skirvin has defined elegance in Oklahoma City. The hotel closed in 1988, but a public-private partnership by the city and developers invested $51 million into a renovation, and the grand hotel is grander than ever. From the Red Piano Lounge to the excellent rooms, the hotel leaves a lasting impression. Some locals might say too long—NBA players have blamed losses to the Oklahoma City Thunder on "haunted" stays here. So long as you're not trying to beat the OKC team, you should be fine.

South Carolina

Wentworth Mansion
149 Wentworth Street
Charleston, South Carolina 29401
(888) 466-1886
wentworthmansion.com $$$

The beauty of Charleston lies in its history. You can't swing an old lady pocket book in this town without hitting some sort of antique. So when you visit, don't just bunk in any modern hotel. The huge Wentworth Mansion was once a private residence to a cotton farming family and if you look carefully at the tile in the foyer, you'll see delicate cotton bulbs depicted there. The rooms are simply splendid, with extravagant beds and spacious bathrooms. Be sure to climb to the cupola for breathtaking views of the city.

Tennessee

Hutton Hotel
1808 West End Avenue
Nashville, Tennessee 37203
(615) 340-9333
huttonhotel.com $$

I'll admit it: I've always liked to abscond with hotel bath soaps and miniature shampoos. At the top of any traveler pirate's frothy bounty sits the Hutton's Molton Brown bath products. Their understated luxury fits right in at the Hutton, which is one of those hotels that doesn't need to trumpet their service, location, and style. Everything here is done well, with minimal pretense but maximum attention to detail. Two things stand out as truly Nashville— the bar (where people-watching could be an Olympic sport) and the fact that you can have exercise equipment in your room. I mean, you gotta get your workout in before hitting Broadway, right?

Price Guide: *Hotel rates vary by season, day of the week, and events in town. Still, on average, for each dollar symbol listed, assume about $100 per night for a double-occupancy room. Want a bargain? Ask for off-season dates, check for discounts, and join the hotel's e-mail list. Often the best rates go to the most loyal customers.*

Texas

Hotel Lumen
6101 Hillcrest Avenue
Dallas, Texas 75205
(214) 219-2400
hotellumen.com **$$**

Not everything in Texas is big. This boutique hotel is just the right size. It's so modern and feels vastly more expensive than your statement will read upon checkout. Plus, the Lumen is close to the George W. Bush Presidential Library, Highland Park Village, and a host of fabulous shopping. Don't let all the posh appointments and swimming pool that looks as if it's never seen a floaty, put you off. This is a friendly place. The staff genuinely cares about you and will make every effort to ensure your comfort. I'm betting they'd even find you a floaty if you ask.

Virginia

Keswick Hall
701 Club Drive
Keswick, Virginia 22947
(434) 979-3440
keswick.com **$$$$**

Decorated in what I call "grand Southern baroque," Keswick Hall is America's answer to Downton Abbey. It is a repository of polished silver, gleaming furniture, and plenty of Mr. Carsons to keep you full of sherry and port. The majestic 48-room mansion commands 600 acres of

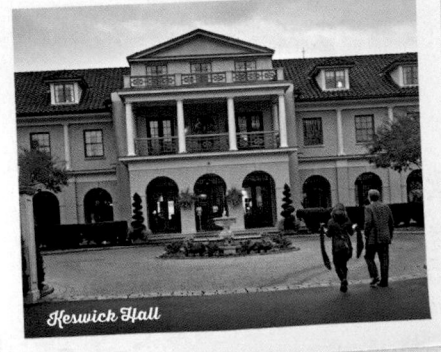

Keswick Hall

prime Virginia real estate, and has a long history dating back to a fine Alabamian named Robert Crawford. The estate became a country club after many years of private ownership, and in 1993 was converted into the elegant hotel. That splendor doesn't come cheap, but I say if you're going to go to debtor's prison, at least do it with style.

West Virginia

Stonewall Resort
940 Resort Drive
Roanoke, West Virginia 26447
(888) 278-8150
stonewallresort.com **$**

Take a wine tour, play a round of golf, head out on the lake, or simply relax in the spa—it's all available at this large, family resort in Roanoke. The hotel has a long list of activities, ranging from hiking and fishing to Segway tours. Perhaps that's because Charleston is an hour-and-a-half away and most of the original town of Roanoke is, um, well, under the lake. No matter, the Stonewall Resort (named for Confederate General Stonewall Jackson, who was from the region) makes a wonderful escape from the bustle of urban life.

Metric Equivalents

The recipes that appear in this cookbook use the standard U.S. method for measuring liquid and dry or solid ingredients (teaspoons, tablespoons, and cups). The information in the following charts is provided to help cooks outside the United States successfully use these recipes. All equivalents are approximate.

Metric Equivalents for Different Types of Ingredients

A standard cup measure of a dry or solid ingredient will vary in weight depending on the type of ingredient. A standard cup of liquid is the same volume for any type of liquid. Use the following chart when converting standard cup measures to grams (weight) or milliliters (volume).

Standard Cup	Fine Powder (ex. flour)	Grain (ex. rice)	Granular (ex. sugar)	Liquid Solids (ex. butter)	Liquid (ex. milk)
1	140 g	150 g	190 g	200 g	240 ml
3/4	105 g	113 g	143 g	150 g	180 ml
2/3	93 g	100 g	125 g	133 g	160 ml
1/2	70 g	75 g	95 g	100 g	120 ml
1/3	47 g	50 g	63 g	67 g	80 ml
1/4	35 g	38 g	48 g	50 g	60 ml
1/8	18 g	19 g	24 g	25 g	30 ml

Useful Equivalents for Liquid Ingredients by Volume

1/4 tsp				=	1 ml
1/2 tsp				=	2 ml
1 tsp				=	5 ml
3 tsp	= 1 Tbsp		= 1/2 fl oz	=	15 ml
	2 Tbsp	= 1/8 cup	= 1 fl oz	=	30 ml
	4 Tbsp	= 1/4 cup	= 2 fl oz	=	60 ml
	5 1/3 Tbsp	= 1/3 cup	= 3 fl oz	=	80 ml
	8 Tbsp	= 1/2 cup	= 4 fl oz	=	120 ml
	10 2/3 Tbsp	= 2/3 cup	= 5 fl oz	=	160 ml
	12 Tbsp	= 3/4 cup	= 6 fl oz	=	180 ml
	16 Tbsp	= 1 cup	= 8 fl oz	=	240 ml
	1 pt	= 2 cups	= 16 fl oz	=	480 ml
	1 qt	= 4 cups	= 32 fl oz	=	960 ml
			33 fl oz	=	1000 ml = 1 l

Useful Equivalents for Dry Ingredients by Weight

(To convert ounces to grams, multiply the number of ounces by 30.)

1 oz	=	1/16 lb	=	30 g
4 oz	=	1/4 lb	=	120 g
8 oz	=	1/2 lb	=	240 g
12 oz	=	3/4 lb	=	360 g
16 oz	=	1 lb	=	480 g

Useful Equivalents for Length

(To convert inches to centimeters, multiply the number of inches by 2.5.)

1 in			=	2.5 cm		
6 in	= 1/2 ft		=	15 cm		
12 in	= 1 ft		=	30 cm		
36 in	= 3 ft	= 1 yd	=	90 cm		
40 in			=	100 cm	=	1 m

Useful Equivalents for Cooking/Oven Temperatures

	Fahrenheit	Celsius	Gas Mark
Freeze water	32° F	0° C	
Room temp	68° F	20° C	
Boil water	212° F	100° C	
Bake	325° F	160° C	3
	350° F	180° C	4
	375° F	190° C	5
	400° F	200° C	6
	425° F	220° C	7
	450° F	230° C	8
Broil			Grill

Index

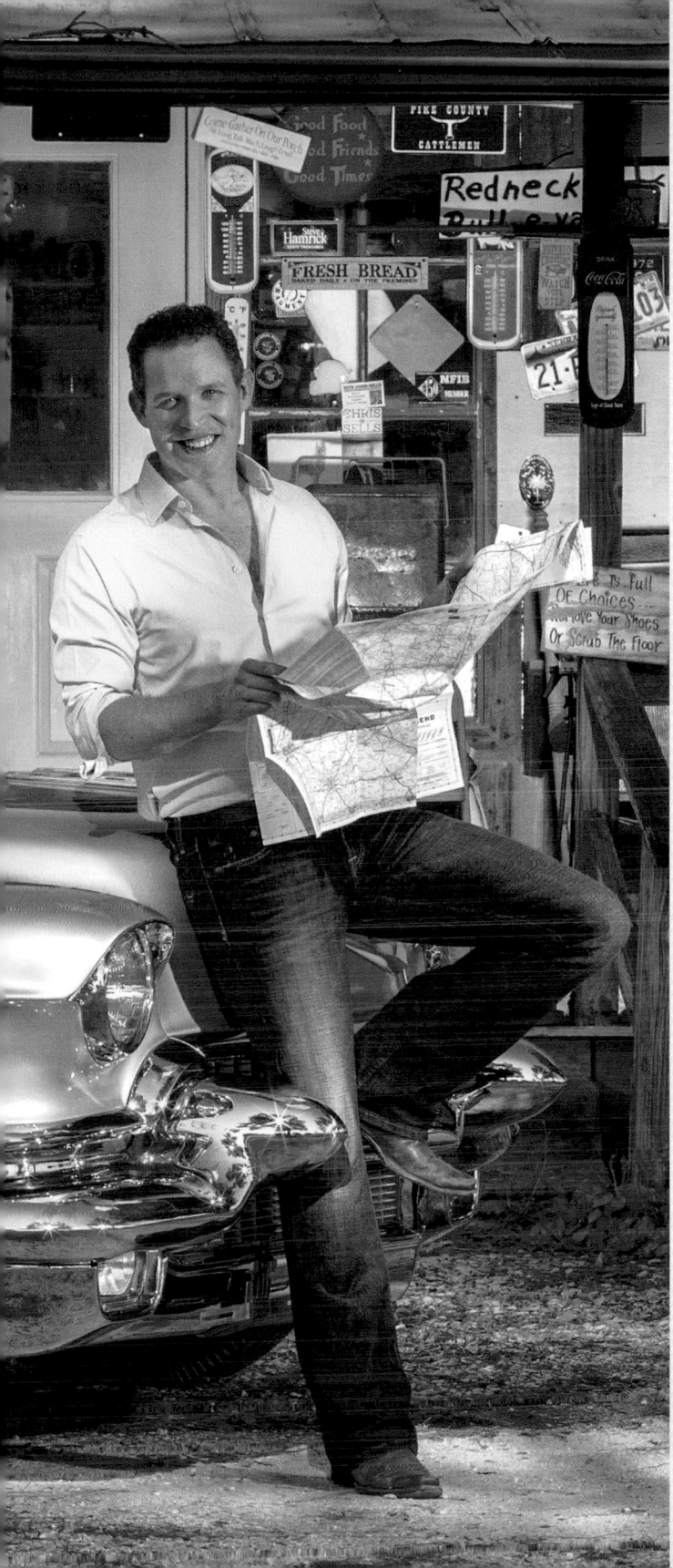

People I owe some pie:

I'm grateful to my colleagues at Oxmoor House, *Southern Living* magazine, and Time Inc.: Margot Schupf, Sid Evans, and Felicity Keane. Thanks, also, to the Oxmoor House Test Kitchen for figuring how to break down recipes that started with 20 gallons of chicken stock or a pound of butter. This book would not be possible without the team at Murphy Media: Nordan Dembitsky, Mike Murphy, Anne Adams, Kristen Ellis, Erin Brown, Kaitlin Alexander, Nushy Rose, and Alex Krook. Lastly, and most importantly, I am deeply indebted to, and humbled by, those restaurateurs who dedicate themselves to feeding their communities and enriching our lives with their creativity in the kitchen.

About Morgan Murphy

The author ventures to 100-plus restaurants annually and has appeared on the Travel Channel, *TODAY*, *Fox & Friends*, and Sirius/XM. Morgan has contributed to *Vanity Fair*, *Forbes*, *Esquire*, and *Southern Living*.

He is a graduate of the University of Oxford and serves as a commander in the U.S. Navy Reserve, where he is assigned to the chairman of the Joint Chiefs of Staff. Commander (sel.) Murphy is a veteran of the war in Afghanistan, where he was awarded the Defense Meritorious Service Medal and the Afghanistan Campaign Medal, among others.

Other books by Morgan Murphy:
Bourbon & Bacon, *Off the Eaten Path: Second Helpings*, *Off the Eaten Path*, and *I Love You, Now Hush*

ISBN 10: 0-8487-4444-6
ISBN 13: 978-0-8487-4444-1
Library of Congress Control Number: 2015932678

Printed in the United States of America
First Printing 2015

Oxmoor House
Creative Director: Felicity Keane
Art Director: Christopher Rhoads
Executive Photography Director: Iain Bagwell
Executive Food Director: Grace Parisi
Managing Editor: Elizabeth Tyler Austin
Assistant Managing Editor: Jeanne de Lathouder

Off the Eaten Path: On The Road Again

Editor: Sarah A. Gleim
Project Editor: Emily Chappell Connolly
Editorial Assistant: April Smitherman
Senior Designer: Melissa Clark
Assistant Designer: Allison Sperando Potter
Assistant Test Kitchen Manager:
    Alyson Moreland Haynes
Recipe Developers and Testers: Stefanie Maloney,
    Callie Nash, Karen Rankin
Food Stylists: Nathan Carrabba, Victoria E. Cox,
    Margaret Monroe Dickey, Catherine Crowell Steele
Photo Editor: Kellie Lindsey
Senior Photographer: Hélène Dujardin
Senior Photo Stylists: Kay E. Clarke,
    Mindi Shapiro Levine
Senior Production Manager: Sue Chodakiewicz
Assistant Production Manager: Diane Rose Keener

Contributors
Writer: Morgan Murphy
Executive Editor: Katherine Cobbs
Copy Editor: Donna Baldone
Proofreaders: Lauren Brooks, Adrienne Davis
Indexer: Mary Ann Laurens
Fellows: Laura Arnold, Kylie Dazzo, Nicole Fisher,
    Loren Lorenzo, Anna Ramia, Caroline Smith,
    Amanda Widis
Recipe Developers and Testers: Leah Van Deren,
    Tamara Goldis, R.D.
Recipe Editor: Julie Christopher
Food Stylist: Ana Kelly
Photographer: Art Meripol (front cover)
Photo Stylists: Mary Clayton Carl,
    Missie Neville Crawford

Time Home Entertainment Inc.
Publisher: Margot Schupf
Vice President, Finance: Vandana Patel
Executive Director, Marketing Services: Carol Pittard
Publishing Director: Megan Pearlman
Assistant General Counsel: Simone Procas

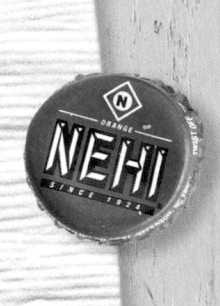

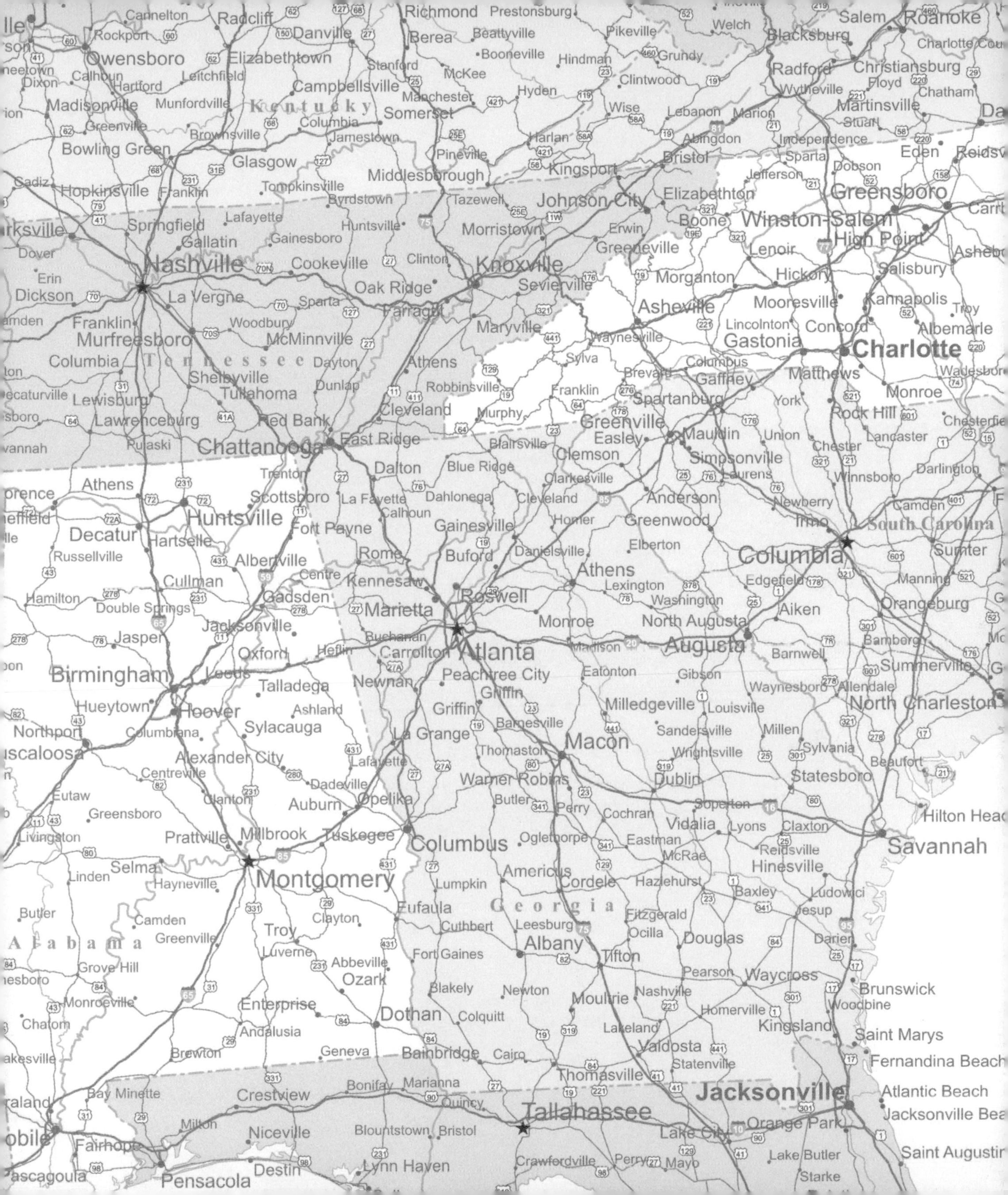
Kentucky
Tennessee
Alabama
Georgia
South Carolina
Cannelton
Radcliff
Richmond
Prestonsburg
Welch
Salem
Roanoke
Rockport
Owensboro
Danville
Berea
Beattyville
Pikeville
Blacksburg
Elizabethtown
Booneville
Hindman
Grundy
Radford
Christiansburg
Charlotte Court
Calhoun
Dixon
Leitchfield
Stanford
McKee
Clintwood
Floyd
Hartford
Campbellsville
Hyden
Wytheville
Chatham
Madisonville
Munfordville
Manchester
Somerset
Wise
Lebanon
Marion
Martinsville
Greenville
Columbia
Stuart
Brownsville
Jamestown
Harlan
Abingdon
Independence
Bowling Green
Pineville
Sparta
Eden
Glasgow
Bristol
Dobson
Kingsport
Jefferson
Middlesborough
Cadiz
Hopkinsville
Franklin
Tompkinsville
Byrdstown
Tazewell
Johnson City
Elizabethton
Greensboro
Springfield
Lafayette
Huntsville
Morristown
Boone
Winston-Salem
High Point
Dover
Gallatin
Gainesboro
Erwin
Greeneville
Lenoir
Nashville
Cookeville
Clinton
Knoxville
Hickory
Salisbury
Erin
Dickson
La Vergne
Sparta
Oak Ridge
Sevierville
Morganton
Farragut
Asheville
Mooresville
Kannapolis
Troy
Murfreesboro
Woodbury
Maryville
Waynesville
Lincolnton
Concord
Albemarle
McMinnville
Gastonia
Charlotte
Columbia
Dayton
Athens
Sylva
Columbus
Shelbyville
Brevard
Gaffney
Matthews
Wadesboro
Tullahoma
Dunlap
Robbinsville
Franklin
Spartanburg
York
Monroe
Lewisburg
Cleveland
Murphy
Rock Hill
Chesterfield
Lawrenceburg
Red Bank
Greenville
Mauldin
Union
Lancaster
Easley
Chester
Pulaski
Chattanooga
East Ridge
Blairsville
Clemson
Simpsonville
Trenton
Dalton
Blue Ridge
Laurens
Winnsboro
Darlington
Athens
Clarkesville
Florence
Scottsboro
La Fayette
Dahlonega
Cleveland
Anderson
Newberry
Camden
Calhoun
Huntsville
Fort Payne
Homer
Greenwood
Irmo
Decatur
Hartselle
Gainesville
Elberton
Russellville
Rome
Buford
Danielsville
Columbia
Sumter
Albertville
Centre
Athens
Cullman
Kennesaw
Lexington
Edgefield
Manning
Hamilton
Gadsden
Roswell
Washington
Aiken
Orangeburg
Double Springs
Marietta
Monroe
North Augusta
Jacksonville
Jasper
Buchanan
Madison
Augusta
Bamberg
Oxford
Heflin
Carrollton
Atlanta
Barnwell
Birmingham
Leeds
Eatonton
Gibson
Summerville
Talladega
Newnan
Peachtree City
Waynesboro
Allendale
Hueytown
Griffin
Milledgeville
Louisville
North Charleston
Hoover
Ashland
Barnesville
Sandersville
Millen
Northport
Columbiana
Sylacauga
La Grange
Tuscaloosa
Thomaston
Macon
Wrightsville
Sylvania
Alexander City
Lafayette
Beaufort
Centreville
Warner Robins
Dublin
Statesboro
Dadeville
Eutaw
Clanton
Auburn
Opelika
Butler
Perry
Soperton
Greensboro
Cochran
Hilton Head
Livingston
Prattville
Millbrook
Tuskegee
Vidalia
Lyons
Claxton
Columbus
Oglethorpe
Eastman
Reidsville
Savannah
Selma
McRae
Hinesville
Linden
Hayneville
Montgomery
Lumpkin
Americus
Cordele
Hazlehurst
Baxley
Ludowici
Eufaula
Jesup
Butler
Clayton
Fitzgerald
Camden
Cuthbert
Leesburg
Ocilla
Douglas
Darien
Troy
Greenville
Albany
Luverne
Tifton
Fort Gaines
Abbeville
Grove Hill
Pearson
Waycross
Brunswick
Ozark
Blakely
Newton
Nashville
Woodbine
Monroeville
Moultrie
Enterprise
Homerville
Dothan
Colquitt
Kingsland
Chatom
Andalusia
Lakeland
Saint Marys
Valdosta
Brewton
Geneva
Bainbridge
Cairo
Statenville
Fernandina Beach
Thomasville
Bonifay
Marianna
Bay Minette
Crestview
Quincy
Jacksonville
Atlantic Beach
Tallahassee
Jacksonville Beach
Milton
Niceville
Blountstown
Bristol
Lake City
Orange Park
Mobile
Fairhope
Lake Butler
Saint Augustine
Crawfordville
Perry
Mayo
Destin
Lynn Haven
Pascagoula
Pensacola
Starke

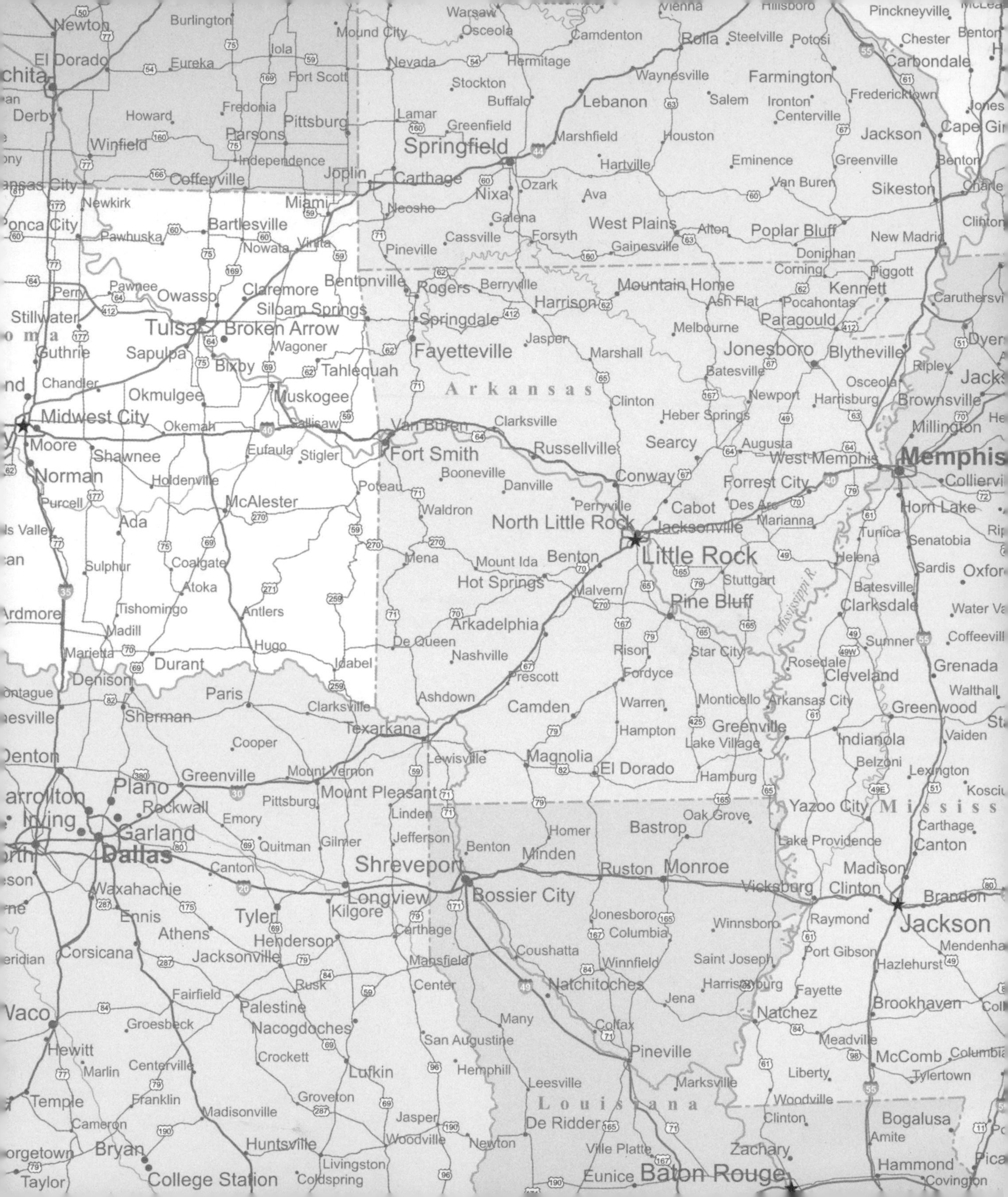

Newton
Burlington
El Dorado
Eureka
Iola
Fort Scott
Derby
Howard
Fredonia
Pittsburg
Winfield
Parsons
Independence
Coffeyville
Joplin
Carthage
Warsaw
Osceola
Mound City
Nevada
Hermitage
Camdenton
Stockton
Buffalo
Lamar
Greenfield
Springfield
Marshfield
Lebanon
Rolla
Steelville
Potosi
Waynesville
Salem
Farmington
Houston
Ironton
Centerville
Fredericktown
Jackson
Cape Gi
Hartville
Eminence
Greenville
Benton
Sikeston
Van Buren
Carbondale
Chester
Pinckneyville
Newkirk
Ponca City
Miami
Bartlesville
Pawhuska
Nowata
Vinita
Neosho
Nixa
Ozark
Ava
Galena
Cassville
Forsyth
West Plains
Alton
Poplar Bluff
Gainesville
Doniphan
New Madrid
Pineville
Perry
Pawnee
Owasso
Claremore
Bentonville
Rogers
Berryville
Harrison
Mountain Home
Ash Flat
Corning
Piggott
Pocahontas
Kennett
Paragould
Stillwater
Siloam Springs
Springdale
Tulsa
Broken Arrow
Guthrie
Sapulpa
Wagoner
Fayetteville
Jasper
Marshall
Melbourne
Jonesboro
Blytheville
Bixby
Tahlequah
Chandler
Batesville
Ripley
Okmulgee
Muskogee
Arkansas
Clinton
Newport
Osceola
Harrisburg
Brownsville
Midwest City
Okemah
Sallisaw
Van Buren
Clarksville
Heber Springs
Millington
Moore
Shawnee
Eufaula
Stigler
Fort Smith
Russellville
Searcy
Augusta
West Memphis
Memphis
Collierville
Norman
Holdenville
Booneville
Danville
Conway
Forrest City
Poteau
Purcell
McAlester
Waldron
Perryville
Cabot
Des Arc
Marianna
Horn Lake
North Little Rock
Jacksonville
Tunica
Senatobia
Ada
Mena
Mount Ida
Benton
Little Rock
Helena
Sardis
Oxford
Sulphur
Coalgate
Hot Springs
Stuttgart
Atoka
Malvern
Pine Bluff
Batesville
Ardmore
Tishomingo
Antlers
Arkadelphia
Clarksdale
Madill
Hugo
De Queen
Rison
Star City
Sumner
Marietta
Durant
Idabel
Nashville
Mississippi R.
Rosedale
Grenada
Denison
Prescott
Fordyce
Cleveland
Paris
Ashdown
Camden
Warren
Monticello
Arkansas City
Sherman
Clarksville
Greenwood
Texarkana
Hampton
Greenville
Lake Village
Indianola
Cooper
Lewisville
Magnolia
El Dorado
Hamburg
Belzoni
Lexington
Denton
Greenville
Mount Vernon
Mount Pleasant
Plano
Rockwall
Pittsburg
Linden
Oak Grove
Yazoo City
Bastrop
Irving
Garland
Emory
Jefferson
Homer
Carthage
Canton
Quitman
Gilmer
Lake Providence
Dallas
Benton
Minden
Shreveport
Ruston
Monroe
Madison
Canton
Longview
Vicksburg
Clinton
Brandon
Waxahachie
Bossier City
Kilgore
Jackson
Ennis
Tyler
Jonesboro
Winnsboro
Raymond
Athens
Henderson
Carthage
Columbia
Corsicana
Jacksonville
Coushatta
Saint Joseph
Port Gibson
Hazlehurst
Mansfield
Winnfield
Fairfield
Rusk
Center
Natchitoches
Harrisonburg
Fayette
Waco
Palestine
Jena
Brookhaven
Groesbeck
Nacogdoches
Many
Natchez
Colfax
Meadville
Hewitt
Crockett
San Augustine
Pineville
McComb
Columbia
Marlin
Centerville
Lufkin
Hemphill
Liberty
Tylertown
Temple
Franklin
Groveton
Leesville
Marksville
Woodville
Louisiana
Cameron
Madisonville
Jasper
De Ridder
Clinton
Bogalusa
Bryan
Huntsville
Woodville
Newton
Amite
Zachary
Georgetown
Ville Platte
Livingston
Hammond
Taylor
College Station
Coldspring
Eunice
Baton Rouge
Covington